Case Studies in

NURSE
ANESTHESIA

Case Studies in
NURSE ANESTHESIA

SASS ELISHA, EdD, CRNA, FAAN
Assistant Director, School of Anesthesia
Kaiser Permanente/California State University Fullerton
Southern California Permanente Medical Group
Pasadena, California

ELSEVIER

Elsevier
3251 Riverport Lane
St. Louis, Missouri 63043

CASE STUDIES IN NURSE ANESTHESIA   ISBN: 978-0-323-68143-8

Notice

Practitioners and researchers must always rely on their own experience and knowledge in evaluating and using any information, methods, compounds or experiments described herein. Because of rapid advances in the medical sciences, in particular, independent verification of diagnoses and drug dosages should be made. To the fullest extent of the law, no responsibility is assumed by Elsevier, authors, editors or contributors for any injury and/or damage to persons or property as a matter of products liability, negligence or otherwise, or from any use or operation of any methods, products, instructions, or ideas contained in the material herein.

International Standard Book Number: 978-0-323-68143-8

Executive Content Strategist: Sonya Seigafuse
Senior Content Development Manager: Lisa Newton
Senior Content Development Specialist: Laura Selkirk
Publishing Services Manager: Julie Eddy
Project Manager: Grace Onderlinde
Senior Project Manager: Jodi Willard
Design Direction: Patrick Ferguson

Printed in India

Last digit is the print number: 9 8 7 6 5 4 3 2 1

Working together
to grow libraries in
developing countries

www.elsevier.com • www.bookaid.org

This book is dedicated to the CRNAs who reside all over the world. I admire your strength, your intellect, your work ethic, and your compassion. It is my humble desire that this book can help serve you and the future students of our profession in your never-ending quest for knowledge and perfection in anesthesia care.

Foreword

My colleagues—Sass Elisha, CRNA, EdD, FAAN, and Jeremy Heiner, CRNA, EdD—and I have been editing textbooks and writing about the scientific foundations of anesthesia for the last 20 years. With each publication, it is our hope that we are able to provide the most updated, concise, and practical information for certified nurse anesthetists (CRNAs), student registered nurse anesthetists (SRNAs), and other health care professionals. Our motivation has always been genuine and stems from the idea that knowledge is powerful. In a complex and rapidly changing specialty such as anesthesia, being academically and clinically prepared is essential.

Elsevier is the publisher of our three books. *Nurse Anesthesia* is the core textbook used by CRNAs, SRNAs, and nurse anesthesia educators in our profession. The rigorous scientific detail and current information are written by over 100 prominent CRNA clinicians, educators, and scholars, who share their expertise on the pages of each chapter. Our new publication, *Current Anesthesia Practice: Evaluation and*

Certification Review, was designed to meet the academic needs of CRNAs as they prepare for recertification and to provide a review of essential academic content. The topic outlines, bulleted format, and 150 review questions make this publication applicable to everyone. Lastly, *Case Studies in Nurse Anesthesia* meets the requests of many CRNAs and SRNAs who want to learn and relearn practical anesthesia information in a case study format. Each chapter highlights a surgical procedure and patient data and then discusses the appropriate anesthetic considerations for management.

Lifelong learning requires dedication and discipline. Our goal is to support your educational needs from the time one begins learning anesthesia and throughout an anesthetist's entire career. We have an immense feeling of satisfaction knowing that we provide the highest-quality evidence-based information so that you can consistently achieve superior patient care outcomes.

John Nagelhout, CRNA, PhD, FAAN

Reviewers

Marc R. Bentz, CRNA, DNAP
Assistant Professor
Graduate Program in Nurse Anesthesia
Department of Pharmacology, Physiology,
    and Neuroscience
University of South Carolina School of Medicine
Columbia, South Carolina

Mark H. Gabot, CRNA, MSN
Didactic and Clinical Educator
School of Anesthesia
Kaiser Permanente
Pasadena, California

Sarah E. Giron, CRNA, PhD
Academic and Clinical Instructor
Kaiser Permanente School of Anesthesia
Pasadena, California

Catherine Gutshall, CRNA, DNAP
Assistant Professor
Graduate Program in Nurse Anesthesia
University of South Carolina
Columbia, South Carolina

Winston T. King, CRNA, MHS
Assistant Professor
Graduate Program in Nurse Anesthesia
University of South Carolina
Columbia, South Carolina

Virginia C. Muckler, CRNA, DNP, CHSE-A, FAAN
Associate Clinical Professor
NLN Simulation Leader
Director, Nurse Anesthesia Program
Duke University
Durham, North Carolina

Jessica D. Szydlowski Pitman, CRNA, DNP, MS
Assistant Professor
Duke University
Durham, North Carolina

Catherine B. Rhea, CRNA, DNAP, MBS
Faculty
Nurse Anesthesia Program
University of South Carolina School of Medicine
Columbia, South Carolina

Andi N. Rice, CRNA, DNP
Consulting Associate
Duke University School of Nursing
Durham, North Carolina

Richard P. Wilson, CRNA, MNA
Assistant Program Director
Graduate Program in Nurse Anesthesia
University of South Carolina School of Medicine
Greenville, South Carolina

Acknowledgments

Paul Aguiar, CRNA, MSN
Travis Allen, CRNA, MSN
Jessica Bair, CRNA, MSN
Deborah T. Bergstein, CRNA, MSN
Tatiana Bevans, CRNA, PhD
Pamela Binns-Turner, CRNA, PhD
Sandra K. Bordi, CRNA, DNP
Greta Bray, CRNA, MSN
Gayne Brenneman, MD
Joseph F. Burkard, CRNA, PhD
John Cavitt, CRNA, MSN
Michael Churchin, CRNA, MSN
Gary D. Clark, EdD, CRNA
Joan Cornachio, CRNA, DNAP
Nicholas C. Curdt, CRNA, MS
Veronica Davis, CRNA, MSN
Matthew D'Angelo, CRNA, DNP
Mark Gabot, CRNA, DNP
Marjorie A. Geisz-Everson, CRNA, PhD
Sarah E. Giron, CRNA, PhD
Mark Goelz, CRNA, MSNA
Charles Griffis, CRNA, DNP
C. Wayne Hamm, CRNA, MSN
Jeremy S. Heiner, CRNA, EdD
Yoo Eun Emily Hwang, CRNA MSN
Donna Jasinski, CRNA, PhD
Vickie S. Jordan, CRNA, DNP

Joseph A. Joyce, CRNA, BSN
Mary C. Karlet, CRNA, PhD
Loretta Kitabjian, CRNA, MSN
Lynn L. Lebeck, CRNA, PhD
Hamid Mahmood, CRNA, DNAP
Erica J. McCall, CRNA, MSN
Shaun Mendel, CRNA, DNP
Nancy A. Moriber, CRNA, PhD
Sandra E. Morris, CRNA, MSN
Greg Nezat, CRNA, PhD
Lisa Osborne, CRNA, PhD
Timothy Palmer, CRNA, PhD
Garrett Peterson, CRNA, DNP
Rachel Polazzi, CRNA, MSN
Michael Rieker, CRNA, DNP, FAAN
Cliff Roberson, CRNA, DNP
Bernadette T. Higgins Roche, CRNA, PhD
Becky Rubin, CRNA, MSN
Michael Rubin, CRNA, MSN
Allan Schwartz, CRNA, DDS
Dennis Spence, CRNA, PhD
Henry Talley, CRNA, PhD
Edward Waters, CRNA, DNP
Dawn C. Welliver, CRNA, MS
Mark D. Welliver, CRNA, DNP
Molly Wright, CRNA, DNP

Contents

1

Tonsillectomy

KEY POINTS

- Tonsillectomy, with or without adenoidectomy, is one of the most commonly performed pediatric surgeries in the United States.
- Indications for tonsillectomy include chronic tonsillitis, recurrent peritonsillar abscess, enlarged tonsils that cause upper airway obstruction, tonsil asymmetry with suspected malignancy, and recurrent tonsillar hemorrhage.

- Patients having a tonsillectomy are at high risk for postoperative nausea and vomiting (PONV).
- Postoperative hemorrhage remains the most serious complication after tonsillectomy.
- Postoperative pain management is vitally important to reduce prolonged recovery and hospitalization.

Case Synopsis

A 7-year-old female presents with a 3-year history of recurrent tonsillitis. Her symptoms have become significantly worse, resulting in difficulty breathing at night and snoring. She has been treated with antibiotic therapy that ended 1 week ago, and her situation has not improved. Currently, she is scheduled for a tonsillectomy.

Preoperative Evaluation and Demographic Data

Past Medical/Surgical History

- Chronic tonsillitis

List of Medications

- No medications

Diagnostic Data

- No preoperative laboratory tests

Height/Weight/Vital Signs

- 120 cm, 21 kg
- Blood pressure, 112/62; heart rate, 88 beats per minute; respiratory rate, 22 breaths per minute; temperature, 36.9°C; room air oxygen saturation, 100%

Pathophysiology

Tonsillitis occurs most often in children 4 to 7 years of age, and it is an infection that involves the pharyngeal

tonsils. This pathologic process is caused by a virus or a bacterial pathogen. A viral tonsillitis is usually self-limiting, whereas a bacterial pathogen will require antibiotic treatment and it can produce more severe systemic complications. Bacterial tonsillitis is primarily caused by group A beta-hemolytic streptococcus (GABHS). The type of tonsillitis (acute, recurrent, or chronic) is determined by the symptomatology and the frequency with which the infection recurs. Acute tonsillitis is characterized by fever, dysphagia, lymphadenopathy, red or exudative tonsils, and sore throat. Mouth breathing, snoring, and obstructive sleep apnea (OSA) may also occur due to tonsillar enlargement. Recurrent tonsillitis is diagnosed when there are 7 episodes of acute tonsillitis in 1 year, 5 episodes in 2 consecutive years, or 3 episodes per year in 3 years. When tonsillitis is recurrent or chronic, a definitive treatment such as a tonsillectomy is recommended. Relative and absolute indications associated with tonsillectomy are outlined by the American Academy of Pediatrics and are listed in Box 1.1.

Surgical Procedure

Surgical removal of the tonsils, with or without adenoidectomy, can be accomplished using a variety of techniques. The method that is used may be determined by the extent of the surgery (partial tonsillectomy or complete tonsillectomy) and preference of the surgeon. Partial tonsillectomy is performed in patients with tonsillar hypertrophy resulting in OSA or airway obstruction. This procedure involves excising approximately 90% of the tonsillar tissue. In a complete tonsillectomy, the entire tonsillar tissue is excised, exposing the underlying pharyngeal constrictor muscle of the throat. Tonsillectomy techniques involve excising the tonsils through the mouth by use of a scalpel, scissors, or curettes. Other techniques include the use of monopolar or bipolar cautery, radiofrequency ablation, harmonic scalpel, carbon dioxide laser, and microdebrider coblation.

Anesthetic Management and Considerations

Preoperative Period

1. *Describe the important elements of the preoperative evaluation for a tonsillectomy.*

    Preoperative evaluation for the patient undergoing a tonsillectomy depends on physical assessment and history. Upper respiratory tract infections (URIs) are commonly associated with patients who present with chronic tonsillitis, recurrent tonsillitis, or a peritonsillar abscess. This may result in airway hyperactivity and potentially increase the incidence of perioperative bronchospasm or laryngospasm. Depending on the severity of URI symptoms, surgery may be postponed approximately 7 to 14 days until its resolution. There is controversy whether a URI in pediatric patients increases the incidence of adverse airway reactions during anesthesia.

    Adult patients who have tonsillar enlargement may display signs of OSA. A STOP-Bang questionnaire should be assessed to determine the presence of OSA and the severity, if present. If OSA is severe, further diagnostic studies are warranted, such as an electrocardiogram and chest radiograph, to determine whether cardiac involvement exists. An oral examination may reveal that the tonsils encroach on airway structures, which can potentially cause difficulty with mask ventilation or direct laryngoscopy. Patients having a tonsillectomy should be asked if they have bleeding disorders or tendencies. Evaluating a complete blood count, prothrombin time, or activated partial thromboplastin time is justified if there is a reason to believe that a coagulopathy is present. Patients with coexisting medical conditions and facial abnormalities, specifically Down syndrome (trisomy 21) and Treacher Collins syndrome, are of concern due to the increased risk of airway obstruction, difficult intubation, and presence of coexisting disease states.

2. *Explain the blood supply and the sensory innervation of the palatine tonsils.*

    The blood flow to palatine tonsils arises via the external carotid and its branches: ascending pharyngeal artery, facial artery, dorsal lingual artery, and palatine branch of the maxillary artery. Sensory innervation to the palatine tonsils is supplied by the glossopharyngeal and lesser or posterior palatine nerve.

3. *Discuss premedication for a patient having a tonsillectomy.*

    Premedication for a child undergoing tonsillectomy should be aimed at decreasing anxiety and providing analgesia. Depending on the child's age and cooperation, an oral anxiolytic (most frequently midazolam) may be administered 30 minutes before surgery to alleviate anxiety and to provide sedation. Premedication should be administered sparingly or not at all for patients who have a history of OSA, facial anomalies, or anticipated difficult mask ventilation and/or intubation. Postoperative analgesia can also be initiated preoperatively by administering rectal or oral analgesic medication (acetaminophen). Lastly, an antisialagogue may be considered to assist with drying of secretions in the pharynx during the intraoperative period, to improve visualization of oral structures due to a decrease in the amount of secretions, and to inhibit vagotonic reflexes.

Intraoperative Period

4. *Discuss anesthetic considerations regarding positioning for a tonsillectomy.*

    Patients are positioned supine with shoulders elevated (with a rolled towel) and head extended. Overextension of the neck may cause postoperative neck pain and can potentially result in atlantoaxial subluxation and displacement of the C1–C2 vertebrae. The head of the operating table is most frequently turned 90 degrees away from the anesthetist. A mouth gag is inserted by the surgeon to open and suspend the mouth for visualization. Special attention to the airway during insertion, positioning, and removal of the mouth gag is imperative, as the endotracheal tube (ETT) may become kinked, advance into the right mainstem bronchus, or inadvertent extubation can occur. Fig. 1.1 depicts a mouth gag and its relationship to the ETT.

5. *Discuss the type of anesthesia most often administered during a tonsillar resection.*

    General anesthesia with an ETT is the optimal technique and airway management strategy for a tonsillectomy. The type of anesthetic induction is dependent on the cooperation of the child. If intravenous (IV) access is accomplished, then an IV induction can be initiated.

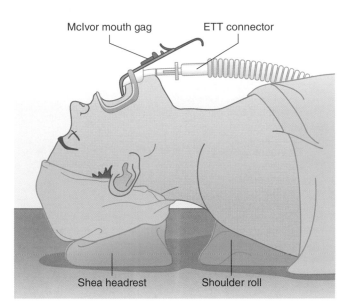

• **Fig. 1.1** Representation of patient position for tonsillectomy. *ETT,* Endotracheal tube.

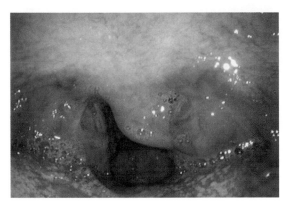

• **Fig. 1.2** View of hypertrophied tonsils. (From Sistla SK, Paramasivan VK, Agrawal V: Anatomic and pathophysiologic considerations in surgical treatment of obstructive sleep apnea, *Sleep Medicine Clinics* 14[1]: 21-31, 2019.)

Otherwise, an inhalation induction is acceptable for most patients, and IV access is established after the patient loses consciousness and an adequate depth of anesthesia is achieved. The intraoperative goals are to ensure unconsciousness, inhibit sympathetic reflexes, obtund oropharyngeal reflexes during direct laryngoscopy and placement of the oral gag, and prevent patient movement during the surgical procedure. These objectives can be achieved by administering inhalation agents alone or in combination with propofol, dexmedetomidine, and possibly neuromuscular blockade. Unfortunately, upon induction of anesthesia, relaxation of the pharyngeal muscles and tissues may cause airway obstruction in those patients who present with facial anomalies, OSA, severe tonsillar hypertrophy (Fig. 1.2), and other medical conditions, resulting in partial or complete airway obstruction.

6. *Discuss the intraoperative anesthetic management during a tonsillectomy.*

The average surgical time required for a tonsillectomy is approximately 30 minutes. Even though this is a short procedure, a high degree of physiologic stimulation occurs due to manipulation of the airway and removal of the tonsils. Therefore a deeper plane of anesthesia is required to adequately blunt the sympathetic reflexes that may elicit hypertension, tachycardia, and arrhythmias. This can be accomplished by increasing the inhalation agent alone or in combination with propofol and/or dexmedetomidine. Hypertension will also increase the volume of blood loss.

7. *During surgical manipulation of the mouth gag, the anesthesia machine alarms "low tidal volume." What action(s) should be taken by the anesthetist?*

A diagnosis to confirm or exclude the potential causes of the situation is essential. The following information is gathered during the assessment of the problem:

- Assessment of bilateral, equal, and clear breath sounds: no breath sounds present
- Assessment of chest rise and fall: no chest rise, but fall is present
- Assessment of end tidal carbon dioxide ($ETCO_2$): no $ETCO_2$ present
- Assessment of anesthesia bag compliance: no compliance present, large air leak present with bag ventilation
- Assessment of tidal volume: no tidal volume present
- Assessment of the depth of the ETT: The ETT was placed at a depth of 17 cm after intubation, and breath sounds were bilaterally equal and clear. The ETT depth is currently at 12 cm.
- The anesthetist smells the odor of inhalation anesthetic agent.

The anesthetist has determined that the patient has been inadvertently extubated.

The anesthetist should immediately ensure mask ventilation with 100% oxygen and prepare for reintubation. Because the operating room table is frequently positioned 90 degrees away from the anesthetist, the anesthetist will initially maintain the mask seal while a second provider ventilates the patient while the table is repositioned. After assurance of adequate mask ventilation, the anesthetist can deepen the patient with an inhalation agent and/or an IV induction agent to help attenuate the sympathetic effects associated with direct laryngoscopy.

8. *During the surgical procedure, the machine alarms "high peak pressure." What action(s) should be taken by the anesthetist?*

A diagnosis to confirm or exclude the potential causes of the situation is essential. The following information is gathered during the assessment of the problem:

- Assessment of bilateral, equal, and clear breath sounds: breath sounds bilaterally equal, wheezing is present
- Assessment of chest rise and fall: chest rise and fall are present

- Assessment of $ETCO_2$: $ETCO_2$ present, sloped expiratory waveform
- Assessment of anesthesia bag compliance: bag compliance is decreased
- Assessment of tidal volume: tidal volume is decreased
- Assessment of the depth of the ETT: The ETT was placed at a depth of 17 cm after intubation, and breath sounds were bilaterally equal and clear. The ETT depth is currently at 20 cm.

The anesthetist has determined that the patient is having a bronchospasm due to several observations. First, the breath sounds indicate bilateral wheezing. Also, the ETT has migrated 3 cm deeper, possibly stimulating the carina. Also, the $ETCO_2$ waveform shows a sloped expiratory limb, which is also suggestive of mild to moderate bronchospasm.

If desaturation is occurring, the surgery should be stopped, and the patient should be ventilated by hand with 100% oxygen. The ETT should be incrementally pulled back to its original position while assessing bilateral breath sounds. Deepening the anesthesia with an inhalation agent and administering albuterol frequently relieves mild to moderate bronchospasm.

9. *Discuss prophylactic treatment strategies used to decrease the incidence of PONV.*

   Patients having a tonsillectomy are at increased risk for PONV due to the ingestion of blood that occurs during excision. The administration of serotonin antagonists (ondansetron) and corticosteroids (dexamethasone) alleviates PONV. Even though dexamethasone has the added benefit of reducing swelling and inflammation in the region of the surgical site, controversy exists as to the antiinflammatory benefits.

10. *Discuss the anesthetic management for emergence.*

   In preparing for emergence, gentle suctioning of blood and secretions from the mouth and oropharynx minimizes laryngospasm with extubation. Suctioning is preferably accomplished while the patient is in a deep plane of anesthesia. The main goal for emergence is to minimize bucking, coughing, or straining of the patient to reduce postsurgical bleeding.

   The most commonly utilized emergence technique is to extubate the patient when fully awake and the protective airway reflexes are intact. A smooth emergence can also be accomplished with a deep extubation. Lidocaine 1 mL/kg can be administered 60 to 90 seconds before extubation to attenuate the airway responses while maintaining spontaneous respirations. The disadvantage of performing a deep extubation is that there is the potential for aspiration due to obtunded protective airway reflexes and laryngospasm associated with upper airway surgery. Also, a deep extubation is not recommended in those patients that were difficult to ventilate or intubate or those with facial anomalies.

Postoperative Period

11. *Discuss the most serious complication associated with tonsillectomy.*

• BOX 1.2 Postoperative Complications Associated With a Tonsillectomy

- Hemorrhage
- Infection
- Dehydration
- Aspiration of blood/mucus
- Airway obstruction due to:
  1. Retained throat pack
  2. Laryngospasm
  3. Bronchospasm
  4. Edema of the uvula
  5. Hematoma
- Pulmonary edema
- Glossopharyngeal nerve injury
- Subcutaneous emphysema
- Pneumomediastinum
- Pneumothorax
- Atlantoaxial subluxation
- Nasopharyngeal stenosis (more common with adenotonsillectomy)
- Velopharyngeal insufficiency (VPI; more common with adenoidectomy)

The most serious complication associated with tonsillectomy is postoperative hemorrhage. Postoperative bleeding occurs in 0.1% to 3% of patients, and 75% of those patients hemorrhage within 6 hours postoperatively. The remaining 25% have bleeding 24 hours after surgery and up to 6 days postoperatively. Postoperative bleeding occurs insidiously due to oozing of the tonsillar bed site; an immeasurable large amount of blood can be swallowed. Often, signs of hypovolemia such as tachycardia and hypotension are evidence of hemorrhage. Other postoperative complications regarding tonsillectomy are summarized in Box 1.2.

12. *Explain the anesthetic management of the patient who hemorrhages posttonsillectomy.*

   If attempts made to maintain hemostasis by nonsurgical means (with pharyngeal packs) have failed, the patient will return to the operating room for exploration of the site and surgical control of bleeding. The initial concern for the anesthetist should focus on restoring intravascular volume in those patients exhibiting signs of hypovolemia. IV access should be obtained, and hydration given before induction. A hemoglobin and hematocrit count is warranted for patients with immeasurable blood loss, as well as a type and screen with the possibility of blood transfusion. These patients are considered to have a full stomach due to the blood that they have swallowed. Therefore a rapid-sequence intubation with cricoid pressure is recommended. Consideration for using video laryngoscopy with continuous suction is warranted. However, in patients with difficult airways or facial anomalies, an awake fiber-optic intubation (to maintain airway reflexes) is an alternative method.

13. *Discuss the postoperative pain management for tonsillectomy.*

   Postoperative tonsillectomy is associated with a high incidence of pain. Unrelieved pain may result in a prolonged recovery and subsequent hospitalization due to dehydration from limited oral intake. Strategies that can be used to relieve postoperative pain include local infiltration of anesthetics and administering opioid analgesics, nonsteroidal antiinflammatory drugs (NSAIDs), dexamethasone, dexmedetomidine, and N-methyl-D-aspartate (NMDA) receptor antagonists (ketamine), either IV or instilled subcutaneously in the operative site. NSAIDs such as ibuprofen and ketorolac are effective analgesics; however, their use in treating pain posttonsillectomy is controversial due to their potential for increasing the risk of bleeding. Commonly, severe pain is treated with IV opioid analgesics (fentanyl, hydromorphone, or morphine). Unfortunately, nausea, vomiting, and respiratory depression are common side effects after opioid administration.

Once patients can drink liquids, moderate to severe posttonsillectomy pain can be treated with oral opioid analgesics (codeine or oxycodone) or an oral opioid combined with acetaminophen. This regimen is routinely started in the recovery room before discharge, and it is the most common practice of pain management posttonsillectomy. The administration of local anesthesia (bupivacaine or ropivacaine) may be injected in the peritonsillar fossa at the end of the surgical procedure to alleviate posttonsillectomy pain. The risks that are associated with localization of the peritonsillar fossa include loss of pharyngeal reflexes and intravascular injection.

Other adjuvant medications that may decrease posttonsillectomy pain include antibiotics. It is believed that after tonsillectomy the exposed tonsillar fossa allow oral bacterial flora to colonize, causing a severe localized inflammatory reaction resulting in pain. The NMDA antagonist ketamine, when administered at a subanesthetic dose (0.2 to 0.5 mg/kg IV), has been used to decrease postoperative analgesic requirements and postoperative pain. Ketamine may cause emergence delirium. Subcutaneous injection of ketamine in the tonsillar beds also decreases pain. Ketamine is advantageous because it does not depress laryngeal protective reflexes or respirations. However, it does increase salivary gland production, and an anticholinergic (glycopyrrolate) should be administered in conjunction with ketamine to decrease oropharyngeal secretions.

Review Questions

1. Bacterial tonsillitis is most commonly caused by:
   a. Influenza A.
   b. Epstein–Barr.
   c. Group B streptococci.
   d. Group A beta-hemolytic streptococci.
2. The initial concern for posttonsillectomy hemorrhage includes:
   a. Obtaining a hemoglobin and hematocrit.
   b. Administering an antiemetic medication.
   c. Fluid administration.
   d. Preparing for an awake fiber-optic intubation.
3. The primary intraoperative goal for a patient having a tonsillectomy is to:
   a. Obtund oropharyngeal reflexes and prevent patient movement.
   b. Maintain a light plane of anesthesia.

   c. Prevent kinking of the endotracheal tube by hyperextension of the patient's head.
   d. Administer an antiemetic prophylactically.
4. An absolute indication for tonsillectomy includes:
   a. Recurrent hemorrhagic tonsillitis.
   b. Recurrent tonsillitis.
   c. Recurrent peritonsillar abscess.
   d. Recurrent otitis media.
5. Which postoperative pain medication may be associated with increased bleeding when repeated doses are administered?
   a. Fentanyl
   b. Acetaminophen
   c. Ketamine
   d. Ketorolac

Suggested Readings

Discolo CM, Darrow DH, Koltai PJ. Infectious indications for tonsillectomy. *Pediatr Clin North Am* 2003;50:445–458.

Gill CJ. Anesthesia for ear, nose, throat, and maxillofacial surgery. In: Nagelhout JJ, Elisha S, eds. *Nurse Anesthesia*, 6th ed. St. Louis, MO: Elsevier, 2018:904–924.

Gigante J. Tonsillectomy and adenoidectomy. *Pediatrics in Review* 2005;26(6):199–203.

Levin B, Sacks R. Post-tonsillectomy bleeding. *Otolaryngology Head and Neck Surgery* 2007;136:S56–S58.

Hong B, Lim CS, Kim YH, Lee JU, Kim YM, Jung C, et al. Comparison of topical ropivacaine with and without ketamine on post-surgical pain in children undergoing tonsillectomy: a randomized controlled double-blind study. *J Anesth* 2017;31(4):559–564.

Piltcher OB, Scarton FB. Antibiotic use in tonsillectomies: therapeutic or prophylactic? Required or excessive? *Brazilian Journal of Otorhinolaryngology* 2005;71(5):686–690.

Pop RS, Manworren RC, Guzzetta CE et al. Perianesthesia nurses' pain management after tonsillectomy and adenoidectomy: pediatric patient outcomes. *J Perianesth Nurs* 2007;22(2):91–101.

Schmidt R, Herzog A, Cook S, et al. Complications of tonsillectomy. *Archives Otolaryngology Head and Surgery* 2007;133(9):925–928.

Tolska HK, Hamunen K, Takala A, Kontinen VK. Systematic review of analgesics and dexamethasone for post-tonsillectomy pain in adults. *Br J Anaesth* 2019;123(2):e397–e411.

Tsui B, Wagner A, Cave D, et al. The incidence of laryngospasm with a "no touch" extubation technique after tonsillectomy and adenoidectomy. *Anesth Analg* 2004;98:327–329.

Walker P, Gillies D. Post-tonsillectomy hemorrhage rates: are they technique-dependent? *Otolaryngology Head and Neck Surgery* 2007;136:S27–S31.

2
Radical Neck Dissection

KEY POINTS

- Lymph node metastasis reduces the survival rate of patients with squamous cell carcinoma by half. The survival rate is less than 5% in patients who previously underwent surgery and have a recurrent metastasis in the neck.
- The greatest risk of a radical neck dissection (RND) is damage to nerves, muscles, and veins in the neck.
- The outcome of neck dissection depends on the stage of cancer, type of metastasis, and quality of the surgery.
- Patients undergoing RND often present with difficult airway management challenges. Physical examination before the surgery may reveal minor or even no distortions to the airway. A meticulous airway examination must be performed, and any abnormal findings should heighten the concern for difficult ventilation and intubation.

- Assurance of adequate analgesia is essential because RND procedures are performed on highly reflexogenic areas. Increasing intraoperative hemodynamic stability and reliably blunting the physiologic reaction to the endotracheal tube (ETT) is desirable.
- A timely and smooth anesthetic emergence must be accompanied by hemodynamic stability and enables the anesthetist to assess the presence of neurologic deficits.
- Antihypertensive medications may be warranted to avoid postoperative hemorrhage and to minimize hemodynamic variability.

Case Synopsis

A 75-year-old man had been diagnosed with squamous cell carcinoma of the neck and suspected lymph node metastasis. Four years after undergoing a left RND and radiation therapy, the patient presents with a recurrence of the cancer. He is scheduled by his otolaryngologist to have a right RND procedure.

Preoperative Evaluation and Demographic Data

Past Medical/Surgical History

- Tobacco smoking with 50 pack/year history
- Hypertension
- Left-sided RND and radiation therapy for squamous cell carcinoma of the neck 4 years before surgery

List of Medications

- Hydrochlorothiazide

Diagnostic Data

- Hemoglobin, 11.1 g/dL; hematocrit, 33.2%
- Electrolytes: sodium, 139 mEq/L; potassium, 4.5 mEq/L; chloride, 106 mEq/L

Height/Weight/Vital Signs

- 170 cm, 70 kg
- Blood pressure, 130/81; heart rate, 61 beats per minute; respiratory rate, 14 breaths per minute; temperature, 36.8°C; room air oxygen saturation, 97%
- Electrocardiogram (ECG): normal sinus rhythm, 62 beats per minute, no abnormalities

Pathophysiology

Squamous cell carcinoma can invade the upper aerodigestive tract resulting from dysfunction in cellular proliferation and differentiation. The primary sites most commonly involved include the mucosal areas of the upper aerodigestive tract, particularly the larynx, oropharynx, hypopharynx, and oral cavity. Metastasis into the regional lymph nodes and vascular channel invasion can occur and seed other parenchymal sites if tumor invasion is not controlled at the lymphatic level. The most likely sites for metastasis to occur include the lungs, liver, bone, brain, and adjacent as well as other sites, depending on the tumor histology.

Furthermore, the most important prognostic factor in patients with squamous cell carcinoma of the head and neck is the status of the neck nodes. The extent of cervical lymphadenopathy is also the strongest and most dominant predictor for the overall prognosis, rate of recurrence, and potential for metastasis in head and neck squamous cell carcinoma. Lymph node metastasis reduces the survival rate of patients with squamous cell carcinoma by half, and the survival rate is less than 5% in patients who previously underwent surgery and develop a recurrent metastasis in the neck.

The risk of lymph node involvement by metastasis varies depending on the site of origin, the size of the primary tumor, the histologic grade of the primary tumor, perineural and perivascular invasion, and extracapsular spread. Poorly differentiated tumors at the primary site are also more aggressive and associated with a higher risk of neck metastasis. Moreover, the prognosis is poor when multiple levels of neck lymph nodes are involved. The cervical lymph nodes are divided into superficial and deep chains. Superficial lymph nodes are involved in a late stage of cancer; therefore they have less oncologic importance. Deep cervical lymph nodes receive drainage from areas of the oral cavity, pharynx, larynx, salivary glands, thyroid, and skin of the head and neck. These deep cervical lymph nodes accompany the internal jugular (IJ) vein and its branches. The greater number of lymph nodes that are involved (greater than four) results in a decreased rate of survival. In addition, posterior triangle and contralateral involvement and node fixation to the carotid artery or a muscle are indications of poor prognosis.

The degree and invasiveness related to the disease process must be discussed collaboratively with the surgeons because the type, size, location, and presence of impingement on other anatomic structures will influence the anesthetic management. Advances in surgical techniques, radiation therapy, and chemotherapy have allowed for more aggressive treatment of advanced head and neck cancers. The goal is to attempt to preserve organ function using either primary radiotherapy or concurrent chemotherapy and radiotherapy, with surgery reserved for oncologic salvage. The outcome of an RND is dependent on the stage of cancer, type of metastasis, and quality of the surgery. Advanced deeply attached neck metastasis, recurrence after radiation or chemoradiation, and metastatic neck abscess pose several technical challenges for the head and neck surgeon in the salvage operation. Conversely, no single standardized treatment for cervical metastasis exists. It has been observed repeatedly that management of the same medical or surgical condition varies enormously between physician, institution, and even geographic region, often without evidence of better outcomes.

Surgical Procedure

An RND is performed for the surgical control of metastatic neck disease in patients with squamous cell carcinomas of the upper aerodigestive tract, salivary gland tumors, and skin cancer of the head and neck. Surgical time averages 1.5 to 3 hours for primary resection and 3 to 6 hours for reconstruction. The resection consists of a complete cervical lymphadenectomy, together with resection of the sternocleidomastoid muscle, the IJ vein, the spinal accessory nerve

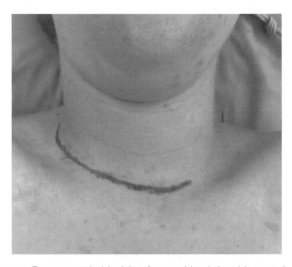

• **Fig. 2.1** Recommended incision for combined thyroid, central, and left lateral neck dissection with vertical limb placed behind the shadow of the sternocleidomastoid muscle. The vertical limb extends about one-third of the distance from the clavicle to the mastoid, allowing sufficient exposure of level II of the neck and minimizing the length of the incision. (From Randolph GW: *Surgery of the thyroid and parathyroid glands*, ed 3, St. Louis, 2021, Elsevier.)

(cranial nerve XI), and the submandibular gland. In attempting to remove as much cancerous tissue as possible, much of the local lymphatic system and some muscles, arteries, veins, and glands are resected.

Neck dissections are seldom performed as isolated surgical procedures and are frequently combined with resection of the primary lesion, which may involve the tongue, pharynx, larynx, etc. As depicted in Fig. 2.1, an apron incision is made along the posterior border of the sternocleidomastoid muscle, curving medially above the clavicles and extending to the contralateral side. Transection of the sternocleidomastoid muscle at its sternal attachment occurs, and the IJ vein is isolated, cut, and tied. The inferior portion of the dissection includes the identification and preservation of the carotid arteries, the vagus nerve, the hypoglossal nerve, the brachial plexus, and the phrenic nerve. As the dissection specimen is swept superiorly, the cervical sensory branches are divided.

To maximize oncologic efficacy and to minimize morbidity, modifications to the classic neck dissection occur. One such modification is the preservation of one or more nonlymphatic structures (e.g., spinal accessory nerve, IJ vein, sternocleidomastoid muscle). The spinal accessory nerve (cranial nerve XI), the hypoglossal nerve (cranial nerve XII), and the lingual nerve are preserved. The defect is closed either primarily, with a split-thickness skin graft, or with a chest flap (pectoralis major or deltopectoral). More recently, free flaps may be created for closure and revascularized using the facial artery or superior thyroid artery.

Although common in the 1950s and 1960s, simultaneous bilateral neck dissections are rarely done because of the associated complications, including facial edema, laryngeal edema, blindness, and cerebral edema, stemming from the

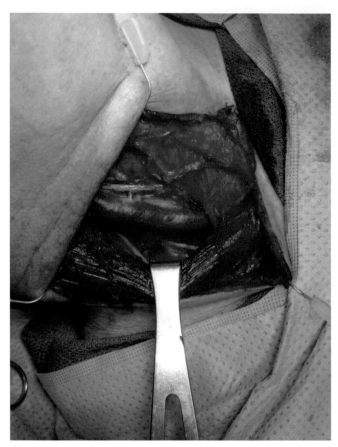

• **Fig. 2.2** A right modified neck dissection with retraction of the right sternocleidomastoid muscle exposing cranial nerves and jugular vein. (From Rothrock JC: *Alexander's care of the patient in surgery*, ed 16, St. Louis, 2019, Elsevier.)

TABLE 2.1	Types of Neck Dissection
Radical neck dissection	• Tissue is removed from an area in front of the trapezius muscle at the side of the neck. Included in this tissue, which extends from the clavicle inferiorly to the mandible superiorly, are dozens of lymph nodes. • The submandibular gland, sternocleidomastoid muscle, internal jugular vein, and spinal accessory nerve are also removed.
Modified radical neck dissection	• Refers to anything that is less than a radical neck dissection. • The sternocleidomastoid muscle, jugular vein, spinal accessory nerve, or even all three structures can be safely preserved.
Selective neck dissection	• Preservation of the sternocleido-mastoid muscle, the spinal accessory nerve, and the jugular vein. • Removes less extensive amounts of lymph nodes and surrounding tissue.

removal of both IJ veins. The operation should not be performed if the cancer has spread beyond the head and neck region, when surgery will not control the primary tumor, or if the cancer invaded the bones of the cervical vertebrae or skull. This is particularly true when invasive cancers such as squamous cell carcinoma, a slow-growing malignant tumor with cells of a distinctive shape, is involved. A modified neck dissection removes less tissue, and a selective neck dissection even less, as is shown in Fig. 2.2. Depending on the extent of the cancer, these variations on neck dissections exist as depicted in Table 2.1.

Anesthetic Management and Considerations

Preoperative Period

1. *Describe the patient population who may likely present for an RND procedure.*

   Tumors of the head and neck are most commonly discovered in elderly patients and are frequently associated with tobacco smoking and alcohol consumption.

Organ pathology in these patients includes pulmonary and hepatic dysfunction, respectively. The presentation of a patient for an RND procedure often includes a high incidence of coronary artery disease, hypertension, bronchitis, pulmonary emphysema, chronic renal insufficiency, and chronic obstructive pulmonary disease. If the tumor interferes with the person's ability to eat, then weight loss, malnutrition, anemia, dehydration, and electrolyte imbalance can be significant. Thus a careful history and physical must be performed to assure that no current exacerbations of preoperative morbidities exist and the patient's functional status is optimized.

2. *Discuss the laboratory studies, imaging techniques, and other tests completed to collect appropriate data for patients presenting for an RND.*

   • **Laboratory studies:** In cases of malignancy or chronic disease, anemia or coagulopathies may be present. Therefore a complete blood count with differential and coagulation studies are useful tests, as patients with advanced cancers of the head and neck may present with preexisting anemia. Prothrombin time (PT), activated partial thromboplastin time (aPTT), and international normalized ratio (INR) measures are also especially important in patients with preexisting bleeding diathesis, with hepatitis, or who are on anticoagulation drug therapy. Furthermore, many patients present with other medical problems or take medications that affect their electrolyte status. Squamous cell carcinoma may cause paraneoplastic syndromes, most commonly syndrome of inappropriate secretions of antidiuretic hormone (SIADH). In addition, liver function tests, glucose tests, blood urea nitrogen (BUN), and creatinine testing are useful. Moreover, a blood type and screen may be beneficial. Although refinements in the surgical technique have significantly reduced blood loss in these procedures, either typing and screening or typing and cross-matching for two units of packed red blood cells are necessary in situations in which blood loss is expected to be significant.

- **Imaging techniques:** Imaging is an integral part of clinical diagnosis and staging, and the results are helpful in deciding treatment. Extensive tests are done before the operation to try to determine the location and the degree of metastasis. Among these techniques are computed tomography (CT) scanning, magnetic resonance imaging (MRI), lymph node biopsies, and barium swallows. CT scanning and MRI scanning provide information as to the presence of lymph node abnormalities, which will help to guide further treatment. These diagnostic data may be crucial in delineating the extent of body structures, deep cervical musculature, and carotid artery circumferential involvement. MRI reveals tumor necrosis and extracapsular spread of the nodal capsule with less precision than CT scan, but MRI is better for assessing enlarged lymph nodes that are not metastatic. Some institutions also use ultrasonography and ultrasound-guided aspiration cytology to determine whether metastasis to the cervical region of the neck has occurred. Further, positron emission tomography (PET) is an adjunct in the diagnosis of lymph node metastasis. Providing information about the metabolic activity of the tissues, PET scanning has shown the ability to differentiate active tumors from chronic fibrotic changes. Thus PET scan results can provide early diagnosis of recurrent head and neck cancer, as well as indicate the status of the neck after chemoradiotherapy.
- **Histologic examination:** The standard to detect lymph node metastasis in the neck is the histologic examination of all nodes. Biopsies of the primary site reveal the etiology of the initial mass and the characteristics of the tumor involved, such as squamous cell carcinoma of the upper aerodigestive tract, nasopharyngeal carcinoma, thyroid carcinomas, and skin cancer of the head and neck. Fine needle aspiration cytology of the neck confirms the pathologic conclusions of the primary tumor. Detection and accurate staging of neck metastasis are extremely important because staging has major implications for prognosis and treatment.
- **Balloon occlusion test:** Since the development of newer surgical procedures minimizing surgical morbidity, the treatment of patients undergoing carotid vessel management remains controversial. Many have advocated for preoperative evaluation of these patients by a balloon occlusion test, which includes the balloon occlusion test and a four-vessel cerebral angiography to evaluate the status of the contralateral carotid, intracerebral circulation, and carotid back pressure.

Patients who are able to tolerate the occlusion of the ipsilateral carotid artery without any evidence of neurologic dysfunction may be candidates for carotid resection. Further, if tumor involvement of the carotid artery is possible, a complete preoperative evaluation assessing the patency of the carotid arteries is indicated.

- **Miscellaneous tests:** A chest radiograph may be performed to exclude metastatic disease. A complete physical examination is mandatory and includes evaluation of neurologic, cardiovascular, and respiratory status. A thorough airway assessment includes palpation of the patient's neck to define size, location, mobility, and degree of softness or hardness of any mass. An ECG is also performed as determined by the patient's condition. A preoperative arterial blood gas analysis in patients with advanced chronic obstructive pulmonary disease, carbon dioxide retention, and oxygen dependence is indicated. Pulmonary flow-volume loops may also be helpful in patients with symptoms associated with obstructive lung disease.

3. *Discuss the physical examination and findings that should be noted on the patient's record before performing surgery.*
   - Physical examination of the head and neck and the findings should be noted. Evaluation of the airway and dentition is essential. A meticulous airway examination must be performed, and any abnormal findings should heighten the concern for difficult ventilation and intubation.
   - Medical history (e.g., hypertension, diabetes, cardiopulmonary disease, and other chronic illnesses; previous surgeries; radiation therapy). A thorough assessment of cardiac risk factors and functional status, identification of asymptomatic carotid bruits or existing carotid artery stenosis, and assessment of neurovascular integrity is vital.
   - All diagnostic data, including those from imaging studies.

4. *Describe the importance of the airway examination and specific concerns with airway planning and management in the patient presenting for RND.*

   Patients undergoing RND often present with the potential for difficult airway. The preoperative physical examination may not reveal the presence of a significant neck mass or other tracheal abnormality. The anesthetist should evaluate the ability of the patient to open the mouth adequately for intubation, reports of airway edema, indications of difficulty with breathing, evidence of tracheal deviation, or changes in the quality of the voice. A history of stridor and hoarseness suggests airway narrowing and possible vocal cord dysfunction. Further, patients with head and neck cancer often have had previous surgery or radiation therapy, and these treatments may further complicate airway management by significantly decreasing tissue compliance.

Radiation therapy alters tissue structure and diminishes the flexibility of native tissues. The cervical spine range of motion may be limited due to prior surgery and radiation scarring. Prior radiation therapy may cause extensive fibrosis of tissues, increased intraoperative bleeding, and ankylosis of the temporomandibular joint, rendering tracheal intubation extremely difficult or impossible.

One must diagnose alterations in the anatomy of the upper airway because of a tumor. Inflammatory or neoplastic growths of the upper aerodigestive tract can occur anywhere within the airway and may achieve significant size with little evidence of airway penetration or obstruction. In 15% of these patients, a metastatic neck mass is present without a distinct primary lesion. These tumors may cause fixation of tissues secondary to expansion and are often fragile and bleed readily even during atraumatic airway management maneuvers. Thus issues of the pathology must be discussed through effective communication and collaboration with the surgeon. Consultation with a surgeon as to parameters, such as the type, nature, extent, and location of the tumor; potential bleeding; and the review of appropriate radiographs and prior therapy administered (e.g., radiation or chemotherapy), has a strong influence on outcome and remains important in determining techniques for airway management.

Multiple plans must be devised to decrease the possibility of a "failed airway." The anesthetist must have experience with the alternative airway management techniques and devices. Establishing a sequence of interventions is also imperative.

- Extraglottic device: Laryngeal mask airway
- Fiber-optic devices: Adult fiber-optic scope
- Video laryngoscopy
- Surgical airway options: Cricothyrotomy, tracheostomy
- A rigid ventilating bronchoscope should be present and assembled.

Prevention and planning before induction are mandatory. If the anesthetist decides to proceed with the conventional means of securing the airway by performing an orotracheal intubation, the patient's head positioning should be optimized carefully, and intubating aids (e.g., stylets, gum elastic bougie) and ETTs of different sizes should be available. If a difficult intubation is foreseen, an awake fiber-optic intubation or tracheostomy under local anesthesia before induction of general anesthesia may be the necessary technique. The use of video laryngoscopy allows for a greater field of vision, and the anesthetists can determine any abnormalities in the upper airways.

Additional considerations include that the patient's airway and operative field is not only shared with the surgeon but immediate access to the airway is difficult because the patient is turned 180 degrees away from the anesthetist. Further, the ETT must be secured, and its positioning should be monitored carefully during surgery to avoid supraglottic or endobronchial migration. Nasal intubation may be desirable to facilitate surgical access, and a surgeon should be consulted. In the difficult airway, good communication and understanding between the surgeon and the anesthetist is a priority.

5. *Explain the anesthetic concerns associated with patients who have had a previous RND.*

Although operation for head and neck cancers carries an increased likelihood for airway obstruction immediately after surgery, this complication can occur after RND and during surgery for another reason. Bilateral RND, even when staged over a period of years, may pose a significant risk to the patient. For patients with previous neck dissection, lymphatic drainage patterns are altered, creating the potential for postoperative edema. This diminishes the ability of tissues within the larynx to tolerate an iatrogenically induced insult that produces edema and swelling, thereby placing this patient at a heightened risk for postoperative airway compromise. Therefore significant postoperative laryngeal edema and neuronal imbalance may ensue, necessitating a tracheostomy.

In addition, one cause of delayed awakening and failure to breathe is associated with cephalic venous obstruction (e.g., significant facial edema, facial cyanosis despite normal pulse oximetry reading, rhinorrhea). Cerebral venous congestion may be a result of central apnea secondary to acutely elevated intracranial pressure (ICP). The treatment if this situation were to arise is to employ measures aimed at reducing ICP and to protect cerebral blood flow.

Intraoperative Period

6. *Describe the monitoring to be utilized in an RND.*

In an RND, the required monitors include standard intraoperative measures, such as ECG, pulse oximetry, end-tidal carbon dioxide monitoring, and body temperature. An arterial line may be indicated in patients with severe cardiopulmonary disease, chronic renal insufficiency, symptoms of cerebrovascular insufficiency, the location of a tumor near the carotid artery, or in patients presenting for lengthy procedures, including any microvascular flap reconstruction. In addition, a nerve integrity monitor may be used by the surgeons to aid in identifying and preserving specific nerves in the neck.

7. *Recognize the physiologic considerations associated with patient positioning during RND.*

Patients are placed in the supine position with the upper half of the operating table elevated to a 30-degree angle. The head is turned to the opposite side of the surgical site, and a shoulder roll extending the neck is placed. It is important for the anesthetist to ensure that the patient's head is adequately supported and padded to avoid hyperextension, which can result in postoperative neck discomfort, brachial plexus injury, and pressure sores. The head-up tilt during such procedures is not done simply to improve the surgical field and expedite the procedure—it is an important measure to ameliorate the effects of jugular venous ligation, increasing the venous return and decreasing blood loss. Thus elevation of the head should continue into the postoperative period.

8. *Discuss relevant nonlymphatic structures in the neck. Investigate the incidence and significance of intraoperative damage to nerves and vasculature in an RND.*

The greatest risk associated with RND is damage to nerves, muscles, and veins in the neck. The neck region has multiple sensory nerves that are sacrificed during an RND. Therefore nerve damage can result in numbness and loss of sensation to different regions on the neck and a temporary or permanent loss of function to multiple parts of the neck, throat, posterior occiput, external ear, mandibular region, lateral shoulder, deltoid area, and upper pectoral area. For instance, it is common after RND for a person to have stooped shoulders, limited ability to lift the arm, and limited head and neck rotation and flexion as a consequence of the removal of nerves and muscles during surgery. Therefore neuromuscular relaxation must be omitted to isolate the nerves and avoid surgical trauma. On occasion, formation of a neuroma at the end of a nerve that has been dissected may cause chronic paresthesias and pain. Sacrifice of the cervical sympathetic chain can produce Horner syndrome, which involves ptosis, anhidrosis, and miosis. The phrenic nerve may also pass into the surgical field, and respiratory problems may develop if diaphragmatic paralysis occurs.

Many arteries and veins are encountered during an RND, including the jugular veins, superior and inferior thyroid artery, and carotid artery. Although the region is highly vascular, major vessel trauma, laceration, tear, or transaction is a rare occurrence. When hemorrhage occurs, the vessel injury is immediately ligated or repaired.

- **Spinal accessory nerve (SAN):** Surgical trauma to the SAN results in painful "shoulder syndrome." Signs and symptoms include shoulder drop or shrug weakness, limitations in active shoulder abduction or flexion, limited range of motion of the arm, lateral scapular winging at rest, and local pain, typically across the upper border of the trapezius muscle. Because electrophysiologic integrity of the SAN does not completely correlate with clinical outcome measures for "shoulder syndrome," trapezium weakness can occur even when the SAN is preserved.
- **Hypoglossal nerve:** Unilateral resection of the hypoglossal nerve is usually well tolerated without serous sequelae. However, bilateral hypoglossal nerve resection

causes serious difficulties with eating, swallowing, and speaking.
- **Facial nerve:** The superficial origin of the facial nerve is located at the level of the tragus of the ear. A small branch of the facial nerve is encountered and preserved when performing a neck dissection. Transection of the marginal mandibular branch of the facial nerve produces lower lip weakness.
- **Vagus nerve:** The vagus nerve in the neck is closely approximated to the carotid sheath and may be injured during the dissection and division of the lower portion of the IJ vein. During RND, dissection around the carotid bulb or surgical manipulation affecting the carotid sinus may elicit a vagal reflex, inducing profound bradycardia, hypotension, or cardiac arrest. The afferent neural pathway involved with carotid sinus or carotid baroreceptor stimulation involves transmission from the carotid sinus to Hering nerve to the glossopharyngeal nerve (CN IX) and then to the brain. Parasympathetic nervous system predominance to the heart results from efferent stimulation via the vagus nerve (CN X), which causes vagotonic effects.

The treatment for severe bradycardia or cardiac arrest includes having the surgeon stop carotid sinus manipulation. For persistent severe bradycardia, atropine should be administered. The reflex can also be diminished by injection of local anesthetic in the region of the carotid sinus. Additionally, postoperative hypertension and a loss of hypoxic drive after a bilateral neck dissection may indicate denervation of the carotid sinuses and bodies. The lower or middle neck of the vagus nerve also carries motor and sensory branches to the larynx and pharynx, and resection will cause vocal cord paralysis and sensory dysfunction.
- **Carotid artery:** The carotid artery rarely needs to be resected or reconstructed. In addition, careful dissection around the carotid arterial system in the neck with gentle retraction, ligation, and manipulation may help prevent the dislodgment of arteriosclerotic plaques from the internal carotid system, decreasing the potential for a stroke.
- **IJ vein:** The IJ vein is frequently nonfunctional, either due to invasion or compression resulting in blockage by the mass. Ligation or transfixation-ligation is feasible because drainage is provided by other veins in the neck. However, injury to the IJ vein at the upper or lower ends may cause significant bleeding postoperatively and may require surgical reintervention. Occasional uncontrollable bleeding requires assistance of a thoracic surgeon to enter the superior mediastinum. Furthermore, major disruptions in venous flow during surgery and venous stasis may result in laryngeal edema and obstruction. Therefore venous thrombus is commonly seen in patients who are undergoing RND.
- **Venous air embolus:** An air embolism can occur when a large vein in the neck is inadvertently

opened. A large volume of air enters rapidly into the open vein by negative pressure and passes directly into the right atrium, causing an airlock at the level of the superior vena cava and the right atrium, leading to decreased or total cessation of blood flow through the heart. Clinically, cyanosis, hypotension, dysrhythmias, a decrease in end-tidal carbon dioxide, an increase in end-tidal nitrogen, ST-segment elevation, and a loud churning mill-wheel murmur over the precordial area may appear suddenly. If a venous air embolus is suspected, the surgeon must be notified immediately to compress the open neck veins, flood the field with normal saline, and pack or clamp the offending vein to stop the entrainment of air. The anesthetist must administer 100% oxygen, turn the patient onto the left side with the head down, and provide circulatory support with intravenous fluids and vasopressors, as indicated. In addition, a disappearance of peripheral pulses may indicate cardiac arrest, requiring aspiration of air from the heart via a central venous catheter, cardiac massage, and standard resuscitation procedures.

9. *Discuss factors that affect the estimated blood loss during an RND.*

    The duration of an RND frequently lasts for more than 6 to 8 hours, but the procedure is rarely associated with significant blood loss. Partly due to the benefits of hemostasis with the electrocautery unit or bipolar forceps and the use of clamps and suture ligation, the average estimated blood loss (EBL) is 150 to 200 mL. The total blood loss, however, is highly variable and is related to the patient history and possible events during the procedure. For instance, patients who have had radiation therapy are likely to lose 200 to 400 mL of blood. If a primary tumor is also resected, the EBL may be 400 to 700 mL. Although rare, uncontrolled bleeding of the IJ vein at the skull base can result in a sudden large amount of blood loss; this can be controlled by the surgeon with digital pressure, allowing the anesthetist to administer fluid or blood as needed.

10. *Examine additional considerations and clinical techniques to optimize operating conditions during head and neck surgery.*

    - **Anesthetic technique:** The anesthetic that is provided for a patient who is undergoing RND must be individualized depending on the surgical procedure and the degree of pathophysiology. A balanced technique using intravenous and inhalational agents is commonly used for RND. Maintenance of general anesthesia frequently includes an inhalational agent blended in air and oxygen. Inspired gases should be humidified to minimize a decrease in temperature and incidence of mucus accumulation. Deep and superficial cervical plexus blocks, as well as a cervical epidural anesthetic, have been used. The doses of anesthetic and hypnotic agents frequently must be reduced due to the patient's age and preexisting medical conditions.

    - **Opioid-based technique:** Assurance of adequate intraoperative and postoperative analgesia is an essential anesthesia requirement, as RND procedures are performed on highly reflexogenic areas. Omission of muscle relaxation is necessary in order for the surgeon to assess nerve function during resection. Therefore an opioid-based technique may be especially advantageous and is acknowledged to more easily maintain hemodynamic stability, to reliably blunt the patient reaction to the ETT, and to facilitate emergence from anesthesia. Due to the invasive nature of the surgical procedure and the degree of postoperative pain that is experienced, opioids such as fentanyl or sufentanil are ideal choices. A continuous infusion of opioids may offer potential advantages over intermittent boluses, resulting in a decrease in total dose, greater hemodynamic stability, more rapid recovery of consciousness, less pain in the immediate postoperative period, and a decreased time to discharge.

    - **Hypotensive anesthesia:** Maintaining relative hypotension (systolic blood pressure 80 to 100 mm Hg and mean arterial pressure $\geq$60 mm Hg) reduces blood loss, resulting in faster surgery and less patient morbidity. This controlled decreased blood pressure is widely employed unless contraindicated secondary to concomitant medical conditions such as cardiovascular or neurovascular disease. Deliberate decreased blood pressure can be accomplished by using a variety of anesthetic and sympatholytic agents such as inhaled anesthetics, narcotics, beta-blockers, and vasodilators.

11. *Analyze the specific concerns related to airway management and emergence from anesthesia after an RND. Compile a list of recommended safe practice standards to promote a safe and smooth anesthetic recovery.*

    Airway protection and maintenance is the primary concern for the anesthetist. Most importantly, the patient must have an intact airway, must have adequate respiratory function, and must be well oxygenated before extubation. The recovery of spontaneous ventilation and airway reflexes is required. In addition to standard extubation criteria, patient characteristics that must be considered before tracheal extubation after an RND procedure include the patient's preoperative physiologic status and airway assessment, and existing comorbidities require a close evaluation. After a major surgical procedure, the need for a prompt emergence and patient cooperation with an immediate postoperative neurologic examination is intended to help assess for the presence of hematoma formation, cerebral ischemia, and nerve injuries. Under these circumstances, residual anesthesia may give the false impression of neurologic deficit. Therefore the patient must be awake, follow verbal commands, and demonstrate appropriate neurologic function before extubation. The patient must be able to sustain spontaneous respirations and maintain normal arterial blood gas values. Additionally, vocal cord inspection before anesthetic emergence through laryngoscopy or a fiber-optic scope should prove unremarkable.

The anesthetist must be familiar with the surgeon's preferences and the surgical procedure that was accomplished before extubation. Surgical determinants of requirement for postsurgical mechanical ventilation include the duration and difficulty of surgery and the degree of edema that has developed. Any intraoperative complications, such as swelling, injury to cranial nerves, hematoma formation, ischemia, or bradycardia associated with operative manipulation, can have a deleterious effect on the patient's outcome. Airway edema due to retraction, surgical trauma, and intravenous fluid administration can result in postoperative respiratory distress.

Of all patients undergoing general endotracheal anesthesia for RND, up to 20% will develop some form of increased laryngeal resistance after extubation. The reduction of airflow results from either anatomic narrowing (e.g., edema) of the glottis (e.g., epiglottis and aryepiglottic folds) or neuronal imbalance of the abductor and adductors of the vocal cords. However, several factors may contribute to laryngeal dysfunction despite an apparently intact vocal cord function. Radiation therapy alters tissue structure and diminishes the flexibility of native tissues. Macroglossia (swelling of the tongue) is a potentially fatal complication of premature extubation. Surgical patients with an unprotected airway are at even greater risk for airway obstruction, hypoxemia, hypercapnia, and aspiration. Reintubation may be impossible, and attempts to secure the airway may cause airway collapse.

A smooth emergence from anesthesia is essential, and every attempt should be made to avoid or minimize the patient's reaction to the ETT. Straining, bucking, coughing, or gagging during emergence will cause an increase in venous pressure that may provoke postoperative bleeding or disruption of delicate suture lines. Prompt emergence and hemodynamic stability are imperative. Excessive bucking or coughing can result in cerebral venous congestion.

Delayed anesthetic recovery has been advocated to limit airway risks linked to awakening from anesthesia. In some patients, elective postoperative ventilation is indicated because of existing neurologic deficits, intraoperative complications, respiratory or hemodynamic alterations, or swelling. By generating a comprehensive list of criteria for early extubation, anesthesia providers can make an educated decision on whether a particular patient would benefit from immediate extubation.

Hematoma formation in the neck most often occurs within the first few hours after surgery has been completed. The mass can impinge upon the trachea and adjacent airway structures and can cause complete airway obstruction. Immediate intervention is necessary

and includes the surgeon evacuating the hematoma and achieving hemostasis followed by airway maintenance. Hematoma evacuation is a definitive treatment and must occur expeditiously. The materials, equipment, and ability to perform an emergency tracheostomy are essential.

Strategies that can be used to decrease the possibility of postoperative respiratory distress caused by airway edema include examination of the degree of edema or tracheomalacia using fiber-optic examination, deflating the ETT cuff to determine if a leak occurs during positive pressure ventilation, and inserting a pediatric ETT exchange device and temporarily leaving it in place after tracheal extubation.

An elective tracheostomy may be accomplished before the end of surgery, in which the patient may be subject to a reintervention procedure to avoid edema. Postoperative sedation and prolonged mechanical ventilation are warranted only in patients with physiologic or pathologic disturbances requiring correction before recovery. This decision is contingent on prominent factors such as the invasiveness and duration of surgery, the patient's prior physical condition, concurrent respiratory disease, and the degree of edema generated intraoperatively.

12. *Recognize the specific physiologic and hemodynamic changes during emergence from anesthesia and tracheal extubation.*

Anesthetic drugs that are compatible with the surgical procedure must be selected. If muscle relaxant medications were administered, residual neuromuscular blockade must be completely reversed, anesthetic drugs discontinued, and no further respiratory depressant drugs administered. The incidence of nausea and vomiting after a radical neck dissection is high. Thus routine antiemetic prophylaxis most commonly is achieved by the intravenous administration of a 5-HT3 blocker and dexamethasone.

Postoperative Period

13. *List the potential postoperative complications that can occur after RND.*

The postoperative complications associated with RND are present in Table 2.2. An RND is associated with low morbidity and mortality rates; however, associated composite resection and ablation of a large surface of mucosal area adjacent to the neck markedly increases the rate of complications. Other factors, such as poor health, chronic malnutrition, alcoholism, diabetes mellitus, advanced age, systemic illness, and radiation therapy, also increase the likelihood for postoperative complications such as wound infection, fistula, flap necrosis, osteoradionecrosis, and carotid artery rupture.

TABLE 2.2 **Postoperative Complications Associated With RND**

Complication	Presentation	Prevention and Treatment
Hematoma formation	1. A hematoma is usually evident in the first few hours after the operation and is best found with inspection. 2. Blood under the flap accumulates rapidly. 3. If the hematoma is recognized and treated early, no adverse consequences occur. However, if the hematoma is found late, airway compromise, infection, or flap necrosis may occur.	1. Meticulous hemostasis during the surgical procedure is mandatory. 2. Suction drains are used to avoid blood accumulation under the skin flap. Ensure that the Hemovac or drains are functioning properly and maintained on continuous suction until they drain less than 20 mL in 24 hours. 3. With unilateral neck dissections, some surgeons use a floppy, moderately compressive dressing. The disadvantage is that the dressing leaves the flaps unavailable for inspection. 4. Treatment requires urgent reintubation, which comprises taking the patient to the operating room, opening and elevating the neck flaps, and evacuating the hematoma. 5. Any source of bleeding is found, ligated, sutured, or electrocauterized.
Facial edema	1. Unilateral RND may result in ipsilateral swelling of the lower face and neck. 2. Bilateral RND performed simultaneously with ligation or resection of both IJ veins results in facial edema, cerebral edema, or both. 3. There is some argument that edema to the face and neck is as much, if not more, a result of lymph stasis as inadequate venous drainage from removal of the IJ vein. 4. Mechanical obstruction of venous drainage and the increase of ICP can cause neurologic deficit and coma. 5. Facial edema commonly appears in patients with previous irradiation and can lead to chemosis. 6. Lid edema may be sufficient to prevent eye opening.	1. Airway management with a tracheotomy is required. 2. Maintain head elevation at a 30-degree angle to promote venous drainage.
Electrolyte disturbances	1. Patients undergoing RND are frequently hypovolemic with electrolyte imbalances. 2. The most common electrolyte disturbance is hyponatremia, usually dilutional; however, it may be related to the secretion of antidiuretic hormone. 3. Occasionally, hypernatremia, hypokalemia, hypercalcemia, and hypophosphatemia are also associated with RND.	1. Obtain serum electrolyte values, and correct abnormal values as deemed necessary. 2. Some fluid replacement and electrolyte balance intraoperatively may be required to maintain cardiovascular stability.
Carotid artery rupture	1. The incidence ranges from 3% to 7%. 2. The precipitating factors include radiation therapy, infection, and salivary fistula; suction catheters that cause erosion of the vessel wall; and exposure by dehiscence of the suture line or necrosis of the dermis. 3. Most patients have prodromal bleeding (i.e., sentinel bleed) within 48 hours of the carotid rupture.	1. Apply direct, firm pressure to the affected area while the operating room is prepared for neck surgery. 2. Two large-bore peripheral intravenous catheters for administration of isotonic crystalloid fluids. Controlling blood pressure and blood volume before the ligation is important. 3. The airway should be adequate and stable. If the patient does not undergo a tracheotomy, orotracheal intubation may be necessary. 4. Type blood and cross-match for 4 to 6 units. 5. If the bleeding cannot be controlled, emergently clamp the common carotid artery after the blood pressure and pulse are within the reference range. 6. Definitive treatment includes ligation of the carotid artery with a silk suture that is reinforced distally and proximally.

TABLE 2.2   Postoperative Complications Associated With RND—cont'd

Complication	Presentation	Prevention and Treatment
Hypertension and tachycardia	1. May be secondary to carotid sinus denervation or pain. 2. Up to 10% of patients may develop sustained hypertensive response early postoperatively, increasing the risk of stroke.	1. Treat this aggressively. Consider beta-blockers. 2. Pain management with patient-controlled analgesia and intravenous opiates.
Lymphatic leak via chylous fistula	1. Major lymph channels are encountered at the lower aspect of the neck, especially on the left side. 2. Apply positive pressure to reevaluate if further leaking occurs.	1. Ligating the thoracic duct is mandatory. 2. A return to the operating room may be required for repair.
Pneumothorax	1. Involves a sudden compromise of the respiratory and circulatory system and causes difficult breathing, bronchospasm, and decrease in oxygen saturation. 2. The pressure of the anesthetic bag does not cause normal expansion of the thorax.	1. Listen to bilateral breath sounds. 2. Obtain a chest radiograph. 3. A large pleural leak with a tension pneumothorax requires immediate aspiration with a 14- or 16-gauge needle in the second intercostal space midclavicular line on the affected side and chest tube placement with an underwater drain.

ICP, Intracranial pressure; IJ, internal jugular; RND, radical neck dissection.

Review Questions

1. The most important factor associated with long-term survival in patients with squamous cell carcinoma of the head and neck is:
   a. Advanced age of the patient.
   b. Positive history of tobacco and alcohol abuse.
   c. Prior surgical history of tonsillectomy and adenoidectomy.
   d. Metastasis to neck lymph nodes.

2. Which is the most common electrolyte disturbance that occurs for patients undergoing RND?
   a. Hyponatremia
   b. Hypernatremia
   c. Hyperkalemia
   d. Hyperphosphatemia

3. Shoulder drop or shrug weakness, limited range of motion of the arm and shoulder, scapular winging, and local pain are associated with:
   a. Internal jugular vein ligation.
   b. Retraction to the sternocleidomastoid muscle.
   c. Surgical trauma to the spinal accessory nerve.
   d. Vagal nerve compression.

4. During which period is the formation of a neck hematoma most likely to occur after an RND procedure?
   a. During surgical wound closure
   b. First few hours after the operation
   c. Four to eight hours postoperatively
   d. Twenty-four hours after the operation

Suggested Readings

Bulbul MG, Zenga J, Puram SV, Tarabichi O, Parikh AS, Varvares MA. Understanding approaches to measurement and impact of depth of invasion of oral cavity cancers: a survey of American Head and Neck Society Membership. *Oral Oncol* 2019;99:104–107.

Burkle CM, Walsh MT, Pryor SG, Kasperbauer JL. Severe post-extubation laryngeal obstruction: the role of prior neck dissection and radiation. *Anesth Analg* 2006;102(1):322–325.

Craig JR, Power K. Apnoea and delayed emergence following staged bilateral radical neck dissection. *Anaesthesia* 2006;61(9):914–915.

de Bree R, Takes RP, Shah JP, Hamoir M, Kowalski LP, et al. Elective neck dissection in oral squamous cell carcinoma: past, present and future. *Oral Oncol* 2019;90:87–93.

Ferrari LR, Gotta AW. Anesthesia for otolaryngologic surgery. In: Barash PG, Cullen BG, Stoelting RK, eds. *Clinical Anesthesia,* 5th ed. Philadelphia: Lippincott Williams & Wilkins, 2006:997–1011.

Gendon EM, Ferlito A, Shaha AR. Complications of neck dissection. *Acta Otolaryngology* 2003;123:795–801.

Gill CJ. Anesthesia for ear, nose, throat, and maxillofacial surgery. In: Nagelhout JJ, Elisha S, eds. *Nurse Anesthesia,* 6th ed. St. Louis, MO: Elsevier, 2018:904–924.

Hutchison IL, Ridout F, Cheung SMY, Shah N, Hardee P, et al. Nationwide randomised trial evaluating elective neck dissection for early stage oral cancer (SEND study) with meta-analysis and concurrent real-world cohort. *Br J Cancer* 2019;121(10):827–836.

Kaplan MJ, et al. Otolaryngology—head and neck surgery. In: Jaffe RA, Schmiesing CA, Golianu B, eds. *Anesthesiologist's Manual of Surgical Procedures,* 5th ed. Philadelphia: Lippincott Williams & Wilkins, 2014:178–258.

Kido K, Shimoda H, Takahashi, M. Bronchoconstriction induced by carotid sinus stimulation during radical neck dissection. *Anesth Analg* 2005;100:1214-1223.

Witt RL, Rejto L. Spinal accessory nerve monitoring in selective and modified neck dissection. *Laryngoscope* 2007;117(5):776–780.

3

Laryngectomy

KEY POINTS

- Squamous cell carcinoma is the primary cause of laryngeal cancer.
- Tobacco use and alcohol misuse combine to cause the vast majority of laryngeal neoplasms.
- Glottic cancer is the most common form of laryngeal malignancy, followed by supraglottic and subglottic cancer.

- TNM (tumor, node, metastasis) cancer staging largely dictates the form of cancer treatment and surgery.
- Thorough diagnostic information and airway assessment determine whether the patient can be safely intubated or the preferred technique for definitive airway management.
- The anesthetist's primary concerns during the intraoperative period are airway protection and massive hemorrhage.

Case Synopsis

A 62-year-old man saw his primary care physician with a complaint of hoarseness for the past 2 weeks. The patient was scheduled to have a diagnostic laryngoscopy with an otolaryngologist. It was discovered that the patient has stage II laryngeal cancer. The patient has received preoperative radiation therapy, and he is currently scheduled for a total laryngectomy.

Preoperative Evaluation and Demographic Data

Past Medical/Surgical History

- Hypertension
- Chronic obstructive pulmonary disease (COPD)
- History of smoking 2 packs of cigarettes per day for the past 45 years
- Daily alcohol consumption averages 2 to 3 beers
- No past surgical history

List of Medications

- Metoprolol
- Hydrochlorothiazide

Diagnostic Data

- Complete blood count (CBC): white blood cells, 5.5/mm^3; hemoglobin, 17 g/dL; hematocrit, 51%; platelets, 150,000/mm^3
- Electrolytes: sodium, 142 mEq/L; potassium, 4.5 mEq/L; chloride, 102 mEq/L; carbon dioxide, 28 mEq/L; calcium, 9.0 mg/dL; magnesium, 2.0 mEq/L
- Blood urea nitrogen (BUN), 22 mg/dL; creatinine, 0.7 mg/dL

- Liver function tests (LFTs), prothrombin time (PT)/partial thromboplastin time (PTT), and basic metabolic panel (BMP) are normal, revealing no sign of hepatorenal disease
- Electrocardiogram (EEG): sinus bradycardia (heart rate, 58 beats per minute) with left atrial enlargement
- Chest x-ray (CXR): mild hyperinflation consistent with emphysema
- Arterial blood gas (ABG), pH 7.36; PaO_2, 95 mm Hg; $PaCO_2$, 45 mm Hg; HCO, 28 mEq/l; O_2 saturation, 99%
- Type and screened for two units of packed red blood cells

Height/Weight/Vital Signs

- 180 cm, 81 kg
- Blood pressure, 128/74; heart rate, 68 beats per minute; respiratory rate, 22 breaths per minute; temperature, 36.8°C; room air oxygen saturation, 96%

Laryngeal Anatomy and Physiology

The larynx provides structural support and protection for airway structures. The larynx consists of three unpaired (epiglottis, thyroid, cricoid) and three paired (two arytenoid, two corniculate, and two cuneiform) cartilages. Anatomically, the larynx is divided into three regions: supraglottic, glottic, and subglottic. The supraglottic region encompasses the epiglottis, arytenoids, and false vocal cords. The glottic region consists of the true vocal cords and glottic opening. The subglottic area extends from beneath the glottic opening to the base of the cricoid cartilage.

The cartilaginous bodies of the larynx are held together by four different ligaments: the thyrohyoid, cricotracheal,

---

• BOX 3.1 Musculature of the Larynx

Extrinsic Muscles of the Larynx

- Sternothyroid
- Thyrohyoid
- Inferior constrictor of the pharynx

Intrinsic Muscles of the Larynx

- Posterior cricoarytenoid
- Lateral cricoarytenoid
- Interarytenoid
- Thyroarytenoid
- Vocalis
- Cricothyroid

• BOX 3.2 Risk Factors Associated With Laryngeal Cancer

- Tobacco
- Alcohol
- Environmental exposure (exposure to wood dust, paint fumes, asbestos)
- Viral infection (oncogenic types of human papillomavirus)
- Dietary factors (lack of A and B vitamins)
- Weakened immune system (AIDS)
- Gender
- Gastroesophageal reflux disease
- Age >50 years
- Ethnicity

• BOX 3.3 TNM System for Cancer Staging

- Tis: Cancer in situ, cancer is completely limited to epithelial layer
- T1: Tumor confined to site of origin
- T2: Tumor is growing into adjacent area
- T3: Tumor is limited to larynx, but vocal cords do not move
- T4a: Tumor extends to tissue beyond larynx
- T4b: Tumor extends into region of cervical spine and chest
- N0: No nodular involvement
- N1: Single lymph node involvement, 3 cm in diameter
- N2: Single lymph node involvement of 6 cm or multinode involvement size between 3 and 6 cm
- N3: Multinodular involvement, 6 cm
- M0: No distant metastasis
- M1: Distant metastasis present
- Stage 0: Tis, N0, M0
- Stage I: T1, N0, M0
- Stage II: T2, N0, M0
- Stage III: T3, N0, M0; T1, T2, or T3, N1, M0
- Stage IVA: T1, T2, or T3, N2, M0 or T4a, N0, N1 or N2, M0
- Stage IVB: T4b, any N, M0, or any T, N3, M0
- Stage IVC: Any T, any N, M1

---

cricothyroid, and hyoepiglottic ligaments. Identification of the cricothyroid membrane is the most important landmark for the anesthetist because it is the site where cricothyroidotomy can be performed.

The muscles of the larynx, which are included in Box 3.1, are divided into the extrinsic and intrinsic muscle groups. The extrinsic muscles shift the larynx upward and downward. The intrinsic muscles are involved in vocal cord tension and relaxation, which are necessary for phonation and extreme exhalation and inhalation.

The recurrent laryngeal nerve and the superior laryngeal nerve supply innervate the airway structures that are housed within the larynx. The recurrent laryngeal nerve provides all sensory innervation below the level of the vocal cords. The internal branch of the superior laryngeal nerve provides sensation to the larynx above the vocal cord level. Motor innervation to the larynx is primarily provided by the recurrent laryngeal nerve, except for the cricothyroid muscle, which is supplied by the external branch of the superior laryngeal nerve. Both the recurrent laryngeal nerve and superior laryngeal nerve are branches of the vagus nerve.

The arterial blood supply to the larynx comes from the superior laryngeal artery, derived from the external carotid artery, and the inferior laryngeal artery, which branches from the subclavian artery. Venous return from the larynx occurs via the superior and inferior laryngeal veins.

Pathophysiology

Laryngeal cancer most frequently affects men between 50 and 70 years of age. Laryngeal cancer accounts for 1% of all malignancies, and it is the eleventh most prevalent carcinoma among men. Men are 10 times more likely to develop this disease compared with women. Squamous cell cancer accounts for 95% of all laryngeal carcinoma, and the overall incidence of laryngeal neoplasm is 3.7 per 100,000.

Multiple risk factors predispose patients to developing laryngeal cancer, and these are listed in Box 3.2. Tobacco use and alcohol consumption are the two most common etiologies for laryngeal malignancy, accounting for 95% of laryngeal carcinomas. The combination of these two risk factors increases the incidence of laryngeal cancer by 15.5 times.

The assessment of laryngeal malignancy depends primarily on its location and the TNM staging of the tumor. Glottic tumors are the most common and comprise 60% of all laryngeal neoplasms. Additionally, 35% of laryngeal cancers involve the supraglottic structures and 5% invade the subglottic region. The TNM system for cancer staging is defined by the following:

- T is *t*umor size.
- N is lymph *n*ode involvement.
- M is the degree of *m*etastasis.

A complete list of the nomenclature that comprises the TNM staging system is present in Box 3.3.

Treatment Options

Radiation therapy is the primary form of treatment for stage I and stage II laryngeal malignancy. The rate of successful treatment ranges from between 80% to 90% for stage I disease and 70% to 80% for stage II disease. A patient will commonly receive radiation 5 days a week for a 7-week duration.

Chemotherapy, radiation treatments, and surgery are strategies that are commonly utilized to treat patients who have developed advanced stage III or stage IV cancers. Chemotherapy is associated with more severe side effects (leukocytopenia, fatigue secondary to anemia, nausea and vomiting) compared with radiation therapy. These side effects are often accentuated when chemotherapy and radiation therapy are combined. Surgery is rarely performed as the sole form of treatment, and it is often combined with radiation and/or chemotherapy for treating laryngeal carcinoma. There are several surgical treatment options for laryngeal cancer, which are listed in Box 3.4.

Surgical Procedure

The goal of laryngeal surgery includes the removal of diseased tissue, preservation or creation of a pathway for air exchange, and maintaining vocal cord function if possible. The definitive surgical procedure that is performed is dependent on the degree of invasion of the tumor, and these variant surgical techniques include the following:

Microlaryngeal surgery is performed for laryngeal cancers that are present in their early stages and can be removed by utilizing an operating microscope, microlaryngeal dissecting instruments, and a carbon dioxide laser. The resection is limited to the diseased tissue, which allows for preservation of adjacent laryngeal structures and superior postoperative laryngeal function.

Hemilaryngectomy involves the removal of one vertical half of the larynx. Unilateral vocal cord reconstruction can be accomplished by using a portion of the strap muscle.

Supracricoid laryngectomy includes the removal of supraglottic structures, true and false vocal cords, and thyroid cartilage while the cricoid and arytenoid cartilages remain. It is performed for lesions that are located in the proximity of the anterior glottis. Preservation of vocal function may be achieved; however, as many as 50% of these patients will continue to be dependent on a tracheotomy.

Supraglottic laryngectomy can be done using an endoscopic approach or a traditional open technique. During this procedure, supraglottic structures, including the false vocal cords, epiglottis, arytenoids, and a portion of the laryngeal cartilage, are resected.

Total laryngectomy is accomplished for patients who have extensive cancerous involvement of the larynx (T3 or T4) and entails the complete removal of the larynx, thyroid cartilage, cricoid cartilage, hyoid bone, and potentially several upper tracheal rings. Total or partial thyroid gland resection may be involved. A permanent tracheostomy is created by connecting the tracheal stump to the lower portion of the neck (Fig. 3.1).

The postoperative course is most dependent on the extent of the cancerous lesion, the type of laryngectomy that was performed, and the physical state of the patient. Potential complications that are associated with a laryngectomy include difficulty with speech, airway complications, diminished sense of taste and smell, pharyngoesophageal stenosis, fistula development between the trachea and esophagus, infection, decreased range of motion caused by fibrosis, hematoma formation, and cranial nerve injury. The intraoperative period for a laryngectomy is highly variable and is dependent on the type of procedure being performed. If a radical neck dissection is to occur in conjunction with a laryngectomy, operative times can exceed 10 hours. The anesthetist's primary initial concern is securing a patent airway (discussed later). Transfusion of packed red blood cells is frequently unnecessary during a laryngectomy because the blood loss is usually less than 300 to 400 mL.

Anesthetic Management and Considerations

Preoperative Period

1. Describe the signs and symptoms associated with laryngeal carcinoma.

This patient had complained of hoarseness to his primary care physician. Hoarseness is a classic sign of laryngeal carcinoma with glottic involvement. Other common signs of laryngeal carcinoma include difficult or painful swallowing, persistent coughing, and dyspnea. A comprehensive list of the signs and symptoms that are associated with this disease is included in Box 3.5. Many of these signs and symptoms do not appear until the disease process is extensive. This is particularly true in cases of supraglottic and subglottic cancer. Approximately 80% of subglottic tumors are diagnosed in late stages (T3 or T4). Careful examination of the neck should be performed to evaluate the patient for the presence of lymph node metastasis and to create a strategy for airway maintenance.

2. Discuss the comorbidities that are associated with laryngectomy.

This patient has a history of both hypertension and COPD. Many of the diseases associated with laryngectomy

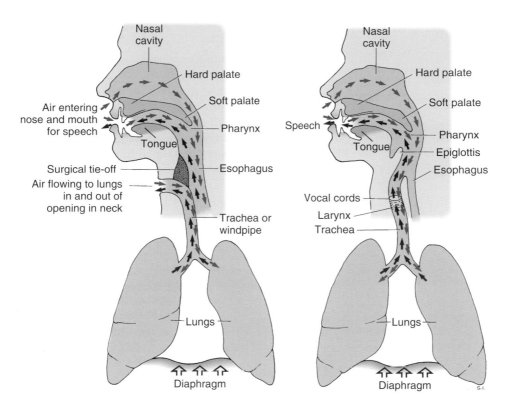

• **Fig. 3.1** Normal airflow in and out of lungs *(left)* and airflow in and out of the lungs after total laryngectomy *(right)*. Clients using esophageal speech trap air in the esophagus and release it to create sound. (From Zerwekh J: *Illustrated study guide for the NCLEX-RN® exam*, ed 12, St. Louis, 2019, Elsevier.)

• BOX 3.5	Signs and Symptoms Associated With Laryngeal Cancer

- Hoarseness
- Muffled voice
- Dysphagia
- Odynophagia (painful swallowing)
- Otalgia (ear ache)
- Cough
- Airway obstruction
- Fixation of the thyroid cartilage
- Neck mass
- Stridor
- Hemoptysis
- Anorexia
- Weight loss

• BOX 3.6	Comorbidities Associated With Patients Having a Laryngectomy

- COPD: a combination of emphysema, chronic bronchitis, and/or asthma
- Cerebrovascular accident
- Lung cancer
- Intermittent claudication
- Coronary artery disease
- Myocardial infarction
- Atherosclerosis
- Hypertension
- Alcohol abuse
- Hepatic failure
- Renal failure
- Tobacco use

are a result of the constellation of diseases associated with cigarette smoking and advanced age. The most common comorbidities that are associated with patients having a laryngectomy are listed in Box 3.6. This patient's hypertension (preoperative blood pressure, 110/64) is well controlled with metoprolol (a beta-blocker) and amlodipine (a calcium channel blocker). His COPD is managed by using an ipratropium inhaler (an anticholinergic), which is administered four times a day, and an albuterol inhaler (a beta-2 agonist), which he uses as a rescue inhaler.

3. *Describe the preoperative diagnostic testing performed for laryngectomy.*

The definitive diagnostic test that is used to assess the presence and degree of laryngeal carcinoma is laryngoscopy and evaluation of tissue removed for biopsy. Upon visual inspection with the laryngoscope, this patient's cancer, although primarily a glottic mass, began to spread to the supraglottic region. Computed tomography (CT) scan was used to identify tumor size and lymph node involvement, and a positron emission tomography (PET) scan allowed for the assessment of metastatic disease. Based on these findings, this patient's carcinoma was identified as a stage II cancer: T2, N0, M0. Diagnostic tools that can be used to detect laryngeal cancer are included in Box 3.7. Although a CXR is not used to identify laryngeal malignancy, it can help the physician identify lung metastasis.

4. *Discuss the preoperative laboratory evaluation that is associated with a laryngectomy.*

There are no laboratory tests that are diagnostic for laryngeal cancer. However, given the treatment options and the comorbidities associated with laryngectomy, several laboratory tests should be performed preoperatively. These tests include the CBC, type and screen (T&S), LFTs, coagulation tests (PT/PTT), electrolyte panel, and an ABG. A list and explanation of laboratory tests are included in Box 3.8. Polycythemia is a common finding caused by COPD. This compensatory change increases the oxygen-carrying capacity that occurs due to chronically decreased PaO_2 that is associated with pulmonary pathology. The bradycardia is likely due to his beta-blocker therapy with metoprolol, and the left atrial enlargement is a common result of chronic hypertension.

5. *Identify the importance of a comprehensive airway assessment and plan for airway management.*

Airway evaluation is an essential preoperative assessment performed by the anesthetist. In addition to standard airway assessment parameters, such as Mallampati class and thyromental distance, it is essential that the anesthetist performs a thorough airway examination. In the event of any preexisting airway obstruction, a decision will be made as to whether the patient can be safely intubated under general anesthesia, whether an awake intubation needs to be performed, or whether the patient requires an awake tracheostomy under local anesthesia before start of the laryngectomy surgery. A strong indicator of the degree of airway obstruction that will be encountered after the induction of anesthesia is the patient's ability to lie in the supine position. If the patient is unable to lie flat without dyspnea, this is highly suggestive of the presence of significant airway obstruction. This patient was able to sleep in the supine position while laying his head on a single pillow. In addition, his diagnostic laryngoscopy and CT scan revealed that it was possible to perform an intubation under general anesthesia.

Diagnostic testing such as CT scan and laryngoscopy will dictate whether the patient can be safely intubated or whether an awake tracheostomy with local anesthesia is required. If there are any concerns of impingement and airway distortion that have the potential to cause upper airway obstruction, further definitive investigation should be performed.

Performing an awake intubation or tracheostomy should be considered when there is preexisting obstructive pathology. The anesthetist and surgical team must be prepared to have all necessary equipment available to perform an emergency tracheostomy. In the specific case of laryngeal cancer, a supraglottic device such as a laryngeal mask airway (LMA) may not be helpful in an emergency situation due to the airway pathology. If the patient is considered to be a potentially difficult intubation, or if massive unremitting airway obstruction is judged to be a likely consequence of induction, an awake tracheostomy is the treatment of choice. Tracheostomy can be performed under several regional anesthetic techniques, which are listed in Box 3.9. Tracheostomy can also be performed with or without conscious sedation, using regional anesthetic techniques alone or in combination.

Intraoperative Period

6. *Discuss important factors involved in patient preparation for laryngectomy.*

The patient is placed in the supine position unless there is preexisting airway obstruction, in which case a

- Deep cervical plexus block: local anesthesia is injected into the bilateral transverse processes of C4
- Superficial cervical plexus block: local anesthesia is infiltrated into the area surrounding the Erb point on both sides of the neck
- Superior laryngeal nerve: local anesthesia is injected bilaterally 1 cm below the greater cornu of the hyoid bone
- Translaryngeal block: local anesthesia is injected through the cricothyroid membrane

semi-Fowler or even side-lying position might be required. The considerations necessary for placing the patient in the supine position include the potential for brachial plexus or ulnar nerve damage. Supine positioning reduces functional residual capacity in a patient who may already be suffering from partial airway obstruction. Thorough preoxygenation before intubation is vital.

During laryngoscopy and intubation, trauma to the tissues results in catastrophic swelling or bleeding in the airway. Pressure exerted on cancerous tissue and/or areas of the oral mucosa that have received radiation therapy are at risk of bleeding during airway instrumentation. Video laryngoscopy may be a viable option for the initial attempt at intubation due to the potential for bleeding post radiation therapy. Once ventilation is established, the patient is intubated with an appropriately sized endotracheal tube (ETT). The surgeon may wish to perform a direct laryngoscopy or upper airway examination under anesthesia before ETT placement. Several sizes of ETTs should be available in the event of difficulty with intubation. The ETT will be secured in a manner that has been discussed with the surgeon in advance (taped midline or to one side, may be sutured). The operating table will be turned to a 90- or 180-degree angle away from the anesthetist. Because the anesthetist will not have ready access to the patient's airway, extension tubing for intravenous lines and the breathing circuit will be needed. In many cases, consideration should be given to using a reinforced ETT to further protect the airway. This should also be discussed with the surgeon in advance of the induction.

The patient's arms will be tucked at his side. The difficulty of accessing the patient's arms during surgery and the need for secure access for drug and fluid therapy necessitate the need for two large-bore IVs (no. 16 or no. 18). A central line is not necessarily required for laryngectomy, but if central line placement is indicated due to the patient's condition, it should be placed in the femoral vein to avoid disruption of the surgical field. The patient may be placed on a pillow or shoulder roll, depending on the surgeon's preference, to create head and neck extension to achieve good operative exposure. The patient's head should be adequately supported. The final position of the patient's head should be discussed in advance with the surgeon. Careful attention to safely covering and protecting the eyes should be a priority.

7. *Describe the importance of patient monitors.*

Standard monitors (ECG, noninvasive blood pressure monitoring, pulse oximetry, end-tidal carbon dioxide monitoring, peripheral nerve stimulator, temperature) are required. Arterial line placement is recommended because it will provide for a continuous assessment of the patient's blood pressure to detect hemodynamic changes that are associated with this patient population. Although the surgery takes place in a highly vascular area (close proximity to the carotid and jugular vasculature), blood loss has the potential to become excessive. The average amount of blood loss is estimated to be 200 to 500 mL of blood. The anesthetist must be aware of the potential for hypotension caused by hemorrhage or vagal stimulation caused by baroreceptor or recurrent/superior laryngeal nerve stimulation.

The placement of an esophageal stethoscope allows for accurate core temperature monitoring and simultaneous auscultation of lung and heart sounds. The average duration of this surgical procedure is variable and lasts between 2 and 6 hours. Patient warming should be provided via a lower body or underbody Bair Hugger (Arizant Healthcare, Inc., Eden Prairie, MN) and intravenous fluids should be heated via a fluid warming device.

8. *Discuss intraoperative complications of laryngectomy.*

Intraoperative complications are related to hemorrhage and surgical stimulation of the vagus nerve. Hypotension can be the result of massive blood loss or vagal stimulation. Vagal stimulation can also produce bradycardia. Pulmonary and airway complications of laryngectomy include pneumothorax, airway obstruction, and air embolism. All patients must be carefully evaluated for the presence of surgical complications upon emergence from anesthesia and before extubation.

Postoperative Period

9. *Describe significant postoperative complications associated with laryngectomy.*

Several postoperative complications are associated with a laryngectomy. The inability to phonate (temporary or permanent), dysphagia, and increased risk of aspiration (with partial laryngectomy) are direct results of laryngectomy. The most common postoperative complications are pharyngocutaneous fistula and wound infection. Other postoperative complications include bleeding, hematoma, pneumonia, airway obstruction, chyle leak, and death.

Review Questions

1. Which characteristics most accurately describe the comorbidities associated with a laryngectomy?
   a. A 42-year-old female, 50 pack-year smoking history, blood pressure 190/110
   b. A 67-year-old male, nonsmoker, drinks three glasses of wine daily
   c. A 65-year-old male, 40 pack-year smoking history, drinks a fifth of vodka daily
   d. A 34-year-old male, history of cocaine abuse, drinks one 6-pack of beer daily
2. Which is the correct sequence indicative of the incidence of laryngeal cancer by region from the greatest to the least?
   a. Supraglottic, glottic, subglottic
   b. Glottic, supraglottic, subglottic
   c. Glottic, subglottic, supraglottic
   d. Supraglottic, subglottic, glottic
3. TNM cancer staging is an abbreviation for which of the following?
   a. Tumor, nodule, mass
   b. Tumor, node, mass
   c. Tumor, neoplasm, metastasis
   d. Tumor, node, metastasis
4. Which diagnostic tests best determine the staging associated with laryngeal carcinoma?
   a. CBC and laryngoscopy with biopsies
   b. PET scan and CXR
   c. CXR and CT scan
   d. Laryngoscopy with biopsies and CT scan
5. What are the most important concerns during the intraoperative period?
   a. Airway protection and massive hemorrhage
   b. Airway protection and bradycardia
   c. Hypotension and bradycardia
   d. Hypotension and massive hemorrhage

Suggested Readings

Bharathi MB, Janga RP, Rakesh BS, Babu AR. Laryngectomy with or without partial pharyngectomy: a systematic review. *Indian J Otolaryngol Head Neck Surg* 2019;71(Suppl 1):489–496.

BuSaba NY, Schaumberg DA. Predictors of prolonged length of stay after major elective head and neck surgery. *Laryngoscope* 2007; 117:1756–1763.

Hall FT, O'Brien CJ, Clifford AR, et al. Clinical outcome following total laryngectomy for cancer. *ANZ J Surg* 2003;73:300–305.

Hill-Madsen L, Kristensen CA, Andersen E, Johansen J, Andersen LJ, et al. Subglottic squamous cell carcinoma in Denmark 1971–2015 - a national population-based cohort study from DAHANCA, the Danish Head and Neck Cancer group. *Acta Oncol* 2019;58(10): 1509–1513.

Marioni G, Marchese-Ragona R, Cartei G, et al. Current opinion in diagnosis and treatment of laryngeal carcinoma. *Cancer Treat Rev* 2006;32:504–515.

Mastropietro C. The anesthetic considerations for the patient undergoing total laryngectomy. *J Am Assoc Nurse Anesth* 1987;55(3): 237–244.

McKenna JP, Fornataro-Clerici LM, McMenamin PG, et al. Laryngeal cancer: diagnosis, treatment and speech rehabilitation. *Am Fam Physician* 1991;44(1):123–129.

Noordzij JP, Ossoff RH. Anatomy and physiology of the larynx. *Otolaryngol Clin North Am* 2006;39:1–10.

Rinaldo A, Ferlito A. Open supraglottic laryngectomy. *Acta Otolaryngology* 2004;124:768–771.

Saraniti C, Speciale R, Santangelo M, Massaro N, Maniaci A, et al. Functional outcomes after supracricoid modified partial laryngectomy. *J Biol Regul Homeost Agents*. 2019;33(6):1903–1907.

Vahl JM, Schuler PJ, Greve J, Laban S, Knopf A, Hoffmann TK. Laryngectomy-still state of the art? *HNO* 2019;67(12):955–976.

Young VVN, Mangus BD, Bumpous JM. Salvage laryngectomy for failed conservative treatment of laryngeal cancer. *Laryngoscope* 2008;118:1561–1568.

4

Vocal Cord Polyp Removal With Laser

KEY POINTS

- Vocal cord polyps usually do not compromise airway patency.
- Gastroesophageal reflux disease (GERD) may be a concomitant condition.
- A laser (light amplification by stimulated emission of radiation) is an intensified beam of energy that can ignite fires.

- Perioperative complications that are associated with vocal cord polyp removal with laser include airway laceration, laryngospasm, burns, and eye injury.

Case Synopsis

A 33-year-old female singer is scheduled for laser removal of a left-sided vocal cord polyp.

Preoperative Evaluation and Demographic Data

Social History

- Cigarette smoker ½ pack per day for 15 years

Past Medical/Surgical History

- Patient denies any past medical or surgical history

List of Medications

- Multivitamin supplement daily

Diagnostic Data

- Hemoglobin, 15 g/dL; hematocrit, 45%
- Glucose, 90 mg/dL
- Blood urea nitrogen, 10 mg/dL; creatinine, 0.5 mg/dL
- Electrolytes: sodium, 140 mEq/L; potassium, 4.2 mEq/L; chloride, 99 mEq/L; carbon dioxide, 25 mEq/L
- Electrocardiogram, normal sinus rhythm (heart rate, 70 beats per minute)

Height/Weight/Vital Signs

- 170 cm, 80 kg
- Blood pressure, 128/88; heart rate, 74 beats per minute; respiratory rate, 18 breaths per minute; room air oxygen saturation, 98%; temperature, 36.8°C

Pathophysiology

Vocal cord polyps, nodules, and cysts have a similar clinical presentation and a slight histologic difference. Vocal cord polyps, nodules, and cysts are most often benign, well-defined, hyperplastic tissue. It has been suggested that vocal cord polyps may represent a chronic response to airway stress compared with an acute pathologic process associated with vocal cord nodules. There is a higher incidence of vocal cord polyps in people who are smokers and those who use their voice in a strenuous manner. Singers and orators may be at greater risk for developing these lesions due to frequent stress that is placed on the vocal cord.

The incidence of vocal cord polyps has been found to be evenly distributed between the sexes. Vocal cord polyps usually do not interfere with vocal cord movement, but larger polyps may alter phonation. Laser ablation of vocal cord polyps is most successful when it is a part of therapy that includes vocal therapy (retraining) and, if present, treating GERD. Fig. 4.1 illustrates a view during laryngoscopy of this patient's vocal cord polyp.

Surgical Procedure

Laser removal of a vocal cord polyp is accomplished using a low-intensity-energy laser directed onto the tissue to be ablated. A low-intensity laser beam is able to ablate the polyp with minimal transfer of energy to deeper and surrounding tissues. Polyp removal by laser is conducted under direct laryngoscopy or microlaryngoscopy to focus the energy beam. Laser ablation is most often accomplished adjacent to an endotracheal tube (ETT) during mechanical

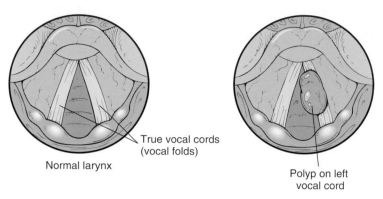

True vocal cords
(vocal folds)

Normal larynx

Polyp on left
vocal cord

• **Fig. 4.1** Laryngoscopic view of airway and vocal cord polyp. (From Frazier MS, Drzymkowski JW: *Essentials of human diseases and conditions*, ed 6, St. Louis, 2016, Elsevier.)

ventilation. A rigid bronchoscope can be used along with jet ventilation. The ETT may be removed during the use of the laser to prevent possible ignition and then reinserted.

Anesthetic Management and Considerations

Preoperative Period

1. *Describe the concerns regarding airway assessment for a patient who has a vocal cord polyp.*

    Performing a standard airway assessment is essential. Unlike tumors, polyps remain relatively small. Polyps are not usually associated with difficult mask ventilation or intubation. Vocal cord polyps may alter phonation and possibly be irritating but do not interfere with ventilation. Polyps are not usually excessively large and infrequently displace or obstruct the trachea. However, the anesthetist should be prepared for a difficult airway if the polyp is large, multiple polyps are present, edema formation has occurred, or other pathologic conditions exist.

2. *What preoperative medications are beneficial for a patient scheduled for laser airway surgery?*

    Midazolam can be administered to decrease anxiety during the preoperative period. Anticholinergics, such as atropine or glycopyrrolate, should be given intravenously to decrease airway secretions. Airway secretions may impair a thorough visualization of the vocal cords, and water molecules in the secretions absorb laser energy. Less vocal cord moisture (mucus, phlegm, saliva) improves the ability of the surgeon to focus and control the laser beam during intraoperative ablation.

Intraoperative Period

3. *Analyze the need for general endotracheal anesthesia for laser vocal cord polyp removal surgery.*

    An ETT maintains a patient's airway during the surgical procedure, which includes placement of throat packs, airway manipulation, focused laser energy, and tissue destruction. The ETT protects the airway from debris and secretions while isolating the glottic opening; higher inspired oxygen concentrations increase the potential for ignition caused by the laser. All three components of general anesthesia—amnesia, analgesia, and immobility—are required for laser surgery on the vocal cords. Analgesia is required to attenuate the sympathetic discharge associated with airway stimulation and manipulation. Short-acting and ultra-short-acting narcotics (remifentanil) are beneficial to blunt the stimulation from the airway manipulation during the procedure. Longer-acting narcotics will cause narcosis after the procedure has concluded, which may contribute to hypoventilation and bradypnea. Dexmedetomidine can be used to increase anesthetic depth and enhance postoperative analgesia without respiratory depression. Immobility is essential to decrease the possibility of injury to other tissues or disruption of the ETT by the endoscope and laser.

4. *Discuss alternatives to placement of an ETT for airway management.*

    The surgeon may want the ETT removed before the laser is used. Mask ventilation or reintubation and ventilation may be done between intermittent laser applications. This approach allows for complete vocal cord visualization but leaves the airway unprotected. Manual or high-frequency ventilation may also be done via a supraglottic small-bore ETT or high-frequency jet ventilation through a transtracheal catheter. A side stream ventilation port on the surgical endoscope may also be used for ventilation. There is an increased risk of fire if the airway management technique does not employ the use of a cuffed ETT due to the presence of supraphysiologic concentrations of oxygen that contact the laser. The surgeon and operating room personnel will also be exposed to anesthetic waste gases. The fraction of inspired oxygen concentration (FiO_2) should be maintained between 21% and 30%. Heliox, a mixture of helium and oxygen, has been successfully employed to lower the potential for combustion. A total intravenous anesthetic technique can also be used.

5. *Explain the associated risks during laser ablation.*

Fire, burns, eye injury, and noxious laser plume are all risks that are associated with the use of a laser. Lasers are a highly focused beam of intense energy that is able to ablate biologic tissues as well as ignite combustible materials. Fire is always a risk when lasers are in use. Burns to the patient or operating room staff may occur directly from the laser beam or by fire ignited by the laser. Surgical drapes, sponges, many prep solutions, and ETT are flammable. The oxygen-rich environment administered during anesthesia increases the risk of fire. Anesthetists must always remain vigilant of these risks and be prepared to respond in the event of a fire.

Eye injuries can occur to the patient or staff when the laser's beam is directed toward an unprotected face. The by-products of tissues ablated with a laser can contain contagious, mutagenic, and carcinogenic substances. Transmission of viruses such as human papilloma can occur. Methods that are used to protect operating room personnel from inhaling the by-products of tissue ablation include each member wearing a small micron particulate facemask (laser mask) and having the surgical assistant suction the laser plume exhaust with a vacuum system.

6. *Describe appropriate preparations an anesthetist can make for a laser vocal cord polyp removal case.*

All personnel that are present during surgical cases that utilize a laser should be trained in its safe operation. Signs warning "laser in use" and "protective eyewear required" should be displayed at all entrances to the operating room. All operating room personnel must wear appropriate laser glasses for the type of laser in use. Saline-soaked eye patches, with or without laser goggles, should be placed on the patient to protect their eyes from the laser's beam.

Preparation to prevent and treat fires and burns is necessary. A liter bottle of saline or water should be kept immediately available to saturate flames in case of fire. The lowest possible concentration of oxygen should be used. It is preferential to administer a blend of air and oxygen to maintain the FiO_2 between 21% and 30%. Helium, which is nonflammable, is useful as a carrier gas to decrease the FiO_2 when mixed with oxygen. Helium also has a lower density, which promotes laminar flow, as demonstrated by the Reynolds equation. Oxygen and nitrous oxide are both oxidizers, and they are associated with rapid combustion of flammable materials. Delivered carrier gases may collect under surgical drapes and may be ignited by a laser placed in close proximity. The laser should be switched into the standby mode or the off position when not in use. It should never be placed on the patient or surgical drapes.

7. *Provide a rationale for considering the use of Heliox for ventilation.*

Heliox is a mixture of helium and oxygen. Helium is nonflammable and possesses a lower density than nitrogen and oxygen, the main constituents of air. Helium allows the use of lower oxygen levels during laser surgery, thus lowering the risk of combustion while improving flow dynamics. Improved laminar flow is described by a lower calculated Reynolds number, as shown in Equation 4.1. A calculated Reynolds number greater than 2000 reflects a predominantly turbulent flow. A calculated Reynolds number less than 2000 will reflect a predominantly laminar flow. The lower the value, the greater the degree of laminar airflow, which can also be described as decreased resistance to airflow.

8. *Describe special precautions necessary for airway management during a general endotracheal anesthetic for laser airway surgery.*

The close proximity of the laser's beam to the ETT and the oxygen-enriched environment of ventilation increase the potential for fire. Oxygen supports combustion, and if the integrity of the ETT becomes breached, explosive ignition may occur. Lower FiO_2 levels lessen the explosive potential of laser fire ignition but do not remove it all together. Many anesthetists fill the ETT cuff with saline and a dye to be able to visually identify perforation of the ETT cuff if it occurs. Frequently, specially manufactured "laser tubes" are used, which are covered in a reflective material to lessen the chance of ignition by the laser energy. In addition, some anesthetists use adhesive-backed aluminum foil that is wrapped around the ETT, providing a reflective surface for the laser's energy.

$$\text{Reynolds number} = 5\ vpd/\eta$$

v is the linear velocity of fluid, **p** is the density of fluid, **d** is the diameter of the tube, and η is viscosity.

Maintenance

9. *Construct an organized systematic response for treatment of an airway fire.*

A quick systematic response to this medical emergency is an absolute necessity to limit injury.

1. Immediately discontinue ventilation and oxygen flow
2. Douse the airway with sterile saline
3. Extubate the patient
4. Verify that the fire is extinguished
5. Mask ventilate
6. Perform direct laryngoscopy, remove any remnants of the ETT or throat packs
7. Reintubate
8. Perform fiber-optic bronchoscopy to visualize and document the degree of injury
9. Corticosteroids and antibiotics will likely be required along with continued intubation

10. *Discuss the choice of volatile anesthetic agents.*

The desirable pharmacokinetic and pharmacodynamic profiles associated with sevoflurane make it desirable to use as the main anesthetic during laser polyp removal because it does not cause irritation to the airway and it is easily titrated. Isoflurane and desflurane cause airway irritation that may contribute to excessive coughing during emergence. Laser surgery on the airway for vocal cord polyp removal is usually a short procedure (15 minutes), and therefore saturation of the muscle and fat compartments with inhalation agent does not significantly delay emergence. The low blood–gas solubility of sevoflurane, along with its lack of pungency, promotes quick and smooth emergence during these procedures.

11. *Provide a rationale for total intravenous anesthesia during laser polyp removal surgery.*

Total intravenous anesthesia (TIVA) using propofol is an appropriate choice for maintenance of anesthesia, especially if intermittent ventilation or a significant leak during mechanical ventilation exists intraoperatively. Interrupting the administration of the inhaled agent during periods of extubation and laser ablation makes controlling the anesthetic depth difficult. Providing TIVA is also beneficial to decrease the exposure of the operating room personnel to anesthetic gases.

12. *Discuss the use of neuromuscular blocking agents during laser surgery on the airway.*

Immobility is necessary, and therefore neuromuscular blocking agents may be administered. The patient must not move during the use of a rigid endoscope to prevent injury. Coughing or "bucking" during laser surgery of the airway can be disastrous, as laceration, perforation, and inadvertent laser injury to normal tissues may occur. Short- or intermediate-duration muscle relaxants are best, as laser surgery of vocal polyps is a relatively short procedure. The ability to reverse muscle relaxants with cholinesterase inhibitors requires a degree of spontaneous recovery of neuromuscular blockade. Sugammadex may be desirable to reverse neuromuscular blockade due to the relatively short length of the procedure and the risk of residual skeletal muscle weakness.

13. *Describe the nervous system innervation to the larynx.*

The larynx is innervated by two branches of the vagus nerve. The superior laryngeal nerve (SLN) bifurcates into the internal superior laryngeal nerve (sensory) and the external superior laryngeal nerve (motor). The internal superior laryngeal nerve provides sensory innervation above the vocal cords. The external superior laryngeal nerve provides motor innervation to the cricothyroid muscle, a vocal cord tensor. The recurrent laryngeal nerve (RLN) innervates all other intrinsic laryngeal muscles to provide motor function and sensory innervation below the level of the vocal cords. The sensory and motor innervation to the larynx is listed in Box 4.1.

14. *Discuss the reason that the surgeon may request visual confirmation of vocal cord movement after removal of the vocal cord polyp.*

It is possible that the surgeon may request to visualize the vocal cords using direct laryngoscopy or a fiber-optic method. This assessment is done to confirm that the recurrent laryngeal nerve, which is primarily responsible for vocal cord movement, remains intact. To accomplish

---

• **BOX 4.1** | **Sensory and Motor Nerve Innervation to the Larynx**

Superior Laryngeal Nerve (SLN)

1. Sensory function: internal branch of the SLN—sensation between the epiglottis and vocal cords
2. Motor function: external branch of the SLN cricothyroid muscle (tenses vocal cords)

Recurrent Laryngeal Nerve (RLN)

1. Sensory function: sensation below the level of the vocal cords
2. Motor function: innervation of seven intrinsic laryngeal muscles
   a. Posterior cricoarytenoid (opens vocal cords)
   b. Lateral cricoarytenoid (closes vocal cords)
   c. Thyroarytenoid (shortens/relaxes vocal cords)
   d. Transverse arytenoid (closes vocal cords)

---

this task, the patient is allowed to spontaneously breathe and then extubated while in a surgical plane of anesthesia to avoid laryngospasm and sympathetic nervous system hyperreactivity.

Injury to the SLN is possible with laser surgery on the vocal cords. Unilateral or bilateral injuries to the SLN may cause hoarseness and fatigue during phonation. Because the motor function of the SLN results in vocal cord tension via the cricothyroid muscle, denervation should not result in airway compromise. Injury to the RLN is unlikely during vocal cord laser polyp removal. The motor function of the RLN innervates all other intrinsic muscles of the larynx. If unilateral injury to the RLN occurs, paralysis of that vocal cord will result. Airway patency is rarely compromised, but vocal function and tone would be affected. Bilateral RLN injury causes bilateral vocal cord paralysis, and unopposed cricothyroid tension closes the glottic opening. Negative inspiratory pressure pulls the vocal cords together, further occluding the glottic opening. The vocal cords will remain in the midline position, and airway obstruction, stridor, and eventual respiratory distress will occur. Intubation or tracheostomy is required to maintain a patent airway with bilateral vocal cord paralysis.

15. *Describe the anesthetic goals during emergence and extubation.*

The goals for emergence and extubation include maintaining adequate analgesia, decreasing airway irritation, and avoiding laryngospasm and airway compromise. Extubation that occurs while the patient is deeply anesthetized will help decrease the risk of laryngospasm. Lidocaine administered intravenously has been used successfully to attenuate laryngeal reflexes.

Postoperative Period

16. *Analyze the physiologic mechanism and causes responsible for laryngospasm.*

Sensory stimulation of the internal branch of the SLN causes an afferent reflex arc at the level of the spinal cord. The efferent reflex from the brain travels via the external branch of the laryngeal nerve to the cricothyroid muscle, causing contraction. The cricothyroid muscle is attached to the cricoid and thyroid cartilages. When contracted, this muscle tenses (adducts) the vocal cords. Laryngospasm is a spasm (sustained contraction) of the cricothyroid muscles. Vocal cord stimulation by the laser, irritation, inflammation, and light anesthesia during the emergence phase all contribute to the increased risk of laryngospasm.

17. *Construct a systematic plan to treat laryngospasm.*

Light anesthesia (stage II), inadequate analgesia, and airway stimulation contribute to the incidence of laryngospasm. Application of positive pressure (10 to 20 cm H_2O) via mask pushes on the vocal cords and stretches the cricothyroid muscle. Stretching a muscle in spasm allows the contraction to be relaxed. Additionally, manual digital pressure on the pressure point in front of the mastoid process by the angle of the mandible aids in attenuating laryngospasm. The exact mechanism is unknown but may be related to an acupressure or pain reflex. Delay in treating laryngospasm

allows persistent cricothyroid contraction and may be resistant to positive pressure maneuvers. Succinylcholine 10 to 20 mg intravenously will relax the cricothyroid muscle when positive pressure does not relieve the laryngospasm. It is important to note that succinylcholine given after reversal of neuromuscular blockade with a cholinesterase inhibitor will have an extended duration of action due to inhibition of pseudocholinesterase. Prolonged paralysis will require assisted ventilation.

18. *Discuss postoperative care for a patient after vocal cord polyp removal.*

Adequate pain control and relieving airway irritation are important postoperative considerations. Intravenous narcotics titrated to patient comfort and respiratory adequacy attenuate irritation, coughing, and laryngospasm. Postoperative delivery of humidified oxygen, aerosolized racemic epinephrine, and intravenous corticosteroids help treat airway hyperreactivity. Stridor is indicative of airway narrowing and may be caused by edema, vocal cord nerve injury, or laryngospasm.

Review Questions

1. Which is true regarding vocal cord polyps?
   a. Frequently malignant
   b. Contribute to a high incidence of airway obstruction
   c. Usually do not interfere with airway patency and ventilation
   d. Occur from an acute response to airway stress
2. Which is not a risk associated with the use of lasers in the operating room?
   a. Fire
   b. Burns
   c. Eye injury
   d. High-dose radiation exposure
3. Which is not a necessary component for fire to occur?
   a. Oxidizer
   b. Carbon dioxide
   c. Ignition source
   d. Fuel
4. Which precautions should be taken during laser surgery that involves the airway?
   a. Eye protection for the patient and the operating room personnel
   b. Administering the highest possible FiO_2
   c. Administering nitrous oxide
   d. Having suction available
5. Which is not a treatment for laryngospasm?
   a. Positive airway pressure
   b. Digital pressure at the angle of the ramus and mastoid process
   c. Cricothyrotomy
   d. Intravenous succinylcholine

Suggested Readings

American Society of Anesthesiologists. Practice advisory for the prevention and management of operating room fires. *Anesthesiology* 2008;108:786–801.

Bigony L. Risks associated with exposure to surgical smoke plume: a review of the literature. *AORN Journal* 2007;86:1013–1023.

Bourgain JL, Desruennes E, Fischler M, et al. Transtracheal high frequency jet ventilation for endoscopic airway surgery: a multicentre study. *Br J Anaesth* 2001;87:870–875.

Heiner JS. Airway management. In: Nagelhout JJ, Elisha S, eds. *Nurse Anesthesia*, 6th ed. St. Louis, MO: Elsevier, 2018:397–440.

Jones TS, Black IH, Robinson TN, Jones EL. Operating room fires. *Anesthesiology* 2019;130(3):492–501.

Singh S, Kate S, Bhan S, Suhag V. Surgical site fire during surgery in operating room under general anaesthesia. *Indian J Anaesth* 2019; 63(10):865–866.

Spiess BD, Ivankovich AD. Anesthetic management of laser airway surgery. *Semin Surg Oncol* 1990;6:189–193.

Werkhaven JA. Microlaryngoscopy-airway management with anaesthetic techniques for CO_2 laser. *Pediatr Anesth* 2004;14:90–94.

White A. Management of benign vocal fold lesions: current perspectives on the role for voice therapy. *Curr Opin Otolaryngol Head Neck Surg* 2019;(3):185–190.

5

Uvulopalatopharyngoplasty

KEY POINTS

- Obstructive sleep apnea (OSA) is characterized by chronic, frequent episodes of upper airway obstruction during sleep, which results in hypoxia and hypercarbia. This condition is associated with increased risk of cardiovascular, neuropsychologic, and endocrine disorders and impaired quality of life.
- It is estimated that up to 93% of women and 82% of men with moderate to severe OSA are undiagnosed.
- OSA is associated with increased perioperative morbidity and mortality because of an increased risk

- of difficult intubation, coexisting diseases, and life-threatening apnea.
- Perioperative risk is based on severity of OSA, invasiveness of surgery, and requirements for postoperative opioids.
- Anesthetic considerations for patients presenting for uvulopalatopharyngoplasty (UPPP) include identifying and managing potentially difficult airways, closely observing for airway obstruction and bleeding, and carefully titrating opioids in the postoperative period.

Case Synopsis

A 45-year-old man with a history of OSA is scheduled by his ear, nose, and throat (ENT) surgeon to have a UPPP.

Preoperative Evaluation and Demographic Data

Past Medical/Surgical History

- Severe OSA
- Obesity
- Non–insulin-dependent diabetes
- Hypertension
- Smoked 1 pack a day for 10 years
- Bilateral myringotomy age 3; no anesthetic complications

List of Medications

- Atenolol

Diagnostic Data

- Hemoglobin, 15 g/dL; hematocrit, 42%
- Blood urea nitrogen, 15 mg/dL; creatinine, 1.1 mg/dL
- Glucose,160 mg/dL
- Electrolytes: sodium, 140 mEq/L; potassium, 3.9 mEq/L; chloride, 104 mEq/L; carbon dioxide, 24 mEq/L
- Sleep study
  - Precontinuous positive airway pressure (pre-CPAP): apnea–hypopnea index (AHI), 50 events/hour; lowest oxygen saturation (LSAT), 75%
  - Post-CPAP: AHI, 38 events/hour; LSAT, 83% at 10 cm H_2O. The titration of CPAP was stopped due to patient intolerance.

- Electrocardiogram (ECG): normal sinus bradycardia (heart rate 58 beats per minute), left ventricular hypertrophy

Height/Weight/Vital Signs

- 175 cm, 113 kg
- Body mass index (BMI), 36.6; blood pressure, 152/80; heart rate, 59 beats per minute; respiratory rate, 20 breaths per minute; room air oxygen saturation, 95%; temperature, 36°C

Airway Examination

- Mallampati (MP) Class III; 13 tonsillar hypertrophy; thyromental distance and mouth opening 3 finger-breadths; short, thick neck (18 inches); and teeth intact

Pathophysiology

OSA is a significant problem that is associated with serious physical consequences. It is characterized by chronic, frequent episodes of upper airway obstruction during sleep that result in hypoxia and hypercarbia and significant morbidity. It is estimated that 2% of women and 4% of men in the United States have OSA. However, surveys suggest that as many as 21% of women and 31% of men may be at risk for OSA and that up to 93% of women and 82% of men with moderate to severe OSA are undiagnosed. Additionally, patients with moderate to severe OSA have a higher incidence of difficult intubation, postoperative respiratory complications (e.g., severe oxygen desaturation, SaO_2 <90%), unplanned intensive care admission, and prolonged hospital stay.

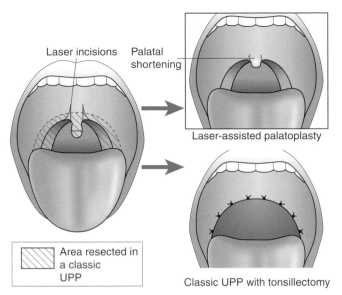

Laser incisions   Palatal shortening

Laser-assisted palatoplasty

Area resected in a classic UPP

Classic UPP with tonsillectomy

• **Fig. 5.1** Uvulopalatopharyngoplasty reduces upper airway obstruction by shortening the uvula, trimming the soft palate, and suturing back the anterior and posterior pharyngeal pillars. (From Dhillon RS, East CA: *Ear, nose, and throat and head and neck surgery*, ed 4, Edinburgh, 2013, Churchill Livingstone.)

Surgical Procedure

The gold standard treatment for OSA is CPAP or bilevel positive airway pressure (BiPAP). Even though it is extremely effective, tolerance of and compliance with the device are difficult for some patients. Patients who cannot tolerate CPAP may be candidates for surgery to alleviate anatomic sites of the obstruction with UPPP. UPPP involves surgical enlargement of the retropalatal airway by trimming and reorienting the posterior and anterior lateral pharyngeal pillars, as shown in Fig. 5.1. The procedure may be combined with adenotonsillectomy or combined with advancement, limited resection, or radiofrequency ablation of the tongue base to achieve maximal enlargement of the retrolingual and retropalatal airway.

Anesthetic Management and Considerations

Preoperative Period

1. Describe the mechanism that causes airway obstruction and diagnostic criteria for OSA.

OSA is a syndrome associated with periodic, partial, or complete obstruction of the upper airway during sleep that leads to episodes of apnea–hypopnea, frequent arousals, oxygen desaturation, and daytime hypersomnolence. Apnea is defined as a cessation of airflow for longer than 10 seconds. The event is obstructive if there is effort to breathe during apnea. Hypopnea is an abnormal respiratory event with at least 30% reduction in thoracoabdominal movement or airflow compared with

Severity of OSA	Apnea–Hypopnea Index
None	0–5
Mild	6–20
Moderate	21–40
Severe	>40

TABLE 5.1 Severity of Obstructive Sleep Apnea

baseline lasting at least 10 seconds and with 4% oxygen desaturation. The formal diagnosis of OSA is made by polysomnography, and the severity is based on the AHI (number of times apnea–hypopnea occurs per hour of sleep). The criterion that is based on the AHI is presented in Table 5.1. Patients with OSA have significantly higher arousal index, lower SaO_2, and decreased slow wave sleep, respectively, compared with non-OSA patients. The typical patient with OSA is a loud snorer who has a BMI 35 kg/m², age 50, neck circumference 17 inches, and is male.

2. Describe the pathophysiologic factors and physiologic consequences associated with OSA.

The pathophysiology of OSA is multifactorial, involving upper airway anatomy, motor control of the pharyngeal dilator muscles, ventilatory control stability, and arousal threshold. The upper airway contains three segments: the nasopharynx, the oropharynx, and the hypopharynx. The inspiratory patency of these segments is controlled by contraction of the tensor palatini, the genioglossus, and the hyoid muscles, respectively. The three segments are prone to collapse because of the lack of bony support in the anterior and lateral walls. During wakefulness, the action of these pharyngeal dilator muscles is important in keeping the airway patent. However, during deep non–rapid eye movement (NREM) and rapid eye movement (REM) sleep, there is a generalized loss of muscle tone, which may result in airway collapse in susceptible patients, as is depicted in Fig. 5.2.

Several factors contribute to the pathophysiologic changes that are present with OSA:

• When OSA is associated with obesity, there is a larger deposition of adipose tissue in the uvula, tonsils, tonsillar pillars, tongue, aryepiglottic folds, and lateral pharyngeal walls, and possibly externally, which can contribute to airway obstruction during sleep.

• There is poor upper airway motor control during sleep in patients with OSA, which is associated with substantial decrements in pharyngeal dilator muscle activity; over time, these muscles may develop neural/muscle damage, which further exacerbates airway obstruction.

• Instability in the control of ventilation results in increases and decreases in respiratory output to pharyngeal dilator muscles, which when combined with increased fat deposition in the airway and poor upper

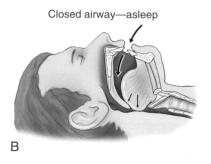
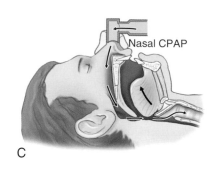

Open airway—awake
Tongue
Epiglottis

Closed airway—asleep

Nasal CPAP

A   Oropharynx   Soft palate

B

C

• **Fig. 5.2** How sleep apnea occurs. (A) The patient predisposed to obstructive sleep apnea (OSA) has a small pharyngeal airway. (B) During sleep, the pharyngeal muscles relax, allowing the airway to close. Lack of airflow results in repeated apneic episodes. (C) Continuous positive airway pressure *(CPAP)* splints the airway open, preventing airflow obstruction. (Modified from Modified from LaFleur Brooks M: *Exploring medical language: A student-directed approach*, ed 8, St. Louis, 2012, Elsevier.)

airway motor control, may further contribute to episodes of obstruction.

Episodes of apnea, hypoxemia, and hypercarbia develop and lead to progressive increases in respiratory effort. These triggers increase neural stimulation into the reticular activating system, which arouses the individual to a lighter stage of sleep, which then activates the pharyngeal dilator muscles to open the airway. Upon arousal, there is increased electroencephalogram activity, and patients may demonstrate vocalization, extremity twitching, turning, gasping, or snoring on airway opening. Ventilation resumes and the hypoxemia and hypercarbia are corrected. However, relief of the obstruction is associated with a short period of hyperventilation, which may significantly decrease the CO_2 and respiratory drive and may contribute to episodes of apnea that are followed by hyperpnea. These repeated obstructive and hypoxemic/hypercarbic events cause sleep fragmentation, sympathetic hyperactivity, systemic inflammation with higher C-reactive protein and interleukin-6 levels, endothelial dysfunction, and metabolic dysregulation, all of which can increase the risk for cardiovascular, neuropsychologic, and endocrine disorders.

3. *Discuss the coexisting diseases that are associated with patients presenting for UPPP and OSA.*

OSA affects the cardiovascular, neuropsychologic, and endocrine systems because of the repeated cycles of apnea and airway obstruction during sleep. Systemic vasoconstriction results in hypertension and may contribute to left ventricular failure. In fact, OSA has been found to be an independent risk factor of essential hypertension after controlling for age, sex, BMI, and antihypertensive agents. Arrhythmias that are caused by hypoxia and hypercarbia such as atrial fibrillation, bradycardia, and atrioventricular block can occur. Sympathetic hyperactivity, inflammation, and endothelial dysfunction contribute to an increased incidence of nocturnal angina and myocardial infarction (MI).

Cerebrovascular disease (CVD) and stroke are associated with OSA. Pulmonary hypertension secondary to frequent hypoxia over many years may lead to right-sided heart failure. Neuropsychologic symptoms include daytime somnolence, impaired cognitive function, increased accidents because of decreased vigilance, depression, and anxiety. The endocrine system manifestations include obesity, glucose intolerance and diabetes, and decreases in testosterone and growth hormone. Table 5.2 summarizes coexisting diseases associated with OSA.

4. *Describe the preoperative evaluation and preparation for a patient with OSA presenting for UPPP.*

Patients with OSA require a thorough preoperative evaluation to identify and minimize perioperative complications. A complete history and physical examination should be performed, with special attention to the airway examination, because patients with OSA have a higher incidence of difficult intubation.

For patients suspected of having OSA, a STOP-BANG questionnaire should be completed. The STOP-BANG assessment has been shown to be highly sensitive for patients that have OSA. The component of this preoperative tool is included in Box 5.1.

Anatomic factors that can complicate direct laryngoscopy and intubation are included in Box 5.2. A history of difficult intubation associated with previous anesthetic experiences, as well as any other complications, should be elicited. Review of systems should focus on the presence, severity, and effectiveness of current management of coexisting diseases associated with OSA. Preoperative testing is dependent on the individual patient's situation and may include electrocardiogram (ECG), stress testing, chest x-ray, electrolyte, complete blood counts, and a coagulation panel.

Sleep study results, if available, should be reviewed and documented. If a sleep study is not available, such patients should be treated as having moderate OSA. They should be considered to have severe OSA if they have markedly increased BMI or neck circumference, episodes of apnea, or the patient falls asleep within minutes if unstimulated. CPAP settings should be documented, and patients should be instructed to bring the machines on the day of surgery.

TABLE 5.2	Coexisting Diseases/Symptoms Associated With Obstructive Sleep Apnea	
Cardiovascular	**Neuropsychologic**	**Endocrine/Other**

• Hypertension
• Arrhythmias:
  • Atrial fibrillation
  • Bradycardia
  • Atrioventricular block
• Coronary artery disease
• Nocturnal angina
• Myocardial infarction
• Congestive heart failure
• Pulmonary hypertension
	• Daytime somnolence
	• Cognitive impairment
	• Accident proneness
	• Anxiety
	• Depression
		• Glucose intolerance and diabetes
		• Obesity
		• Gastroesophageal reflux disease

• BOX 5.1 STOP-BANG Obstructive Sleep Apnea Assessment

STOP

1. **S**noring: Do you snore loudly? (Loud enough to be heard through a closed door?) Y/N
2. **T**ired: Do you often feel tired, fatigued, or sleepy during the day? Y/N
3. **O**bserved: Have you been observed to stop breathing during sleep? Y/N
4. Blood **P**ressure: Do you have high blood pressure? Y/N

BANG

1. **B**MI: >35 kg/m²? Y/N
2. **A**ge over 50 years? Y/N
3. **N**eck circumference: >40 cm? Y/N
4. **G**ender: Male? Y/N

High risk for OSA: Yes to ≥3 questions
Low risk for OSA: Yes to <3 questions

• BOX 5.2 Risk Factors Associated With Difficult Intubation

- Mallampati Class III or IV
- Long upper incisors
- Prominent overbite
- Mandibular incisors anterior to maxillary incisors
- <3 fingerbreadths thyromental distance
- >3 cm interincisor distance
- Retrognathia or micrognathia
- Macroglossia
- High arched or very narrow palate
- Stiff, indurated, occupied by mass, or nonresilient mandibular space
- Short, thick neck; neck circumference >40–42 cm
- Limited neck range of motion
- Apnea–hypopnea index >40
- Obesity

The suitability for inpatient or outpatient surgery, extended postoperative monitoring (i.e., monitored settings vs. routine hospital wards), and duration of stay (extended stay in postanesthesia care unit [PACU] vs. no extended stay in PACU; hospital admission vs. no admission) should be determined before surgery. These decisions should be based on the severity of the OSA, anatomic or physiologic abnormalities, status of coexisting diseases, type of anesthesia, need for postoperative opioids, patient age, adequacy of postdischarge observation, and capabilities of the facility.

5. *Utilizing the American Society of Anesthesiologists (ASA) Practice Guidelines for OSA, predict the perioperative risk for this patient.*

The ASA Practice Guidelines for OSA estimate risk of perioperative complications based on:
- **(A) Severity of OSA:** none, 0 points; mild, 1 point; moderate, 2 points; and severe, 3 points—subtract 1 point if CPAP or BiPAP preop and postop, 11 points if $PaCO_2$ >50 mm Hg

- **(B) Invasiveness of surgery:** superficial surgery under local or peripheral nerve block anesthesia without sedation, 0 points; superficial surgery with moderate sedation or general anesthesia, 1 point; peripheral surgery with spinal or epidural anesthesia (with no more than moderate sedation), 1 point; peripheral surgery with general anesthesia or airway surgery with moderate sedation, 2 points; and major surgery or airway surgery with general anesthesia, 3 points
- **(C) Requirements for postoperative opioids:** none, 0 points; low-dose oral opioids, 1 point; high-dose oral, parental, or neuraxial opioids, 3 points
- Estimation of the overall risk is based on the sum of A + B + C (range 0 to 6). Patients with a score of 4 may be at increased perioperative risk from OSA; scores of 5 or 6 significantly increase the perioperative risk from OSA.

This patient has severe OSA (3 points), is having airway surgery under general anesthesia (3 points), and has a low-dose opioid requirement postoperatively (3 points). The patient has been using CPAP preoperatively, and it is anticipated he will use it postoperatively (subtract 1 point). The overall score is 5, which indicates the patient may be at significantly increased perioperative risk from OSA.

Intraoperative Period

6. *Summarize the effects of anesthesia on the airway and respiratory function.*

Patients who have OSA are extremely sensitive to the airway and respiratory depressant effects of anesthetic agents and opioids. Anesthetic agents such as propofol, midazolam, opioids, small doses of neuromuscular blockers, and nitrous oxide diminish the pharyngeal dilator muscle action and promote upper airway collapse. Additionally, most anesthetics and opioids alter the control of breathing by affecting the chemical, metabolic, or behavioral control of respiration. Propofol has been shown to produce a dose-dependent decrease in the genioglossal muscle, which results in greater airway collapsibility. Nasopharyngeal anesthesia with 4% lidocaine is associated with decreased genioglossal muscle function and increased pharyngeal airway collapsibility. Dexmedetomidine is associated with anxiolytic, sedative, and analgesic effects without causing significant respiratory depression.

7. *Describe the effects of anesthesia and surgery on postoperative sleep patterns.*

Patients with OSA who use opioids during the postoperative period for pain relief are at increased risk of life-threatening apnea for approximately a week after surgery. Sleep architecture is altered after surgery with suppression of stage 3 and 4 REM and NREM sleep. Postoperative pain is greatest in the first several days after surgery, and these patients are at increased risk for life-threatening obstructive apnea secondary to respiratory depressive effects of opioids. After the third postoperative day, deep REM sleep rebounds, and patients who have OSA are at risk for life-threatening deep sleep–induced apnea.

8. *Formulate an anesthetic plan for a patient presenting for UPPP with severe OSA and a potentially difficult airway.*

The patient's airway examination, obesity, and severe OSA increase the risk that the patient may be a difficult mask ventilation and intubation, respectively. Given this information, an awake fiber-optic intubation is recommended. Box 5.3 lists considerations for performing an awake fiber-optic intubation. Important points when a fiber-optic intubation is planned include:

- Administration of an antisialagogue such as glycopyrrolate in the preoperative area
- Carefully administering sedation to maintain meaningful contact with the patient
- Adequately anesthetizing the patient's airway
- Utilizing proper technique when manipulating the fiber-optic scope
- Ability to troubleshoot problems

| BOX 5.3 | Procedure for Awake Fiber-Optic Intubation |

1. Discuss need for awake fiber-optic intubation with patient and surgical team.
2. IV access should be obtained as soon as possible and glycopyrrolate 0.2 mg IV (takes up to 20 minutes for peak effect).
3. Difficult airway cart with a fiber-optic bronchoscope (at least 2 mm narrower than the ETT), atomizer, nebulizer, nasal trumpets, viscous lidocaine and lubricant, Ovassapian and Williams airways, sources of oxygen and suction, cotton-tipped applicators, bag valve mask, and additional difficult intubation equipment should be in room.
4. Bronchoscope should be verified for proper functioning and attached to a light source and camera if present. Practice rotating, antiflexing, and retroflexing the scope.
5. Adequate airway topicalization is critical. Techniques include:
   - 4% lidocaine by atomizer or nebulizer.
   - 5% lidocaine ointment on top of tongue depressor placed in the back of mouth near posterior pharynx.
   - If nasal intubation is needed, the nares should be sprayed with Neo-Synephrine spray, then may use 4% lidocaine in a syringe or atomizer to spray in the nose; 2% lidocaine jelly in a 10-mL syringe can be injected into the nose.
   - Glossopharyngeal and superior laryngeal nerve blocks with 1–2 mL of lidocaine 1%–2%. Glossopharyngeal nerve block provides anesthesia to the posterior third of the tongue, anterior epiglottis, posterior and lateral walls of the pharynx, and the tonsillar pillars. The superior laryngeal nerve block abolishes the gag reflex by providing anesthesia of the larynx down to but excluding the vocal cords.
6. If oral intubation is done, a Williams or Ovassapian airway should be used to keep the scope midline. The ETT can then be slid close to the cords then past the fiber-optic scope; alternatively, the scope may be passed first. If nasal intubation, then pass the tube first into the posterior pharynx.
7. Before passing the scope through the cords, additional lidocaine can be injected onto the cords via the side port on the scope. Alternatively, a transtracheal injection of local anesthetic can be performed to block the recurrent laryngeal nerve.
8. Suction and oxygen can be attached to the scope and used if needed.
9. If pink tissue is seen, pull the ETT and scope back until the vocal cords can be seen. An assistant may also provide a jaw thrust or cricoid pressure to help open the airway and improve visualization/guidance.
10. Once fiber-optic scope is passed through the vocal cords, advance and avoid touching the carina. Next, slide the ETT over the fiber-optic scope. If resistance is met, pull the tube back and rotate the ETT 90 degrees counterclockwise—this turns the tip away from the arytenoids.
11. After placement is confirmed, general anesthesia may be induced.

ETT, Endotracheal tube; IV, intravenous.

Sedation for the procedure may include anxiolytics such as Versed titrated to effect and opioids such as fentanyl or alfentanil. Extreme caution should be used when determining to give opioids to patients with severe OSA while in the preoperative area. Other sedatives include dexmedetomidine and ketamine. Once the patient is intubated by a fiber-optic approach, an intravenous and/or inhalation induction may be performed. Agents chosen should be based on the patient's coexisting diseases. Placement of a mouth gag that is used to keep the jaw in the open position is stimulating, and boluses of propofol or an opioid may be needed to blunt the airway response. Dexamethasone is frequently given to decrease the degree of edema formation in the oral cavity, although there is a lack of scientific evidence to support this intervention.

The anesthetic can be maintained by administering short-acting agents such as desflurane with or without nitrous oxide, remifentanil, or alfentanil and subtherapeutic doses of intermediate-acting neuromuscular blockers. Because blood that enters the stomach is highly emetogenic, antiemetics such as ondansetron should be considered. Based on surgeon preference and the presence of adequate hemostasis, ketorolac may be given for postoperative analgesia. This patient was identified as having a difficult intubation, and the fiber-optic scope and airway cart/adjuncts should be immediately available if the need for emergent reintubation should arise. The patient should respond to commands appropriately and meet other extubation criteria before removal of the endotracheal tube (ETT). Hemostasis should be confirmed before extubation. The patient may need to be extubated over a tube changer if there was difficulty or concern with the airway. Extubation should occur in the semi-recumbent or the reverse Trendelenburg position to minimize compression of the diaphragm by the abdomen.

Postoperative Period

9. *List the potential postoperative complications/events and frequency that can occur after UPPP.*
   - Respiratory 1.1% to 11% (i.e., laryngospasm, postobstructive pulmonary edema, airway obstruction and oxygen desaturation, emergent tracheotomy, reintubation, and pneumonia)
   - Hemorrhage 0.3% to 14% (biphasic occurrence; immediate postoperatively or several days after surgery)
   - Hypertension 2% to 70%
   - Cardiovascular 0.3% (i.e., arrhythmias, cardiac arrest, angina, MI, cerebrovascular accident, or pulmonary embolism)

10. *Describe the postoperative management for patients after UPPP with severe OSA.*

    Anesthetic considerations in the postoperative period include:
    - Decreasing postoperative pain
    - Ensuring adequate oxygenation
    - Observing for airway obstruction
    - Positioning the patient in a lateral or semi-recumbent position
    - Using CPAP

    Patients with severe OSA are at high risk for opioid-induced airway obstruction in the postoperative period and should not be discharged from the recovery room to an unmonitored setting. This is especially important because UPPP surgery is associated with moderate postoperative pain, and patients may require intravenous narcotics and have an increased susceptibility to airway obstruction, given the type of surgery. Nonsteroidal antiinflammatory agents have an opioid-sparing effect and should be considered. Supplemental oxygen and continuous pulse oximetry should be continued until patients can maintain room air oxygen saturation at baseline or 90% and not develop airway obstruction when left undisturbed. Patients should be positioned either in the lateral or semi-recumbent position, and CPAP should be restarted in the postoperative period. Finally, patients with severe OSA should be admitted to an intensive care setting for airway observation for up to 24 hours.

Review Questions

1. Obstructive sleep apnea is associated with periodic, partial, or complete obstruction of the upper airway during sleep and is not associated with:
   a. Apnea–hypopnea and frequent arousals.
   b. Oxygen desaturation.
   c. Daytime hypersomnolence.
   d. Hypocarbia.
2. Which classification of OSA is associated with a preoperative apnea–hypopnea index of 25?
   a. None
   b. Mild
   c. Moderate
   d. Severe
3. Which statement is true regarding the pathophysiologic changes associated with obstructive sleep apnea?
   a. Poor upper airway motor control
   b. Increased upper airway motor control
   c. Ventilatory control stability
   d. Increased pharyngeal dilator muscle activity
4. Repeated obstructive and hypoxemic/hypercarbic events do not result in:
   a. Sleep fragmentation.
   b. Parasympathetic nervous system stimulation hyperactivity.
   c. Metabolic dysregulation.
   d. Systemic inflammation.

5. Postoperative narcotic administration and airway obstruction can increase the risk for life-threatening apnea because of:
   a. Stability of the sleep architecture, postoperative pain, and rebound of light REM sleep.
   b. Alteration of the sleep architecture alteration, postoperative pain, respiratory depressant effect of opioids, and rebound of deep REM sleep.
   c. Alteration of the sleep architecture alteration, decreased postoperative pain, and rebound of deep REM sleep.
   d. Inhibition of the airway reflexes, stimulation of the sympathetic nervous system, and increased myocardial oxygen consumption.

Suggested Readings

Chung F, Yegneswaran B, Liao P, et al. Validation of the Berlin questionnaire and American Society of Anesthesiologists checklist as screening tools for obstructive sleep apnea in surgical patients. *Anesthesiology* 2008;108(5):822–830.

Chung SA, Yuan H, Chung F. A systemic review of obstructive sleep apnea and its implications for anesthesiologists. *Anesth Analg* 2008;107(5):1543–1563.

Dickerson SC. Perioperative guidelines in anesthesia. *Otolaryngol Clin North Am* 2019 Dec;52(6):981–993.

Gross JB, Bachenberg KL, Benumof JL, et al. Practice guidelines for the perioperative management of patients with obstructive sleep apnea: a report by the American Society of Anesthesiologists Task Force on Perioperative Management of Patients with Obstructive Sleep Apnea. Anesthesiology 2006;104(5):1081–1093; quiz 1117–1118.

Kezirian EJ, Weaver EM, Yueh B, et al. Risk factors for serious complication after uvulopalatopharyngoplasty. *Arch Otolaryngol Head Neck Surg* 2006;132(10):1091–1098.

McNicholas WT, Ryan S. Obstructive sleep apnea syndrome: translating science to clinical practice. *Respirology* 2006;11(2):136–144.

Mechanick JI, Apovian C, Brethauer S, Garvey WT, Joffe AM, Kim J, Kushner RF, et al. Clinical practice guidelines for the perioperative nutrition, metabolic, and nonsurgical support of patients undergoing bariatric procedures - 2019 update: cosponsored by American Association of Clinical Endocrinologists/American College of Endocrinology, The Obesity Society, American Society for Metabolic and Bariatric Surgery, Obesity Medicine Association, and American Society of Anesthesiologists - executive summary. *Endocr Pract* 2019;25(12):1346–1359.

Moos DD, Prasch M, Cantral DE, et al. Are patients with obstructive sleep apnea syndrome appropriate candidates for the ambulatory surgical center? *AANA J* 2005;73(3):197–205.

Pawlik MT, Hansen E, Waldhauser D, et al. Clonidine premedication in patients with sleep apnea syndrome: a randomized, double-blind, placebo-controlled study. *Anesth Analg* 2005;101(5):1374–1380.

Santer P, Eikermann M. Unrecognized obstructive sleep apnea in patients undergoing surgery. *JAMA* 2019;322(12):1211.

Subramani Y, Nagappa M, Wong J, Mubashir T, Chung F. Preoperative evaluation: estimation of pulmonary risk including obstructive sleep apnea impact. *Anesthesiol Clin* 2018;36(4):523–538.

Tamisier R, Fabre F, O'Donoghue F, Lévy P, Payen JF, Pépin JL. Anesthesia and sleep apnea. *Sleep Med Rev* 2018;40:79–92.

6

Exploratory Laparotomy for Bowel Resection

KEY POINTS

- Hemodynamic variability is possible and can be attributed to factors such as preoperative dehydration, evaporative fluid loss from the surgical site, sepsis, and blood loss.
- Electrolyte and acid–base abnormalities may occur during the intraoperative management.

- Extensive third-space expansion due to extravasation of fluid from the intravascular space and from perforated viscera may prohibit abdominal closure at the end of surgery.
- The patient's history and intraoperative course contribute to decisions regarding postoperative management.

Case Synopsis

A 48-year-old woman is scheduled to have an exploratory laparotomy. She has a 3-day history of increasing episodes of vomiting. A nasogastric tube is inserted, and 300 mL of gastric secretions are suctioned. The patient is complaining of severe abdominal pain.

Preoperative Evaluation and Demographic Data

Past Medical/Surgical History

- Hypertension
- Cholecystectomy (open): 2 years ago, no anesthetic complications
- Total abdominal hysterectomy: 12 years ago, no anesthetic complications

List of Medications

- Zestril (lisinopril)
- Nexium (esomeprazole magnesium)

Diagnostic Data

- Hemoglobin, 13 g/dL; hematocrit, 39%
- Electrolytes: sodium, 132 mEq/L; potassium, 2.8 mEq/L; chloride, 96 mEq/L; carbon dioxide, 22 mEq/L
- Arterial blood gases: pH, 7.46; $PaCO_2$, 32 mm Hg; HCO_3, 20 mEq/L; base excess +6

Height/Weight/Vital Signs

- 163 cm, 72 kg
- Blood pressure, 96/62; heart rate, 112 beats per minute; respiratory rate, 28 breaths per minte; room air oxygen saturation, 94%; temperature, 38.5°C
- Electrocardiogram (ECG): sinus tachycardia, heart rate, 108 beats per minute

Pathophysiology

There are multiple causes for acute abdominal disease with intestinal obstruction. Obstruction can occur in various portions of the bowel, and the etiology of obstruction may be multifactorial—most likely caused by adhesions, strictures, or tumor. Intestinal obstruction may be intraluminal (e.g., due to tumor, sequestration within a hernia, stricture), extraluminal (e.g., cholelithiasis, foreign body), or as part of a process directly involving the bowel tissue (e.g., ulcerative colitis, Crohn disease, ischemic pathology). Pain is the most common initial symptom associated with abdominal disease and is typically present in acute obstructive disease. The etiology of abdominal pain is multifactorial. Pain may initially be localized or nonspecific and referred from one abdominal region to another due to anatomic confluence of common neural pathways from various intraabdominal structures. Abdominal distention may progress dramatically, which strongly suggests the presence of a perforated intraabdominal viscus—a sign that is verified by radiographic findings showing evidence of free air within the abdominal cavity. Associated symptoms include nausea and vomiting, abdominal distention, constipation, and diarrhea.

Other causes of acute bowel obstruction may be attributed to the development of adhesions that occurs as a result of previous abdominal surgery. Incarcerated or strangulated loops of bowel that become trapped within hernias in the abdominal wall may occur. A prior history of abdominal surgery, particularly in the pelvic region, is associated with a greater risk of developing intraabdominal adhesions. Patients who are sedentary, debilitated, and taking chronic medications (e.g., phenothiazines) are at increased risk of developing hypotonic bowel. Such an area may evolve into a strangulated loop of bowel or into a complete bowel obstruction. Bowel obstruction, strangulation, and perforation result in hypovolemia from causes that include vomiting, diarrhea, extravascular fluid losses, and gastric suctioning. Peritonitis and sepsis, which occur from the bacteria and enterotoxins that are released from the perforated bowel, further magnify fluid loss. These processes can dramatically affect intravascular volume, electrolyte balance, and acid–base balance and result in sepsis. Multisystem organ dysfunction syndrome is associated with increased mortality, which is initiated via the inflammatory response and may result in acute respiratory distress syndrome.

Surgical Procedure

Surgical resection of a diseased portion of intestine is accomplished by creating a midline abdominal incision. This surgery is necessary for a variety of reasons, including the presence of a tumor or to remove an ischemic portion of the bowel caused by adhesions, volvulus, or herniation of the intestine. The fascia and the muscle layers are excised, and retractors are placed within the abdomen to improve visualization. The peritoneal cavity is inspected. After the diseased portion of the bowel is identified and resected, the distal and proximal ends of the bowel are excised. An anastomosis is created by inserting a stapling device through a purse-string suture that is made at the distal portion. The abdominal incision is closed and dressed.

Anesthetic Management and Considerations

Preoperative Period

1. *Compare and contrast the clinical considerations associated with a large bowel and small bowel obstruction.*

    Large bowel obstruction typically has a longer prodromal period before acute signs and symptoms occur. It may be associated with fewer acute metabolic derangements because its primary function is storage rather than secretion and absorption. The large bowel is less likely to strangulate than the small bowel, but it can become markedly distended under certain conditions, such as toxic megacolon, which may lead to rupture.

Small bowel obstruction generally occurs with a more acute onset. The progression of small bowel obstruction begins with hypotonia (loss of motility with intraluminal stasis), osmotic disequilibrium leading to transudation of fluids into the peritoneum, accumulation of gas, and eventually electrolyte imbalance. Systemic derangements in organ function may be more dramatic and acute in comparison to large bowel obstruction. A small bowel obstruction is more likely to occur than a large bowel obstruction (75% to 80%).

The risk of gastric aspiration is increased in patients who have a bowel obstruction due to increased gastric volume resulting in increased gastric pressure. The competency of the lower esophageal sphincter is also compromised, and as a result a rapid-sequence induction during induction of anesthesia and tracheal intubation is warranted. Tracheal extubation at the end of surgery is undertaken only after the patient demonstrates awareness and control of airway reflexes.

2. *Discuss the physiologic concerns associated with toxic megacolon.*

    Toxic megacolon occurs more frequently in patients that have ulcerative colitis. This condition can occur in critically ill patients undergoing aggressive antibiotic therapy. In this disease process, acute stasis of the large colon permits bacterial overgrowth, promoting a dramatic increase in intraluminal pressure. This results from overproduction of gas within the lumen of the bowel caused by anaerobic metabolism. The result is mucosal inflammation with loss of bowel wall integrity, which facilitates systemic absorption of bacterial endotoxins. Clinical signs include abdominal distention, fever, tachycardia, pain, and the absence of bowel sounds. Anemia, leukocytosis, hypokalemia, and hypoalbuminemia are typically present. Aggressive resuscitation and emergent colectomy are indicated. The mortality rate associated with this condition may be as high as 30%.

3. *Describe typical signs and symptoms of bowel obstruction.*

    The most common signs and symptoms associated with bowel obstruction are included in Box 6.1.

4. *Describe the physiologic manifestations associated with bowel perforation.*

    Bowel perforation results from decreased blood flow, which causes tissue ischemia and a breakdown of the bowel wall resulting from increased intraluminal pressure. Obstruction to blood flow along with impairment in bowel motility leads to sequestration and accumulation of fluid and gas proximal to the level of obstruction. Absorption of intraluminal fluid is impaired because of increased intraluminal pressure. Furthermore, hypersecretion of fluid occurs, which is enhanced by the release of prostaglandins. Release of bacteria, endotoxins, and intraluminal contaminants from within the bowel lumen into the peritoneum and into the systemic circulation results in sepsis.

• BOX 6.1	Signs and Symptoms Associated With Bowel Obstruction and Perforation

- Pain
- Abdominal distention
- Bloating
- Constipation
- Nausea and vomiting
- Fever
- Leukocytosis
- Hemodynamic variability
- Intraluminal gas and fluid within the lumen of segments proximal to the obstruction
- Free air present within the peritoneum (suggestive of bowel perforation)

5. Describe the cardiovascular abnormalities associated with bowel obstruction.

Profound alterations in cardiovascular functioning and metabolic homeostasis are possible because of disruption in the integrity of the gastrointestinal tract. Hemodynamic function is particularly susceptible to alterations in fluid, electrolyte, and acid–base balance that occur. Cardiovascular function is affected by decreased preload resulting from an intravascular fluid volume deficit. Compensatory sympathetic responses (tachycardia and vasoconstriction) attempt to restore adequate perfusion to tissues; however, there is a point where the compensatory mechanism will no longer support an adequate cardiovascular response and hypotension will occur. If the bowel is perforated and sepsis occurs, bacterial endotoxins enhance the activity of inducible nitric oxide, inhibits vasopressin, or activates adenosine triphosphate (ATP)–sensitive potassium channels in vascular smooth muscle resulting in systemic vasodilation. It is surmised that one or a combination of these mechanisms causes severe hypotension that may or may not be responsive to vasopressor medication during septic shock.

Cardiac conduction abnormalities resulting from hypokalemia during a bowel obstruction can cause ECG abnormalities, which include atrial and ventricular dysrhythmias, ST-T wave depression, prominent U-wave, prolonged PR interval, and increased P-wave amplitude. A rapid progression to shock and systemic organ failure will occur.

6. Define abdominal compartment syndrome (ACS) and the anesthetic implications.

ACS is associated with increased intraabdominal pressure (IAP), which can cause end-organ dysfunction. Increased IAP decreases cardiac output, glomerular filtration, and mesenteric and hepatic perfusion. Decreased respiratory excursion and functional residual capacity can lead to increased peak airway pressures and hypoxia. Because of pressure on the venous and arterial vasculature within the abdominal cavity, increases in intracranial pressure occur.

Normal IAP approximates atmospheric pressure. Progressive impairment on organ dysfunction occurs as IAP exceeds 25 mm Hg. ACS is associated with abdominal trauma, infarction with necrosis of abdominal viscera, repair of a ruptured abdominal aortic aneurysm, and pancreatitis. A large infusion of colloid and/or crystalloid intravenous (IV) solutions during emergent resuscitation can cause ACS. Fulminant ACS is associated with an approximate mortality rate of 50%.

Intraoperative Period

7. Discuss the use of invasive intraoperative monitoring for bowel resection.

The clinical decision to employ invasive monitoring is dependent on numerous factors, including the magnitude of the surgical procedure, the length of surgical time anticipated, the degree to which fluid shifts may become problematic, the extent of preoperative preparation of the patient, and the presence of comorbid patient factors.

An arterial line and pressure monitoring allow for beat-to-beat assessment of arterial blood pressure and allow the anesthetist to obtain blood for intraoperative analysis. The use of central venous pressure (CVP) monitoring may be considered. The CVP is used to assess volume status and to administer fluids, blood, or vasoactive medications. CVP values have been determined to be unreliable in the presence of both right and left ventricular dysfunction, pulmonary hypertension, valvular dysfunction, and abdominal distention. When utilized, the CVP should be used to monitor trends and responses to fluid boluses used to correct hypovolemia related to hypotension. Central venous catheterization may increase the risk of infection. Noninvasive cardiovascular monitoring allows the anesthetist to assess the arterial waveform contour analysis, stroke volume, and stroke volume variation (SVV) as real-time parameters of cardiac performance and volume status. Data that have been obtained support these indicators of cardiac performance in comparison with single, point-in-time measurement of cardiac output as obtained by a pulmonary artery catheter.

8. Discuss the complexities regarding fluid management for a patient having a bowel resection.

Implementation of a fluid management strategy is based on assimilated preoperative data and the patient's preexisting comorbidities (e.g., cardiovascular disease, renal insufficiency, pulmonary disease, advanced age). Laboratory values are also pertinent in estimating the magnitude of deficit necessitating replacement, as well as in selection of appropriate resuscitative fluid. Fluid losses caused by vomiting and diarrhea are associated with electrolyte losses, which may warrant concurrent replacement in addition to restoration of circulating intravascular volume.

In the presence of bowel obstruction, third-space loss occurs into the interstitium within the intestinal wall. Fluid may also be sequestered within the lumen of the bowel. Both examples result in bowel dilation leading to failure in barrier function. With the loss of bowel wall integrity, hypoalbuminemia occurs because of loss of protein-rich exudate into the peritoneum. An aberrant osmolar gradient facilitates continued fluid loss into this space.

Patients undergoing elective intraabdominal surgery may undergo a preoperative mechanical bowel preparation (MBP), which is administered orally or via enema. The potential benefits of this intervention include lower wound infection rates and lower rates in peritoneal contamination and anastomotic breakdown. Oral antibiotics in combination with MBP is more effective than MBP alone at decreasing surgical site infections. No clinically reliable method is available that can accurately account for this fluid loss. The potential magnitude of volume and electrolyte loss can be extreme. Preoperative assessment of volume deficit and electrolyte balance must therefore not only consider losses mediated by diarrhea, vomiting, third-space loss, and fasting but also as secondary to bowel preparation. In patients who are in relatively good health, the effects of bowel preparation are generally well tolerated; however, the physiologic consequences in patients who are malnourished or medically compromised may result in tachycardia, hypotension, decreased renal blood flow, and possible increased morbidity. An adequate amount of urine output is 0.5 to 1 mL/kg/hr.

Indiscriminate infusion of excessive volumes of crystalloid can damage the endothelial glycocalyx (EG). The EG layer is composed of glycoprotein and proteoglycan that closely adheres to the lumen of the vascular endothelium, where it acts as a barrier. It is believed that the EG layer is responsible for maintaining fluid vascular permeability. IV fluids and possibly pressure ventilation can damage the EG and predispose to the development of edema formation and acute lung injury.

9. *Discuss the advantages and contraindications associated with laparoscopic bowel resection compared with a traditional open approach.*

Depending on the preoperative patient presentation, a laparoscopic or laparoscopic-assisted technique may be possible. Laparoscopy has evolved into a standard minimally invasive surgical technique with an ever-increasing array of applications. The benefits associated with laparoscopic surgery for bowel resection are listed in Box 6.2. Surgical trauma necessary for exposure and access is associated with inducing an inflammatory response, which results in a variable degree of systemic manifestations. Due to the minimal invasiveness of laparoscopic bowel resection compared with the conventional open approach, surgical morbidity is decreased. The contraindications associated with laparoscopic bowel resection are listed in Box 6.3.

• BOX 6.2 Advantages of Laparoscopic Bowel Resection

- Decreased postoperative pain
- Decreased hospitalization time
- Decreased postoperative ileus
- Rapid recovery of pulmonary function
- Improved cosmetic result
- Decreased overall morbidity

• BOX 6.3 Contraindications to Laparoscopic Bowel Resection

- Intestinal obstruction
- Bulky tumors
- Evidence of metastatic tumor growth in adjacent abdominal organs
- Pregnancy

---

10. *Describe the anesthetic challenges associated with intraoperative ventilation during pneumoperitoneum.*

The creation of a pneumoperitoneum through insufflation of carbon dioxide (CO_2) gas into the abdominal cavity is necessary to perform a laparoscopic bowel resection. The advantages to using CO_2 as an insufflating gas include its nonflammability, its rapidity in movement across lipid membranes, its high degree of solubility within the blood, and its rapid removal by the lungs. The effects on the patient's cardiovascular system and pulmonary ventilatory mechanics can be significant.

Absorption of CO_2 that results from the insufflating gas consistently occurs during laparoscopy as increased end-tidal CO_2 occurs. Thus increased minute ventilation is necessary to achieve normocapnia. Furthermore, insufflation of CO_2 gas under pressure can cause subcutaneous emphysema. If the insufflating trocar is placed inappropriately and/or migrates within the abdominal cavity, then a pathway for CO_2 gas to diffuse into the subcutaneous space develops.

The use of CO_2 has additional disadvantages and can cause hypercarbia, peritoneal irritation, hypertension, and acidosis. The adverse effects of CO_2 insufflation can be further exacerbated by the effects caused by surgery and anesthesia. The mechanics associated with ventilation during laparoscopy cause increased dead-space ventilation, reduction in functional residual capacity, and decreased pulmonary compliance. The lithotomy and Trendelenburg positions further decrease pulmonary compliance causing ventilation–perfusion mismatch.

Ventilatory alterations imposed by anesthesia and pneumoperitoneum can be partially offset by administering positive-end expiratory pressure (PEEP) and pressure-controlled ventilation utilizing a higher ventilatory rate and lower tidal volumes to achieve normocarbia and acceptable peak ventilating pressures. The overall postoperative pulmonary function (forced expiratory volume in 1 second [FEV_1] and forced vital capacity [FVC]) in patients undergoing laparoscopic procedures in comparison with those patients undergoing conventional laparotomy is improved.

11. *Describe the hemodynamic effects of increased intraperitoneal pressure (IAP) caused by a pneumoperitoneum.*

Elevation in IAP causes obstruction of blood flow to the mesentery, liver, and inferior vena cava. Renal function may be compromised due to compression of renal venous flow, as evidenced by decreased urine output. Reduced cardiac preload with consequent reduction in cardiac output and perfusion pressure may also occur. Systemic blood pressure is usually maintained or increased because CO_2 gas exerts pressure within the peritoneum, causing increased sympathetic tone and systemic peripheral resistance. Increased cardiac filling pressures may initially occur with insufflation due to increased intrathoracic pressure. Ventricular wall tension and left ventricular function are generally well preserved in healthy patients, but pneumoperitoneum may have deleterious consequences in patients with compromised cardiac function. Decreased preload and increased afterload can result in decreased cardiac output and myocardial ischemia in patients with limited cardiac reserve.

A CO_2 gas embolism is a rare event but can result in decreased myocardial and cerebral perfusion. As CO_2 gas is inadvertently entrained into venous circulation, an air lock is created at the level of the inferior vena cava and right atrium, within the right atrium or right ventricle. The signs associated with CO_2 air embolism include:

- Hypotension
- Hypoxemia
- Decreased end tidal CO_2
- Dysrhythmias
- Cyanosis

The interventions used to treat a venous air embolus that results in cardiovascular compromise include:

- Immediate exsufflation
- Administer 100% oxygen
- Turn off anesthetic agents
- Call for anesthesia help
  - IV fluid bolus
  - Vasopressors
  - Minimize peak airway pressures
- Positioning in left lateral decubitus position
- Placement and aspiration from a central venous pressure line

12. *Describe the activation of the neuroendocrine stress response caused by bowel surgery.*

Abdominal insufflation, as well as intraabdominal exploration, induces a stress response, as evidenced by increased plasma concentrations of cortisol, renin,

vasopressin, epinephrine, norepinephrine, and angiotensin. The plasma levels of these substances can increase mean arterial pressure (MAP), systemic vascular resistance (SVR), and cardiac output. Methods that can be used to attenuate the hemodynamic responses in the susceptible patient include delivery of a balanced anesthetic using opioids, alpha-2 agonists, dexmedetomidine, and beta-adrenergic receptor blockade.

13. *Discuss the anesthetic options for a laparoscopic bowel resection.*

A balanced anesthetic technique utilizing a volatile inhalation anesthetic agent with opioid and muscle relaxation is effective for laparoscopy. Nitrous oxide is best avoided in laparoscopic surgery due to its potential for causing bowel distention. Nitrous oxide can also delay resolution of a gaseous air embolism and may increase the incidence of postoperative nausea and vomiting (PONV). Laparoscopic surgery is associated with increased PONV, and prophylactic interventions should be used to decrease the incidence.

Extensive intraabdominal procedures requiring significant visceral manipulation and retraction, particularly in the mid and upper abdomen, will dramatically increase the patient's work of breathing. As a result, neuraxial anesthesia is not commonly used as the sole anesthetic technique during bowel resection. However, epidural anesthesia that is combined with general anesthesia is advantageous by decreasing intraoperative medication requirements and providing postoperative analgesia.

Postoperative Period

14. *Discuss strategies that can be used to decrease postoperative pain after laparotomy.*

A number of strategies may be employed for the purpose of providing postoperative analgesia after laparotomy. The degree of postoperative pain will be significantly less if a laparoscopic approach was instituted. Epidural analgesia may be used alone or combined with supplemental IV or oral medications to control pain. Patient-controlled analgesia (PCA) may also be employed effectively as a primary modality or as a supplement to an epidural technique. An epidural infusion may be initiated preoperatively and used as an adjunct in intraoperative anesthetic management and continued to provide an established level of analgesia for postoperative management. The use of N-methyl-D-aspartate (NMDA) antagonists such as ketamine, administered in low IV doses, has been shown to effectively augment the effect of opioids. Nonsteroidal antiinflammatory drugs (NSAIDs) can be used effectively as single therapy or in combination with opiates. Dexmedetomidine has also been shown to have analgesic properties and decrease postoperative opioid requirements. Regional anesthesia utilizing a transverse abdominis plane block anesthetizes sensory nerves of the anterior abdominal wall. Infiltration of the surgical wound edges with local anesthetic may offer valuable analgesic supplementation.

Pain that occurs in one or both shoulders after a laparoscopic bowel resection commonly occurs and is most effectively treated with ketorolac. It is theorized that shoulder pain that is caused by creation of a pneumoperitoneum is due to subdiaphragmatic peritoneal irritation from either blood or residual carbon dioxide gas or due to stretching of intraabdominal tissues. Irrigation of the peritoneal cavity and peritoneal instillation of bupivacaine have been shown to decrease the incidence. Ketorolac should not be administered if the patient is coagulopathic or has asthma, renal insufficiency, or gastric ulcers.

Review Questions

1. Which is not a sign that is associated with an acute bowel obstruction?
   a. Diarrhea
   b. Abdominal distention
   c. Fever
   d. Vomiting
2. Which is an advantage of laparoscopic bowel resection compared with laparotomy?
   a. Increased postoperative pain
   b. Decreased hospitalization time
   c. Increased postoperative ileus
   d. Delayed recovery of pulmonary function
3. Which is not a contraindication to laparoscopic bowel resection?
   a. Intestinal obstruction
   b. Bulky tumors
   c. Evidence of metastatic tumor growth in adjacent abdominal organs
   d. Obesity
4. Which is a sign of CO_2 gas embolism?
   a. Hypertension
   b. Hypoxemia
   c. Increased end tidal CO_2
   d. Decreased hemoglobin
5. Pain that is associated with laparoscopic bowel resection is most likely caused by:
   a. Release of inflammatory mediators.
   b. Trendelenburg positioning.
   c. Subdiaphragmatic peritoneal irritation.
   d. Inflammation of the bowel.

Suggested Readings

Chappell D, Mathias J, Hofmann-Kiefer K, et al. A rational approach to perioperative fluid management. *Anesthesiology* 2008;109:723–740.

Chilkoti GT, Karthik G, Rautela R. Evaluation of postoperative analgesic efficacy and perioperative hemodynamic changes with low dose intravenous dexmedetomidine infusion in patients undergoing laparoscopic cholecystectomy - a randomised, double-blinded, placebo-controlled trial. *J Anaesthesiol Clin Pharmacol* 2020;36(1):72–77.

Church J. Laparotomy for acute colorectal conditions in moribund patients: is it worthwhile? *Dis Colon Rectum* 2005;48:1147–1152.

Collins SB, Johnson CA. Hepatobiliary and gastrointestinal disturbances and anesthesia. In: Nagelhout JJ, Elisha S, eds. *Nurse Anesthesia,* 6th ed. St. Louis, MO: Elsevier, 2018:709–742.

Damadi AA, Lax EA, Smithson L, Pearlman RD. Comparison of therapeutic benefit of bupivacaine HCl transversus abdominis plane (TAP) block as part of an enhanced recovery pathway versus traditional oral and intravenous pain control after minimally invasive colorectal surgery: a prospective, randomized, double-blind trial. *Am Surg* 2019;85(12):1363–1368.

Kang D, Yoo KY. Fluid management in perioperative and critically ill patients. *Acute Crit Care* 2019;34(4):235–245.

Kehlet H, Dahl J. Anaesthesia, surgery, and challenges in postoperative recovery. *Lancet* 2003;362:1921–1928.

Krielen P, Di Saverio S, Ten Broek R, Renzi C, Zago M, et al. Laparoscopic versus open approach for adhesive small bowel obstruction, a systematic review and meta-analysis of short term outcomes. *J Trauma Acute Care Surg* 2020;88(6):866–874.

McSorley ST, Steele CW, McMahon AJ. Meta-analysis of oral antibiotics, in combination with preoperative intravenous antibiotics and mechanical bowel preparation the day before surgery, compared with intravenous antibiotics and mechanical bowel preparation alone to reduce surgical-site infections in elective colorectal surgery. *BJS Open* 2018;2(4):185–194.

Ng A, Smith G. Gastrointestinal reflux and aspiration of gastric contents in anaesthetic practice. *Anesth Analg* 2001;93:494–513.

Sujatha PP, Nileshwar A, Krishna HM, Prasad SS, Prabhu M, Kamath SU. Goal-directed vs traditional approach to intraoperative fluid therapy during open major bowel surgery: is there a difference? *Anesthesiol Res Pract* 2019;2019:3408940. doi: 10.1155/2019/3408940.

7

Laparoscopic Gastric Bypass

KEY POINTS

- As the incidence of obesity continues to increase in the United States, the frequency of bariatric surgery is expected to rise.
- Surgical intervention can attenuate and even resolve the pathophysiologic effects of severe systemic disease that are associated with obesity.
- Successful airway management and intraoperative ventilation present challenges for the anesthetist.
- Patients who present for bariatric surgery frequently have other pathologic conditions that are associated with obesity.

Case Synopsis

A 56-year-old woman who is morbidly obese has consulted with her physician and consented to have a gastric bypass procedure. The surgeon has chosen a laparoscopic Roux-en-Y procedure for this patient based on her individual needs.

Preoperative Evaluation and Demographic Data

Past Medical/Surgical History

- Type 2 diabetes
- She uses a walker and frequently develops shortness of breath. She is unable to walk up a flight of stairs. She is sedentary.
- Hypertension
- Hypercholesterolemia
- Obstructive sleep apnea
- Gastroesophageal reflux disease
- Smoked 1 pack of cigarettes per day for 25 years; however, she stopped 1 year ago
- Appendectomy 20 years ago without associated anesthesia complications

List of Medications

- Glipizide
- Cimetidine
- Hydrochlorothiazide
- Lisinopril

Diagnostic Data

- Hemoglobin, 12.2 g/dL; hematocrit, 36.6%
- Platelet count, 336/mm^3
- Glucose, 156 mg/dL, A1c, 7.2%
- Blood urea nitrogen (BUN), 19 mg/dL; creatinine, 0.9 mg/dL
- Prothrombin time, 10.2 seconds; activated partial thromboplastin time, 29 seconds; international normalized ratio, 1.0
- Electrolytes: sodium, 134 mEq/L; potassium, 4.3 mEq/L; chloride, 100 mEq/L; carbon dioxide, 24 mEq/L
- Electrocardiogram: normal sinus rhythm with nonspecific ST-segment abnormalities
- Liver function: alanine transaminase (ALT), 28 units/L; aspartate transaminase (AST), 31 units/L
- Cardiac echocardiography: left ventricular hypertrophy; normal systolic ventricular function; ejection fraction, 67%
- Chest X-ray within normal limits
- Pulmonary function test: forced expiratory volume in 1 second (FEV$_1$), 70% of predicted

Height/Weight/Vital Signs

- 155 cm, 152 kg; body mass index (BMI) is 63.3 kg/m^2, indicating morbid obesity
- Blood pressure, 158/92; heart rate, 86 beats per minute; respiratory rate, 22 breaths per minute; room air oxygen saturation, 95%; temperature 36.6°C

Pathophysiology

When caloric consumption is greater than the body's physiologic requirements, obesity is likely to occur. However, the cause of obesity is multifactorial, including environmental factors, genetic predisposition, hormonal disorders, behavioral variables, and cultural norms. Obesity has reached epidemic in proportions in the United States, and projections suggest that the rate of this disease process will continue to increase in the future.

Approximately two-thirds of adults in the United States are overweight (BMI ≥25 kg/m^2) and one-third are considered obese (BMI ≥30 kg/m^2). The spectrum continues to include people who are morbidly obese (BMI ≥35 kg/m^2), super obese (BMI ≥55 kg/m^2), and super-super obese (BMI ≥60 kg/m^2). Medications, diet, exercise, and behavioral modification techniques all have poor long-term results and are associated with complications and significant cost. Although risks are associated with bariatric surgery, it is the most successful intervention to achieve long-term weight loss and to improve or resolve the comorbid diseases that are associated with obesity. Patients who are candidates for bariatric surgery generally have a BMI greater than 35 kg/m^2 with one or more comorbid conditions. A comprehensive medical and surgical bariatric program will include a medical evaluation and optimization of all pathologic disease states, psychologic and nutritional counseling, and a weight loss program before surgery will be performed. Significant risks are associated with bariatric surgery, and a list of contraindications is highlighted in Box 7.1.

Surgical Procedure

The goal of bariatric surgery is to reduce the patient's caloric intake by either restricting the amount an individual can consume (restrictive procedure) or by reducing the amount absorbed from the gastrointestinal tract (malabsorptive procedure). It is estimated that between 70% and 80% of excess body weight is frequently lost in patients who undergo gastric bypass. Several gastric bypass procedures can be performed to treat obesity. The most commonly described technique is the Roux-en-Y gastric bypass procedure that restricts the person's ability to consume a large amount of food by partitioning the stomach and creating a small proximal and distal pouch. After gastric bypass surgery, when the person eats a small amount of food, the proximal pouch rapidly becomes distended and afferent impulses to the brain signal that the person is satiated. A decrease in the absorption of calories and nutrients occurs because the anastomosis of the jejunum is to the proximal pouch of the stomach, which bypasses a significant portion of the small intestine. The Roux-en-Y gastric bypass procedure is one of the most common bariatric techniques performed worldwide. An illustration of the Roux-en-Y procedure is presented in Fig. 7.1. An alternative surgical method for bariatric surgery is sleeve gastrectomy, where the stomach from the upper fundus to the lower antrum is resected longitudinally to decrease the size of the stomach and the volume of food and liquid that can be consumed at one time.

Gastric restrictive procedures such as laparoscopic adjustable gastric banding or vertical banded gastroplasty are less invasive and are associated with a shorter surgical duration, but the long-term results and complications such as dietary restrictions, gastric and intestinal erosion, and migration of the restrictive device are factors that will affect daily life. Adjustable gastric banding may become more popular and effective in the future as new and more effective gastric banding devices and surgical techniques are developed. Roux-en-Y gastric bypass has a greater potential for serious complications compared with gastric banding. The complications that are associated with a Roux-en-Y procedure are listed in Box 7.2.

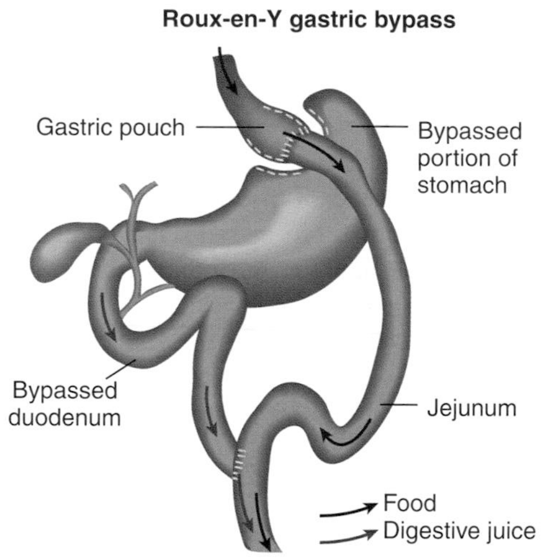

Roux-en-Y gastric bypass

• **Fig. 7.1** Roux-en-Y gastric bypass procedure involves constructing a gastric pouch whose outlet is a Y-shaped limb of small intestine. (From Harding MM, Kwong J, Roberts D, et al: *Lewis's medical-surgical nursing: Assessment and management of clinical problems*, ed 11, St. Louis, 2020, Elsevier.)

• **BOX 7.1** **Contraindications to Bariatric Surgery**

- Severe cardiac disease
- Poor myocardial reserve
- Significant chronic obstructive pulmonary disease or respiratory dysfunction
- Noncompliance with medical treatment
- Psychological disorders prohibiting long-term management
- Eating disorders
- Severe hiatal hernia or gastroesophageal reflux disease

• **BOX 7.2** **Complications Associated With the Roux-en-Y Procedure**

- Hemorrhage
- Respiratory infection
- Deep vein thromboembolism
- Bowel obstruction
- Leakage, stricture, and/or ulcer at the sites of anastomosis
- Infection
- Dumping syndrome
- Nutritional deficiency

Anesthetic Management and Considerations

Preoperative Period

1. *Discuss preoperative preparation for a patient having gastric bypass.*

    Preparation for surgery involves coordination between health care disciplines: psychiatry, internal medicine, surgery, and anesthesia. The procedure is described to the patient, and the risks, benefits, and alternatives must be clearly communicated. The patient has also been extensively counseled regarding the typical postoperative course, expectations for weight loss, and dietary limitations. All chronic pathophysiologic conditions need to be medically optimized before surgery.

2. *Discuss the common coexisting diseases that are associated with patients presenting for bariatric surgery.*

    Morbid obesity and any associated illnesses are medically managed in hopes of optimizing the patient's level of functioning. Frequently, immobility and joint discomfort become the major motivating factors that drive patients to have bariatric surgery. Within 1 year after successful bariatric surgery, many of the pathologic disease states such as diabetes, hypertension, and respiratory difficulty improve or resolve. A list of the pathology that is associated with obesity is included in Box 7.3.

3. *Outline the positive physiologic effects of weight loss after bariatric surgery.*

    Obesity is considered to occur as a result of behavioral factors, and surgery is the final intervention. The outcome data associated with bariatric surgery and weight loss demonstrate advantages for both the individual patient and for society by decreasing future expenses that would be incurred as a result of treating multiple chronic disease states. It has been demonstrated that improvement or complete resolution of following pathologies occurs:

    - 76.8% decrease in type 2 diabetes
    - 70% decrease in hypercholesteremia
    - 61.7% decrease in hypertension
    - 85.7% decrease in obstructive sleep apnea

• BOX 7.3 Commonly Occurring Pathologies Associated With Obesity

- Coronary artery disease
- Atherosclerosis
- Hypertension
- Diabetes mellitus
- Obstructive sleep apnea
- Systemic and pulmonary hypertension
- Gastroesophageal reflux disease
- Nonalcoholic fatty liver disease
- Cholelithiasis
- Deep vein thromboembolic disease
- Degenerative disc disease

The survival rate for morbidly obese patients under 40 years who have bariatric surgery is 13.8% compared with 3.0% for those who did not receive surgical management. The dramatic reduction in body weight is associated with a decreased incidence of cancer, infectious disease, musculoskeletal disorders, respiratory dysfunction, nervous system pathology, psychiatric illness, and reproductive health issues.

4. *Discuss the physiologic concerns for patients having bariatric surgery.*

    Evaluation of the patient presenting for bariatric surgery should focus on optimizing the comorbidities to decrease the perioperative risk.

    - **Cardiac function** should be evaluated via echocardiography, electrocardiogram, exercise, or dobutamine stress testing. The high incidence of hypertension, high cholesterol, and inactivity coupled with the physiologic stress that results from the pneumoperitoneum, surgical procedure, and anesthetic management predisposes the patient to untoward perioperative cardiac events. A higher incidence of congestive heart failure occurs in the obese patient population. A cardiomyopathy resulting in cardiomegaly, left ventricular dilation, and myocyte hypertrophy can cause sudden cardiac death. The demand on the heart is further increased, as there is an associated increase in total blood volume with obesity. This patient's cardiac ultrasound demonstrated left ventricular hypertrophy, which is consistent with myocardial compensation caused by increased afterload over time. She has normal systolic ventricular function and adequate ejection fraction of 67%.

    - **Pulmonary function** must be scrutinized before anesthesia. Due to the excessive adipose tissue present on the chest wall, extrathoracic compliance is decreased, causing restrictive lung disease. Oxygen consumption and carbon dioxide production are increased resulting from excessive tissue. Changes in lung volumes that are associated with obesity include decreased vial capacity, decreased total lung capacity, decreased functional residual capacity (FRC), and decreased expiratory reserve volume. Closing capacity—the volume at which distal airway closure occurs—is increased, facilitating atelectasis and decreased oxygen transport. This patient has a history of a prolonged period of smoking, which causes obstructive lung disease and the potential for airway hyperreactivity. This patient should have a chest x-ray and pulmonary function testing before surgery.

    - **Endocrine function** is important to consider because this patient has type 2 diabetes mellitus and requires insulin to maintain normoglycemia. Excessive adipose tissue results in the increased breakdown of free fatty acids that stimulate gluconeogenesis (breakdown of amino acids and the glycerol portion of fat) in the liver to increase blood glucose. Insulin is released to facilitate movement of glucose into cells; however, over time, the cells' responsiveness to the effects of insulin diminishes and insulin resistance occurs. The pancreas compensates by secreting increased amounts of insulin that can result in beta cell dysfunction and decreased insulin production. Her preoperative blood sugar is 156 mg/dL, but her hemoglobin A1c, a measure of sustained glycemic control, is elevated. The acute increase in blood sugar is frequently a physiologic response to stress. Because the anesthetist appropriately instructed the patient to hold the glipizide on the morning of surgery, a repeat blood sugar check should be instituted before discharge from the postanesthesia care unit (PACU).

- **Hepatic function** as assessed using laboratory data may be abnormally elevated in the obese population; however, there is no correlation between routine liver function tests and the liver's capacity to metabolize medications. Drug clearance is usually unimpaired in this patient population. These patients are at increased risk for developing liver failure. Tests for coagulation are prudent, given the potential for hepatic dysfunction, the invasive nature of the surgery, and the administration of low-molecular-weight heparin for deep vein thrombosis prophylaxis. This patient's liver and coagulation function are within the normal range.
- **Renal function** affects drug excretion, which is often increased in obese patients due to increased renal blood flow and increased glomerular filtration rate. This patient's BUN and creatinine are within normal limits.
- **Gastrointestinal pathology** is believed to exist in patients who are morbidly obese because of increased intragastric pressure and decreased gastric transit time. Additionally, this patient has a history of gastroesophageal reflux disease and is taking cimetidine to control the symptoms. Therefore aspiration prophylaxis should be instituted in the preoperative period.
- **Venous access** is frequently challenging; however, the need for reliable intravenous access is imperative. Central venous access and arterial line placement are used for those patients who are at high cardiovascular risk.

5. *Describe the preinduction preparation for a patient having bariatric surgery.*

Anxiety is common for many patients during the preoperative period. The use of midazolam during this time will help achieve anxiolysis and amnesia, as well as decreasing sympathetic nervous system predominance. However, careful titration of all sedative medications administered is vital because significant respiratory depression may lead to rapid and severe hypoxemia.

It is important to know the weight limit for the specific operating table and to secure the patient to the table once they have moved. Airway management is a critical aspect for any patient; however, for morbidly obese patients, due to the potential for redundant airway tissue, large neck, and decreased FRC, rapid desaturation will occur if the conditions are not optimal. Placement of a ramp under the patient using blankets under their shoulders and then elevating the head will provide optimal "sniffing position," which facilitates the alignment of the oral, pharyngeal, and laryngeal axis. The back of

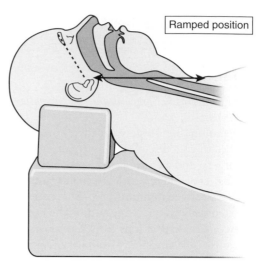

• **Fig. 7.2** Morbidly obese patients are best intubated in a ramped position with elevation of the upper part of the back, neck, and head; the ideal position aligns the external auditory canal and the sternum. (From Roberts JR: *Roberts and Hedges' clinical procedures in emergency medicine and acute care*, ed 7, St. Louis, 2019, Elsevier.)

the table can be elevated to help the anesthetist achieve this position and to facilitate improved respiratory excursion during preoxygenation. Fig. 7.2 depicts proper positioning for an obese patient before the induction of anesthesia.

Preoxygenation of the patient should occur for as long as possible. Patients must be reminded to take vital capacity breaths before induction. Increasing the concentration of oxygen in the blood and also the pulmonary residual volume will increase the time before desaturation occurs after the patient becomes apneic. After induction but before intubation, continuous positive airway pressure (CPAP) can be used to optimize oxygen transfer at the level of the alveoli and help to decrease atelectasis.

A rapid sequence induction is indicated for this patient due to her morbid obesity and history of gastroesophageal reflux. If airway management and intubation prove difficult, then having airway adjuncts available such as a video laryngoscope, Eschmann stylet (elastic gum bougie), and laryngeal mask airway is prudent. The anesthetist should be familiar with and have experience utilizing the American Society of Anesthesiologists' difficult airway algorithm.

The blood pressure cuff should be placed on the patient's upper arm or forearm. Inaccurate blood pressure measurements can occur if the blood pressure cuff is too large or too small. It is necessary to be vigilant regarding positioning and padding of the arms, legs, and pressure points. Continuous assessment of the position and pressure points is imperative because changes in the operating table position or surgical manipulation may cause a shift. Positioning is the responsibility of the entire surgical team, and when it is accomplished properly before the surgical incision, the incidence of a compression injury or nerve palsy can be minimized.

• BOX 7.4 Cardiovascular Effects Associated With a Pneumoperitoneum

- Increased neurohumoral response
- Decreased venous return (preload)
- Increased systemic vascular resistance (afterload)
- Increased heart rate
- Increased blood pressure
- Decreased cardiac output

• BOX 7.5 Respiratory Effects Associated With a Pneumoperitoneum

- Increased carbon dioxide absorption
- Decreased vital capacity
- Increased intrathoracic compliance
- Decreased pulmonary compliance
- Increased peak airway pressure
- Decreased functional residual capacity
- Increased atelectasis
- Increased ventilation/perfusion mismatch

Intraoperative Period

6. *Describe the hemodynamic variability that frequently occurs during a laparoscopic Roux-en-Y procedure.*

Although reverse Trendelenburg positioning is optimal during the induction period and airway management, returning the patient to the supine position facilitates hemodynamic stability and allows the nursing staff to proceed with the surgical preparation. The patient may be given a bowel preparation solution the day before surgery that facilitates removal of fecal material and water from the gastrointestinal system, resulting in dehydration. This process, coupled with preoperative fasting and the use of antihypertensive medications, can exacerbate hypotension. Depending on the patient's cardiovascular status, an intravenous fluid bolus preinduction will decrease the degree and duration of a hypotensive episode that is caused by the anesthetic induction agents.

The creation of a pneumoperitoneum occurs when the abdominal cavity is insufflated with carbon dioxide gas. If intraabdominal pressures exceed 15 mm Hg, cardiovascular compromise can occur. Vasopressors can be used to maintain adequate cerebral and coronary perfusion pressure if hypotension exists. However, the degree of hypotension compared with the patient's preoperative norm, the state of the individual's cardiovascular status, and the degree of surgical stimulation must be considered, as ephedrine and phenylephrine can both increase myocardial oxygen demand. A complete list of the cardiovascular and respiratory physiologic changes that are associated with a pneumoperitoneum is included in Boxes 7.4 and 7.5.

The average blood loss associated with a laparoscopic Roux-en-Y procedure is between 50 and 100 mL; however, as with any laparoscopic surgical intervention, there is always the possibility of inadvertent vascular damage resulting in acute hemorrhage. The anesthetists must be cautious of rapidly developing fluid overload. Attention to the estimated blood loss and urine output is essential. The signs consistent with fluid volume overload for a patient receiving general anesthesia are included in Box 7.6.

7. *Discuss the airway dynamics and ventilation strategy for patients having laparoscopic bariatric surgery.*

A reduction in FRC occurs in obese patients, and this phenomenon presents a host of unique challenges

---

• BOX 7.6 Signs of Fluid Overload in an Anesthetized Patient

- Increased peak inspiratory pressures
- Jugular venous distention
- Increased central venous pressure
- Bilateral rales
- Pink frothy secretions in the endotracheal tube
- Hypoxemia/hypercarbia/acidosis
- Dysrhythmias
- Hypotension/hypertension

---

during anesthetic management and intraoperative ventilation. Respiratory spirometry in morbidly obese patients is similar to patients who have restrictive lung disease. Initial tidal volume settings (ventilation based on volume) or pressure settings (ventilation based on pressure to achieve a specific volume) for ventilation should begin at 5 to 7 mL/kg, and positive-end expiratory pressures (PEEP) of 3 to 7 cm H_2O pressure can be used to decrease the development of atelectasis and improve ventilation–perfusion mismatch. PEEP can decrease venous return by increasing intrathoracic pressure and contribute to barotrauma. Larger tidal volumes can cause barotrauma even if peak pressures are not excessively high, and this maneuver may not improve arterial oxygenation. The tidal volume should be increased or decreased depending on the peak pressure and the oxygen saturation.

Due to the pneumoperitoneum, pressure is exerted on the diaphragm. This fact coupled with the Trendelenburg position that is required during the surgical procedure and morbid obesity dramatically increases peak inspiratory pressures. It is recommended that the initial tidal volume is calculated using the patient's ideal body weight. If peak airway pressures increase significantly greater than 30 mm Hg, then the tidal volume or ventilating pressures can be decreased by 10% to 30%. The respiratory rate can be increased to maintain the end-tidal carbon dioxide within physiologic parameters.

An attempt should be made to extubate the patient while they are positioned in reverse Trendelenburg to facilitate respiratory excursion. Due to this patient population's compromised respiratory function, rapid desaturation will occur unless adequate spontaneous tidal volume breaths occur post-extubation. After the patient moves back to the gurney, they should be placed in a sitting position and supplemental oxygen should be provided for transport. This intervention increases FRC and decreases the incidence of airway obstruction. Atelectasis commonly occurs in obese patients, and alveolar recruitment and distention may be addressed by providing CPAP in the immediate post-operative period.

8. *Cite the pharmacokinetic implications and dose requirements for patients having bariatric surgery.*

Significant increases in the volume of distribution occur due to the high degree of lipid solubility of most of the medications used to provide anesthesia. Doses of lipid-soluble (fat-soluble) medications should be increased by 20% beyond the dose that is calculated for ideal body weight because a portion of the patient's total body weight is lean body mass.

Medications that are lipophilic are sequestered within adipose tissue as distribution of the drug occurs. If a person has a greater percentage of adipose tissue, then a greater percentage of lipid-soluble medications will remain in the body for a prolonged period compared with a lean person. When a drug is bound to adipose tissue, it is not available to undergo hepatic metabolism or renal excretion. Therefore inhalation agents with a low blood–gas solubility coefficient (insoluble) will redistribute to adipose tissue to a lesser degree and, when the medication is discontinued, pulmonary elimination will be more rapid (e.g., desflurane, sevoflurane). Neuromuscular blocking medications are water soluble and do not redistribute to adipose tissue. The pharmacokinetic profile of this drug class in obese patients is similar to that of patients who are ideal body weight. The amount of nondepolarizing medications that is administered for maintenance of paralysis should be assessed using neuromuscular blocking monitoring.

Although BMI provides a more accurate determination of patients' ideal body weight because this formula accounts for height calculated in meters squared, the Broca index helps the anesthetist determine initial drug dosages because the difference is expressed in kilograms. An estimation of ideal body weight can be calculated using the following equation:
- Male, Height (cm) − 100 = ideal kilogram weight
- Female, Height (cm) − 105 = ideal kilogram weight

Many variables affect drug metabolism and excretion, such as individual variability, liver and renal function, and cytochrome P450 induction or inhibition. The safest method of dosing when considering these factors is to titrate medications as determined by the physiologic response.

9. *Identify key aspects of anesthetic maintenance.*
- **Cardiovascular function** and titration of anesthetic medication, antihypertensive agents, and vasopressors are administered as needed to maintain adequate coronary perfusion. Due to the high incidence of hypertension in this population, these patients may require preoperative-level mean arterial pressure. The coronary artery autoregulation curve is shifted to the right in patients with hypertension, requiring a higher pressure for adequate myocardial perfusion.
- **Intraoperative ventilation** should be titrated to maintain normocarbia, avoid hypoxemia, decrease the development of atelectasis, and minimize peak inspiratory pressures. Awareness of the potential for endotracheal tube migration during changes in the patient position is critical. The immediate result of right mainstem ventilation of a morbidly obese patient in the Trendelenburg position with a pneumoperitoneum is rapidly occurring desaturation.
- **Neuromuscular blockade** should be maintained throughout the surgical procedure to decrease the possibility of patient movement, facilitate the creation and maintenance of the pneumoperitoneum, and ensure ideal operating conditions.
- **Positioning** a patient who is morbidly obese can be difficult, and care to ensure that all pressure points are padded and checking throughout the intraoperative period is essential to decrease the possibility of nerve palsy and the development of pressure sores.
- **Maintenance of normothermia** is imperative for adequate blood coagulation and the metabolism of anesthetic medications. Postoperative hypothermia that results in severe shivering will increase myocardial oxygen consumption by 400% to 600%. The use of a heated air warming blanket, fluid warming system, low fresh gas flow rate, and core temperature monitoring is indicated.
- **Anesthetic medications** that are most commonly used for maintenance during this surgical procedure include inhalation agents, dexmedetomidine, ketamine, and narcotics. Ketamine and dexmedetomidine also have an opioid-sparing effect postoperatively. The anesthetic goal throughout the intraoperative period is inhibition of sympathetic nervous system predominance and maintenance of analgesia and unconsciousness. However, the intraoperative titration of these medications will affect the emergence and postoperative period. It is important that morbidly obese patients are able to breathe effectively postoperatively, and oversedation should be avoided. Utilizing a transversus abdominis plane block and following enhanced recovery after surgery (ERAS) protocols decreases postoperative pain and narcotic consumption, while facilitating discharge.
- **Antibiotic prophylaxis** using a broad-spectrum agent is to be administered within 60 minutes before surgical incision to decrease the potential for infection. The antibiotic regimen should be continued during the postoperative period.

10. *Describe the anesthetic concerns associated with emergence and extubation.*

The inhalation agents are lipid-soluble medications and are sequestered in adipose tissue. Incremental decreases of the volume percent concentration of the agent before complete surgical closure will help facilitate a more rapid emergence from anesthesia. Reversal of neuromuscular blockade should be accomplished and guided using a nerve stimulator. Ketorolac can be given before emergence to decrease postoperative pain. Relative contraindications to the use of ketorolac include impaired renal function, bleeding, and hyperreactive airway. Narcotics can also be carefully titrated if pain persists in the postoperative area. A combination of medications used as prophylaxis for nausea and vomiting may include antidopaminergics (e.g., metoclopramide), serotonin receptor antagonists (e.g., ondansetron), steroids (e.g., dexamethasone), NK1 inhibitors (aprepitant), butyrophenones (e.g., droperidol), and anticholinergics (scopolamine). Once the patient has been moved back to the gurney, the head of the bed should be elevated and supplemental oxygen provided during the transportation to the postoperative area.

Postoperative Period

11. *Describe the common complications associated with bariatric surgery.*

Intestinal leakage at the site of the surgical anastomosis is the most frequent complication associated with bariatric surgery. The development of a deep vein thrombosis that may or may not develop into a pulmonary embolus occurs in approximately 2% of these patients. Low-molecular-weight heparin is routinely administered during the postoperative period to decrease the potential for deep vein thrombosis. Strictures that develop within the gastrointestinal tract resulting from surgical intervention range from 3% to 8%. The mortality rate for this surgical specialty ranges from 0.1% to 2%. Overall, the postoperative complication rate for laparoscopic Roux-en-Y procedure is 13%; however, incidence of mortality is less than 1%. A complete list of the complications associated with the Roux-en-Y procedure is included in Box 7.2.

Review Questions

1. A common complication associated with bariatric surgery includes:
   a. Cardiovascular collapse.
   b. Pitting edema formation.
   c. Congestive heart failure.
   d. Deep venous thrombosis.
2. Which disease state frequently resolves after significant weight reduction?
   a. Gastroesophageal reflux disease
   b. Osteoarthritis
   c. Diabetes mellitus
   d. Chronic obstructive pulmonary disease
3. Diagnostic abnormalities that would be unexpected in a morbidly obese patient include:
   a. Pulmonary function test.
   b. Creatinine.
   c. Cardiac echocardiography.
   d. Blood glucose.
4. What respiratory changes are associated with morbid obesity? (Choose two.)
   a. Decreased functional residual capacity
   b. Decreased residual volume
   c. Obstructive lung disease
   d. Increased total lung capacity
5. Which range of abdominal insufflation pressure is most likely to significantly reduce cardiac output?
   a. 20 to 30 mm Hg
   b. 1 to 5 mm Hg
   c. 6 to 10 mm Hg
   d. 10 to 18 mm Hg

Suggested Readings

Chand B, Gugliotti D, Schauer P, et al. Perioperative management of the bariatric surgery patient: focus on cardiac and anesthesia considerations. *Cleve Clin J Med* 2006;73(S1):51–56.

de Raaff CAL, de Vries N, van Wagensveld BA. Obstructive sleep apnea and bariatric surgical guidelines: summary and update. *Curr Opin Anaesthesiol* 2018;31(1):104–109.

Golembiewski J. Considerations in selecting an inhaled anesthetic agent. *Am J Health-System Pharmacy* 2004;61(20):S10–S17.

Hassani A, Kessell G. Neck circumference and difficult intubation. *Anesth Analg* 2008;107(5):1756–1757.

Jia W. Obesity, metabolic syndrome and bariatric surgery: a narrative review. *J Diabetes Investig* 2020;11(2):294–29.

Kaya C, Bilgin S, Cebeci GC, Tomak L. Anaesthetic management of patients undergoing bariatric surgery. *J Coll Physicians Surg Pak* 2019;29(8):757–762.

Lee CW, Kelly JJ, Wassef WY. Complications of bariatric surgery. *Curr Opin Gastroenterol* 2007;23(6):636–643.

McCarthy RJ, Ivankovich KG, Ramirez EA, Adams AM, Ramesh AK, et al. Association of the addition of a transversus abdominis plane block to an enhanced recovery program with opioid consumption, postoperative antiemetic use, and discharge time in patients undergoing laparoscopic bariatric surgery: a retrospective study. *Reg Anesth Pain Med* 2020;45(3):180–186.

Rao SL, Kunselman AR, Schuler HG, et al. Laryngoscopy and tracheal intubation in the head-elevated position in obese patients: a randomized, controlled, equivalence trial. *Anesth Analg* 2008; 107:1912–1918.

Trotta M, Ferrari C, D'Alessandro G, Sarra G, Piscitelli G, Marinari GM. Enhanced recovery after bariatric surgery (ERABS) in a high-volume bariatric center. *Surg Obes Relat Dis* 2019;15(10): 1785–1792.

Varner KL, March AL. Prevention of nausea and vomiting after laparoscopic sleeve gastrectomy: are we doing enough? *AANAJ* 2020;88(2):142–147.

Zeeni C, Aouad MT, Daou D, Naji S, Jabbour-Khoury S, et al. The effect of intraoperative dexmedetomidine versus morphine on postoperative morphine requirements after laparoscopic bariatric surgery. *Obes Surg* 2019;29(12):3800–3808.

8

Open and Laparoscopic Appendectomy

KEY POINTS

- The definitive treatment for acute appendicitis is an appendectomy.
- Techniques that are used include laparoscopic appendectomy (LA) and open appendectomy (OA).
- Timely surgery, intravenous (IV) fluids, and antibiotic administration significantly decrease the overall morbidity and mortality associated with acute appendicitis.

- The Trendelenburg position and the creation of a pneumoperitoneum used during LA cause physiologic changes that affect anesthetic management.
- Patients who have experienced a ruptured appendix will develop sepsis. The degree of sepsis encountered by the patient will affect the anesthetic technique and medications that are used.

Case Synopsis

A 33-year-old woman who is treated in the emergency department complains of a 3-day history of abdominal pain that is localized in the right lower quadrant (RLQ), persistent nausea and vomiting, and a low-grade fever. She has been scheduled for an LA.

Preoperative Evaluation and Demographic Data

Past Medical/Surgical History

- Asthma as a child; no current problems with asthma

List of Medications

- Multivitamins
- Birth control pills

Diagnostic Data

- Hemoglobin, 13.5 g/dL; hematocrit, 39.8 g/dL; white blood cells, 15,000 mm^3
- Electrolytes: sodium, 139 mEq/L; potassium, 3.5 mEq/L; chloride, 104 mEq/L; carbon dioxide, 24 mEq/L
- Computed tomography (CT) scan reveals inflammation of a large tubular structure with slight bowel wall thickening; impression, acute appendicitis.

Height/Weight/Vital Signs

- 173 cm, 74 kg
- Blood pressure, 112/68; heart rate, 95 beats per minute; respiratory rate, 18 breaths per minute; room air oxygen saturation, 100%; temporal artery temperature, 38.2°C

Pathophysiology

There are more than 250,000 new cases of acute appendicitis in the United States every year, with an overall incidence of 7% to 8% in the US population. Demographically, males between the ages of 10 and 30 years have a higher incidence than females of developing the disease. Appendicitis occurs most often in the second decade of life, and the median age is 22 years. Patients with higher fiber intake have a lower incidence of developing appendicitis due to a decreased formation of hard stool, also known as *fecalith*. Appendicitis can occur at any age but is rare in infants and octogenarians. Appendectomy is one of the most common surgical procedures performed in the pediatric population.

The appendix is a blind-ended loop of bowel that arises from the cecum 3 to 4 cm below the ileocecal valve. Appendicitis is inflammation of the appendix, and it is most commonly caused by a bacterial invasion of an obstructed appendiceal lumen. As the bacteria multiply, the appendix becomes distended, congested, and inflamed. Peritonitis may occur and, if the condition remains untreated, arterial blood flow to this portion of the intestine is compromised and tissue ischemia can develop, which can result in necrosis of the appendiceal wall. A perforation of the appendix can occur, which causes the release of fecal contents into the peritoneal cavity. Other less common causes of appendicitis include obstruction resulting from foreign bodies or fecalith, inflammatory strictures, and parasitic infections.

Morbidity and mortality significantly increase if immediate recognition and treatment are not instituted. Once appendicitis has developed, surgery to remove the appendix is necessary, along with IV fluids and antibiotics.

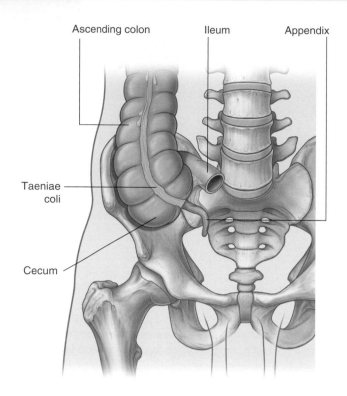

• **Fig. 8.1** Anatomic position of the appendix and the surrounding structures. (From Drake RL, Vogl AW, Mitchell WM: *Gray's anatomy for students*, ed 4, Philadelphia, 2020, Elsevier.)

The appendix has been thought to be a remnant of a digestive organ that has disappeared as a result of evolution in humans. Interestingly enough, the appendix is made of lymph tissue; it may have played a role in immune function. Located at the proximal aspect of the large intestine, the appendix is thought to be a reserve for bacteria. Fig. 8.1 depicts the anatomic position of the appendix and the surrounding structures.

The clinical presentation associated with appendicitis includes epigastric or periumbilical pain that migrates to the RLQ. Direct pain and rebound tenderness may occur at the McBurney point, which is known as the *McBurney sign*. It is located on the RLQ of the abdomen, two-thirds the distance between the umbilicus and the anterosuperior iliac spine. Abdominal tenderness in this region does not always occur in patients with acute appendicitis. Other physical signs include Rovsing sign (pain felt in the RLQ when palpating the left lower quadrant [LLQ]), psoas sign (an increase in pain from passive extension of the right hip that stretches the iliopsoas muscle), and a fever of >38°C. Retractable pain upon palpation of the abdominal wall frequently parallels the severity of the inflammatory process. A leukocyte count >10,000 cells/mL and an increase in C-reactive protein commonly occur. A normal white blood cell count should not exclude appendicitis. A contrast-enhanced CT scan is recognized as a useful and accurate method to diagnose appendicitis. A positive CT scan indicating the presence of appendicitis may show a distended appendix, appendiceal or bowel wall thickening, peri-appendiceal abscess formation, or inflammation of a large tubular structure. The CT scan can also assist with the differential diagnosis by revealing other causes of acute abdominal pain such as ovarian cyst, tubal pregnancy, acute salpingitis, mesenteric adenitis, and perforated duodenal ulcer.

Surgical Procedure

Open Approach

Through a right paramedian 2- to 4-inch incision in the abdomen, the cecum is exposed and removed through the wound. The appendix is identified, separated from the surrounding tissue, ligated, crushed, and then transected at its base and removed. The surgical site is irrigated, then the layers including the peritoneum, muscle, and fascia are sutured closed. In some instances, when the appendix is perforated and infection has occurred, the wound is sometimes left open, and a soft Penrose drain is inserted to facilitate drainage out of the surgical site.

Laparoscopic Approach

An LA is performed using three to four trocar sites, with an initial 10-mm trocar placed at the umbilicus and subsequent trocars placed in the lower abdomen according to the surgeon's preference. After insufflation of the abdomen or establishing a "pneumoperitoneum," the patient is placed in Trendelenburg position with left tilt to facilitate exposure of the appendix. The base of the cecum is identified, the appendix is mobilized, and the base of the appendix is stapled. After stapling the mesoappendix, the appendix is freed from the intestine, placed in a bag, and removed through the 10-mm trocar. Fig. 8.2 illustrates the laparoscopic approach for an appendectomy. The umbilical fascia is closed, and the skin is approximated.

Anesthetic Management and Considerations

Preoperative Period

1. *List the advantages and disadvantages associated with an LA compared with an OA.*

   Since the introduction of LA in 1983, the debate continues over the potential advantages and disadvantages comparing LA with the traditional OA. Clear advantages to an LA technique include improved aesthetic result due to smaller incisions, decreased pain, less blood loss and postoperative pulmonary impairment, a reduction in postoperative ileus, shorter hospital stays, faster postoperative recovery, and fewer wound infections. LA has become a standard surgical approach in medical centers; however, the disadvantages associated with LA include longer operative times (related to the surgical experience and skill of the surgeon with laparoscopic techniques), increased postoperative nausea and vomiting

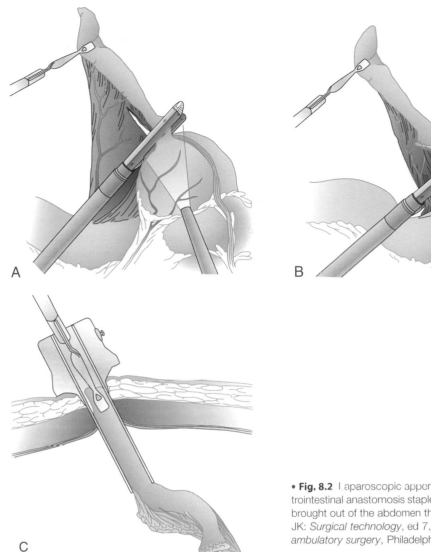

A

B

C

• **Fig. 8.2** Laparoscopic appendectomy. (A) The appendix is amputated with the gastrointestinal anastomosis stapler. (B) The mesoappendix is divided. (C) The appendix is brought out of the abdomen through one of the operative ports. (**A** and **B**, From Fuller JK: *Surgical technology*, ed 7, St. Louis, 2018, Elsevier; **C**, From Moody FG: *Atlas of ambulatory surgery*, Philadelphia, 1999, Saunders.)

(PONV), and higher incidence of postoperative intraabdominal abscess and bowel perforation.

The most often utilized surgical approach is laparoscopic removal of the appendix. The OA technique was once considered the gold standard for appendectomy and is still an alternative if LA is unsuccessful. A surgeon may consider an open procedure or convert intraoperatively to an OA for patients with a history of complicated perforated appendicitis, previous abdominal surgery with dense scar tissue or adhesions, morbid obesity, inability to gain adequate surgical access to the appendix, or when excessive bleeding occurs intraoperatively.

2. *List the anesthetic options available for an OA procedure.*

General endotracheal anesthesia (GETA) using a rapid sequence induction is most frequently employed. Patients who have appendicitis generally do not have significant comorbidities. These patients usually have abdominal pain and may have recently eaten, making it prudent to consider that aspiration prophylaxis may be necessary. Administration of metoclopramide (gastrokinetic),

cimetidine, ranitidine, or famotidine (H_2 antagonists) and Bicitra (sodium citrate, a nonparticulate antacid) decreases the risk of aspiration and assists in the control of PONV. It is worth noting that if the patient may have a bowel obstruction, metoclopramide should be avoided, as the gastrokinetic effects of this drug can enhance the potential for perforation of the bowel. A combination of air–oxygen with inhalation agents, narcotics, and a muscle relaxant is frequently used during the maintenance period. An orogastric tube can be inserted after induction to drain gastric residual secretions. It has not been conclusively determined that by decompressing the stomach during surgery, the risk of PONV is decreased, and antiemetic medications (5-HT3 antagonist) are customarily ideally administered 15 to 30 minutes before the end of surgery.

The administration of regional anesthesia is an option and should be discussed with the patient. Local anesthesia using ilioinguinal, iliohypogastric nerve blocks, and injections at the incision site supplemented with sedation can be accomplished for OA. Neuraxial blockade, subarachnoid, and epidural blocks can be provided if the patient is normovolemic and does not exhibit signs of septicemia. When neuraxial anesthesia and local anesthesia are placed at the surgical incision site, it has been demonstrated to decrease both postoperative pain and the incidence of PONV. Transversus abdominal plane blocks decrease postoperative pain and have an opioid-sparing effect after LA.

3. *List possible complications associated with LA.*

The pneumoperitoneum is accomplished by insufflating carbon dioxide gas, which allows the surgeon to perform a laparoscopic procedure. Complications that can arise include:

- The use of pressurized gas increases the possibility of extravasation of CO_2 along the tissue planes, resulting in subcutaneous emphysema, pneumomediastinum, or pneumothorax. Nitrous oxide is highly diffusible and will enter the bowel lumen and possibly cause distention and increase the difficulty of the surgical procedure. If nitrous oxide is administered, it should be discontinued, and insufflation pressures must be decreased if subcutaneous emphysema occurs.
- The pneumoperitoneum creates a cephalad displacement of the diaphragm, which results in decreased functional residual capacity and pulmonary compliance, which promotes the development of atelectasis.
- The celiac reflex can be elicited during the creation and maintenance of the pneumoperitoneum. Pressure in the abdominal cavity causes vagal nerve stimulation that can result in mild, moderate, or severe bradycardia. The immediate treatment for severe bradycardia is to have the surgeon immediately release the pneumoperitoneum, administer 100% oxygen, check the blood pressure, and consider the use of an anticholinergic (glycopyrrolate, atropine) or ephedrine if severe bradycardia is unrelieved.
- Shoulder tip pain can occur, and this phenomenon is thought to be caused by diaphragmatic irritation as a result of residual CO_2 gas.

4. *Identify the challenges during anesthetic management for patients who have experienced a perforated appendix.*

When the appendix ruptures, intestinal bacteria infect the peritoneal cavity and cause sepsis. The severity of sepsis will depend on the amount of time that the patient has endured the infection. The signs and symptoms associated with a ruptured appendix are reflective of bacteremia and hypermetabolism and include leukocytosis, fever, vomiting, hypovolemia, tachycardia, pain, and possibly compensated or uncompensated metabolic acidosis. The anesthetist should assess all these factors and the patient's immediate condition before making the decision to use a particular type of anesthetic technique and to administer anesthetic medications. Due to the fever and decreased fluid intake, providing hydration is indicated. Depending on the patient's condition and kilogram weight, a 10 to 20 mL/kg fluid bolus will help decrease the tachycardia and hypotension that may occur upon induction of anesthesia.

Administration of antibiotics is required, and a third-generation cephalosporin given within 1 hour of surgical incision provides maximal coverage. If the appendix has ruptured, a multidose IV antibiotic regimen is required, and the patient is admitted to the hospital.

Intraoperative Period

5. *Describe the anesthetic technique that is best suited for LA.*

Rapid sequence induction GETA with balanced air–oxygen inhalation, narcotic, and muscle relaxation is the preferred anesthetic choice, as this technique minimizes the risk of aspiration from increased intraabdominal pressures during insufflation. Muscle relaxation allows for lower insufflation pressures, provides better visualization, and prevents unexpected patient movement. The duration of the surgical procedure is dependent on the expertise of the surgeon, but this surgical procedure is frequently brief, approximately 30 minutes. Therefore careful titration of medications is necessary to ensure a timely emergence from anesthesia.

It is possible to provide neuraxial anesthesia during OA; however, with LA, the pneumoperitoneum can cause visceral discomfort, as well as making spontaneous respiration difficult; thus general anesthesia is most commonly employed.

6. *Identify the reasons that CO_2 is used to create a pneumoperitoneum.*

Carbon dioxide is the insufflating gas of choice for laparoscopy because it is nonflammable, readily diffuses across membranes, and is rapidly degraded.

7. *Describe the physiologic manifestations associated with a CO_2 embolus that can occur during an LA.*

A CO_2 gas embolism may also result from unintended insufflation of gas into an open vein. This may lead to hypoxemia, pulmonary hypertension, pulmonary edema, and cardiovascular collapse. A "gas lock" is created at the level of the vena cava, right atrium, right ventricle, and pulmonary artery that disrupts blood flow through the heart. Treatment includes immediate release of the pneumoperitoneum, placing the patient on 100% FiO_2, administration of a fluid bolus, administration of a vasopressor, and utilizing the Durant maneuver (patient's head down in a left lateral decubitus position) and insertion of a central venous catheter to aspirate the air from the right side of the heart.

8. *List the hemodynamic and pulmonary changes that occur with pneumoperitoneum and Trendelenburg positioning during LA.*

The patient is placed in the supine and in the Trendelenburg position with both arms tucked at their sides. The patient's body is rotated to the left to increase visualization of the lower abdomen and pelvis. Because gravity promotes blood flow in a cephalad direction, an increase in venous return, central blood volume, and cardiac output occurs. This change increases the myocardial workload and may cause cardiac ischemia or infarction in those patients with cardiovascular disease.

The patient's functional residual capacity and vital capacity decrease secondary to diaphragmatic and abdominal contents displacement, leading to a decrease in pulmonary compliance, increase in ventilation–perfusion mismatch, increase in peak inspiratory pressure (PIP), and increase in $ETCO_2$. In addition to these altered pulmonary dynamics, CO_2 will be absorbed into the systemic circulation resulting from the pneumoperitoneum. Lastly, patients who are hypermetabolic have an increased rate of CO_2. Ventilation should be adjusted to normalize $ETCO_2$ ($PaCO_2$) by increasing the minute ventilation. Right mainstem intubation and hypoxemia may occur with this position because the endotracheal tube is secured proximally at the mandible and does not move with the trachea as the diaphragm displaces the lungs and carina cephalad.

Postoperative Period

9. *Explain the difference in the length of hospitalization when comparing LA with OA.*

LA offers advantages over OA by decreasing the postoperative wound infection rate, decreasing the need for postoperative pain medications, shortening the days of hospitalization, decreasing postoperative bowel and pulmonary complications, and decreasing the amount of time before the patient can return to work.

Review Questions

1. Which is not considered an advantage of a laparoscopic approach for an appendectomy?
   a. Decreased wound infections
   b. Decreased incidence of pulmonary complications
   c. Decreased length of stay in the hospital
   d. Decreased antibiotic administration
2. The intraoperative use of nitrous oxide:
   a. Increases the minimum alveolar concentration of the volatile agent.
   b. Decreases the necessity for an oral gastric tube.
   c. Increases the degree of bowel distention.
   d. Decreases the amount of CO_2 needed for creation of the pneumoperitoneum.
3. During insufflation, the patient's heart rate abruptly decreases to 35 beats per minute. Your initial intervention includes:
   a. Call a code, start cardiopulmonary resuscitation, administer atropine.
   b. Stop insufflation, deliver 100% oxygen, administer an anticholinergic if bradycardia continues.
   c. Obtain a blood pressure, deliver 100% oxygen.
   d. Administer atropine before insufflation begins.

4. Physiologic changes that occur during prolonged Trendelenburg positioning include:
   a. Metabolic alkalosis.
   b. Metabolic acidosis.
   c. Respiratory acidosis.
   d. Respiratory alkalosis.
5. Durant position is indicated for a:
   a. CO_2 gas embolus.
   b. Massive hemorrhage.
   c. Pneumothorax.
   d. Cardiac tamponade.

Suggested Readings

Brogi E, Kazan R, Cyr S, Giunta F, Hemmerling TM. Transversus abdominal plane block for postoperative analgesia: a systematic review and meta-analysis of randomized-controlled trials. *Can J Anaesth* 2016;63(10):1184–96.

Corneille MG, Steigelman MB, Myers JG, et al. Laparoscopic appendectomy is superior to open appendectomy in obese patients. *Am J Surg* 2007;194:877–881.

Fujishiro J, Watanabe E, Hirahara N, Terui K, Tomita H, Ishimaru T, Miyata H. Laparoscopic versus open appendectomy for acute appendicitis in children: a nationwide retrospective study on postoperative outcomes. *J Gastrointest Surg* 2020 Mar 3. doi: 10.1007/s11605-020-04544-3

Ninh A, Wood K, Bui AH, Leitman IM. Risk factors and outcomes for sepsis after appendectomy in adults *Surg Infect* 2019;20(8):601–606.

Norton JA, Oberlhelman HA, Malott KA. Intestinal surgery. In Jaffe R, Samuels S, eds. *Anesthesiologist's Manual of Surgical Procedures*, 5th ed. Philadelphia: Lippincott Williams and Wilkins, 2014:520–536.

Schick KS, Hüttl TP, Fertman JM, et al. A critical analysis of laparoscopic appendectomy: how experience with 1,400 appendectomies allowed innovative treatment to become standard in a university hospital. *World J Surg* 2008;32:1406–1413.

Talha A, El-Haddad H, Ghazal AE, Shehata G. Laparoscopic versus open appendectomy for perforated appendicitis in adults: randomized clinical trial. *Surg Endosc* 2020;34(2):907–914.

Wang D, Dong T, Shao Y, Gu T, Xu Y, Jiang Y. Laparoscopy versus open appendectomy for elderly patients, a meta-analysis and systematic review. *BMC Surg* 2019;19(1):54.

9

Cholecystectomy: Open and Laparoscopic Approaches

KEY POINTS

- The open technique is utilized in less than 10% of patients having a cholecystectomy.
- It is estimated that less than 5% of these procedures will require conversion to an open technique.
- Many benefits are associated with the laparoscopic surgical technique compared with the traditional open technique, including decreased postoperative respiratory dysfunction,

  decreased postoperative pain, and decreased postoperative analgesic requirements, which reduce lethargy, nausea, vomiting, and constipation.
- Alterations in normal physiologic functioning occur as a result of the creation of a pneumoperitoneum during laparoscopic cholecystectomy.

Case Synopsis

A 40-year-old man presents to the emergency room vomiting with severe upper right abdominal pain. The patient is evaluated by a general surgeon with a diagnosis of cholecystitis and prepared for emergency cholecystectomy.

Preoperative Evaluation and Demographic Data

Past Medical/Surgical History

- Cholelithiasis
- Alcohol abuse
- Left knee anterior cruciate ligament repair; no anesthetic complications

List of Medications

- Thiamin
- Folic acid

Laboratory Tests

- Hemoglobin, 14.8 g/dL; hematocrit, 44%; white blood cells, 7.9/mm³; platelet count, 270/mm³
- Blood urea nitrogen (BUN), 20 mg/dL; creatinine, 1.1 mg/dL
- Electrolytes: sodium, 142 mEq/L; potassium, 4.0 mEq/L; chloride, 101 mEq/L; carbon dioxide, 28 mEq/L
- Coagulation: prothrombin time, 10.4 seconds; partial thromboplastin time, 41.1 seconds; international normalized ratio, 1.03
- Liver function: bilirubin, 1.0 mg/dL; aspartate aminotransferase (AST), 28 units/L; alanine aminotransferase

  (ALT), 30 units/mL; alkaline phosphatase (ASP), 1.9 units/mL; and albumin, 3.9 g/dL

Height/Weight/Vital Signs

- 173 cm, 85 kg; body mass index (BMI), 28.4
- Blood pressure, 168/86; heart rate, 95 beats per minute; respiratory rate, 22 breaths per minute; room air–oxygen saturation, 98%; temperature, 37.6°C
- Electrocardiogram: normal sinus rhythm

Pathophysiology

The gallbladder is a hollow, pear-shaped organ that is located on the underside of the right lobe of the liver. Bile that is produced within the liver is stored in the gallbladder until it is released into the intestine. The cystic duct connects the gallbladder to the common hepatic duct, forming the common bile duct. The gallbladder concentrates and acts as a reservoir for bile. Bile salts, bile pigments, cholesterol, and calcium are component parts that comprise bile. The role of bile is to aid in the intestinal absorption and breakdown of dietary fat.

When the gallbladder becomes full, the sphincter of Oddi will relax, allowing bile to be released into the duodenum. Cholecystokinin, a hormone secreted by the duodenum in response to acid contents, causes contraction of the gallbladder and relaxation of the sphincter of Oddi. Normally, 500 to 1000 mL of bile are secreted per day.

Cholelithiasis results in hard masses formed within the gallbladder. Gallstones are formed from bile, which is composed of bile acids, bile pigments, cholesterol, and calcium.

These stones can become lodged in the cystic duct, resulting in obstruction. Cholecystitis occurs as a result of infection, inflammation, and from the blockade of bile flow through the cystic duct or common bile duct. This result can cause severe right upper abdominal pain that characteristically radiates to the right shoulder. Patients with cholecystitis typically present with an acute, severe mid-gastric pain that radiates to the right abdominal quadrants. Patient factors that increase the risk for developing cholecystitis include female gender, obesity, parity, and age.

A diagnostic evaluation called *Murphy sign* can be used to assess for the presence of cholecystitis. During an abdominal examination, the patient is asked to exhale while the practitioner places their hand over the approximate location of the gallbladder. The patient is instructed to inhale, and if the patient stops breathing, this sign may be indicative of abdominal tenderness resulting from gallbladder disease.

The blood test results in patients that have cholecystitis include increased plasma bilirubin, ALP, and amylase. Ileus and localized tenderness may indicate a gallbladder perforation with associated peritonitis. If complete obstruction of the cystic duct occurs, jaundice may occur. Confirmation of cholecystitis is accomplished by cholescintigraph, a contrast study of the gallbladder that is accomplished by ultrasonography.

Patients who have cholecystitis are frequently dehydrated caused by decreased oral intake, vomiting, or nasogastric tube evacuation. Unless other pathophysiologic conditions exist that preclude fluid resuscitation, it is warranted to correct volume depletion. Ileus should be treated with a nasogastric tube. Free air that is determined to be present within the abdomen causes fever, ileus, abdominal rigidity and pain, vomiting, and dehydration. It is estimated that 20% of patients who develop cholecystitis will become symptomatic and develop pain when biliary obstruction occurs. Fig. 9.1 shows the anatomy of the gallbladder and biliary tree. Notice the gallstones present within the gallbladder and lodged within the cystic duct.

Surgical Procedures

A cholecystectomy can be performed as an open procedure or by a laparoscopic approach. For patients who have undergone previous abdominal surgeries, adhesions around the past surgical field can increase the complexity of the surgical procedure. Significant medical problems such as obesity, cardiac and pulmonary pathology, and coagulopathy will complicate the anesthetic management. The open technique is utilized in less than 10% of cholecystectomy procedures performed. It is estimated that less than 5% of laparoscopic cholecystectomy procedures will be converted to the open approach.

Open Cholecystectomy

An open cholecystectomy is performed by making a right subcostal or midline incision into the abdominal wall. Dissection into the peritoneal cavity occurs, and traction is

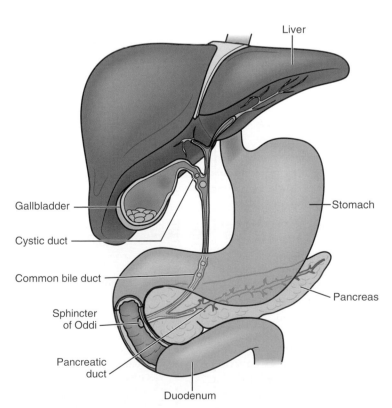

• **Fig. 9.1** Gallstones within the gallbladder with obstruction of the common bile and cystic ducts. (From Stromberg HK: *deWit's medical-surgical nursing: Concepts and practice*, ed 4, St. Louis, 2021, Elsevier.)

placed on the liver and the duodenum until maximum exposure of the gallbladder, cystic duct, cystic artery, and common bile duct is achieved. The gallbladder is excised from the liver bed, followed by isolation of the cystic artery and cystic duct. Alternative techniques include isolation of the cystic duct and cystic artery first, followed by retrograde removal of the gallbladder from the liver bed.

Laparoscopic Cholecystectomy

A laparoscopic cholecystectomy is initiated through insufflation of carbon dioxide (CO_2) into the patient's peritoneum in order to create a pneumoperitoneum. A Veress needle is inserted just below the umbilicus and then introduced into the peritoneal cavity. Correct needle placement is confirmed in several ways. The most common method is for the surgeon to feel and hear a distinct "pop" that occurs when the needle pierces the fascia and peritoneum. A more scientific and safe approach is accomplished by placing a drop of water on the hub of the Veress needle. Due to the negative pressure that is present in the peritoneal cavity, a drop of water will be drawn inward when placed in the hub of the Veress needle, confirming proper placement. An alternative method, the Hasson technique, involves creating a small incision through the abdominal fascia in order to place the trocars in the abdomen. Confirmation of proper location is further demonstrated by percussion of the CO_2 in the abdomen during insufflation. Once correct needle placement is confirmed, it is replaced with a cannula or trocar, which allows for a video laparoscope to visualize the operative field and instruments to be inserted.

Anesthetic Management and Considerations for Cholecystectomy

Preoperative Period

1. *Identify the associated disease states that commonly occur in patients having a cholecystectomy.*

    Patients who present for a cholecystectomy often have associated pathologic conditions, including gastrointestinal disorders including paralytic ileus, cirrhosis, hemolytic disorders, choledocholithiasis, and active pancreatitis.
2. *Describe the alteration in respiratory dynamics that occurs in patients who have cholecystitis.*

    Patients presenting with symptomatic cholecystitis may exhibit splinting secondary to pain resulting from an acute abdominal process. This may lead to an impaired respiratory function resulting in atelectasis, decreased functional residual capacity, and hypoventilation. The respiratory changes associated with a pneumoperitoneum are discussed later in this chapter. A patient with a history of impaired pulmonary function or chronic pneumonitis may be at increased risk for desaturation and barotrauma during the intraoperative period. Preoperative testing for patients with pulmonary disorders should include a chest x-ray.

3. *Describe the potential decreased intravascular volume status and management for patients having a cholecystectomy.*

    A patient who presents for a cholecystectomy may be dehydrated from vomiting and decreased oral intake. Preoperative evaluation of the patient's hemodynamic status must include blood pressure measurement, heart rate, and the presence of orthostatic hypotension. Fluid resuscitation is recommended for those patients who present with the signs and symptoms of hemodynamic compromise. Preoperative testing for patients with cardiac pathology should include an electrocardiogram (ECG).
4. *Describe the benefits of using laparoscopic surgery versus open procedures.*

    Many benefits are related to the use of a laparoscopic surgical technique compared with the traditional open technique. Box 9.1 presents the advantages of a laparoscopic approach for surgical procedures.
5. *Describe the potential for renal insufficiency for patients having a cholecystectomy.*

    Occasionally, these patients will present with obstructive jaundice that requires the preoperative administration of bile salts, which may cause postoperative renal insufficiency. Preoperative testing should include a urinalysis (UA) and BUN and creatinine. These patients' BUN and creatinine are considered to be within the high-normal range. The presence of bilirubin in the urine is indicative of a bile duct obstruction.
6. *Describe the potential for gastrointestinal pathology for patients having a cholecystectomy.*

    Patients may present with peritonitis, which may result in abdominal distension and paralytic ileus. Preoperative laboratory testing should include bilirubin, AST, ALT, ALP, and albumin. These patients' liver function tests are considered to be within the normal limits. Increased bilirubin, AST, ALT, and ALP and decreased albumin are consistent with hepatic dysfunction.
7. *Discuss premedication for the cholecystectomy patient.*

    Preoperative medications to consider include drugs that will reduce spasm of the sphincter of Oddi. These include anticholinergic medications such as glycopyrrolate.

• BOX 9.1 Advantages Associated With a Laparoscopic Approach for Surgical Procedures

- Faster return to normal activities
- Decreased time of hospitalization
- Decreased incidence of ileus and adhesions resulting from less bowel exposure and fewer manipulations
- Early postoperative ambulation
- Decreased postoperative pain
- Decreased postoperative physiologic stress
- Decreased need for analgesic medication
- Decreased postoperative respiratory dysfunction
- Improved cosmetic result

Vitamin K administration is indicated if the patient has a prolonged prothrombin time. For those patients who are at increased risk of gastric aspiration, a histamine-2 antagonist such as cimetidine, a gastrokinetic such as metoclopramide, and a nonparticulate antacid such as sodium citrate (Bicitra) should be administered.

Intraoperative Period

8. *Describe the anesthetic technique used for laparoscopic cholecystectomy.*

   The anesthetic technique of choice utilized for cholecystectomy is general anesthesia. Providing general anesthesia and an endotracheal tube used for airway maintenance allows for airway protection and provides the ability to control and manage CO_2 during artificial ventilation. The use of muscle relaxation will help minimize abdominal insufflation pressures and expedite surgical exposure of the gallbladder. Because cholecystectomy is frequently accomplished as an outpatient procedure and the degree of postoperative discomfort is rarely extreme, the use of a significant amount of narcotic is not warranted.

9. *Which gas is utilized for insufflation during laparoscopic surgical procedures?*

   Many gases have been utilized during laparoscopic insufflation, including helium, argon, nitrous oxide (N_2O), and CO_2. All of these gases, with the exception of CO_2, possess properties that can cause untoward physiologic effects. Carbon dioxide is noncombustible and therefore it can be used in conjunction with electrocautery. Additionally, CO_2 is rapidly and easily eliminated from the lungs by increasing minute ventilation.

   Absorption of CO_2 can occur through the intraperitoneal route, which is common as a result of normal laparoscopic insufflation, which will result in increased end tidal CO_2. Inadvertent extraperitoneal insufflation can occur and CO_2 can accumulate in the subcutaneous tissues, between the fascia and the peritoneum, and in the pericardium or mediastinum.

   End tidal CO_2 ($ETCO_2$) is an estimate of the $PaCO_2$ levels. In healthy patients, the $PaCO_2$–$ETCO_2$ gradient is typically 3 to 5 mm Hg. However, in patients with severe cardiovascular disease or prolonged laparoscopic surgeries, the $PaCO_2$–$ETCO_2$ gradient will be increased. It is important to attempt to maintain normocapnia throughout the procedure because hypercapnia causes coronary and cerebral vascular dilation as well as sympathetic nervous system stimulation.

10. *Explain the effect of a pneumoperitoneum during laparoscopic cholecystectomy on the following body systems: cardiovascular, pulmonary, cerebral, renal, and hepatic.*

    A pneumoperitoneum that is created during insufflation of CO_2 gas results in a variety of physiologic changes that are thought to result from three distinct mechanisms: a direct mechanical effect caused by compression, the presence of a neurohumoral response, and the effects of CO_2 absorption. Insufflation of gas into the peritoneal cavity allows the surgeon to visualize, expose, and manipulate the intraabdominal contents. Other factors that contribute to physiologic changes include anesthetic medication, artificial ventilation, patient positioning, and surgical stimulation.

    Cardiovascular: Creation of a pneumoperitoneum causes several hemodynamic changes during a laparoscopic cholecystectomy. Increases in systemic vascular resistance (SVR) or afterload occur because of mechanical compression on the arterial system and from sympathetic nervous system stimulation. As a result, mean arterial blood pressure increases. Patients undergoing laparoscopic cholecystectomy have elevated levels of dopamine, vasopressin, epinephrine, norepinephrine, renin, and cortisol levels. Hemodynamic changes occurring in these patients have been most often associated with the release of vasopressin. Catecholamine levels are slightly increased and may be the result of the stress response to the surgical procedure.

    Venous return to the heart (preload) is decreased from increased venous resistance, compression of the inferior vena cava, and peripheral pooling of blood in the lower body. This effect is accentuated when intraabdominal pressure exceeds 20 Torr. The position used during laparoscopic cholecystectomy is reverse Trendelenburg. This position can further result in decreased venous return to the heart.

    As SVR increases, a reduction in stroke volume that results in a decrease in cardiac output occurs. A pneumoperitoneum increases cardiac workload and myocardial oxygen requirements, which is the reason laparoscopic procedures are relatively contraindicated for patients who have a severely limited cardiac reserve. Interventions that can be used to minimize the associated reductions in stroke volume include intravenous fluid administration and compression of the patient's lower extremities. Upon discontinuation of the pneumoperitoneum and return of the patient to the supine position, the stroke volume will increase. Box 9.2 summarizes the hemodynamic effects associated with laparoscopic cholecystectomy.

    Respiratory: Patients having laparoscopic surgery have a decrease in postoperative pulmonary complications compared with an open procedure. However,

---

• BOX 9.2 Hemodynamic Effects Associated With Laparoscopic Cholecystectomy

1. Neurohumoral response: Activated
2. Venous return (preload): Decreased
3. Systemic vascular resistance (afterload): Increased
4. Heart rate: Increased
5. Blood pressure: Increased
6. Cardiac output: Decreased

creation of a pneumoperitoneum causes intraoperative pulmonary dysfunction. The use of CO_2 displaces the diaphragm cephalad, resulting in altered pulmonary dynamics, which are listed in Box 9.3. Insufflation compresses the basilar lobes of the lungs resulting in atelectasis, decreased functional residual capacity (FRC), decreased vital capacity, and increased dead-space ventilation. After creation of a pneumoperitoneum, $PaCO_2$ levels will plateau within 40 minutes after insufflation. Inadvertent CO_2 insufflation in the extraperitoneal space can result from a misplaced trocar or lack of CO_2 sequestration into the intraperitoneal space. Extraperitoneal CO_2 insufflation results in a rapid increase in $ETCO_2$.

Surgical patients that have pulmonary dysfunction, such as obstructive lung disease, require careful monitoring of CO_2 levels during laparoscopic surgery. In patients with normal pulmonary physiology, utilization of $ETCO_2$ monitoring provides a proportional relationship between $ETCO_2$ and CO_2. Patients with preexisting pulmonary disease may have an inaccurate $ETCO_2$–$PaCO_2$ relationship, ultimately underestimating the $PaCO_2$ values. The direct measurement of $PaCO_2$ with blood gas analysis may be necessary in this patient population.

Neurologic: Absorption of CO_2 during laparoscopy results in hypercarbia, leading to an increase in cerebral blood flow and intracranial pressure. Pneumoperitoneum itself will also increase intracranial pressure with or without any increase in the $PaCO_2$ levels due to the pressure exerted on the major venous structures within the abdominal cavity. Increased intracranial pressure leads to a decrease in cerebrospinal fluid drainage. Laparoscopic surgery is contraindicated in patients with increased intracranial pressure.

Renal: Abdominal insufflation affects the kidneys and causes oliguria as a result of compression of the renal vasculature, compression of the inferior vena cava causing decreased CO_2, and increased antidiuretic hormone secretion. Decreased renal blood flow leads to decreased glomerular filtration rate, urine output, and creatinine clearance sodium excretion; as a result, there is a potential for fluid overload. The anesthetist should avoid extreme hypotension in patients who have preoperative renal impairment. The patient's plasma vasopressin, renin, and aldosterone levels increase during CO_2 insufflation and remain elevated for up to 1 hour after removal of the pneumoperitoneum. The renal effects that are associated with a pneumoperitoneum are listed in Box 9.4.

Hepatic: Decreases in hepatic and splanchnic blood flow are associated with a pneumoperitoneum. Use of low insufflation pressures can help maintain normal hepatic and splanchnic blood flow.

11. *Discuss the effects of CO_2 absorption during laparoscopic procedures.*

    Carbon dioxide can be absorbed during laparoscopic surgeries in various parts of the body and may lead to untoward effects. Direct effects of CO_2 absorption result in decreases in heart rate, contractility, and SVR. The body reacts to these effects with sympathetic nervous system stimulation, resulting in increased heart rate, contractility, and SVR. High levels of CO_2 can cause vagal nerve stimulation, producing bradycardia and cardiac arrest.

12. *Examine the effects of steep reverse Trendelenburg positioning for laparoscopic cholecystectomy.*

    Patients undergoing a laparoscopic cholecystectomy are placed into the reverse Trendelenburg position and tilted with their left side downward to facilitate visualization of the gallbladder. When the patient is placed into this position, the bowels shift downward away from the liver, which is located in the right upper quadrant. Lung and chest compliance are improved; however, there is the potential for hypotension as gravity pulls blood downward away from the heart. The anesthetist must also be cautious regarding the possibility of endotracheal tube migration or dislodgement.

13. *During insufflation of CO_2, the patient's heart rate abruptly decreases from 82 to 36 beats per minute. Identify the cause and treatment of this situation.*

    Stretching of the abdominal cavity during insufflation can initiate the celiac reflex. The parasympathetic nervous system innervation to the abdominal cavity is via the vagus nerve. The stretching of the abdominal viscera is sensed and transmitted to the brain as an afferent visceral response. The efferent response from the brain to the heart increases vagal tone, resulting in decreased heart rate, decreased contractility, and decreased rate of cardiac impulse conduction.

The treatment for the celiac reflex depends on the severity of bradycardia and the degree of hypotension that ensues. In this particular case, cardiac output is inadequate in most patients whose heart rate decreases to 36 beats per minute. The immediate initial intervention would be to tell the surgeon to rapidly remove the CO_2 gas from the peritoneal cavity. If severe bradycardia persists, an anticholinergic such as atropine should be administered. If the bradycardia is not as dramatic and cardiac output is adequate, then assessing the blood pressure to determine if perfusion is adequate is acceptable. Cardiac arrest can be caused by parasympathetic nervous system predominance as a result of CO_2 insufflation.

14. *What are the potential complications associated with open cholecystectomy?*
   • Injury to the common bile duct
   • Hemorrhage
   • Infection of the surgical wound
   • Injury to intraperitoneal organs or major abdominal blood vessels
   • Postoperative respiratory insufficiency

15. *List the potential complications associated with laparoscopic cholecystectomy.*
   • Deep vein thrombosis
   • Injury to intraperitoneal organs or major abdominal blood vessels
   • Hemorrhage
   • Increased intracranial pressure
   • Increased risk of regurgitation
   • Postoperative nausea and vomiting
   • Pneumothorax
   • Pneumopericardium
   • Pneumomediastinum
   • Shoulder pain
   • Subcutaneous emphysema
   • Carbon dioxide venous gas embolism

Subcutaneous emphysema: Subcutaneous emphysema is a known complication of laparoscopic surgery. It is sometimes unavoidable, and it is caused by accidental extraperitoneal insufflation. This situation develops as crepitus occurs over the abdominal wall and causes an increase in $ETCO_2$. The CO_2 gas can migrate upward into the head and neck region resulting in airway edema. The crepitus will resolve in time after exsufflation, but the patient should be kept intubated until the presence of hypercarbia is resolved. The severity of crepitus is dependent on the amount and the speed of extraperitoneal CO_2 gas extravasation.

Pneumothorax: A pneumothorax is a rare but life-threatening complication that can occur during a laparoscopic cholecystectomy. This situation results from CO_2 gas traversing the thorax through a tear in the visceral peritoneum, a disruption of the parietal pleura during dissection, or a congenital defect in the diaphragm. Patients may be asymptomatic or exhibit rapid desaturation, unilateral breath sounds, bronchospasm, increased $ETCO_2$, increased peak airway pressures, and

severe hypotension. After removal of the pneumoperitoneum, spontaneous resolution of the pneumothorax may occur within 30 to 60 minutes. If the pneumothorax is large, a thoracentesis should be performed. Correction of hypoxemia is paramount, and ventilation with 100% oxygen is vital while adding positive-end expiratory pressure (PEEP) may be necessary.

Carbon dioxide gas embolism: A CO_2 gas embolism is a rare but potentially fatal complication associated with laparoscopic surgery. It typically occurs shortly after creation of a pneumoperitoneum, especially in those patients who have had previous abdominal surgery. Carbon dioxide gas enters into the venous system through a disruption created in a vein within the abdominal wall or peritoneum and then it travels into the heart and pulmonary circulation via the inferior vena cava. If a significant amount of gas is entrained over a short period, a venous gas embolism can result in significant hemodynamic compromise. An air lock at the level of the right atrium decreasing blood flow through the heart results in hypotension, decreased cardiac output, tachycardia, pulmonary edema, hypoxemia, hypercarbia, increased peak airway pressure, jugular venous distention, and facial cyanosis.

Treatment of a patient who develops a carbon dioxide gas embolism includes immediate evacuation of the pneumoperitoneum, ventilation with 100% oxygen, administering fluid, and vasopressors. The patient should be placed in the left lateral decubitus position with the head oriented downward to prevent gas bubble entry into the pulmonary and arterial circulation. If a central venous catheter is placed, the gas embolism may be removed by aspiration.

Postoperative Period

16. *Identify the key aspects of postoperative anesthetic management for a patient having an open cholecystectomy or laparoscopic cholecystectomy.*

Hemodynamic stability: Emergence phenomena can occur during emergence and extubation. However, the hemodynamic effects can persist throughout the initial postoperative phase. The anesthetist should determine whether the patient is experiencing pain, which is a potent stimulus of the sympathetic nervous system. Extreme hypertension and tachycardia should be treated with vasodilators, beta-blockers, or calcium channel medications. The specific treatment plan should be tailored to the individual patient.

Respiratory status: A rapid assessment of the patient's postoperative respiratory function is imperative. The head of the patient's bed should be elevated to promote respiratory excursion, and supplemental oxygen should be administered. Abdominal splinting can occur with pain and results in an inadequate tidal volume and contributes to the development of atelectasis and ventilation–perfusion mismatch. Hypoventilation is more often associated with an open cholecystectomy due to the pain caused by the surgical incision. Analgesic medications should be administered to alleviate discomfort and promote adequate respiratory function.

Postoperative pain: The severity of postoperative pain that is experienced is highly variable and is dependent on the individual patient. As stated previously, patients who undergo an open cholecystectomy frequently have more pain compared with the laparoscopic approach due to the right upper quadrant incision and retraction of the skin and abdominal contents. However, a specific character of pain occurs during a laparoscopic cholecystectomy, and it is described as shoulder tip pain. It is believed that this discomfort is caused by diaphragmatic irritation as a result of the CO_2 gas used to create the pneumoperitoneum.

A variety of intravenous or oral analgesic medications can be administered. Ketorolac decreases postoperative pain without inhibiting ventilation or causing sedation, which is desirable for outpatient surgery.

Nausea and vomiting: The incidence of nausea and vomiting for patients after the administration of anesthesia ranges from 30% to 70%. Multimodal drug therapy has been shown to be more effective in treating this event compared with monotherapy. Medications that can be used to inhibit nausea and vomiting include propofol, steroids (dexamethasone), serotonin receptor antagonists (ondansetron), and dopamine receptor antagonists (droperidol/metoclopramide). *Aprepitant,* a neurokinin type 1 receptor antagonist, has been shown to be effective at decreasing nausea and vomiting.

Review Questions

1. Which gas is routinely used during laparoscopic surgery to create a pneumoperitoneum?
   a. Argon
   b. Carbon dioxide
   c. Helium
   d. Nitrous oxide
2. Which is not a hemodynamic change associated with a pneumoperitoneum?
   a. Decreased venous return to the heart
   b. Increased afterload
   c. Increased mean arterial pressure
   d. Increased stroke volume
3. Which respiratory effect occurs during carbon dioxide insufflation for laparoscopic surgery?
   a. Decreased functional residual capacity
   b. Decreased pulmonary compliance
   c. Increased intrathoracic pressure
   d. Increased vital capacity

4. Which renal effect occurs during carbon dioxide insufflation for laparoscopic surgery?
   a. Decreased aldosterone levels
   b. Decreased antidiuretic hormone levels
   c. Decreased urine output
   d. Increased glomerular filtration
5. Which preoperative laboratory test is not indicated for a patient having a cholecystectomy?
   a. Alanine aminotransferase (ALT)
   b. Aspartate aminotransferase (AST)
   c. Bilirubin
   d. Cholesterol

Suggested Readings

Bablekos GD, Michaelides SA, Roussou T, et al. Changes in breathing control and mechanics after laparoscopic vs open cholecystectomy. *Arch Surg* 2006;141:16–22.

Bourgouin S, Mancini J, Monchal T, Bordes J, Balandraud P. Response to "individualized care in patients undergoing laparoscopic cholecystectomy". *Am J Surg* 2019;218(5):1029.

Collins SB, Johnson CA. Hepatobiliary and gastrointestinal disturbances. In: Nagelhout JJ, Elisha S, eds. *Nurse Anesthesia*, 6th ed. St. Louis, MO: Elsevier, 2018:709–742.

Cunningham AJ, Brull SJ. Laparoscopic cholecystectomy: anesthetic implications. *Anesth Analg* 1993;76:1120–1133.

Gangakhedkar GR, Monteiro JN. A prospective randomized double-blind study to compare the early recovery profiles of desflurane and sevoflurane in patients undergoing laparoscopic cholecystectomy. *J Anaesthesiol Clin Pharmacol* 2019;35(1):53–57.

Goel A, Gupta S, Bhagat TS, Garg P. Comparative analysis of hemodynamic changes and shoulder tip pain under standard pressure versus low-pressure pneumoperitoneum in laparoscopic cholecystectomy. *Euroasian J Hepatogastroenterol* 2019;9(1):5–8.

Joris JL, Noirot DP, Legrand MJ, et al. Hemodynamic changes during laparoscopic cholecystectomy. *Anesth Analg* 1993;76:1067–1071.

Kim SS, Donahue TR. Laparoscopic cholecystectomy. *JAMA* 2018;319(17):1834.

McIntyre C, Johnston A, Foley D, Lawler J, Bucholc M, Flanagan L, Sugrue M. Readmission to hospital following laparoscopic cholecystectomy: a meta-analysis. *Anaesthesiol Intensive Ther* 2020;52(1):47–55.

Raval AD, Deshpande S, Koufopoulou M, Rabar S, et al. The impact of intra-abdominal pressure on perioperative outcomes in laparoscopic cholecystectomy: a systematic review and network meta-analysis of randomized controlled trials. *Surg Endosc* 2020;34(7):2878–2890.

Ros A, Carlsson P, Rahmqvist M, et al. Non-randomised patients in a cholecystectomy trial: characteristics, procedures and outcomes. *BMC Surgery* 2006;6:17.

Yi NJ, Han HS, Min SK. The safety of a laparoscopic cholecystectomy in acute cholecystitis in high-risk patients older than sixty with stratification based on ASA score. *Minim Invasive Ther Allied Tech* 2006;15(3):159–164.

10

Liver Failure and Nonalcoholic Steatohepatitis

KEY POINTS

- Hepatic dysfunction is often multifactorial and can be categorized as prehepatic, intrahepatic (hepatocellular), or posthepatic (cholestatic) based on measurement of serum bilirubin, aminotransferases, and alkaline phosphatase.
- Orthotropic liver transplantation (OLT) has emerged as a definitive treatment option for patients with end-stage hepatic disease, and this is largely attributable to advances in surgical technique, immunosuppressive therapy, and donor organ procurement.

- Anesthesia-related concerns for patients undergoing OLT are consistent with those for patients undergoing major surgery with severe cirrhosis.
- There is no single anesthetic technique that has been proven superior during anesthetic management of OLT.
- Anesthetic management is strongly influenced by the various hemodynamic manifestations presented during the three major phases of the procedure.

Case Synopsis

A 38-year-old woman with a history of nonalcoholic steatohepatitis presents with end-stage liver disease and is scheduled for a liver transplant. She was recently hospitalized because of jaundice, fever, confusion, urine incontinence, and progressive abdominal pain and swelling. Two months before admission the patient noted pain and swelling of her elbows. One month later she developed malaise, weakness, and irritability. The patient's clinical status has stabilized with diuretic and albumin therapy, administration of parenteral nutrition, and salt restriction. The patient has been on the liver transplant list for 8 months.

Preoperative Evaluation and Demographic Data

Past Medical/Surgical History

- Nonalcoholic steatohepatitis
- Acute renal failure
- Smoked an average of 1 pack per day for 10 years, stopped 1 year ago
- Jaundiced with multiple spider angiomas of the face and trunk
- Abdominal distention due to ascites
- Hematoma present on the anterior wall after a recent paracentesis

List of Medications

- Lisinopril
- Zosyn
- Lasix

Diagnostic Data

Test Name	Result		Normal Range
White blood cell (WBC)	30.2 K/CUMM	(High)	4.8–10.8 K/CUMM
Blood urea nitrogen (BUN)	47.14 mmol/L	(High)	2.9–7.1 mmol/L
Creatinine	411.53 umol/L	(High)	61.9–114.9 umol/L
Bilirubin	110.34 mcmol/L	(High)	1.7–5.1 mcmol/L
Aspartate aminotransferase (AST)	260 unit/L	(High)	12–38 unit/L
Alanine aminotransferase (ALT)	59 unit/L	(High)	10–45 unit/L
Albumin	17 g/L	(Low)	35–48 g/L
Protein (serum)	70 g/L	(Normal)	60–80 g/L
Protein (urine)	30	(Positive)	Negative trace
Urinalysis (bacteria)	Many	(Positive)	None

Height/Weight/Vital Signs

- 168 cm, 64 kg
- Blood pressure, 150/88 mm Hg; heart rate, 100 beats per minute; respiratory rate, 22 breaths per minute; room air oxygen saturation, 96%; temperature, 38.1°C

Pathophysiology

When hepatic dysfunction (jaundice) occurs, an analysis of historical data, clinical signs, and symptoms; serial liver function tests; and a search for extrahepatic causes of hepatic dysfunction facilitate development of a differential diagnosis. Table 10.1 lists the causes of hepatic dysfunction and can be categorized as prehepatic, intrahepatic (hepatocellular), or posthepatic (cholestatic) based on measurement of serum bilirubin, aminotransferases, and alkaline phosphatase. Hepatic dysfunction is often multifactorial. Box 10.1 describes factors that can be used to develop a differential diagnosis for hepatic dysfunction.

Surgical Procedure

OLT has emerged as a definitive treatment option for patients with end-stage hepatic disease. This is largely attributable to advances in surgical technique, immunosuppressive

---

• BOX 10.1 Factors Used to Develop a Differential Diagnosis for Hepatic Dysfunction

1. Review all drugs administered
2. Check for sources of sepsis
3. Evaluate the possibility of an increased exogenous bilirubin load such as a blood transfusion
4. Rule out occult hematoma formation
5. Rule out hemolysis
6. Assess for evidence of hypotension, hypoventilation, and hypovolemia
7. Assess for congestive heart failure and renal insufficiency
8. Consider the possibility of immune-mediated hepatotoxicity

---

therapy, and donor organ procurement. Other contributing factors have greatly attenuated the previously formidable morbidity and mortality associated with this procedure, including advances in technologic and perioperative management.

Patients with end-stage hepatic disease who experience progressive life-threatening complications that become increasingly refractory to medical intervention are candidates for OLT. Transplantation may also be considered a therapeutic option in patients with certain viral infections who respond poorly to medical management but are nevertheless deemed physiologically salvageable. In the adult population, postnecrotic (nonalcoholic) cirrhosis constitutes the most common indication for OLT.

The refinement of immunosuppressive therapy has been instrumental in the increasingly impressive survival rates in patients undergoing OLT. A vital component has been the use of cyclosporine, which interferes with helper T-cell activity and inhibits interleukin (IL)-2 and other proinflammatory cytokines. Cyclosporine is often used concurrently with azathioprine and corticosteroids. Anti-OKT3, a monoclonal antibody directed toward lymphocytes, has also shown efficacy in preventing acute rejection, particularly if it is steroid refractory. Tacrolimus (FK-506) is an effective alternative to cyclosporine. Technical refinements in the procedure and development of more precise support modalities have also contributed to the overall improved outcome in patients undergoing OLT.

Anesthesia-related concerns for patients undergoing OLT are consistent with those for patients undergoing major surgery with severe cirrhosis. The multisystem effects of cirrhosis are underscored. Profound hemodynamic derangements may preexist and are likely to be exacerbated by the numerous stressors imposed during particular phases of the procedure. These include the hemodynamic consequences of clamping and unclamping the portal vein and vena cava, as well as alterations in metabolism. Hyperkalemia and venous air embolism may be encountered with perfusion of the transplanted graft.

TABLE 10.1 Causes of Hepatic Dysfunction Based on Liver Function Tests

Hepatic Dysfunction	Bilirubin	Aminotransferase Enzymes	Alkaline Phosphatase	Causes
Prehepatic	Increased unconjugated fraction	Normal	Normal	Hemolysis, hematoma, bilirubin overload
Intrahepatic	Increased conjugated fraction	Markedly increased	Normal to slightly increased	Viral, drugs, sepsis, hypoxemia, cirrhosis
Posthepatic	Increased conjugated fraction	Normal to slightly increased	Markedly increased	Biliary tract stones, sepsis

Anesthetic Management and Considerations

Preoperative Period

1. List various causes that result in cirrhosis of the liver.

Cirrhosis can result from a large variety of chronic, progressive liver diseases. Most often cirrhosis is the result of excessive chronic alcohol ingestion or chronic viral hepatitis due to hepatitis B virus (HBV) or hepatitis C virus (HCV) infection. Scarring of the liver results in disruption of normal liver architecture, and regenerating parenchymal nodules are typically seen. A percutaneous liver biopsy establishes the diagnosis of cirrhosis. Computed tomography (CT), magnetic resonance imaging (MRI), and hepatic ultrasonography with Doppler flow studies may reveal findings consistent with cirrhosis (splenomegaly, ascites, irregular liver surfaces). Fatigue and malaise are common with all forms of cirrhosis as well as with almost all forms of acute and chronic liver disease. Characteristic but nondiagnostic physical findings of cirrhosis include palmar erythema, spider angioma, gynecomastia, testicular atrophy, and evidence of portal hypertension (splenomegaly, ascites). A decreased serum albumin concentration and a prolonged prothrombin time are characteristic of cirrhosis. An increase in serum aminotransferase and alkaline phosphate concentration is common. Hepatic and extrahepatic complications of hepatic cirrhosis develop predictably in patients afflicted with progressive liver scarring. Acute hepatic failure is characterized by an increased expression of these complications and includes a list for differential diagnosis found in Box 10.2.

2. Discuss the major features of nonalcoholic steatohepatitis (NASH).

NASH is a common, often "silent" liver disease. This condition resembles findings that are consistent with alcoholic liver disease but occurs in people who drink little or no alcohol. The major feature in NASH is fat in the liver, along with inflammation and damage.

• BOX 10.2 Pathologic Consequences Associated With Acute Hepatic Failure

- Portal hypertension
- Esophagogastric varices
- Ascites
- Hyperdynamic circulation
- Anemia
- Coagulopathy
- Arterial hypoxemia
- Hepatorenal syndrome
- Hypoglycemia
- Gallstones
- Hepatic encephalopathy
- Hepatic carcinoma

Most people with NASH feel well and are not aware that they have a liver problem. Nevertheless, NASH can be severe and can lead to cirrhosis, in which the liver is permanently damaged and scarred and no longer is able to function properly. NASH affects 2% to 5% of Americans. An additional 10% to 20% of Americans have fat in their liver but no inflammation or liver damage, a condition called "fatty liver." NASH is becoming more common, possibly because of the greater number of Americans who are obese. In the past 10 years, the rate of obesity has doubled in adults and tripled in children. Obesity also contributes to diabetes and high blood cholesterol, which can further complicate the health of someone with NASH. NASH is initially suspected in a person who is found to have elevations in liver tests that are included in routine blood test panels, such as alanine aminotransferase or aspartate aminotransferase. When further evaluation shows no apparent reason for liver disease and x-rays or imaging studies of the liver indicate the presence of fat deposition, NASH is suspected. The only confirmatory test for NASH is a liver biopsy, which will show fat and inflamed tissues. NASH is usually a silent disease with few or no symptoms.

Patients generally do not develop symptoms in the early stages; however, fatigue, weight loss, and weakness occur once the disease is more advanced or cirrhosis develops. The progression of NASH can take years to develop, and as fibrosis develops and becomes more severe, cirrhosis occurs (Fig. 10.1). The liver becomes scarred and hardened, and as a result, hepatic function is impaired. Currently, no specific therapies are used to treat NASH. The most important recommendations given to persons with this disease are to:
1. Reduce their weight
2. Follow a balanced and healthy diet
3. Increase physical activity
4. Avoid alcohol
5. Avoid unnecessary medications

People with NASH often have other medical conditions, such as diabetes, high blood pressure, or elevated cholesterol. Once cirrhosis and liver damage develop, liver transplantation is considered.

Intraoperative Period

3. Identify the anesthetic management and monitoring considerations for liver surgery.

Invasive monitoring modalities are mandatory for OLT. These include intraarterial pressure monitoring and central venous or pulmonary artery catheterization. Due to the profound fluid shifts and blood loss encountered in these procedures, direct measurement of central filling pressures is vital for guiding volume and blood-product replacement. Large-bore (14- to 16-gauge) intravenous catheters are needed for administration of large volumes using rapid infusion devices. Intravenous fluids should be warmed to prevent hypothermia in

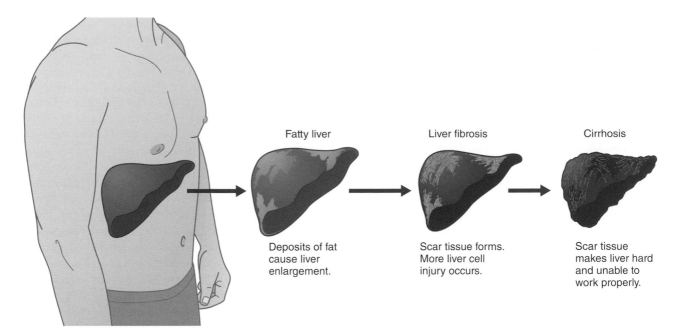

Fatty liver

Liver fibrosis

Cirrhosis

Deposits of fat cause liver enlargement.

Scar tissue forms. More liver cell injury occurs.

Scar tissue makes liver hard and unable to work properly.

• **Fig. 10.1** Degenerative changes that progress toward cirrhosis. (Adapted from National Institute of Diabetes and Digestive and Kidney Diseases, National Institutes of Health. Retrieved from https://www.niddk.nih.gov/news/media-library/9459.)

order to avoid the untoward effects on coagulation, pharmacokinetics, and other metabolic processes. Other measures used to maintain normothermia include forced-air surface warming and possibly increased ambient room temperature. All airway gases should be humidified. Urinary output, as measured via indwelling urinary catheter, should be maintained at a minimum of 0.5 mL/kg/hr.

4. *Identify the serial laboratory results that must be assessed during anesthetic management for OLT.*

Patients with severe cirrhosis are typically coagulopathic (deficient in coagulation factors and thrombocytopenic). Massive blood loss should be anticipated. Red blood cells, fresh frozen plasma (FFP), platelets, and cryoprecipitate should be readily available. Blood-salvaging technology should also be used. Infusion of antifibrinolytics such as aminocaproic acid may also be useful perioperatively in efforts to control hemorrhage. Serial laboratory measurements are performed throughout surgery, which include arterial blood gases, electrolytes, hemoglobin and hematocrit levels, and metabolic studies assessing ionized calcium and serum glucose. Coagulation parameters are also closely assessed via activated partial thromboplastin time, prothrombin time, fibrinogen, and platelet count.

5. *Discuss the anesthetic technique of choice for OLT.*

No single anesthetic technique has been shown to be superior during anesthetic management of OLT. Patients undergoing OLT are considered at increased risk for aspiration of stomach contents because of the likelihood of abdominal distention or history of upper gastrointestinal

bleeding. General anesthesia is therefore induced via rapid-sequence technique with cricoid pressure. Premedication may be administered but may be curtailed in the presence of marked encephalopathy. Ketamine, propofol, and etomidate are all suitable hypnotic agents, but the requisite doses may be modified based on the patient's preexisting mental and hemodynamic status. Succinylcholine is used for rapid onset of neuromuscular blockade; however, rocuronium may also be used if no difficulty with intubation is anticipated. Maintenance of anesthesia is accomplished using inhalation agent and intravenous opioid by bolus administration or infusion. Patients with severe encephalopathy may have increased intracranial pressure requiring hyperventilation. The minimum alveolar concentration of volatile agent should also be reduced in these patients. The use of nitrous oxide is limited or avoided because of concerns pertaining to its capability to expand air bubbles that may reside in the nonperfused donor liver. Bowel distension is also a consideration with prolonged usage. Patients undergoing OLT typically remain intubated and mechanically ventilated in the intensive care unit postoperatively.

6. *Describe the three phases during OLT and the associated anesthetic management.*

Intraoperative anesthetic management is strongly influenced by the various hemodynamic manifestations presented during the three major phases of the procedure. During the preanhepatic (dissection) phase, a wide subcostal incision is used to provide optimal surgical exposure. Prior abdominal surgeries may have resulted in adhesion formation, thereby potentially increasing blood loss. The liver remains attached to the portal vein, inferior vena cava, biliary tract, and hepatic artery. During the anhepatic phase, the vena cava is clamped above and below the liver. The portal vein, common bile duct, and hepatic artery are also ligated. Total excision is then undertaken. Venovenous bypass is generally reserved for patients with pulmonary hypertension or significant cardiovascular disease. Removal of the liver may result in hypocalcemia because of loss of the liver's role in the metabolic removal of citrate from blood products that may have been administered. Citrate is a preservative used in banked blood that binds calcium, and the associated hypocalcemia that occurs may also result in cardiac depression. Ionized calcium levels should be regularly assessed and should guide exogenous replacement (200 to 500 mg). Loss of hepatic clearance of acid metabolites from the gastrointestinal tract results in progressive acidosis. Sodium bicarbonate is administered judiciously to prevent hypernatremia, hyperosmolality, and metabolic alkalosis. Should large amounts of sodium bicarbonate be needed, tromethamine should be considered as an alternative. Hyperglycemia may be encountered more commonly than hypoglycemia because of the increased glucose load presented from large amounts of transfused blood products. In general, dextrose-containing intravenous fluids are avoided. Air emboli may result from air entrapped in venous sinusoids and released when the donor liver is reperfused. The incidence of air embolism is reduced by infusing cold crystalloid solution through the venous structures as the graft is being anastomosed. After the portal and suprahepatic caval anastomoses but before infrahepatic caval anastomosis is completed, the liver is flushed by portal blood through the incomplete infrahepatic anastomosis.

Caval clamping is associated with profound hemodynamic changes, particularly decreased cardiac output and hypotension. Renal perfusion may be adversely affected as well. Increased venous back pressure may also increase bleeding and impair splanchnic perfusion. The technique of venovenous bypass consists of cannulation of the inferior vena cava and portal vein and an axillary vein with the intention of diverting blood away from the liver and delivering it directly to the heart. Venovenous bypass is used to minimize hypotension, maintain renal and splanchnic perfusion, and prevent gut edema and ischemia. Heparinization is not necessary because of circuit design technology. Venovenous bypass is associated with an element of risk, however. Venovenous bypass may lengthen operative time and subject the patient to increased risk of air embolic and thromboembolic events. Brachial plexus injury and hypothermia are also recognized side effects. Cannulation of the internal jugular vein rather than the axillary vein as a return circuit also has been used and has been shown to attenuate several side effects of venovenous bypass. Percutaneous methods for establishing venous bypass also have been described. Prophylactic measures for preservation of

renal perfusion include the use of mannitol and low-dose dopamine infusion (2 to 3 mcg/kg/min). Ultimately renal perfusion, as well as overall systemic organ perfusion, is best accomplished by optimizing cardiac output and systemic blood pressure. For this, any of several vasoactive and inotropic agents should be available and used as needed.

7. *Construct a plan to manage intraoperative electrolyte imbalances.*

Hypocalcemia and myocardial depression associated with removal of the liver are managed with periodic administration of calcium chloride, which is guided by assessment of serum ionized calcium concentration. Hyperkalemia may be a consequence of the progressive acidosis frequently encountered during the anhepatic stage. Symptomatic hyperkalemia may lead to cardiac dysrhythmias and refractory asystole. Treatment consists of the administration of calcium chloride, sodium bicarbonate, and glucose and insulin and the application of hyperventilation. Maintaining adequate diuresis throughout surgery is crucial to controlling hyperkalemia.

8. *Discuss the fluid of choice for perioperative fluid replacement.*

Fluid management presents a formidable perioperative challenge because of its unpredictability and variability. This is influenced in large part by the extent and magnitude of portal hypertension, the challenges in dissection, and the coagulation status. Ongoing goals include maintaining normovolemia, sustaining organ system perfusion, and optimizing oxygen-carrying capacity. Selection of crystalloid is based on these goals and preservation of electrolyte and acid–base balance. Lactated Ringer's solution may increase serum lactate levels and contribute to hyperkalemia. Normal saline may cause hyperchloremic metabolic acidosis. Isotonic solutions with greater compatibility to normal osmolality are therefore preferred. Rapid transfusion devices that allow the infusion of large volumes of warmed fluids and blood products should be used. Correction of acidosis may be accomplished by optimizing systematic perfusion, hyperventilation, and sodium bicarbonate. Excessive sodium bicarbonate may result in hyperosmolality, hypernatremia, central pontine myelinolysis, and metabolic acidosis. Before reperfusion of the grafted donor liver, correction of electrolyte and acid–base abnormalities should be undertaken. Central filling pressures should also be allowed to increase, and hyperventilation should be instituted. Preparation for rapid infusion of warmed blood products, as well as for administration of indicated inotropic and vasoactive agents, allows prompt retrieval of hemodynamic parameters secondary to reperfusion hypotension.

During the *postanhepatic* (revascularization–biliary reconstruction) phase, the venous anastomoses are completed and circulation to the new liver is accomplished via the anastomosed hepatic artery. A Roux-en-Y choledochojejunostomy connects the bile duct to the recipient gastrointestinal tract. The reperfusion phenomenon can result in acidosis, hypotension, and electrolyte abnormalities, particularly hyperkalemia.

9. *Discuss the management of electrocardiographic aberrations during liver transplantation.*

Electrocardiographic aberrations may occur and most typically manifest as bradycardia. Management is largely supportive and consists of volume restoration by colloid or crystalloid (as directed by laboratory findings, central filling pressures, and urinary output), calcium chloride, and sodium bicarbonate. Inotropic and vasoactive support may be indicated. To optimize the activity of these agents, acidosis must be corrected. Postperfusion coagulopathy is commonly encountered after reperfusion. This may be attributable to the release of sequestered heparin in the donor liver or to activity of an endogenous heparinoid.

10. *Describe the laboratory technique that is utilized to monitor intraoperative fibrinolysis.*

Hyperfibrinolysis is frequently encountered subsequent to increased release of tissue plasminogen activator inhibitor during the anhepatic phase. The use of thromboelastography (TEG) allows for accurate detection of fibrinolysis and abnormalities in platelet activity and is valuable, in addition to laboratory findings, in directing blood and blood-component resuscitation. Platelets and FFP should be available. Cryoprecipitate may also be used for restoration of an adequate fibrinogen level in the presence of fibrinolysis. Desmopressin (DDAVP) may be administered to help improve platelet function. Overtransfusion with blood components and crystalloid should be avoided to prevent pulmonary edema, decreased oxygenation, peripheral edema, and prolonged intubation and ventilation and their attendant risks.

Postoperative Period

11. *Identify postoperative complications that are associated with OLT.*

Postoperative complications may include:
- Persistent hemorrhage
- Fluid volume overload
- Metabolic and electrolyte abnormalities (hyperglycemia, hyperkalemia, metabolic alkalosis)
- Infection
- Neurologic (encephalopathy, seizures, cyclosporine neurotoxicity, cerebrovascular hemorrhage)

12. *Discuss the surgical complications that require surgical reintervention.*

Surgical complications that may require surgical reintervention include anastomotic leak or stricture of the biliary reconstruction or dehiscence or thrombosis of the hepatic or portal vessels. Prophylactic antibacterial and antifungal agents are administered in addition to the immunosuppressive agents. The incidence of infection is high. The locus of infection may be an intraabdominal source, an indwelling catheter, the surgical wound, the urinary tract, or an intrapulmonary source. Numerous infective entities may be causative. Commonly encountered are fungi, gram-negative bacteria, viruses, and parasites. Postoperative hepatitis may be caused by herpes virus, Epstein–Barr virus, cytomegalovirus, adenovirus, or hepatitis B or C virus. Reactivation of a preexisting viral infection is also a causative possibility. Potential organ rejection is closely monitored and differentially determined by live biopsy. The most common period in which rejection occurs is during weeks 1 to 6 after transplantation. Laboratory findings usually reflect a prodromal period before this occurs.

13. *Discuss the anesthetic considerations for patients undergoing retransplantation.*

Considerations for patients with hepatic failure apply to patients who undergo retransplantation. These patients are immunosuppressed and sensitized to antibodies, which makes blood type and cross-matching more complex. A variable degree of renal insufficiency and hypertension secondary to cyclosporine toxicity may also be present. Patients on immunomodulatory steroids who undergo retransplantation are considered steroid dependent and require steroid supplementation before surgery. Strict aseptic technique is mandatory for all patients who are immunocompromised.

Living donor hepatic transplantation is currently being undertaken in select centers and accounts for approximately 10% of all hepatic transplants. This modality has been made possible through research and experience-based advances in surgical, medical, and perianesthetic techniques and strategies. In living donor hepatic transplantation, the recipient typically receives the healthy right hepatic lobe from the donor. Besides the advantage of a closer graft match and decreased waiting time between donor and recipient, intraoperative ischemic time of the liver graft is significantly minimized. Recipient and donor hepatectomy are performed nearly simultaneously to reduce the time from donation to transplant. Anesthetic concerns for the donor will focus on perioperative management for hepatectomy while attempting to minimize the degree of potentially complicating comorbidities. Posttransplant regeneration of liver tissue within the donor is noted to occur within a year. Return of hepatic function to preoperative levels correlates with the amount of donor liver mass resected. The relative risk for complications in the donor is consistent with the degree of resection (right lobe donor, 32%; left lateral segment, 9%; left lateral lobe, 7.5%). Biliary complications (stricture and leakage), infection, and blood-product transfusion factors are major postoperative donor complications. Reoperation for complications (4.5%) may be necessary.

In cadaveric liver transplantation, the time from retrieval to transplantation is limited to less than 6 hours, even under the most rigorous cooling and preservative protocols. Anesthetic considerations for the recipient of a cadaveric graft are consistent with those of the patient with end-stage liver disease.

Review Questions

1. Which class of medications is instrumental for survival of patients undergoing OLT?
   a. Antibiotics
   b. Narcotics
   c. Immunosuppressants
   d. Beta-adrenergic antagonists
2. Which disease process causes cirrhosis of the liver due to the infiltration of fat?
   a. Hepatitis
   b. Alcohol
   c. Diabetes
   d. Nonalcoholic steatohepatitis (NASH)
3. Which electrolyte imbalance is caused by progressive acidosis resulting from cirrhosis?
   a. Hyperkalemia
   b. Hypercalcemia
   c. Hyponatremia
   d. Hypoglycemia
4. Administration of which of the following substances improves platelet function?
   a. Packed red blood cells (PRBC)
   b. Desmopressin (DDAVP)
   c. Fresh frozen plasma (FFP)
   d. Cryoprecipitate
5. The most common period for rejection of the liver is within:
   a. The first 72 hours.
   b. The first week.
   c. 1 to 6 weeks after the transplant.
   d. 6 months after the transplant.

Suggested Readings

Brentjens T, Weyker PD. Diseases of the liver and biliary tract. In: Hines RL, Marschall KE, eds. *Stoelting's Anesthesia and Co-Existing Disease,* 7th ed. St. Louis, MO: Elsevier, 2018:345-358.

Collins SB, Johnson CA. Hepatobiliary and gastrointestinal disorders and anesthesia. In: Nagelhout JJ, Elisha S, eds. *Nurse Anesthesia,* 6th ed. St. Louis, MO: Elsevier, 2018:709–742.

Hawkins RB, Raymond SL, Hartjes T, Efron PA, Larson SD, Andreoni KA, Thomas EM. Review: the perioperative use of thromboelastography for liver transplant patients. *Transplant Proc* 2018;50(10): 3552–3558.

Herbert MF, Wacher VJ, Roberts JP, et al. Pharmacokinetics of cyclosporine pre- and post-liver transplantation. *J Clin Pharmacol* 2003; 43:38–42.

Merritt WT. Living donor surgery: overview of surgical and anesthesia issues. *Anesthesiol Clin North Am* 2004;22(4):633–650.

Olivo R, Guarrera JV, Pyrsopoulos NT. Liver transplantation for acute liver failure. *Clin Liver Dis* 2018;22(2):409–417. doi: 10.1016/j.cld.2018.01.014.

Saner FH, Bezinover D. Assessment and management of coagulopathy in critically-ill patients with liver failure. *Curr Opin Crit Care* 2019;25(2):179–186.

Schmidt AE, Israel AK, Refaai MA. The utility of utility of thromboelastography to guide blood product transfusion. *Am J Clin Pathol* 2019;152(4):407–422.

Sonny A. Cardiovascular adverse events after liver transplantation: a long road ahead for improvement. *Eur Heart J Qual Care Clin Outcomes* 2020;6(4):227–228. pii: qcaa031. doi: 10.1093/ehjqcco/qcaa031.

Spring A, Saran JS, McCarthy S, McCluskey SA. Anesthesia for the patient with severe liver failure. *Anesthesiol Clin* 2020;38(1):35–50.

Webb K, Shephard L, Day E, et al. Transplantation for alcoholic liver disease: report of a consensus meeting. *Liv Transplant* 2006; 12(2):301–305.

Xu Q, Zhu M, Li Z, Zhu JK, Xiao F, Liu FY, Wang YD, Liu CZ. Enhanced recovery after surgery protocols in patients undergoing liver transplantation: a retrospective comparative cohort study. *Int J Surg* 2020;78:108–112. pii: S1743-9191(20)30306-X. doi: 10.1016/j.ijsu.2020.03.081.

11

Hepatic Resection

KEY POINTS

- A common cancer that occurs within the liver is due to hepatocellular carcinoma and metastasis from colorectal cancer.
- Most hepatic resections are performed for the removal of cancerous tissue.
- Bleeding and hemorrhage are major risks associated with hepatic resection.

- Advances in equipment and technology, perioperative management, and modern surgical techniques have decreased the morbidity and mortality associated with liver resections.
- Epidural analgesia can be used to attenuate the stress response and decrease postoperative pain.

Case Synopsis

A 65-year-old white man with liver cancer is scheduled for surgery. The planned procedure includes a right hepatic lobectomy for removal of hepatocellular carcinoma (HCC).

Preoperative Evaluation and Demographic Data

Past Medical/Surgical History

- Colon resection
- Laparoscopic cholecystectomy
- Hernia repair
- Hypertension
- Gastroesophageal reflux disease
- Colon cancer

List of Medications

- Metoprolol
- Lipitor
- Pepcid
- Aspirin

Diagnostic Data

- Hemoglobin, 13.3 g/dL; hematocrit, 39.7%
- Platelet count, 109,000 cells/mm^3
- Glucose, 100 mg/dL
- Electrolytes: sodium, 140 mEq/L; potassium, 3.8 mEq/L; chloride, 103 mEq/L; carbon dioxide, 27 mEq/L
- Prothrombin time (PT), 22.5 seconds; partial thromboplastin time, 40 seconds; international normalized ratio, 2.1

- Liver function: aspartate transaminase, 120 units/L; alanine transaminase, 205 units/L; albumin, 2.1 g/dL; bilirubin, 1.2 mg/dL
- Transthoracic echocardiography: ejection fraction of 50%; no evidence of wall motion abnormalities or hypertrophy
- Electrocardiogram: normal sinus rhythm, heart rate 78 beats per minute
- Lungs are clear to auscultation

Height/Weight/Vital Signs

- 175 cm, 84 kg; body mass index (BMI), 27.36
- Blood pressure, 155/89 mm Hg; heart rate, 90 beats per minute; respiratory rate, 14 breaths per minute; room air oxygen saturation, 99%; temperature, 37.1°C

Anatomy and Physiology

The liver is a versatile organ weighing about 1.5 kg and it is located in the right upper quadrant of the abdominal cavity. It extends from the fifth rib to the lower border of the thoracic cage. It is divided into four anatomic lobes and performs many functions that maintain homeostasis. The basic functional unit of the liver is the liver lobule, which is composed of hepatocytes, sinusoids, and Kupffer cells in a triangular arrangement around a central vein (Fig. 11.1). Liver lobules are connected via an intricate network of arteries, veins, and a unique drainage system. In the average adult, normal hepatic blood flow is estimated to be approximately 1500 mL/min or 25% to 30% of cardiac output.

The liver produces and excretes bile into the small intestine, where bile is used to emulsify fats. Bile is also stored in

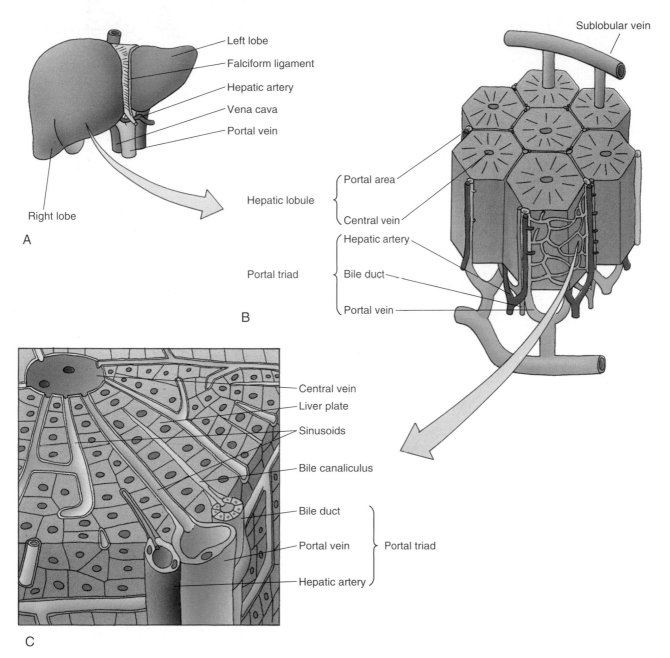

• **Fig. 11.1** Schematic diagram of the liver. (A) Gross anatomy of the liver. (B) Liver lobules displaying the portal areas and the central vein. (C) Portion of the liver lobule displaying the portal area, liver plates, sinusoids, and bile canaliculi. (From Gartner LP: *Textbook of histology*, ed 5, Philadelphia, 2021, Elsevier.)

the gallbladder and released as needed. Another function of the liver is the breakdown of carbohydrates, fats, and proteins. Metabolism of carbohydrates includes gluconeogenesis (synthesis of glucose from amino acids, lactate, and glycerol), glycogenesis (formation of glycogen from glucose), glycogenolysis (breakdown of glycogen to glucose), and breakdown of insulin and other hormones. Lipid metabolism includes cholesterol synthesis and lipogenesis or the production of triglycerides (fats). Other metabolic functions include drug metabolism via phase 1 (oxidation, reduction, and hydrolysis) and phase 2 (conjugation) reactions.

The liver synthesizes plasma proteins, such as albumin and alpha-1 antitrypsin, that help maintain plasma osmotic pressure. Other plasma proteins that are created in the liver include clotting factors I (fibrinogen), II (prothrombin), V, VII, IX, and XI; proteins C and S; and antithrombin. The liver functions as a storage site for folate, glycogen, fat-soluble vitamins (B$_{12}$, A, D, E, and K), and minerals such as iron and copper. Hemoglobin from the red blood cells is broken down to bilirubin and is converted to biliverdin by the liver to facilitate excretion. Blood is also filtered for ammonia, and the ammonia is subsequently converted to urea. A list of

• BOX 11.1 **Physiologic Functions Performed by the Liver**

- Carbohydrate metabolism
- Protein metabolism
- Lipid metabolism
- Drug metabolism
- Breaks down hemoglobin
- Produces and excretes bile
- Converts ammonia to urea
- Produces plasma proteins
- Produces factors for coagulation

TABLE 11.1	Lobes in Relation to the Segments of the Liver	
Lobe	**Segment**
Caudate	1
Lateral	2, 3
Medial	4a, 4b
Right	5, 6, 7, 8

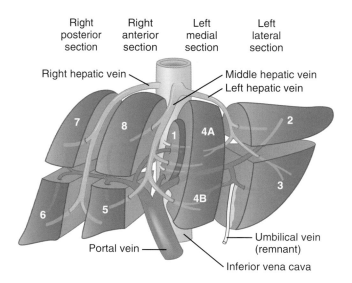

• **Fig. 11.2** Anatomy of the liver and associated vasculature. (From Hertzberg BS, Middleton WD: *Ultrasound: The requisites*, ed 3, Philadelphia, 2016, Elsevier.)

the physiologic functions associated with the liver is included in Box 11.1.

The classic description of the liver is based on the external appearance of four anatomic lobes or segments: right, left, caudate, and quadrate. The right and left lobes are separated by the falciform ligament, which is positioned anteriorly. The ligamentum venosum and ligamentum teres divide right and left lobes on the posterior aspect of the liver. The transverse fissure divides the caudate and quadrate lobes, as well as internal features such as vessels and biliary duct branching that are vital for hepatic surgery. Therefore the more common functional anatomic model, the Couinaud classification, is used for anatomic liver resections.

The Couinaud classification used during liver resection divides the liver into eight functionally independent segments, with each segment having an independent vascular system, as illustrated in Fig. 11.2. The middle hepatic vein divides the liver into the right and left lobes, or hemiliver. The left hepatic vein divides the left hemiliver into a lateral part (corresponding to segments 2 and 3) and a median part (corresponding to segment 4 that can be further divided into 4a, superior, and 4b, inferior). The right hepatic vein

divides the right hemiliver into an anterior section (corresponding to segments 5 and 8) and a posterior section (corresponding to segments 6 and 7). Table 11.1 describes the lobes in relation to the segments of the liver.

Pathophysiology

HCC is the most common primary malignancy affecting the liver. It is also known as *primary liver cancer* or *hepatoma*, which is primarily caused by chronic hepatitis B or C and cirrhosis due to chronic alcohol abuse. The initial symptoms of HCC are variable, with abdominal pain being the most common symptom accompanied by unexplained weight loss. In addition, patients with cirrhosis may develop jaundice, ascites, esophageal varices, or portal hypertension.

In those patients who have HCC without evidence of cirrhosis, liver resection is the treatment of choice. However, when cirrhosis is the cause of HCC, liver resectability is limited and may be unsuitable in those patients exhibiting a low platelet count ($<80,000$ cells/mm^3), a decreased albumin (<3.5 g/dL), ascites, portal hypertension with esophageal varices, and a prolonged PT due to a high risk for postoperative liver failure. Therefore nonsurgical therapies such as percutaneous ethanol injection and radiofrequency ablation may be an option for treatment. Ultimately, liver resectability is judged by liver function, stage of liver cancer, and overall condition of the patient.

Surgical Procedure

Hepatic resection can be performed traditionally via laparotomy or laparoscopically in which one or more complete anatomic segments are removed or a specific nonanatomic division of the liver is resected (wedge resection). The type of resection performed depends on the size, site, and number of tumors and their relation to vascular and biliary structures.

Segmental anatomic surgery involves dissecting the porta hepatis or transverse fissure with mobilization and ligation of the extrahepatic branches of the hepatic artery, portal vein, bile duct, and hepatic vein before resecting the liver parenchyma. Nonanatomic division of the liver, or wedge resection, involves ligating and resecting branches of the vessels and hepatic ducts as they are encountered during the resection of the liver parenchyma; only the tumor with a margin of 1 to 2 cm is removed.

Anesthetic Management Considerations

Preoperative Period

1. List the components of a thorough preanesthetic evaluation.

- A comprehensive preanesthetic assessment and interview
- Review of pertinent laboratory data: electrolytes, glucose, liver function tests (LFTs), PT/partial thromboplastin time/international normalized ratio, hemoglobin/hematocrit, and type and cross
- Review chest X-ray, computed tomography (CT) scan, echocardiogram, and results of an abdominal ultrasound.
- Obtain consent for general anesthesia, central line, and arterial line placement
- Obtain intravenous (IV) access, and placement of an arterial line and a central line
- Attempt to treat/optimize the status of those patients who are coagulopathic by administering blood products/antifibrinolytic medication
- Prepare to administer packed red blood cells and albumin
- A rapid fluid-infusing device should be immediately available in the room
- Consider placement of an epidural catheter for intraoperative and postoperative management unless a coagulopathy is present

2. Explain the surgical interventions used during hepatic resection.

Three-dimensional (3D) imaging in the surgical planning for hepatic resection is gaining popularity. A 3D visualization of the tumor is possible. A major advantage of 3D mapping is that it can help determine whether a resection is feasible without invasive exploration. Another practice that provides visualization is the intraoperative ultrasound (IOUS), which allows the surgeon to determine the relationship of the tumor and major intrahepatic vessels. Surgeons may use dye injection to stain the segment of choice into the segmental portal vein to aid in the transection of the parenchyma.

Intraoperative blood loss is the most important determinant of survival in the first few days postoperatively. The typical range of blood loss is between 250 mL and 2000 mL. Blood loss can be significant during liver resection, and most technologies are focused on reducing blood loss. The introduction of hemostatic stapling has revolutionized hepatic surgery, as well as thoracic and gastrointestinal surgery. During a liver resection, staplers can be used to gain vascular control or to transect parenchyma. Another transection method, ultrasonic dissection using the Cavitron Ultrasonic Surgical Aspirator (CUSA), has become popular.

3. Describe the use of the Pringle maneuver during liver resection.

The Pringle maneuver is a commonly used technique to prevent intraoperative blood loss that involves occlusion of the main blood vessels that enter the liver. Prolonged application of this procedure can cause significant ischemia and have a detrimental effect on liver function. Most patients can tolerate a repeated 15- to 20-minute clamp time followed by a 5-minute period of reperfusion. Total vascular occlusion is another technique that can be used, which involves occlusion of arterial blood flow into the liver and the venous blood flow out of the liver.

4. Identify anesthetic interventions used to treat low central venous pressure (CVP).

Managing CVP appropriately to reduce blood loss is a major goal in the anesthetic management for liver resection. This is typically achieved by fluid restriction, postural changes, vasodilators, and/or diuresis. Maintaining CVP at <5 mm Hg generally facilitates the goal of achieving a lower blood loss, but can predispose to acute renal failure. Higher CVP measurements result in greater bleeding and increased incidence of blood transfusion. Intravenous nitroglycerine and furosemide are used to pharmacologically manage CVP, although other vasodilators and diuretics may be employed. Reverse Trendelenburg can also help in decreasing CVP. Oliguria may occur, but the rate of postoperative renal failure does not increase when systolic blood pressure is maintained above 90 mm Hg. At the completion of the liver resection, volume resuscitation is initiated with crystalloid and albumin to normalize the hemodynamic profile and to help the surgeon discover unrecognized areas of bleeding.

Maintaining a low CVP during anesthesia is vital during liver resection. However, by decreasing venous pressure, this intervention increases the risk for developing a venous air embolism. Venous air embolism is a common occurrence during liver resection, although it usually does not result in physiologic compromise. If the patient exhibits signs of a venous air embolism, immediate interventions include:

- Flooding the surgical field with normal saline
- Ventilation with 100% oxygen
- Attempt to aspirate the air from the right atrium via the central line
- Trendelenburg and left lateral decubitus position
- Administer intravenous fluids
- Administer vasopressors to help increase the blood pressure

These measures should be utilized in conjunction with advanced cardiac life support (ACLS) resuscitation as appropriate.

5. List the advantages associated with laparoscopic liver resection.

Liver surgeries are commonly performed via an open incision, but in selected circumstances a laparoscopic approach can be utilized. Laparoscopic liver resections are performed for cancers that are present on the surface of the liver where the larger blood vessels are not affected. The advantages of laparoscopic surgeries include absence of a large abdominal incision, decreased postoperative pain, decreased length of stay, and decreased recovery time.

Intraoperative Period

6. Discuss the considerations for anesthetic induction and maintenance for patients having a liver resection.

Considerations for Induction

- Routine monitors: electrocardiogram, arterial line and cuff blood pressure monitoring, CVP, temperature, FiO_2, $ETCO_2$, and pulse oximeter
- Consider pharmacologic interventions to reduce gastric volume and increase pH
- Consider performing a rapid sequence induction (RSI) with cricoid pressure
- Consider the patient's individual hemodynamic status before choosing an induction agent

Considerations for Maintenance

Although all muscle relaxants have been used, the most acceptable would be those that do not undergo hepatic or renal metabolism. For example, cisatracurium is degraded by Hoffmann elimination and plasma hydrolysis by nonspecific red blood cell esterases, and its pharmacokinetic profile is unchanged in patients with hepatic dysfunction. The anesthetist may choose to avoid using nitrous oxide due to the risk of a venous air embolism. Administration of a narcotic, dexmedetomidine, and ketamine are acceptable choices for liver resection, and these medications will attenuate intraoperative sympathetic nervous system responsiveness as well as provide for postoperative analgesia.

Glucose levels should be controlled to avoid hypoglycemia and hyperglycemia. Hypothermia inhibits the coagulation cascade and contributes to intraoperative blood loss. The patient's temperature should be maintained within normal limits via a forced-air warming blanket and

---

> **• BOX 11.2 Postoperative Complications Associated With Liver Resection**
>
> - Hemorrhage
> - Respiratory complications (atelectasis, effusion, and pneumonia)
> - Electrolyte abnormalities
> - Hypothermia
> - Hypoglycemia
> - Disseminated intravascular coagulation

fluid warmer. Coagulation factors should be monitored, and platelets, fresh frozen plasma, and cryoprecipitate should be administered as needed. Antifibrinolytics such as aminocaproic acid and tranexamic acid should also be considered.

Postoperative Period

7. Discuss the postoperative anesthetic management after liver resection.

The postoperative complications associated with liver resection are included in Box 11.2. Postoperative pain control for the patient who has undergone hepatic resection is challenging. Providing epidural analgesia remains controversial with liver resection, mainly due to the associated coagulopathy and epidural hematoma formation. Patient-controlled analgesia (PCA) is also an option to treat postoperative pain. Injection of liposomal bupivacaine into the abdominal wall or transversus abdominis plane blocks help decrease postoperative opioid usage, and both have been shown to be effective methods to decrease postoperative pain.

Review Questions

1. Which intervention can be used to inhibit bleeding caused by decreased coagulation factors?
   a. Administering packed red blood cells
   b. Administering dexamethasone
   c. Administering aminocaproic acid
   d. Administering vitamin K
2. Which is not a physiologic function associated with the liver?
   a. Glycogenesis
   b. Storage of iron and copper
   c. Synthesis of alpha-1 antitrypsin
   d. Corticosteroidogenesis
3. Segments 2, 3, 4a, and 4b constitute the _____ lobe of the liver.
   a. Caudate
   b. Quadrate
   c. Right
   d. Left
4. Which intraoperative factor is associated with increased early postoperative mortality after liver resection?
   a. Severe blood loss
   b. Mean arterial pressure >90 mm Hg
   c. Urine output less than 1 mL/kg/hr
   d. Presence of metastatic cancer
5. Which is not a postoperative event associated with hepatic resection?
   a. Pneumonia
   b. Hemorrhage
   c. Electrolyte imbalance
   d. Hyperglycemia

Suggested Readings

Amundson AW, Olsen DA, Smith HM, et al. Acute benefits after liposomal bupivacaine abdominal wall blockade for living liver donation: a retrospective review. *J Gastrointest Surg* 2018;22(6): 981–988.

Bennett S, Ayoub A, Tran A, English S, Tinmouth A. Current practices in perioperative blood management for patients undergoing liver resection: a survey of surgeons and anesthesiologists. *Transfusion* 2018;58(3):781–787.

Collins SB, Johnson CA. Hepatobiliary and gastrointestinal disorders and anesthesia. In: Nagelhout JJ, Elisha S, eds. *Nurse Anesthesia*, 6th ed. St. Louis, MO: Elsevier, 2018:709–742.

Egger ME, Gottumukkala V, Wilks JA, Soliz J, et al. Anesthetic and operative considerations for laparoscopic liver resection. *Surgery* 2017;161(5):1191–1202.

Katz SC, Shia J, Liau KH, et al. Operative blood loss independently predicts recurrence and survival after resection of hepatocellular carcinoma. *Ann Surg* 2009;249(4):617–623.

Kıtlık A, Erdogan MA, Ozgul U, Aydogan MS, Ucar M, Toprak HI, Colak C, Durmus M. Ultrasound-guided transversus abdominis plane block for postoperative analgesia in living liver donors: a prospective, randomized, double-blinded clinical trial. *J Clin Anesth* 2017;37:103–107.

Lillemoe HA, Marcus RK, Day RW, Kim BJ, Narula N, Davis CH, Gottumukkala V, Aloia TA. Enhanced recovery in liver surgery decreases postoperative outpatient use of opioids. *Surgery* 2019 Jul;166(1):22–27.

Redai I, Emond J, Berntjens T. Anesthetic considerations during liver surgery. *Surg Clin N Am* 2004;84:401–411.

Saint-Marc O, Cogliandolo A, Piquard A, et al. Early experience with laparoscopic major liver resections: a case comparison study. *Surg Laparosc Endosc Percutan Tech* 2008;18(6):551–555.

So SK, Oberheleman HA, Lemmens HJ. Hepatic surgery. In: Jaffe RA, Schmiesing CA, Golianu B. *Anesthesiologist's Manual of Surgical Procedures*, 5th ed. Philadelphia: Lippincott Williams & Wilkins, 2014:564–570.

Thornblade LW, Seo YD, Kwan T, Cardoso JH, Pan E, Dembo G, Yeung RSW, Park JO. Enhanced recovery via peripheral nerve block for open hepatectomy. *J Gastrointest Surg* 2018;22(6): 981–988.

Wang W, Liang L, Haung X, Yin X. Low central venous pressure reduces blood loss in hepatectomy. *World J Gastroenterol* 2006; 12:935–939.

Yu L, Sun H, Jin H, Tan H. The effect of low central venous pressure on hepatic surgical field bleeding and serum lactate in patients undergoing partial hepatectomy: a prospective randomized controlled trial. *BMC Surg* 2020;20(1):25.

12

Anesthesia Case Management for Excision of a Pheochromocytoma

KEY POINTS

- The meaning of pheochromocytoma is dusky-colored tumor (*phios* means dusky, *chroma* means color, and *cytoma* means tumor), and the neoplasm is derived from chromaffin cells.
- A pheochromocytoma is most commonly located within the adrenal medulla but can also be localized within extraadrenal sites.
- Approximately 90% of pheochromocytomas cause a massive amount of norepinephrine to be produced and released into systemic circulation. Epinephrine can also be the predominant catecholamine that is produced.
- The most common triad of symptoms include headache, diaphoresis, and tachycardia.
- Excessive and prolonged alpha-1 receptor stimulation can result in intravascular volume depletion, renal insufficiency, hemorrhagic cerebral infarct, myocardial irritability,

ischemia, and infarction. Congestive heart failure and cardiomyopathy can occur if hypertension remains untreated.
- Preoperative management includes adrenergic receptor blockade (alpha-receptor blockade followed by beta-receptor blockade), intravascular volume replacement, and assessment of end-organ damage.
- Intraoperative surges in catecholamine release can occur at the time of laryngoscopy, intubation, and manipulation of the tumor and during ligation of the adrenal vein.
- Postoperative anesthetic concerns include treating pain and stabilizing blood pressure. Prompt diagnosis and treatment of a pneumothorax, hypoglycemia, and hypoadrenocorticism should also be considered.

Case Synopsis

A 38-year-old woman presents to the emergency room complaining of severe headaches and palpitations several times a day. She has become increasingly anxious and diaphoretic. Her blood pressure, heart rate, and respiratory rate are elevated. Plasma tests reveal elevated plasma metanephrine levels. An endocrinologist reviews her case and orders further diagnostic testing that includes a computed tomography (CT) scan and a 24-hour urine sample to assess for metanephrines and normetanephrines. The CT scan reveals a right adrenal mass. An iodine-123 meta-iodobenzylguanidine (MIBG) scan, which is specific for endocrine tumors such as pheochromocytoma, is positive. Medical management of a pheochromocytoma is initiated, and she is scheduled for a right-sided adrenalectomy in 2 weeks.

Preoperative Evaluation and Demographic Data

Past Medical/Surgical History

- Depression
- Cesarean section; no anesthetic complications

List of Medications

- Phenelzine sulfate (Nardil) 15 mg TID (monoamine oxidase [MAO] inhibitor)

Diagnostic Data

- Hemoglobin, 16.5 g/dL; hematocrit, 49.5%
- Glucose, 170 mg/dL
- Blood urea nitrogen, 33 mg/dL; creatinine, 1.5 mg/dL
- Electrolytes: sodium, 147 mEq/L; potassium, 3.4 mEq/L; chloride, 95 mEq/L; carbon dioxide 24 mEq/L
- Electrocardiogram (ECG): sinus tachycardia, nonspecific T-wave changes, occasional premature ventricular contraction (PVC)
- Echocardiogram (ECHO): mild left ventricular hypertrophy, ejection fraction 55%

Catecholamines and Metabolites

- Urinary vanillylmandelic acid (VMA), 32 mg/24 h (normal value 2 to 7 mg/24 h)
- Urinary metanephrine, 6.8 mg/24 h (normal value <1.3 mg/24 h)
- Urinary norepinephrine, 458 mcg/24 h (normal value <100 mcg/24 h)

- Plasma norepinephrine, 1109 pg/mL (normal value 150 to 450 pg/mL)
- Plasma epinephrine, 37 pg/mL (normal value <35 pg/mL)

Height/Weight/Vital Signs

- 165 cm, 68 kg
- Blood pressure, 146/80; heart rate, 92 beats per minute; respiratory rate, 24 breaths per minute; room air oxygen saturation, 98%; temperature, 37.3°C

Pathophysiology

A pheochromocytoma is a catecholamine-secreting tumor that originates within the adrenal gland in approximately 90% of cases. These unique tumors can also arise anywhere along the paravertebral sympathetic chain and are known as *extraadrenal pheochromocytomas*. The tumors are composed of chromaffin cells that can produce, store, and secrete catecholamines. The majority of extraadrenal pheochromocytomas exist within the abdominal cavity. These tumors most frequently affect a unilateral adrenal gland, and most are benign. Familial pheochromocytomas occur in bilateral adrenal glands in 50% of cases and are frequently benign. Pheochromocytomas are associated with only 0.2% of all patients who have hypertension. This disease affects males and females equally and most frequently manifests between 30 and 50 years of age. There is an association between pheochromocytoma and multiple endocrine neoplasia type II A and B, neurofibromatosis, tuberous sclerosis, Sturge–Weber syndrome, and von Hippel–Lindau disease.

Sympathetic nervous system (SNS) stimulation in patients with pheochromocytoma causes a massive release of catecholamines, predominantly norepinephrine, which stimulates alpha-adrenergic receptors. Subsequently, common clinical manifestations associated with a pheochromocytoma include headache, diaphoresis, tachycardia, arrythmias with palpitations, anxiety, pallor, hypertension, hyperglycemia, and paresthesias to the extremities. Orthostatic hypotension and polycythemia occur due to intravascular volume depletion resulting from extreme peripheral vasoconstriction. Cerebral hemorrhage, myocardial infarction, cardiomyopathy, congestive heart failure, and renal insufficiency can occur.

A pheochromocytoma is not directly innervated by the autonomic nervous system, and therefore is not controlled by neural stimulation. Consequently, stimulation of the tumor resulting in catecholamine release is not completely understood, and the precipitating factors are not clearly defined and vary per individual. However, events that are associated with causing tumor activation include hypotension, hypothermia, defecation, physiologic stress, medication, intubation, and surgery.

Surgical Procedure

Adrenalectomy for removal of pheochromocytoma is traditionally accomplished by performing an open transperitoneal approach. The patient is placed in the supine position and the incision is made in the subcostal or midline regions. The adrenal vein is located and ligated. The adrenal gland is then excised and removed.

Laparoscopic adrenalectomy has become the most common surgical technique for removal of a pheochromocytoma. The patient is placed in the lateral decubitus position for maximal exposure to the surgical site. The close proximity of the inferior vena cava to the adrenal veins increases the potential for rapid and uncontrolled hemorrhage. Because the patient's cardiovascular system may be compromised due to long-standing untreated hypertension, the potential for cardiovascular compromise caused by prolonged insufflation should be considered. The adrenal glands are anatomically located on the superior aspect of each kidney, and there is a potential for developing a pneumothorax during the surgical dissection. The advantage of a laparoscopic approach compared with a traditional open technique is the small incision that results in decreased postoperative pain. The adrenal glands are surrounded by a layer of fat and a thin fibrous capsule, which make the resection complicated and tedious.

Anesthetic Management and Considerations

Preoperative Period

1. *Describe the signs and symptoms associated with a pheochromocytoma.*

    A triad of signs and symptoms that is most commonly associated with a pheochromocytoma include headache, diaphoresis, and tachycardia. A list of physiologic signs and symptoms is included in Box 12.1. Hypertension associated with tachycardia is most common; however, the physiologic response is directly proportional to the concentration of catecholamines that are released. It is possible that the patient can develop bradycardia caused by the baroreceptor activation in response to extreme hypertension. Arrythmias, ST-segment changes, nervousness, and anxiety may also be observed.

2. *Identify various methods that can be used to diagnose pheochromocytoma.*

    The initial diagnosis of pheochromocytoma is difficult to make because the symptoms are nonspecific, can occur in a

> **• BOX 12.1 Signs and Symptoms Associated With Pheochromocytoma**
>
> - Headache
> - Diaphoresis
> - Tachycardia
> - Chest pain
> - Bradycardia
> - Anxiety
> - Blurred vision
> - Seizures

variety of disease states and vary among individuals, and because pheochromocytoma is a rare disease. A thorough history and physical is essential and vital in order to correctly diagnose a pheochromocytoma. Further diagnostic tests include plasma free metanephrines, urine catecholamine and metanephrine levels, and a clonidine suppression test.

- **24-hour urine test:** Three urine samples are collected within a 24-hour period, and the concentration of metanephrines is analyzed. It is estimated that 95% of patients with pheochromocytomas have increased levels of urinary metanephrines. If urine metanephrine levels are elevated, then three 24-hour urine samples are tested for free catecholamines. If all three samples are within normal limits, the patient is not considered to have a pheochromocytoma.
- **Plasma test:** Elevations in the concentration of norepinephrine in plasma may be indicative of a pheochromocytoma. The plasma test is extremely sensitive to factors such as exercise, stress, and medications—all of which may increase catecholamines within the blood.
- **Clonidine suppression test:** Clonidine 0.2 mg is administered by mouth, and within 3 hours, the patient's blood pressure should decrease. Clonidine causes centrally mediated alpha-2 agonism, which decreases catecholamine output from the brain. A patient with a pheochromocytoma will remain hypertensive despite the actions of clonidine because the catecholamine release from the tumor is not centrally controlled.
- **Imaging studies:** A CT scan, positron emission tomography (PET) scan, or magnetic resonance imaging (MRI) is obtained to identify the presence of a tumor and the tumor's size and location.
- **MIBG scintigraphy:** This chemical possesses a high affinity for secretory granules present in chromaffin cells. The chemical structure of MIBG is similar to norepinephrine, and when injected, it concentrates within these granules as a result of reuptake. The sensitivity and specificity of this test for confirming the presence of a pheochromocytoma are 85% and 97%, respectively.

3. *Discuss the preoperative pharmacologic preparation for a patient with a pheochromocytoma.*

Preoperative pharmacologic management of these patients includes alpha-receptor blockade, beta-receptor blockade, and volume expansion. Alpha-receptor blockade is always instituted before beta-receptor blockade and is usually accomplished by the administration of phenoxybenzamine, a noncompetitive alpha-1 receptor and alpha-2 receptor antagonist. The patient will take phenoxybenzamine 10 to 100 mg orally mg/day for 10 to 14 days preoperatively. Once adequate alpha-receptor blockade is established, beta-receptor blockade can begin. Initiation of beta-receptor blockade before alpha-receptor blockade can cause a hypertensive crisis and can lead to the development of congestive heart failure. The tachycardia that is either caused by excessive beta-receptor activity or vasodilation caused by phenoxybenzamine is managed with beta-receptor blockade, most often

propranolol. In order to judge the adequacy of volume resuscitation, a decrease of 5% from the baseline hematocrit level is indicative of adequate hydration. Note that this patient is polycythemic before adrenergic receptor blockade and fluid resuscitation. Another method that can be used to assess the adequacy of fluid management is to determine if the patient develops orthostatic hypotension associated with a decline in the systolic blood pressure greater than or equal to 15%, while maintaining a systolic pressure of at least 80 mm Hg.

Another medication that can be administered preoperatively is metyrosine. This medication has an inhibitory effect on the creation of catecholamines, which occurs in adrenergic nerves. This drug decreases the concentration of tyrosine hydroxylase, an enzyme that is necessary during the biosynthesis of catecholamines, and this process is shown in Fig. 12.1.

This patient has been taking phenelzine sulfate, a nonspecific MAO inhibitor. MAO is present within the synaptic cleft of adrenergic nerves, and its function is to enzymatically degrade catecholamines. As a result, inhibition of MAO increases the concentration of catecholamines within the synaptic junction in adrenergic nerves. Phenelzine sulfate administration in a patient with a pheochromocytoma can result in an uncontrolled hypertensive response. She will have to discontinue taking this medicine 1 to 2 weeks before surgery.

4. *Explain the optimal preoperative cardiovascular criteria that should be achieved before surgery.*

The goal of preoperative therapy for a patient with a pheochromocytoma includes control of excessive catecholamine release that causes extreme physiologic aberrations. The following criteria must be met before surgical intervention and anesthesia administration:

- Blood pressure must remain less than 160/90 mm Hg within 48 hours before surgery.
- Orthostatic hypotension must occur; however, the blood pressure must be greater than 80/45 mm Hg.
- The ECG must not have ST/T-wave abnormalities for at least 1 week and have no more than one PVC within 5 minutes.
- Adequate hydration is achieved by a decrease in the hematocrit by approximately 5% from the baseline value.

5. *Identify the factors that increase the morbidity and mortality associated with removal of a pheochromocytoma.*

Factors that increase the potential for morbidity and mortality include:

- The activity of the pheochromocytoma. A highly active tumor is associated with increased concentrations of catecholamines and a more dramatic physiologic response.
- Inadequate preoperative alpha-receptor and then beta-receptor blockade.
- Advanced end-organ damage (cardiovascular, renal failure).
- Whether the pheochromocytoma is malignant or benign. The 5-year survival rate for a patient with a benign tumor is approximately 90%. However, if the pheochromocytoma is malignant, the survival rate

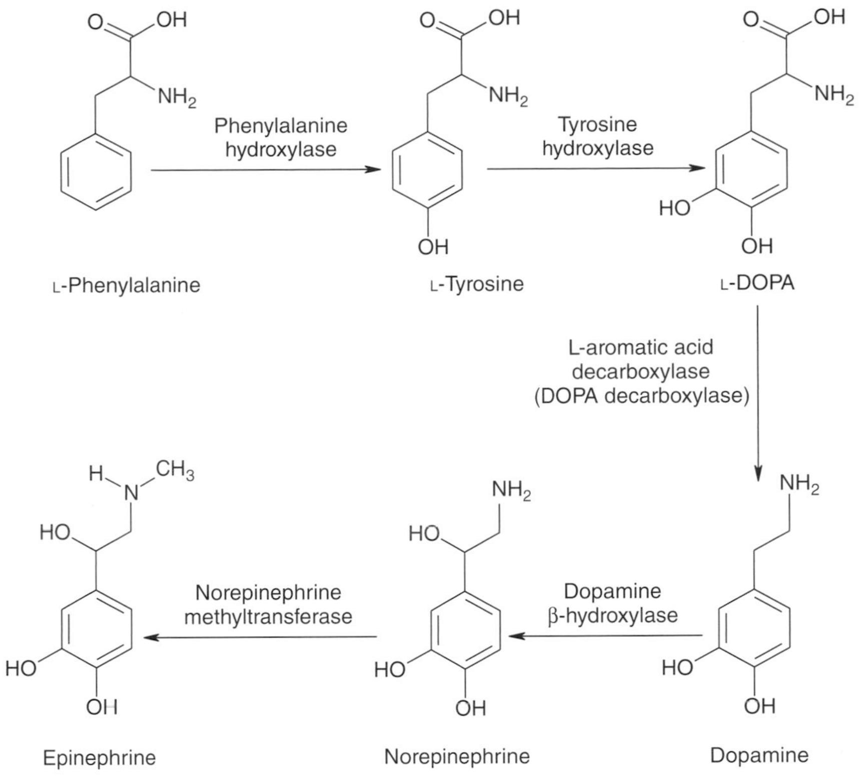

• **Fig. 12.1** Biosynthesis of catecholamines.

dramatically decreases to 10% due to metastasis resulting from the high amount of blood flow that courses through the adrenal glands.
• Prolonged surgical duration

Intraoperative Period

6. *List the medications that should be avoided during intraoperative management.*

Administration of any medications that can cause an increase in blood pressure or heart rate or cause the release of histamine should be avoided. Alternative drugs that stimulate the release or inhibit the breakdown of catecholamines should be used. A complete list of anesthetic medications that should be avoided for these patients is included in Box 12.2.

7. *Discuss the anesthetic considerations for a patient with a pheochromocytoma.*

General anesthesia and endotracheal intubation are necessary, and an epidural placed preoperatively can be used to provide anesthesia during the surgery and analgesia during the postoperative period. The concern when dosing an epidural catheter with local anesthetic medications during the intraoperative period is that after the pheochromocytoma is isolated, the concentration of catecholamines dramatically decreases and hypotension commonly occurs. This fact, along with adrenergic receptor downregulation and alpha-receptor blockade,

---

• **BOX 12.2** **Anesthetic Medications that Should Be Avoided in Patients With a Pheochromocytoma**

• Desflurane: Sympathomimetic effects
• Pancuronium: Sympathomimetic effects
• Atracurium: Histamine release
• Succinylcholine: Fasciculation causing catecholamine release
• Morphine: Histamine release
• Droperidol: Antidopaminergic effects – neuroleptic malignant syndrome
• Metoclopramide: Antidopaminergic effects – neuroleptic malignant syndrome
• Phenothiazines: Antidopaminergic effects – neuroleptic malignant syndrome
• Ephedrine: Sympathomimetic effects
• Ketamine: Sympathomimetic effects
• Atropine: Produces tachycardia
• Naloxone hydrochloride: Sympathetic nervous system predominance

---

predisposes to severe hypotension. Preganglionic sympathetic B-fiber blockade that results in vasodilation from neuraxial anesthesia will augment this effect.

Because rapidly developing hemorrhage is a major concern, two large-bore peripheral intravenous lines are indicated. Aside from the American Society of Anesthesiologist basic monitoring modalities, arterial line placement is required for blood pressure monitoring.

A central line is indicated to monitor central venous pressure to assess the patient's volume status.

Anesthetic management for a patient with pheochromocytoma begins with preoperative sedation to decrease anxiety and SNS activity. An adequate anesthetic depth should be achieved before direct laryngoscopy to avoid an exaggerated SNS response. Nitrous oxide should be avoided due to concerns regarding the development of a pneumothorax. The administration of succinylcholine for muscle paralysis is controversial because the resulting fasciculations cause abdominal rigidity and can increase the release of catecholamines from the pheochromocytoma. The anesthetist should expect blood pressure lability throughout the entire perioperative course.

Hypertension most commonly occurs during intubation, incision, manipulation of tumor, and ligation of the venous drainage of the affected adrenal gland. Hypertension is most effectively managed by:
- Increasing the concentration of inhalation anesthetic agent
- Administering narcotics/dexmedetomidine
- Using sodium nitroprusside as an intravenous drip
- Administering clevidipine
- Administering magnesium sulfate

Hypotension is most common after removal of the tumor. It is most effectively treated by:
- Decreasing the anesthetic depth
- Administering crystalloids, colloids, or packed red blood cells

- Administering a direct-acting vasopressor such as phenylephrine

The patient's blood glucose should be assessed preoperatively and incrementally throughout the surgical procedure. Hyperglycemia commonly occurs before the tumor removal due to the inhibition of endogenous insulin release due to SNS predominance and glycogenolysis by the liver. Conversely, hypoglycemia can develop rapidly during the postoperative period. If tachycardia occurs and beta-receptor blockade is necessary, the advantage for administering esmolol is that the metabolism is extremely rapid and persistent blockade is not a concern.

8. *Describe the intraoperative course for a patient having a laparoscopic adrenalectomy for a pheochromocytoma by assessing the hemodynamic variables provided in Fig. 12.2.*
   1. Despite alpha- and beta-adrenergic blockade, note the degree of hypertension and heart rate variability that occur during the periods of induction, endotracheal intubation, and placement of an epidural catheter.
   2. At 10:00 there is an abrupt increase in the blood pressure, most probably due to surgical manipulation of the pheochromocytoma. An infusion of nitroprusside is started and titrated to the degree of hypertension that occurs. Notice that the heart rate abruptly decreases to less than 50 beats per minute during the extreme hypertensive response, which was most likely caused by the baroreceptor response or by the administration of labetalol.

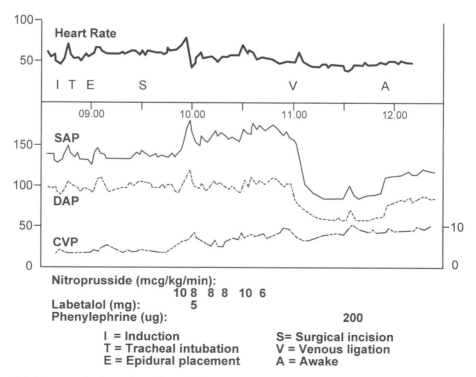

• **Fig. 12.2** Intraoperative hemodynamic profile during excision of a pheochromocytoma. *CVP*, Central venous pressure; *DAP*, diastolic arterial pressure; *SAP*, systolic arterial pressure. (Modified from Prys-Roberts C: Phaeochromocytoma - recent progress in its management, *British Journal of Anaesthesia* 85[1]:44-57, 2000.)

3. At approximately 11:00 the venous drainage from the adrenal gland is ligated. High concentrations of catecholamines are present in the venous system, which are forced into systemic circulation before ligation. Notice the rapid speed with which the blood pressure decreases as the catecholamines are metabolized. The hypotension is also caused by the administration of anesthesia and the preoperative adrenergic blockade. The blood pressure is supported by decreasing the anesthetic depth and by administering fluids, as is reflected by an increase in the central venous pressure.

4. At 11:45 the inhalation anesthetic concentration is decreased, and local anesthetic is given in incremental boluses through the epidural catheter.

Postoperative Period

9. *Identify potential complications after an adrenalectomy for a pheochromocytoma.*
   - Hypertension may result from residual pheochromocytoma, pain, hypoglycemia, hypervolemia, and hypoxia.
   - Hypotension can result from residual alpha-adrenergic receptor blockade, hypovolemia, myocardial ischemia or infarction, bleeding, or sepsis.
   - Pneumothorax
   - Hemorrhage
   - Sepsis
   - Hypoglycemia
   - Hypoadrenocorticism
   - Acute renal failure

Review Questions

1. The classic triad of symptoms associated with pheochromocytoma include:
   a. Elevated systolic pressure/swelling/anxiety.
   b. Headache/diaphoresis/tachycardia.
   c. Elevated diastolic pressure/diaphoresis/tachycardia.
   d. Mood swings/increased pulse pressure/arrhythmias.
2. The majority of extraadrenal pheochromocytomas are located in which region of the body?
   a. Thorax
   b. Cranium
   c. Mediastinum
   d. Abdomen
3. Which is true regarding pheochromocytoma excretion of endogenous catecholamines?
   a. Norepinephrine > epinephrine
   b. Norepinephrine < epinephrine
   c. Dopamine > norepinephrine
   d. Epinephrine < dopamine

4. Which of the preoperative vital signs are reflective of adequate for surgery and anesthetic management for a patient scheduled for adrenalectomy for pheochromocytoma?
   a. Heart rate 101, blood pressure 138/66, hematocrit 27
   b. Heart rate 83, blood pressure 149/82, hematocrit 36
   c. Heart rate 96, blood pressure 165/66, hematocrit 48
   d. Heart rate 62, blood pressure 138/112, hematocrit 51
5. Which sign, symptom, or diagnostic test is most sensitive to diagnose a pheochromocytoma?
   a. T-wave changes on a 12-lead ECG
   b. Idiopathic hypertension
   c. Elevated urinary metanephrine levels on a 24-hour urine collection
   d. Chronic headache

Suggested Readings

Araki S, Kijima T, Waseda Y, Komai Y, Nakanishi Y, et al. Incidence and predictive factors of hypoglycemia after pheochromocytoma resection. *Int J Urol* 2019;26(2):273–277.

Buisset C, Guerin C, Cungi PJ, Gardette M, Paladino NC, et al. Pheochromocytoma surgery without systematic preoperative pharmacological preparation: insights from a referral tertiary center experience. *Surg Endosc* 2020 Feb 18. doi: 10.1007/s00464-020-07439-1. [Epub ahead of print]

Higashi YS. Excess norepinephrine impairs both endothelium dependent and independent vasodilation in patients with pheochromocytoma. *Hypertension* 2002;39(2):513–518.

Karlet MC. The endocrine system. In: Nagelhout JJ, Elisha S, eds. *Nurse Anesthesia*, 6th ed. St. Louis, MO: Elsevier, 2018:782–822.

Kenny L, Rizzo V, Trevis J, Assimakopoulou E, Timon D. The unexpected diagnosis of phaeochromocytoma in the anaesthetic room. *Ann Card Anaesth* 2018;21(3):307–310.

Lodin M. Laparoscopic adrenalectomy: keys to success: correct surgical indications, adequate preoperative preparation, surgical team experience. *Surg Laparosc Endosc Percutan Tech* 2007;17(5):392–395.

Naranjo J, Dodd S, Martin YN. Perioperative management of pheochromocytoma. *J Cardiothorac Vasc Anesth* 2017;31(4):1427–1439.

Naruse M, Satoh F, Tanabe A, Okamoto T, Ichihara A, et al. Efficacy and safety of metyrosine in pheochromocytoma/paraganglioma: a multi-center trial in Japan. *Endocr J* 2018;65(3):359–371.

Pacak, K. Preoperative management of the pheochromocytoma patient. *J Clin Endocrinol Metab* 2007;92(11):4069-4079.

Park J, Lin DT, Greco RS, Nikrivan S, Mihm F. Endocrine surgery. In: Jaffe RA, Schmiesing CA, Golianu, eds. *Anesthesiologist's Manual of Surgical Procedures,* 5th ed. Philadelphia: Lippincott Williams & Wilkins, 2014:683–692.

Prys-Roberts C. Phaeochromocytoma-recent progress in management. *Br J Anesth* 2000;85:44–57.

Sesay M. Real time heart rate variability and its correlation with plasma catecholamines during laparoscopic adrenal pheochromocytoma surgery. *Anesth Analg* 2008;106(1):164–170.

Sonntagbauer M, Koch A, Strouhal U, Zacharowski K, Weber CF. Catecholamine crisis during induction of general anesthesia: a case report. *Anaesthesist* 2018;67(3):209–215.

13

Thyroidectomy

KEY POINTS

- Indications for thyroidectomy include increased thyroid function (hyperthyroidism), cancer is present or suspected, decreased thyroid function (hypothyroidism) with a goiter that causes respiratory difficulty, and enlargement of the thyroid gland (idiopathic hypertrophy without increased thyroid hormone synthesis and release).
- Ideally, patients should be rendered euthyroid before surgery.
- The systemic effects of hyperthyroidism are manifested as exaggerated sympathetic nervous system responses.

- Perioperative care should focus on avoiding stimulation of the sympathetic nervous system.
- Hemodynamic stability is essential and should be maintained by providing adequate fluid resuscitation, preoperative administration of antithyroid medications, and avoidance of excessive sympathetic stimulation.
- Thyroid storm is a potentially fatal complication that can occur during the intraoperative and postoperative period.

Case Synopsis

A 31-year-old African American woman with a history of Graves disease and toxic multinodular goiter is scheduled by her surgeon to have a total thyroidectomy.

Preoperative Evaluation and Demographic Data

Past Medical/Surgical History

- Hyperthyroidism
- No past surgical history

List of Medications

- Propranolol prescribed 10 days preoperatively
- Propylthiouracil prescribed 6 weeks preoperatively
- Sodium iodide prescribed 10 days preoperatively

Diagnostic Data

- Hemoglobin, 13.1 g/dL; hematocrit, 38.2%; white blood cell count, 4100/mm³; platelet count, 155,000/mm³
- Thyroid studies: total T_4, 11.6 mcg/dL (normal value 5.0 to 12.0 mcg/dL); free T_3, 176 ng/dL (normal value 70 to 195 ng/dL); thyroid-stimulating hormone (TSH), 0.6 mU/L (normal value 0.4 to 5.0 mU/L)
- Glucose, 125 g/dL
- Electrocardiogram (ECG): sinus tachycardia; heart rate, 86 beats per minute
- Airway evaluation: Mallampati 2, thyromental distance 7 cm, full range of motion of cervical spine and temporomandibular joint. A 3-cm palpable nodule present on the left side of the neck approximating the cricoid cartilage. She denies changes in the quality of her voice or difficulty in breathing while lying flat.

Height/Weight/Vital Signs

- 173 cm, 68 kg
- Blood pressure, 136/82; heart rate, 84 beats per minute; respiratory rate, 14 breaths per minute; room air oxygen saturation, 100%; temperature, 37.2°C

Anatomy and Physiology of Thyroid Gland

The thyroid gland consists of two lobes connected by an isthmus. It is bound to the anterior and lateral aspects of the trachea by the superior border of the isthmus located just below the cricoid cartilage. Two pairs of parathyroid glands, which regulate plasma calcium levels, are located on the posterior aspect of each lobe, one pair that is superior and one pair that is inferior on each lobe. The posterior aspects of the thyroid gland run alongside the carotid sheath and the esophagus.

The recurrent laryngeal nerve (RLN) and the external superior laryngeal nerve (SLN) are branches of the vagus nerve that innervate the intrinsic muscles of the larynx that serve a variety of functions, including adducting and abducting the vocal cords. These nerves exist in proximity to the thyroid gland, and they can be damaged during resection of the thyroid gland.

Arterial blood is supplied by the superior and inferior thyroid arteries. A venous plexus is formed by the superior, middle, and inferior thyroid veins. In addition, the thyroid gland lies adjacent to the common carotid artery and the anterior jugular vein, which are potential sources of rapid and massive blood loss. Fig. 13.1 illustrates the anatomic

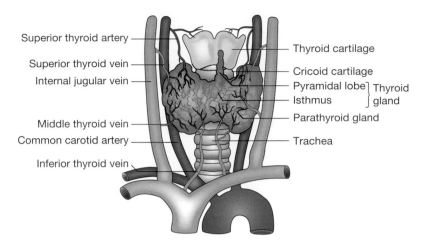

• **Fig. 13.1** Anatomy of the thyroid gland and adjacent structures. (From Kallenbach JZ: *Review of hemodialysis for nurses and dialysis personnel*, ed 10, St. Louis, 2021, Elsevier.)

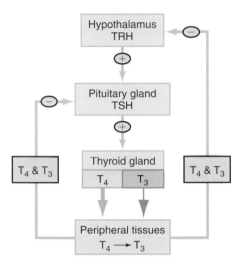

• **Fig. 13.2** Physiologic control of thyroid hormone secretion. *TRH*, Thyrotropin-releasing hormone; *TSH*, thyroid-stimulating hormone. (From Hall RM, Hockberger RS, Gausche-Hill M: *Rosen's emergency medicine: concepts and clinical practice*, ed 9, St. Louis, 2018, Elsevier.)

complexity associated with the thyroid gland and its adjacent structures.

The hypothalamus secretes thyrotropin-releasing hormone (TRH) that circulates within the hypophyseal portal system and stimulates the anterior pituitary gland to create TSH. The biosynthesis of thyroid hormone created by the thyroid gland is solely controlled by TSH. The thyroid functions to produce and secrete thyroid hormones T_3 (triiodothyronine) and T_4 (tetraiodothyronine [thyroxine]) in a ratio of 1:10, respectively. When the concentration of thyroid hormone is sufficient, T_3 and T_4 have an inhibitory effect on the hypothalamus and anterior pituitary gland, creating a negative-feedback loop. This process is illustrated in Fig. 13.2. Although T_3 is found in smaller concentrations compared with T_4, it is approximately four times more potent. Table 13.1 compares the physiologic effects of thyroid hormones. In addition to T_3 and T_4, the thyroid gland produces calcitonin from parafollicular C cells, which

in addition to the parathyroid glands helps regulate serum calcium levels.

Thyroid hormones regulate the metabolic rate of numerous physiologic processes, including tissue growth, oxygen consumption, and the rate at which tissues utilize energy for catabolic processes. The symptomatology associated with thyroid dysfunction is directly related to the increase or decrease in metabolic rate that occurs with hyperthyroid or hypothyroid disease states, respectively. The symptomatology associated with these disease states is presented in Box 13.1.

Pathophysiology

Hyperthyroidism is a pathologic state in which the thyroid gland secretes an excessive amount of T_3 and T_4 resulting in hypermetabolism. Most cases are a result of Graves disease, toxic multinodular goiter, or toxic adenoma. Common signs and symptoms that are associated with hyperthyroidism are consistent with hypermetabolism and include:

- Weight loss
- Exophthalmos
- Heat intolerance
- Tachycardia
- Muscle weakness
- Hyperglycemia
- Increased deep tendon reflexes
- Fatigue

The cardiac manifestations associated with hyperthyroidism include tachycardia, dysrhythmias (atrial fibrillation is most common), and increased cardiac output caused by adrenergic hyperactivity. Ideally, surgical intervention should be postponed until the patient has taken antithyroid medications and is euthyroid, but if this is not possible, the patient will often receive beta-adrenergic antagonists to maintain hemodynamic stability.

Patients with low levels of T_3 and T_4 are hypothyroid, which can be caused by an autoimmune disease such as Hashimoto thyroiditis, radioactive iodine, antithyroid medications, or iodine deficiency, among others. The

TABLE 13.1 Comparison of the Physiologic Effects of T₃ and T₄

Name	Triiodothyronine (T₃)	Tetraiodothyronine (T₄) thyroxine
Amount in circulation	5%–10%	90%–95%
Degree of protein binding	99.80%	99.98%
Potency	4 times > T_4	
Onset	6–12 hours	2–3 days
Half life	1–2 days	6–7 days
Activity	80%	20%

• BOX 13.1 Comparison of Signs and Symptoms of Hyperthyroidism and Hypothyroidism

Hyperthyroidism
- Heat intolerance
- Weight loss
- Anorexia
- Frequent bowel movements
- Muscle weakness/fatigue
- Tremors
- Tachydysrhythmia (atrial fibrillation)

Hypothyroidism
- Cold intolerance
- Weight gain
- Depression
- Constipation
- Fatigue
- Mood swings
- Pericardial effusion
  - Coronary artery disease
  - Hypoglycemia
  - Peripheral vascular disease

TABLE 13.2 Normal Laboratory Values for Thyroid Function Tests

TSH	0.4–5.0 mU/L
Total T_4	5.0–12.0 mcg/dL
Free T_4 (F T_4)	0.9–2.4 ng/dL
Free T_3 (F T_3)	70–195 ng/dL
Free thyroxine index (F T_4 index)	1.2–4.9 ng/dL
T_3 resin uptake (R T_3U)	24%–39%

clinical presentation associated with hypothyroidism reflects a decrease in metabolic rate. Decreased cardiac output is caused by a decrease in both heart rate and stroke volume. Although patients who develop hyperthyroidism are at increased risk for perioperative complications, mild hypothyroidism is not considered a contraindication to surgery. Because a range of severity is associated with thyroid disease, patients with severe hypothyroidism (myxedema coma) may have an increased risk for perioperative complications associated with the physiologic stress of surgery and anesthesia.

Surgical Procedure

Removal of the thyroid gland is performed via a transverse neck incision through the platysma and strap muscles, exposing the thyroid gland and its blood supply. Once hemostasis is achieved, resection can begin. Depending on the pathologic condition, a subtotal thyroidectomy or lobectomy (one lobe of the thyroid gland is removed) can be accomplished. The amount of thyroid gland tissue that is removed depends on the severity of thyroid disease and the intraoperative findings. The muscle and fascia layers are sutured closed using dissolvable material, and the wound edges are approximated and then sutured or stapled.

Anesthetic Management and Considerations

Preoperative Period

1. *Discuss the key findings that should be evaluated preoperatively in a patient presenting for thyroidectomy.*

   All elective cases should be postponed until antithyroid medications can allow the patient to achieve a euthyroid state. Serum thyroid levels should be within normal limits as these values are shown in Table 13.2. The patient should be evaluated for signs and symptoms such as tachycardia, fever, dysrhythmias, or agitation. Airway assessment and management may be complicated in patients having a thyroidectomy. The anesthetist must be aware that a potentially difficult intubation may occur in a patient with an enlarged thyroid gland. A nodule or goiter may displace the larynx and distort the normal airway anatomy, thus obscuring the view during laryngoscopy. Additionally, one should note the quality of the patient's voice and if changes have occurred, as hoarseness may indicate RLN palsy caused by compression from the enlarged thyroid gland. Lastly, if the patient states that it is difficult to breathe in the supine position, pressure from the thyroid gland can cause tracheal compression and occlusion.

2. *Describe the mechanism of action and indications for medications used to achieve a euthyroid state for patients who are hyperthyroid.*
   - **Thioamides:** Propylthiouracil (PTU) and methimazole (Tapazole) are thioamide medications that decrease

the formation of thyroid hormone by inhibiting thyroid peroxidase, which catalyzes the conversion of iodide to iodine in the thyroid follicle cell. Additionally, these medications inhibit the organification process by decreasing the iodination of iodine onto tyrosine, decreasing diiodotyrosine and monoiodotyrosine. Methimazole is 10 times more potent compared with PTU. The patient will be prescribed one of these medications.

- **Iodides:** Sodium iodide or potassium iodide inhibits the organification process, the production and release of thyroid hormone, and the size and vascularity of the thyroid gland if hyperplasia exists. Because 60% of T_3 and T_4 is composed of iodine, it would seem counterintuitive to administer iodide. However, the Wolff–Chaikoff effect is an autoregulatory process that inhibits thyroid activity for several days to weeks if excessive quantities of iodide are present.
- **Radioactive iodine:** The isotope I^{131} is administered orally, collects within the follicle, and emits radiation that destroys the thyroid cells. Patients can achieve a euthyroid state within several weeks after treatment.
- **Beta-adrenergic blockade:** Beta-blocking medications that do not possess intrinsic sympathomimetic activity inhibit the peripheral conversion of T_4 to T_3 and decrease the cardiac manifestations consistent with enhanced sympathetic nervous system activity.
- **Corticosteroids** Steroids have an inhibitory effect on TSH. These medications can be used in conjunction with others to achieve a euthyroid state.

Intraoperative Period

3. *Identify anesthetic induction agents that can be administered for a patient having a thyroidectomy.*

Propofol and, if indicated, etomidate are acceptable medications to use for induction. Ketamine is not a reasonable choice for an induction agent due to the potential sympathetic nervous system stimulation. Hyperthyroidism may cause increased systemic vascular resistance, and upon induction, hypotension may occur due to intravascular volume depletion.

4. *Discuss concerns regarding airway management that should be taken before intubation.*

A good understanding of the degree of thyroid pathology from preoperative imaging will help determine if an awake or asleep intubation is necessary. If the thyroid mass or goiter causes significant displacement of normal laryngeal anatomy, an awake intubation using a flexible intubating endoscope (i.e., fiber-optic scope) should be considered. If there is minimal to no laryngeal displacement, a standard induction and intubation using video laryngoscopy (VL) is adequate. A bougie stylet may help with endotracheal tube delivery during VL. Finally, a large thyroid goiter may significantly displace

both the thyroid and cricoid cartilages, making location of the cricothyroid membrane difficult or impossible to identify. Thus it is prudent to locate these landmarks before airway manipulation in the event that a cricothyroidotomy is necessary.

5. *Describe patient positioning for thyroidectomy and associated anesthetic considerations.*

Patients are placed supine with the head elevated 30 degrees and the neck extended. The eyes should be carefully taped, especially for patients who have developed exophthalmos, in order to avoid corneal abrasions. The anesthetist should be aware that there is a possibility of endotracheal tube migration during neck extension and flexion. The surgeon may request a shoulder roll and extend the patient's head to achieve the ideal position for maximal surgical exposure. It is important to support the occiput in order to avoid postoperative neck discomfort or brachial plexus injury. Due to this position, the level of the thyroid gland will be above the level of the heart, and although a rare complication, a venous air embolism is possible.

6. *Discuss the effect of hyperthyroidism on the maintenance of adequate anesthetic depth.*

Maintenance of anesthesia should focus on attenuating sympathetic nervous system stimulation. This can be achieved by obtaining adequate depth of anesthesia to prevent an exaggerated response to surgical stimulation and avoidance of drugs that excite the sympathetic nervous system. Due to its low blood gas solubility and cardiovascular stability, sevoflurane is an acceptable inhalational anesthetic. Some anesthetists avoid the use of desflurane because of the potential for sympathetic nervous system activation. Narcotics and dexmedetomidine can help attenuate the sympathetic nervous system response and provide postoperative analgesia.

Although hyperthyroidism increases metabolic requirements, clinical evidence does not support an increase in minimum alveolar concentration (MAC) requirements for these patients. MAC requirements may be increased in the presence of hyperthermia; on average, a 4% to 5% increase in MAC occurs with every degree that the temperature increases above 37°C. For this reason, continuous temperature monitoring is essential.

7. *Identify measures that can be taken to maintain hemodynamic stability.*

Hemodynamic stability should be closely monitored and appropriately managed to maintain stability and prevent onset of a thyrotoxic crisis. The ECG may reveal atrial fibrillation, a common tachydysrhythmia seen with hyperthyroidism. The onset of tachycardia that is unresponsive to fluid replacement may indicate the need for additional beta-adrenergic receptor blockade. Hypotension that is unresponsive to fluid resuscitation is best treated with a direct-acting vasopressor such as phenylephrine. Ephedrine, an indirect agonist for catecholamine release, is best avoided because patients with hyperthyroidism may have an exaggerated sympathetic nervous system response to catecholamines.

8. *Explain the rationale for the use of a nerve integrity monitoring (NIM) endotracheal tube during a thyroidectomy.*

The NIM endotracheal tube uses electromyographic (EMG) information to determine the real-time integrity of the right and left RLNs. The electrodes that are present on the proximal end of the tube are inserted into a monitor that interprets the signals and allows the surgeon to determine if RLN function remains intact throughout surgery. Neuromuscular blockade and laryngeal tracheal lidocaine have an inhibitory effect on EMG, and their use is contraindicated if this endotracheal tube is used. If the patient must remain intubated for a prolonged period, the NIM endotracheal tube should be replaced with a standard endotracheal tube because of the potential for kinking and rupturing.

9. *Discuss the signs, symptoms, differential diagnosis, and treatment of thyroid storm.*

Early detection and prevention of thyrotoxic crisis (e.g., thyroid storm) are essential, and resuscitative measures should be instituted as soon as possible to prevent circulatory collapse or decompensation of one or more organ systems. Patients who develop thyroid storm are hypermetabolic due to an abrupt increase of circulating thyroid hormone. In most cases, diagnosis of thyroid storm is based on clinical findings alone, as onset is abrupt, and treatment precludes diagnosis with laboratory tests or other screening measures. The signs and symptoms that are most often associated with thyroid storm include hyperthermia, tachycardia and tachydysrhythmia, central nervous system symptoms such as psychosis or altered mental state, and can also include rhabdomyolysis. Although thyrotoxic crisis can occur intraoperatively, the onset more frequently occurs 6 to 18 hours postoperatively. Precipitating factors include infection, surgery, diabetic ketoacidosis, congestive heart failure, pregnancy, and extreme physiologic stress. Without treatment, thyroid storm can be fatal, and mortality ranges from 10% to 75%.

Thyroid storm can be mistaken for other hypermetabolic states caused by different pathologic processes such as malignant hyperthermia or hypertensive crisis resulting from a pheochromocytoma. A comparison of the signs and symptoms associated with various hypermetabolic states is included in Box 13.2. Thyroid storm is most commonly occurring in patients who are not euthyroid preoperatively and is most strongly linked to patients with Graves disease.

Treatment of thyroid storm involves pharmacologic treatment to decrease circulating thyroid hormone, as well as providing supportive interventions, which include:

- Increasing the fraction of inspired oxygen concentration because the increased metabolic rate will lead to increased O_2 consumption.

• BOX 13.2 **Differentiation Between Thyroid Storm, Malignant Hyperthermia, and Pheochromocytoma**

Thyroid Storm	Malignant Hyperthermia	Pheochromocytoma
Hyperthermia	Elevated $ETCO_2$	Paroxysmal extreme hypertension
Tachycardia	Tachycardia	Tachycardia
Dysrhythmia	Dysrhythmia	Dysrhythmia
Hypertension	Hypertension	Headaches
Altered mental status	Hypercarbia	
	Hyperthermia	
	Masseter spasm	

- Fluid resuscitation with cooled intravenous (IV) fluids in the presence of hyperthermia.
- Propylthiouracil or methimazole can be administered to further inhibit the synthesis of thyroid hormone. It is recommended that the use of methimazole for thyroid storm because it acts more rapidly and is associated with fewer side effects than propylthiouracil.
- Sodium iodide is given to block release of hormone from the thyroid gland.
- Acetaminophen is the antipyretic of choice, as aspirin can displace thyroid hormone from proteins, thereby increasing circulating free hormone.
- Beta-adrenergic antagonists should be administered to control the cardiovascular effects associated with sympathetic nervous system predominance. Propranolol or a continuous infusion of esmolol can be administered.
- Steroid administration such as dexamethasone or hydrocortisone may also be considered.
- Serial electrolyte and arterial blood gas analysis.
- Other treatment options include attempts to increase the clearance of circulating thyroid hormone, whether by hemodialysis, plasmapheresis, or administration of cholestyramine, to clear hormone via the gastrointestinal tract.

Postoperative Period

10. *Identify postoperative complications associated with thyroidectomy and discuss prevention and/or treatment.*
- **RLN damage** can be either unilateral or bilateral. Unilateral damage will manifest as hoarseness, whereas bilateral nerve palsy may result in aphonia, stridor, or respiratory distress. The incidence of permanent vocal cord paralysis is rare (0.5% to 2.4%), with incidence of temporary paralysis being 2.6% to 5.9%. This complication can be avoided by surgically identifying the location of the RLN intraoperatively

before resection of the thyroid gland. However, identification may be difficult if extreme hypertrophy or cancer causes distortion of the thyroid anatomy. Vocal cord function can be assessed either via direct laryngoscopy after deep extubation or by having the patient phonate "e" postoperatively. RLN dysfunction, whether unilateral or bilateral, may require reintubation and reexploration of the surgical site for possible nerve compression.

- **Hematoma formation** can cause further compression or collapse of the airway secondary to tracheomalacia (a weakening of the walls of the trachea). The incidence is rare (approximately 1%) and typically occurs within 6 to 24 hours postoperatively. Inadequate surgical hemostasis, coagulopathy, acute hypertension, and straining from postoperative nausea and vomiting can increase the potential for postoperative bleeding. The definitive treatment involves immediate evacuation of the hematoma and reexploration of the surgical site.

- **Pneumothorax** is a rare complication associated with a thyroidectomy. Because the apices of the lungs extend above the level of the clavicles very close to the surgical site, there is the potential for air to enter the thoracic cavity.

- **Acute hypocalcemia** resulting from inadvertent removal of the parathyroid glands. The incidence of postoperative hypocalcemia ranges from 10% to 50%, and for this reason, the anesthetist may be asked to obtain serum calcium and parathyroid hormone levels intraoperatively or immediately postoperatively to help predict the potential for hypoparathyroidism. Hypocalcemia is most likely to occur 24 to 48 hours after surgery is complete. Parathyroid dysfunction is typically transient if all four have not been removed—normal function may return in 4 weeks postoperatively. Inadvertent parathyroid resection will result in permanent dysfunction, and both situations are treated with oral calcium and vitamin.

- **Thyroid storm**, as discussed previously.

Review Questions

1. What is the preoperative goal of pharmacologic prophylaxis for patients with hyperthyroidism?
   a. To maintain a hyperthyroid state via administration of exogenous thyroid hormone
   b. To blunt the sympathetic nervous system by obtaining an adequate depth of anesthesia and avoiding drugs that cause sympathetic stimulation
   c. To stimulate the sympathetic nervous system via administration of cardiac stimulants
   d. To observe complete muscle paralysis via administration of a nondepolarizing neuromuscular blocker

2. Which sign is not commonly observed during thyroid storm?
   a. Hypertension
   b. Hyperthermia
   c. Tachycardia
   d. Hypercarbia

3. Which best describes the physiologic sequence that leads to the biosynthesis of thyroid hormone?
   a. Thyroid-stimulating hormone stimulates the thyroid gland to produce T_3 and T_4.
   b. Thyrotropin-releasing hormone stimulates the thyroid gland to produce thyroid hormone.
   c. T_3 and T_4 directly stimulate the thyroid gland to produce thyroid hormone.
   d. T_3 and T_4 directly stimulate the hypothalamus to produce thyroid-stimulating hormone.

4. Which best describes the relationship between the minimum alveolar concentration (MAC) of an inhalational agent, hyperthyroidism, and a temperature of 38.1°C?
   a. Increased MAC of inhalational agents
   b. Decreased MAC of inhalational agents
   c. MAC of inhalational agents remains unaffected
   d. Increased MAC can precipitate hyperthyroidism

5. Due to its close proximity to the thyroid gland, accidental removal of the parathyroid gland may result in:
   a. Hypokalemia.
   b. Hypomagnesemia.
   c. Hypermagnesemia.
   d. Hypocalcemia.

Suggested Readings

Amathieu R. Difficult intubation in thyroid surgery: myth or reality? *Anesth Analg* 2006;103(4):965–968.

Asari R, Passier C, Kaczirek K, et al. Hypoparathyroidism after total thyroidectomy: a prospective study. *Arch Surg* 2008;143(2):132–137.

Del Rio P, Rossini M, Montana CM, Viani L, et al. Postoperative hypocalcemia: analysis of factors influencing early hypocalcemia development following thyroid surgery. *BMC Surg* 2019;18 (Suppl 1):25.

Elisha S, Heiner J, Nagelhout J, Waters E. Anesthesia case management for thyroidectomy. *AANA J* 2010;78(2):151–160.

Grimes CM. Intraoperative thyroid storm: a case report. *AANA J* 2004;72(1):53–55.

Karlet MC. The endocrine system. In: Nagelhout JJ, Elisha S, eds. *Nurse Anesthesia*, 6th ed. St. Louis, MO: Elsevier, 2018:782–822.

Liu MY, Chang CP, Hung CL, Hung CJ, Huang SM. Traction injury of recurrent laryngeal nerve during thyroidectomy. *World J Surg* 2020;44(2):402–407.

Myssiorek D. Recurrent laryngeal nerve paralysis: anatomy and etiology. *Otolaryngol Clin North Am* 2004;37(1):25–44.

Nisi P, Piva G, Cozzani F, Rossini M, Bonati E, Madoni C. et al. Intraoperative neuromonitoring in traditional and mini-invasive thyroidectomy. A single center experience in 1652 nerve at risk. *Acta Biomed* 2020;91(1):64–69.

Peramunage D, Nikravan S. Anesthesia for endocrine emergencies. *Anesthesiol Clin* 2020;38(1):149–163.

Piantanida E. Preoperative management in patients with Graves' disease. *Gland Surg* 2017;6(5):476–481.

Ponce de León-Ballesteros G, Velázquez-Fernández D, et al. Hypoparathyroidism after total thyroidectomy: importance of the intraoperative management of the parathyroid glands. *World J Surg* 2019;43(7):1728–1735.

Randle RW, Bates MF, Long KL, Pitt SC, Schneider DF, et al. Impact of potassium iodide on thyroidectomy for Graves' disease: implications for safety and operative difficulty. *Surgery* 2018;163(1):68–72.

Shindo M. Incidence of vocal cord paralysis with and without recurrent laryngeal nerve monitoring during thyroidectomy. *Arch Otolaryngol* 2007;133(5):481–485.

Ylli D, Klubo-Gwiezdzinska J, Wartofsky L. Thyroid emergencies. *Pol Arch Intern Med* 2019;129(7-8):526–534.

14

Emergency Airway Management for the Trauma Patient

KEY POINTS

- A traumatic airway injury necessitates rapid assessment and emergency management in critically ill patients.
- Properly executing a rapid sequence induction (RSI) is a vital and fundamental skill. Anesthesia providers must be proficient at performing an RSI during rapid airway maintenance.

- Patients who have sustained a potential or actual cervical spine injury must be intubated using in-line manual axial stabilization.

Case Synopsis

A 38-year-old man who has been assaulted arrives via ambulance to a trauma center. He has sustained multiple stab wounds to the face, neck, and torso. Blood is streaming out of his mouth, and he is combative.

Preoperative Evaluation and Demographic Data

Past Medical/Surgical History

- Unknown. Medical alert bracelet on right wrist reads, "Diabetic."

List of Medications

- Unknown

Diagnostic Data

- None

Height/Weight/Vital Signs

- 193 cm, 87 kg
- Blood pressure, 88/39; heart rate, 126 beats per minute; respiratory rate, 32 breaths per minute; room air oxygen saturation, 88%; temperature, 36.8°C

Physical Examination

The primary trauma assessment is rapidly completed upon arrival. The findings include a patient who is a well-developed male with obvious deep tissue lacerations along his face and neck with multiple 2- to 3-cm punctures along his chest

wall, primarily situated around the right fourth rib at the midclavicular line. He arrived with a cervical collar in place and on a backboard. His initial airway examination indicates the following signs: respiratory stridor, hemoptysis, broken teeth, facial lacerations, and a large hematoma on the right side of his neck near the sixth cervical vertebrae. You are immediately consulted by the trauma team and asked to secure the patient's airway. During laryngoscopy and direct visualization of the oropharyngeal region of the airway, you notice the presence of supraglottic edema and left-sided tracheal deviation.

Traumatic Airway Overview

Endotracheal intubation is a mainstay of anesthesia practice. Despite its routine use during general anesthesia, intubation and airway management can be challenging when caring for an acutely injured patient. Difficult tracheal intubation is the third most common respiratory-related event that leads to brain damage and death. Although many patients who endure a traumatic injury will not have an airway that is difficult to manage, the anesthetist frequently will not have the opportunity to perform an airway examination. Therefore it is vitally important for the anesthetist to have a contingency plan if a difficult airway is encountered.

RSI is the preferred method that should be used for traumatic airway management. One of the greatest differences between performing a routine anesthetic induction and an RSI is the timing of administration of a muscle relaxant. In an RSI, the patient is paralyzed without the anesthetist knowing if the patient can be mask-ventilated. The use of muscle relaxants in this situation increases the risk of a "can't intubate/can't ventilate" scenario. Muscle relaxation is associated with the highest overall rate of successful airway management and provides the greatest possibility for rapidly securing the airway.

Emergency intubation for the trauma patient should adhere to the American Society of Anesthesiologists (ASA) difficult airway algorithm. In addition to requiring a secured airway, trauma patients are assumed to have delayed gastric emptying and are at increased risk for aspiration. The anesthesia provider must be skilled in utilizing a variety of airway adjuncts, including video laryngoscopy and cricothyroidotomy.

Cervical Spine Injuries

Patients who have sustained a blunt or penetrating injury to the neck and face must be considered to have cervical spine instability. Cervical spine injuries remain a significant concern during airway management of the trauma patient. The incidence of cervical spine injury after trauma is approximately 3% to 6% of all trauma patients and approximately 10% for patients who have experienced a traumatic brain injury. It is prudent for the anesthetist to assume that the patient has a cervical spine injury until it can be definitively determined by physical examination and radiography or computed tomography (CT) scan that the spinal cord and cervical vertebrae are intact. Immobilization of the neck is essential, and in-line manual axial stabilization allows for the removal of the front of the cervical collar, allowing jaw and mouth movement necessary to insert the laryngoscope blade, while limiting the risk for further injury.

Cricoid pressure (Sellick maneuver) assists the anesthetist by displacing the larynx posteriorly and providing an improved view of the vocal cords. This procedure may also help to prevent both gastric insufflation during bag–valve–mask ventilation and passive reflux of gastric contents during laryngoscopy. A disadvantage of providing cricoid pressure to a patient with a cervical spine injury is that pressure is exerted on the cervical vertebrae (C5) that could possibly result in spinal cord and vascular injury, and therefore its use in this instance is relatively contraindicated. Patients with actual or suspected cervical spine injuries should be intubated while using in-line manual axial stabilization, as shown in Fig. 14.1.

Rapid Sequence Induction

Patients with traumatic injury present with varying degrees of injury and may not require emergent airway management. The most common indications for endotracheal intubation include inadequate oxygenation/ventilation; loss of airway reflexes; decreased level of consciousness; and, in some cases, the need to secure the airway in order to provide sedation during painful procedures. Once it is deemed

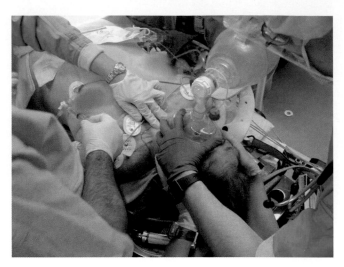

• **Fig. 14.1** Four providers are recommended for securing the airway. Providers are assigned to (1) ventilate with the bag–valve–mask and intubate, (2) maintain in-line cervical stabilization, (3) administer cricoid pressure, and (4) push drugs and assist with airway devices. (From Cameron JL, Cameron AM: *Current surgical therapy*, ed 13, Philadelphia, 2020, Elsevier.)

that the patient must be intubated, it should be accomplished by using an RSI. An RSI is conducted to rapidly control a patient's airway, while reducing the likelihood of gastric aspiration. The procedure consists of five primary components: (1) preoxygenation, (2) cricoid pressure, (3) induction/muscle relaxation, (4) apneic oxygenation, and (5) direct laryngoscopy. Each of these steps is discussed in the following text.

Preoxygenation

Thorough preoxygenation of the patient is imperative before the induction of anesthesia for RSI. Preoxygenation provides an increased period after the patient stops breathing before hypoxemia ensues, which occurs by increasing the concentration of oxygen contained within the functional residual capacity. The procedure is accomplished by administering 100% high-flow (10 to 15 L/min) oxygen via a nonrebreathing facemask or bag–valve facemask. It is estimated that four to eight tidal volume breaths provide an adequate degree of preoxygenation. Quantifying the adequacy of preoxygenation by observing the ETO$_2$ is recommended.

Cricoid Pressure

Cricoid pressure was first described by Sellick in 1961. The goal of this maneuver is to reduce the risk of pulmonary aspiration of gastric contents by compressing the esophagus against the cricoid cartilage and the cervical vertebrae. Cricoid pressure is maintained throughout the RSI and is not released until endotracheal tube (ETT) placement has been confirmed to be bilaterally equal. Aspiration of gastric contents can occur if the ETT cuff is placed too deeply and migrates into the right mainstem bronchus. The application of cricoid pressure is contraindicated for patients with confirmed or suspected cervical spine injury, patients with tracheal and/or cricoid cartilage injury, and patients who are actively vomiting.

Induction Agents

The anesthetic induction that is used for RSI can be achieved by using a variety of agents, but care should be taken when selecting an initial dose. Any induction agent has the potential for causing a dramatic decrease in blood pressure, especially in the presence of hypovolemia. This effect can occur due to the inhibition of high circulating catecholamine levels and because of an increased sensitivity of the brain during shock. The precise dose of induction agent that should be used in a trauma patient is variable and highly individualized. Induction agents should be titrated to response, realizing that sympathetic nervous system (SNS) inhibition can have dramatic cardiovascular effects in patients who have hypovolemic shock. Although there is no induction agent that is contraindicated for this patient, the dose should be reduced to minimize the potential for hemodynamic decompensation. One potential exception is etomidate and the potential for adrenocortical suppression for 24 to 48 hours after use.

The choice to administer succinylcholine or a nondepolarizing muscle relaxant for paralysis may be complex because there are advantages and disadvantages to using these medications. A discussion of inducing paralysis and the type of neuromuscular blocking medication that should be used will occur later in this chapter.

Apneic Oxygenation

Apneic oxygenation is the concept of providing pulmonary ventilation using high-flow oxygen. The purpose of this procedure is to reduce the risk of gastric distension and pulmonary aspiration from positive pressure ventilation while preventing hypoxemia. The principle of apneic oxygenation is based on the Boyle law in which gas leaves the facemask, fills the lungs, and exchanges within the lungs based on the concentration gradient of gases in the alveoli. Unfortunately, optimal gas exchange may not occur, resulting in hypoxemia.

Apneic oxygenation used for RSI is intended to reduce the risk of aspiration for a potential full stomach, yet many trauma patients are unable to inhale deeply and take tidal volume breaths prior to induction, resulting in a reduced functional residual capacity and reduced pulmonary reserve. Avoiding the potential for hypoxemia is important, and clinical modifications have been made to RSI that include bag–valve–mask ventilation through cricoid pressure. There does not appear to be any increase in aspiration by bag–valve–mask ventilation while cricoid pressure is achieved. However, it is prudent to maintain peak inspiratory pressures less than 20 cm/H_2O pressure to avoid gastric insufflation.

Direct Laryngoscopy

There is no evidence to show that there is an optimal laryngoscope blade or size for laryngoscopy to accomplish RSI. The anesthetist should use the equipment with which they are most comfortable. Successful ETT placement is immediately confirmed by the presence of carbon dioxide, bilateral equal and clear breath sounds, the absence of sounds over the stomach, and chest rise and fall. If the initial attempt at laryngoscopy is unsuccessful, a second attempt should incorporate a change in the technique (operator, laryngoscope blade, patient position). When video laryngoscopy was compared with direct laryngoscopy for patients with cervical spine injury during intubation, although there was no observed difference in cervical spine movement, video laryngoscopy provides superior visualization. Supporting oxygenation throughout the intubation process is of paramount importance. An understanding of airway management adjuncts and the ability to be proficient with these techniques is critical to provide safe patient care.

Anesthetic Management and Considerations

1. *Describe the immediate concerns regarding airway management for a patient who has sustained a traumatic injury.*

   This patient is exhibiting signs of significant respiratory distress:

   - **Respiratory compensation:** Respiratory rate is 32 breaths per minute, audible stridor, and oxygen delivered by nonrebreathing oxygen facemask. The patient's oxygen saturation is 88%.

   An increased respiratory rate can occur for a variety of reasons; however, in this scenario, the patient's physiologic compensatory mechanism for hypoxia includes increasing minute ventilation. Despite a supraphysiologic concentration of inhaled oxygen that is being delivered, the patient's SpO_2 remains 88%. The most accurate method of assessing the degree of hypoxemia is by obtaining an arterial blood gas. According to the values present on the oxyhemoglobin dissociation curve, an SpO_2 of 90% is consistent with a PaO_2 of approximately 60 mm Hg, indicating the presence of arterial hypoxemia.

   This patient is exhibiting signs of compensated hypovolemic shock, as determined by the following:

   - **A potential for vascular injury:** Blood pressure, 88/39; heart rate, 126 beats per minute; evidence of a hematoma and edema on the right side of his neck; the presence of hemoptysis; blood is streaming out of his mouth.

   The SNS response associated with hypoxia and hypovolemic shock is powerful and involves the release of major neurovascular mediators such as epinephrine, norepinephrine, and cortisol. By increasing cardiac output and systemic vascular resistance, the physiologic compensatory response should result in increasing blood pressure and thus systemic perfusion, which results in oxygen and substrate delivery and carbon dioxide removal to body tissues. However, this patient's blood pressure remains low, suggesting the possibility of moderate to severe hypovolemic shock.

Blood coming out of his mouth indicates the possibility of intraoral or pharyngeal laceration. This fact, along with his broken teeth and hematoma on his neck, will complicate direct laryngoscopy by obscuring the anesthetist's vision and distorting the structures that comprise the airway anatomy, as seen in Fig. 14.2. It is also necessary to determine if the patient has sustained a pulmonary contusion that is actively bleeding. In this case, lung isolation using a double-lumen ETT or a bronchial blocker is indicated. Hemoptysis and respiratory distress make it unlikely that this patient will cooperate and be able to take tidal volume breaths for adequate preoxygenation. It is imperative to perform a secondary assessment for this patient because there is the possibility that he has sustained other injuries that may be contributing to his state of shock.

This patient should be allowed to sit upright and be permitted to suction his oral pharynx as tolerated. Gravity will likely facilitate movement of fluids from his airway. At the same time, high-flow oxygen should be supplied via a nonrebreathing facemask, face tent, or blow-by oxygen to optimize pulmonary reserve prior to induction. An arterial blood gas, hemoglobin and hematocrit values, and a type and cross should be rapidly obtained. A surgeon should evaluate the type and extent of his vascular injures, and a plan for surgical intervention is necessary. The anesthetist should expect hypotension to occur after induction, and vasopressor

medication should be prepared. Preparation for immediate surgical airway intervention is warranted.

2. *Identify the safest and most efficient method for acute airway management for this patient.*

Airway management for this patient should include an RSI and in-line manual axial stabilization. This patient presents with several unique problems for the anesthetist. Despite the presence of penetrating injuries and the potential for cervical spine injury, he will likely not tolerate lying supine. In this instance, it may be necessary to begin induction in the high-Fowler position. Supplemental oxygen via bag–valve–mask should be placed over the patient's face. Induction should begin when all participants are prepared to provide cricoid pressure (unless cervical spine/tracheal injury is present or suspected), administer induction agents, lower the head of the bed, and hold in-line manual axial stabilization. It would be prudent to have a surgeon or another provider skilled in cricothyrotomy if airway management is unsuccessful. After airway control has been established, in-line manual axial stabilization with use of a cervical spine collar should be maintained.

3. *Discuss the advantages and disadvantages of using succinylcholine or rocuronium to facilitate intubation during RSI.*

Succinylcholine (1.5 mg/kg) provides the most rapid onset of muscle relaxation to facilitate intubation and is the preferred agent in any patient without a specific contraindication to its use. Box 14.1 lists contraindications for the use of succinylcholine. Life-threatening hyperkalemia after the administration of succinylcholine is a risk for patients with neurologic deficits that are caused by spinal cord injuries. Nicotinic cholinergic receptor upregulation occurs within 24 to 48 hours postinjury, and it is after this period that the administration of succinylcholine is absolutely contraindicated. High-dose rocuronium (1.2 mg/kg) can also be used for RSI, and adequate intubating conditions are present

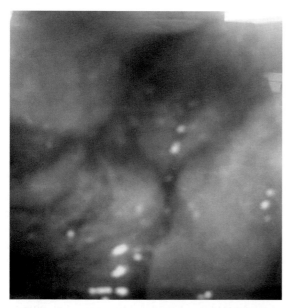

• **Fig. 14.2** Videolaryngoscope (VAL) view of a massively swollen airway. No features were discernible via direct laryngoscopy. (From Fink MP, Vincent JL, Moore FA: *Textbook of critical care*, ed 7, St. Louis, 2017, Elsevier.)

• BOX 14.1 **Contraindications for the Use of Succinylcholine**

- Malignant hyperthermia
- Hyperkalemia
- Spinal cord injury (chronic injury is safe for acute airway management within 24 hours of trauma)
- Crush injury (massive trauma)
- Stroke
- Guillain–Barré syndrome
- Burn injury (>24 hours)
- Muscular dystrophy
- Motor neuron disease
- Mitochondrial myopathies
- Hyperkalemic periodic paralysis
- Pseudocholinesterase deficiency

within 1 minute. Being prepared to administer sugammadex if a "cannot intubate/ventilate" situation occurs is vital.

4. *Describe an appropriate management strategy for a failed attempted direct laryngoscopy.*

The anesthetist must approach every airway management opportunity with several alternative plans in the event of a failed intubation. The ASA difficult airway algorithm helps the anesthetists organize a plan in the event of an airway emergency. However, the algorithm was not designed with the intent for airway management of a trauma patient. As such, alternative airway management strategies may be required. The literature demonstrates a place for the gum elastic bougie (intubating stylet) for traumatic airway management. The gum elastic bougie facilitates nearly blind passage of the ETT. Regardless of any plan, prolonged apnea may necessitate the need for bag–valve–mask ventilation while cricoid pressure is maintained, and in approximately 1% of situations, the creation of a surgical airway is necessary.

5. *Discuss the physiologic implications that occur resulting from a prolonged period of apnea due to failed intubation.*

The failure to secure a patent airway for the trauma patient will rapidly result in physiologic decompensation. Thus airway management for the trauma patient often occurs during an acute, unstable period requiring immediate and lifesaving intervention.

Apnea and hypoventilation cause a variety of pathologic responses related to increases in $PaCO_2$ and decreases in PaO_2. These changes are exacerbated in the trauma patient due to increased metabolic demands. The peripheral chemoreceptors that are located within the aortic and carotid bodies produce an excitatory response caused by decreased PaO_2, increased $PaCO_2$, and decreased pH, which stimulates an increase in SNS outflow. The SNS stimulates increased cardiac excitation and vasoconstriction.

In this patient scenario, a rightward shift of the oxyhemoglobin dissociation curve occurs due to hypercarbia, hypoxemia, and increased 2,3 diphosphoglycerate (DPG). The creation of 2,3 DPG occurs in red blood cells and is a by-product that is associated with metabolism. Increased 2,3 DPG is associated with anaerobic metabolism. This results in a conformational change in the hemoglobin molecule that creates a decreased affinity between oxygen and hemoglobin, which favors the release of oxygen to the tissues.

The rate and increase of arterial carbon dioxide accumulation during apnea is predictable. The average $PaCO_2$ accumulation is 6 mm Hg for the first minute and 3 to 4 mm Hg for each additional minute. Additionally, the metabolic tissue demand for the average adult is approximately 3 mL/kg/min. Assuming that the pulse oximeter reading is accurate, his PaO_2 of 88% SaO_2 would be less than 60 mm Hg. This equates to rapid desaturation and worsening hypoxemia.

Severe hypoxia will rapidly progress to cardiovascular collapse as a result of anaerobic respiration, cellular energy depletion, hydrogen ion and lactate accumulation, and acidosis. If hypoxia continues, the patient will exhibit decompensation, as the cardiac rhythm will progress from tachydysrhythmias or bradydysrhythmias to asystole.

6. *Discuss the appropriate anesthetic management for severe hypotension that occurs after positive pressure ventilation and after successful endotracheal intubation.*

A tension pneumothorax occurs as a result of air becoming trapped in the thorax due to a defect or rupture in the lung tissue. The pathology related to a tension pneumothorax is unique in that it allows gas to escape from the lung into the pleural cavity during inspiration. However, gas is trapped in the thoracic cage due to a flap in the tissue that acts as a one-way valve and decreases the volume of gas that is exhaled. As pressure continues to increase within the thoracic cavity, pressure is exerted on the mediastinum, which impinges on the heart and major vasculature and results in diminished cardiac filling and reduced cardiac output. Typically, a tension pneumothorax will occur shortly after the implementation of positive pressure ventilation. The anesthetist should be aware of the signs associated with a tension pneumothorax, which are listed in Box 14.2.

Release of the thoracic tension via chest tube thoracoscopy or needle decompression is required to manage this complication. Needle decompression is accomplished by placing a 2- to 3-inch angiocatheter into the second intercostal space at the midclavicular line on the affected side of the chest. If cardiac function does not immediately improve, the other side of the patient's chest should be decompressed and the advanced cardiac life support protocol initiated. Once needle decompression occurs, the angiocatheter must remain in place until a chest tube is placed to avoid the reaccumulation of air.

• BOX 14.2 Signs Associated With a Tension Pneumothorax

Pulmonary Manifestations

- Hypoxemia
- Hypercarbia
- Increased peak inspiratory pressures
- Decreased pulmonary compliance
- Absence of breath sound on the affected side
- Tracheal deviation in the opposite direction of the pneumothorax

Cardiac Manifestations

- Hypotension
- Tachycardia
- Mediastinal shift in the opposite direction of the pneumothorax
- Distended neck veins

Review Questions

1. Which patient should receive in-line manual axial stabilization for a rapid sequence induction and emergency airway management?
   a. Sustained a blunt airway injury
   b. Sustained an acute head injury
   c. Involved in a high-speed car accident
   d. All of these patients should receive a rapid sequence induction

2. The administration of succinylcholine during a rapid sequence induction is appropriate for a patient with:
   a. Hypokalemia.
   b. A spinal cord transection that occurred 2 weeks ago.
   c. A history of malignant hyperthermia.
   d. A crush injury to the left thigh.

3. A patient has a $PaCO_2$ of 47 mm Hg before induction. It takes 4 minutes to successfully intubate the patient. The anesthetist should expect the patient's $PaCO_2$ to increase by:
   a. 7 mm Hg.
   b. 18 mm Hg.
   c. 52 mm Hg.
   d. 65 mm Hg.

4. The _____ reflex activates the sympathetic nervous system when hypoxemia or hypercarbia occurs.
   a. baroreceptor
   b. chemoreceptor
   c. oculocardiac
   d. atrial stretch

5. Which best describes correct placement of an angiocatheter for a patient who has a tension pneumothorax?
   a. At the level of the sternal notch
   b. Above the fifth rib at the midaxillary line
   c. In the second intercostal space at the midclavicular line
   d. On the side opposite the direction of the tracheal deviation

Suggested Readings

Allen C, Washington S. The role of etomidate as an anaesthetic induction agent for critically ill patients. *Br J Hosp Med.* 2016;77(5):282–6.

Braz LG, Carlucci MTO, Braz JRC, Módolo NSP, do Nascimento P Jr, Braz MG. Perioperative cardiac arrest and mortality in trauma patients: a systematic review of observational studies. *J Clin Anesth.* 2020;64:109813.

de la Grandville B, Arroyo D, Walder B. Etomidate for critically ill patients. Con: do you really want to weaken the frail? *Eur J Anaesthesiol.* 2012;29(11):511–4.

Goto T, Goto Y, Hagiwara Y, et al. Advancing emergency airway management practice and research. *Acute Med Surg.* 2019;6(4):336–351.

Gronert GA, Theye RA. Pathophysiology of hyperkalemia induced by succinylcholine. *Anesthesiol.* 1975;43(1):89–99.

Heier T, Feiner JR, Lin J, et al. Hemoglobin desaturation after succinylcholine-induced apnea: a study of the recovery of spontaneous ventilation in healthy volunteers. *Anesthesiol.* 2001;94(5):754–759.

Heiner JS. Airway management. In: Nagelhout JJ, Elisha S, eds. *Nurse Anesthesia,* 6th ed. St. Louis, MO: Elsevier, 2018:397–440.

Johnson KB, Egan TD, Kern SE, et al. The influence of hemorrhagic shock on propofol: a pharmacokinetic and pharmacodynamic analysis. *Anesthesiology.* 2003;99(2):409–420.

Kovacs G, Sowers N. Airway management in trauma. *Emerg Med Clin North Am.* 2018;36(1):61–84.

Robitaille A, Williams SR, Tremblay MH, Guilbert F, et al. Cervical spine motion during tracheal intubation with manual in-line stabilization: direct laryngoscopy versus GlideScope videolaryngoscopy. *Anesth Analg.* 2008;106(3):935–941.

Sohn L, Hajduk J, Jagannathan N. Apneic oxygenation as a standard of care in children: how do we get there? *Anesth Analg.* 2020;130(4):828–830

Tobin JM, Barras WP, Bree S, Williams N, et al. Anesthesia for trauma patients. *Anesthesiol Clin.* 2018;36(3):431–454.

15

Craniotomy for the Acute Head Injury

KEY POINTS

- It is estimated that 1.5 million acute head injuries (AHIs) occur every year in the United States, most often caused by motor vehicle accidents, sports injuries, and falls.
- The primary objective for induction and maintenance of anesthesia is to decrease elevated intracranial pressure (ICP) if present, optimize cerebral perfusion and oxygenation, and avoid secondary injury from hypoxia and hypotension.

- Hypotension with systolic blood pressure ≤100 mm Hg is a major contributor to poor outcome after acute brain injury.
- Pupillary abnormalities such as size, light reflex, and symmetry occur in 20% to 30% of patients presenting for craniotomy for AHI.

Case Synopsis

A 21-year-old man developed an epidural hematoma after falling off a skateboard and hitting his head on the ground. He is scheduled by his neurosurgeon to have an emergent craniotomy for evacuation of an epidural hematoma.

Preoperative Evaluation and Demographic Data

Past Medical/Surgical History

- Tonsillectomy at age 10; no anesthetic complications
- No known allergies

List of Medications

- None

Diagnostic Data

- Hemoglobin, 14.0 g/dL; hematocrit, 40.0%
- Glucose, 98 mg/dL
- Prothrombin time, 12 seconds; partial thromboplastin time, 34 seconds; platelets, 350,000/mL
- Electrolytes: sodium, 136 mEq/L; potassium, 4.2 mEq/L; chloride, 107 mEq/L; carbon dioxide, 26 mEq/L
- Blood urea nitrogen, 14 mg/dL; creatinine, 0.9 mg/dL
- Computed tomography (CT) scan of head without contrast demonstrates a large epidural hematoma to the right temporal region. His cervical spine was not injured.
- Glasgow Coma Scale score = 9

Height/Weight/Vital Signs

- 183 cm, 90 kg
- Blood pressure, 170/85; heart rate, 110 beats per minute; respiration rate, 26 breaths per minute; room air saturation, 97%; temperature, 37.28°C

Pathophysiology

An epidural hematoma is considered a focal brain injury in that the damage produced by a direct mechanical impact and the acceleration–deceleration stress onto the skull and brain tissue results in skull fractures and intracranial lesions. Epidural hematoma is often caused by skull fracture and laceration of the middle meningeal artery or anterior cerebral artery, allowing bleeding to occur between the skull and dura. This condition can also result from a closed head injury. In adults, epidural hematomas are most commonly located in the temporoparietal and temporal regions of the brain.

A multitude of physiologic compensatory mechanisms are initiated in order to increase cerebral perfusion. The cardiovascular responses that are typically observed in the compensatory stage of AHI include tachycardia, hypertension, and increased cardiac output. Hypotension and decreased cardiac output are associated with substantial blood loss and/or a progressive or irreversible stage of injury. The respiratory responses that occur as a result of AHI include apnea and abnormal respiratory patterns. Respiratory insufficiency and hyperventilation frequently occur. Cerebral blood flow (CBF) and the cerebral metabolic rate of oxygen consumption ($CMRO_2$) are decreased in the core area of injury. If ICP increases, then a diffuse and more profound hypoperfusion and hypometabolism of the brain will ensue. Acute brain swelling and cerebral edema develop concomitantly after acute brain injury, which further decreases CBF resulting in cerebral ischemia. Cerebrovascular autoregulation is also impaired. The decision to perform a craniotomy for AHI is typically based on the patient's Glasgow Coma Score (GCS), pupillary examination, associated comorbidities, CT scan findings, and ICP values. After the initial injury, secondary neurologic insults such as blood–brain barrier disruption, loss of cerebral autoregulation, release of inflammatory and excitatory mediators, and oxidative stress lead to cell death.

Surgical Procedure

Evacuation of an epidural hematoma will depend on the location of the injury. A frontotemporal craniotomy is performed for most AHIs that require surgical intervention, as shown in Fig. 15.1. Once anesthetized, the patient's head is placed in a headrest of pins, suction cups, or horseshoe, based on the surgeon's preference. The scalp incision begins anterior to the tragus and continues superiorly in a question mark shape to the frontal area. The scalp is then peeled back, and the skull bone is exposed. The skull is punctured using a cranial drill at the temporal site. Additional burr holes are made in the skull, avoiding injury to the major venous structures, with the anterior burr hole being placed above the frontal sinus. A formal bone flap is then removed, allowing access to the dura, and bleeding is controlled. The dura may also be lacerated and in this instance the opening is repaired.

Depending on the degree of cerebral edema, the bone flap may or may not be reapplied at the time of surgical closure. A drain may be placed and extend through a separate incision near the surgical site. An ICP monitor may be placed at the end of surgery to monitor postoperative ICP.

Anesthetic Management and Considerations

Preoperative Period

1. *Describe the importance of establishing a patent airway and providing ventilation for a patient with an AHI presenting for craniotomy.*

    Many patients with AHI exhibit partial or complete airway obstruction caused by the tongue blocking the posterior pharyngeal space. Additionally, patients with an AHI who require a craniotomy often have a full stomach, decreased intravascular volume, and potentially a cervical spine injury. Immediate oxygenation and securing of the airway with an endotracheal tube (ETT) may be necessary during the brief and rapid preoperative assessment. If the patient is found to be hemodynamically stable, rapid sequence induction with in-line neck manual axial stabilization is appropriate; however, intubation may produce an elevation in blood pressure and ICP. In hemodynamically unstable patients, the induction drug dosages are decreased or omitted depending on level of consciousness. Once the airway is secured, a nondepolarizing muscle relaxant should be given and mechanical ventilation initiated to achieve low normocarbia and partial arterial pressure carbon dioxide ($PaCO_2$) of approximately 35 mm Hg. If cerebral edema is extreme, hypoventilation may be instituted to improve operating conditions. Prolonged and aggressive hyperventilation of $PaCO_2$ <30 mm Hg is to be avoided because hypocarbia causes cerebral vasculature constriction, which decreases CBF. CBF decreases by 1 mL/100 g brain tissue/minute for each 1 torr decrease in $PaCO_2$. Hypoxia, if present, should be corrected immediately, as decreased cerebral oxygenation is associated with poor neurologic outcomes.

2. *Discuss the importance of an initial preoperative neurologic evaluation.*

    With a diagnosis of epidural hematoma caused by an AHI, 22% to 56% of patients are comatose immediately before surgery. A lucid period, where there is wakefulness and rapid neurologic deterioration, may also be observed. A quick neurologic assessment must be performed with special attention to the level of consciousness, presence or absence of increased ICP, and extent of focal deficits.

    The GCS is a valid and reliable method for assessing neurologic status and is shown in Table 15.1. Pupillary abnormalities such as size, light reflex, and symmetry

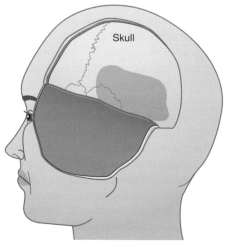

1. Incision

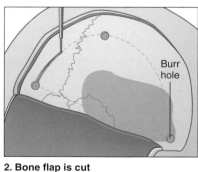

2. Bone flap is cut

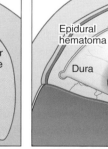

3. Evacuation of epidural hematoma

• **Fig. 15.1** Frontotemporal craniotomy performed to treat a cerebral epidural hematoma.

TABLE 15.1 Adult Glasgow Coma Scale (GCS)

Response	Score
Eye Opening (E)	
Spontaneous, open and blinking	4
To speech	3
To pain	2
None	1
Verbal Response (V)	
Oriented	5
Answers but confused	4
Inappropriate but recognizable words	3
Incomprehensible sounds	2
None	1
Best Motor Response (M)	
Obeys verbal commands	6
Localizes painful stimuli	5
Withdraws from painful stimuli	4
Decorticate posturing (upper extremity flexion)	3
Decerebrate posturing (upper extremity extension)	2
No movement	1

GCS ≤8, deep coma, severe head trauma, poor outcome; GCS 9–12, conscious patient with moderate injury; GCS >12, mild injury.

- Cushing's Triad
  1. Widening pulse pressure (increased systolic blood pressure)
  2. Bradycardia
  3. Irregular respirations
- Headache
- Nausea
- Papilledema
- Unilateral pupillary dilation
- Nystagmus
- Abducens and oculomotor palsies
- Altered level of consciousness
- Seizures

by becoming excited. The result of this excitation is an increase in systemic arterial pressure and heart rate. Cushing's triad, which includes widening pulse pressure (increased systolic blood pressure and decreased diastolic blood pressure), irregular respirations, and bradycardia, is indicative of severely elevated ICP, profound cerebral ischemia, and possible cerebral herniation. If the AHI is accompanied with significant blood loss, additional multiple systemic injuries, or late-stage recognition of injury, hypotension, and decreased cardiac output may be noted during the initial cardiovascular examination. A systolic blood pressure (SBP) of less than <100 mm Hg is associated with poor neurologic outcomes. SBP values ≥100 mm Hg for patients ≥50 years old and ≥110 mm Hg for patients <49 years old are associated with improved outcomes.

Intraoperative Period

4. *Discuss the choice of anesthetic used for induction and maintenance of anesthesia for patients presenting for craniotomy resulting from AHI.*

The primary objective for induction and maintenance of anesthesia is to decrease elevated ICP if present, optimize cerebral perfusion and oxygenation, and avoid secondary injury from hypoxia and hypotension. Laryngoscopy with ETT placement, if not already performed preoperatively, is best achieved using medications that blunt response to stimulation of laryngoscopy and decrease ICP, all while maintaining SBP ≥100 mm Hg.

- Hypnotic agents decrease ICP, $CMRO_2$, CBF, and brain metabolism. Both propofol and etomidate are good choices for induction of anesthesia in the AHI patient, provided the blood pressure at the time of induction is adequate or easily supported with fluids and vasopressors. If hemodynamic instability is present with induction, preservation of the existing blood pressure may best be achieved by administering dexmedetomidine, a potent selective alpha-2 adrenoreceptor agonist.

occur in 20% to 30% of patients presenting for craniotomy for AHI. Other presenting symptoms may include hemiparesis, decerebration, and seizures. Signs of increased ICP are included in Box 15.1. The importance of the preoperative assessment is for initial understanding of the patient's baseline neurologic status and urgency for craniotomy; however, equally important is the evaluation used for comparison of the postoperative neurologic assessment once the craniotomy is completed.

3. *Examine the initial cardiovascular changes in a patient with an AHI.*

The most common early cardiac manifestations associated with AHI include cardiac dysrhythmias, systemic hypertension, and tachycardia, possibly leading to bradycardia. Most patients with AHI initially exhibit hypertension and tachycardia, which is the central nervous system's response to brain ischemia. After AHI, blood flow to the vasomotor center in the brain may be decreased, causing cerebral ischemia. With this decrease in blood flow, the vasoconstrictor and cardioaccelerator neurons in the vasomotor center react to the ischemia

- Due to the sympathomimetic action, the administration of ketamine is relatively contraindicated in patients with increased ICP, as it increases CBF and ICP. Increasing evidence disputes this effect and shows the potentially beneficial effects of antagonism of N-methyl-D-aspartate (NMDA) receptors. Ketamine decreases the release of glutamate, and this substance is neurotoxic.

- Inhalation agents are appropriate to administer for maintaining anesthesia during craniotomy. Dissimilarities between isoflurane, desflurane, and sevoflurane regarding metabolic suppression and CBF are minor, but all have an advantageous effect of decreasing $CMRO_2$. The negative effects associated with inhalation agents are that they cause cerebrovascular dilation and increase CBF, which may further increase ICP. However, this effect is dependent on the dose administered, and with concentrations <1 minimum alveolar concentration (MAC), ICP can be maintained. The use of nitrous oxide (N_2O) is contraindicated. N_2O is a modest cerebrovascular dilator and can increase ICP and CBF. N_2O does not provide cerebral protection and may lessen the protective effects of propofol or other inhalation agents. N_2O may also contribute to expansion of a venous air embolism or pneumocephalus should these complications occur.

- Opioids are a useful part of a balanced anesthesia in craniotomy; all have negligible effects on CBF and a dose-dependent effect on cerebral metabolism. Once laryngoscopy is achieved, opioids for craniotomy due to AHI should be used conservatively, so that respiratory depression causing hypercarbia resulting in increased ICP is avoided upon emergence. Morphine and hydromorphone will be eliminated more slowly based on their fat-soluble properties and have the potential to cause respiratory depression and delay neurologic assessment due to sedation once the craniotomy is completed. Short-acting synthetic opioids, such as a remifentanil infusion used during the craniotomy, may be advocated due to the short duration of action and rapid metabolism, resulting in a shortened period of respiratory depression. This allows the anesthetist to perform a more accurate neurologic assessment at the end of the case.

- Dexmedetomidine decreases blood pressure by acting as a potent and highly selective central alpha-2 agonist. It has a synergistic effect to attenuate the stress response during surgery and anesthesia. Dexmedetomidine also decreases postoperative opioid requirements and may inhibit excitatory mediator release in the brain.

- Muscle relaxants administered during craniotomy can aid in mechanical ventilation and reduce ICP that can be caused by bucking or straining. The use of a succinylcholine in this patient population is controversial because the fasciculations caused by total body depolarization will increase ICP. If succinylcholine is

necessary for emergent control of the airway, a defasciculating dose of a nondepolarizing muscle relaxant should be administered first. If muscle relaxation is required throughout the maintenance period, all muscle relaxant medications, with the exception of pancuronium, are suitable for administration and have nominal effects on ICP, blood pressure, or heart rate. Pancuronium is not recommended due to its vagolytic effect, possibly leading to increased ICP caused by hypertension and tachycardia.

5. *Discuss methods used to decrease elevated ICP during craniotomy for AHI.*

Located within the cranium are three major components that comprise the intracerebral volume: the brain including neurons and glia, the cerebrospinal fluid (CSF) and extracellular fluid, and blood that perfuses the brain. Initially, intracranial volume can rise without causing an appreciable increase in ICP. However, there is a point (critical volume) when the cerebral volume within the cranium has reached maximum size and small increases in intracranial volume produce extreme increases in ICP that must be managed rapidly to avoid reductions in CBF and cerebral herniation. Fig. 15.2 depicts the relationship comparing intracranial volume and ICP. Removal of CSF for acutely increased ICP >22 mm Hg is recommended.

Cerebral perfusion pressure (CPP) is directly related to both mean arterial pressure (MAP) and ICP, as shown in the following equation:

$$CPP = MAP - ICP \text{ or } CVP$$

CPP, cerebral perfusion pressure;
CVP, central venous pressure;
ICP, intracranial pressure;
MAP, mean arterial pressure.

If ICP is increased and becomes greater than MAP, CPP is reduced, resulting in reduced CBF. Normal ICP is equal to or less than 10 mm Hg, and normal CPP varies between 80 and 100 mm Hg. Therefore the major determinant of CBF is MAP. Management of increased

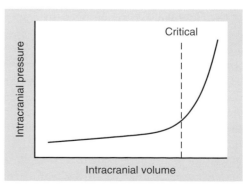

• **Fig. 15.2** Relationship comparing intracranial pressure and intracranial volume. (From Fonseca RJ: *Oral and maxillofacial surgery*, ed 3, St. Louis, 2018, Elsevier.)

ICP during craniotomy is performed using several different techniques. Ideal CPP for patients with increased ICP is between 80 and 100 mm Hg.

- Hyperventilation to a $PaCO_2$ of 25 to 30 mm Hg can be instituted as a rapid and effective method to manage severely increased ICP by decreasing CBF and the blood volume within the brain. However, prolonged hypocarbia is associated with poor neurologic outcome. CBF becomes less sensitive to the effects of hyperventilation within 24 to 48 hours.
- Periodic hyperventilation is recommended for severe increases in ICP as a temporizing measure.
- Hyperventilation should be avoided for the first 24 hours due to decreased blood flow from a loss of cerebral autoregulation.
- Diuretic therapy using mannitol, an osmotic diuretic, can provide effective ICP reduction intraoperatively. Mannitol administered as a bolus 1 g/kg over 10 minutes or slow infusion 0.25 to 1 g/kg over 20 minutes may improve CBF and oxygen delivery by reducing blood viscosity. Hypotension and hypovolemia are possible side effects with mannitol administration, and serum osmolarity must be monitored frequently if multiple doses are administered. Serum osmolarity should not exceed 320 mOsm/L. Furosemide, a loop diuretic, provides a synergistic effect with mannitol and may be administered for persistently increased ICP.
- Increasing the level of the patient's head from 10 to 30 degrees increases cerebral venous and CSF drainage, therefore lowering ICP. This position should be maintained throughout the perioperative period. Severe flexing or turning of the head may obstruct cerebral venous drainage, and increased ICP may result.
- Hypertonic saline pulls fluid from tissues into the intravascular space and can decrease cerebral edema. Hypertonic saline 3%: 250 mL can be infused IV over 30 minutes. The anesthetist should avoid hypertonic saline if the patient's serum sodium is above 160 mEq/L.

6. *Discuss fluid requirements and circulatory management for a patient having a craniotomy.*

Hypotension with SBP $\leq$100 mm Hg is a major contributor to a poor neurologic outcome after acute brain injury. Fluid resuscitation and circulatory management should begin immediately, and inotropic and vasopressor medications should be considered to stabilize blood pressure if hypotension ensues. Administration of dopamine or phenylephrine infusions are recommended to maintain CPP 60 to 110 mm Hg. A bolus dose of a vasopressor must be used cautiously, as a sudden increase in blood pressure can elevate ICP. Hypertension may be caused by the Cushing reflex, which causes sympathetic nervous system hyperactivity in response to increased ICP. This event is associated with profound bradycardia caused by baroreceptor activation. Before treating the hypertension, heart rate along with adequate oxygenation and anesthetic depth should be considered.

Fluid resuscitation should be guided by assessing blood pressure, urinary output, and central venous pressure (CVP) readings if available. Rapid administration of crystalloid and colloid solutions to restore intravascular volume should be monitored to achieve an CPP >60 mm Hg, while trying to avoid additional brain swelling.

Glucose-containing solutions, such as Ringer's lactate, should be avoided in acute brain injured patients undergoing craniotomy because hyperglycemia is associated with poor neurologic outcomes caused by further intracellular acidosis. Ringer's lactate solution, which is slightly hypotonic and contains glucose, promotes swelling in uninjured portions of the brain. Therefore the crystalloid of choice to be given via rapid infusion is isotonic normal saline.

Monitoring the coagulation status should be performed because patients with an AHI are at higher risk for developing coagulopathies. Blood transfusions may be necessary, and although there is not one absolute hemoglobin or hematocrit value that mandates transfusion, patients with hematocrit below 30% may need a transfusion to promote oxygen delivery to the brain. Careful fluid resuscitation using crystalloid solutions and blood products must be assessed to minimize cerebral swelling. Blood pressure, urine output, and CVP readings may become crucial to assess the need for blood product or fluid based on the intravascular volume status.

7. *Describe the effects of temperature on patients with increased ICP.*

Hypothermia is believed to reduce metabolic demand, suppress excitatory neurotransmitters, diminish free radical formation, and reduce edema of the brain. A decrease of each degree Celsius decreases $CMRO_2$ by 7%. The benefits of controlled hypothermia for cerebral protection remain controversial. There is a lack of high-quality evidence that mild to moderate hypothermia improves meaningful long-term outcomes. The potential side effects associated with induced hypothermia include hypotension, cardiac arrhythmias, pneumonia, and coagulopathies. However, hyperthermia is definitively associated with poor neurologic outcome. Hyperthermia depletes adenosine triphosphate (ATP) stores and increases calcium influx into cells. Often, AHI patients' thermoregulatory processes are disrupted, and hyperthermia persists, which can be detrimental to recovery. The secondary effects associated with hypothermia to decrease ICP such as coagulopathy and pneumonia are the reason that it is not routinely recommended.

8. *Identify intraoperative monitoring modalities used during craniotomy for AHI.*

Standard American Society of Anesthesiologists (ASA) monitors are essential for the intraoperative monitoring. Additionally, intraarterial blood pressure measurement, CVP monitoring, and urine output are used.

Intraarterial line measurement is necessary for management of CPP and to assess the correlation between arterial blood gases measurements, especially $PaCO_2$

with the $ETCO_2$ display via capnography. The intraarterial transducer should be placed at the level of the tragus of the ear at the external auditory canal to improve accuracy. Arterial blood pressure monitoring also allows for measurement of hematocrit, electrolytes, glucose, and serum osmolarity.

A CVP catheter is often inserted intraoperatively for a craniotomy for AHI. These patients are at risk for fluid volume deficits, and CVP monitoring allows for intraoperative fluid volume management. The CVP catheter can be placed in an antecubital vein, subclavian vein, or internal jugular vein. Placement depends on the risk of venous air embolism (VAE) during surgery and whether the patient can tolerate their head being placed in a dependent position during the insertion process. If the patient has a possible risk for VAE, the location of choice for the CVP catheter placement is subclavian, with the tip of the CVP catheter located 3 cm below the right atrium–superior vena cava junction in the heart. This is the optimal location to withdraw air from the CVP catheter if a VAE occurs during opening of the venous sinuses of the brain.

Doppler ultrasound is frequently used to monitor for VAE during craniotomy. The Doppler is placed between the third and sixth intercostal spaces on the right sternal border, and auditory classic mill wheel murmur is monitored throughout surgery. During craniotomy for AHI, air can potentially enter the circulation through defects in the skull such as burr holes or pin holes from the head holder and when the head is positioned 10 cm above the midthorax. Doppler ultrasound is a sensitive, noninvasive method for detecting a VAE.

Postoperative Period

The total operative time of the surgical craniotomy for evacuation of epidural hematoma after AHI was 240 minutes. In the operating room, the patient demonstrated the following evaluation: delayed awakening, irregular respiratory pattern, blood pressure of 108/62, respiratory rate of 1/min, inadequately low tidal volume respirations, heart rate of 65 beats per minute, room air saturation of 98%, and temperature of 35.5°C.

9. *List potential postoperative complications and diagnostic criteria after craniotomy for AHI.*

Potential postoperative complications after craniotomy include:

- **Delayed awakening:** Consider preoperative neurologic baseline and residual anesthetic effects, allowing at least 2 hours for residual anesthesia to metabolize and fully reverse muscle paralysis; consider the amount of opioid use intraoperatively and need for naloxone.
- **Hypothermia:** Slow active rewarming with forced-air warming device.
- **Seizures:** This is a significant incidence of postoperative seizure activity after acute head injury and increased ICP. Treatment with an antiseizure drug such as a loading dose of phenytoin 1 g given intravenously slowly can avoid developing hypotension.
- **Postoperative cerebral edema:** Continued administration of mannitol or furosemide postoperatively, limit fluids, monitor CVP readings, position patient with head up 10 to 30 degrees; patients demonstrating hydrocephalus may require a shunt procedure to decrease the volume of CSF within the cerebral ventricles.
- **Metabolic or electrolyte disturbances:** Obtain postoperative electrolytes and carefully correct imbalances such as glucose, sodium, and potassium, especially after mannitol and furosemide administration.
- **Hematoma:** Evaluate with CT scan of head, obtain coagulation studies, and administer fresh frozen plasma and platelets if necessary to correct coagulopathy.
- **Irregular respiratory pattern and inability to extubate:** Consider brainstem ischemia; evaluation of this complication includes a CT scan of the head.

Treatment for this patient postoperatively would include continuous ventilatory support in the intensive care unit, hourly neurologic evaluations, sedation, a CT scan of the head, fluid volume management, and circulatory support to maintain CPP 60 to 70 mm Hg, along with serial blood draws.

Review Questions

1. Which interventions can be used to manage severely increased ICP? (Choose two.)
   a. Administration of mannitol
   b. Hyperventilation
   c. CSF drainage
   d. Administration of etomidate
2. Cerebral perfusion pressure is determined by which two factors?
   a. MAP and urine output
   b. CVP measurement
   c. MAP and ICP
   d. ICP only
3. A systolic value of _____ mm Hg is a major contributor to poor neurologic outcome after craniotomy for AHI.
   a. ≤100
   b. ≤120
   c. ≤80
   d. ≤90

4. Which crystalloid solution should be avoided in acute head injured patients presenting for craniotomy?
   a. Normal saline
   b. Albumin
   c. Ringer's lactate
   d. Packed red blood cells

5. Headache, nausea, papilledema, unilateral pupillary dilation, abducens, and oculomotor palsies are symptoms that are associated with:
   a. Increased ICP.
   b. Decreased cerebral perfusion.
   c. Cervical spine injury.
   d. Hypovolemia.

Suggested Readings

Colton K, Yang S, Hu PF, Chen HH, Stansbury LG, Scalea TM, Stein DM. Responsiveness to therapy for increased intracranial pressure in traumatic brain injury is associated with neurological outcome. *Injury.* 2014;45(12):2084–2088.

Colton K, Yang S, Hu PF, Chen HH, Bonds B, Scalea TM, Stein DM. Intracranial pressure response after pharmacologic treatment of intracranial hypertension. *J Trauma Acute Care Surg.* 2014;77(1):47–53.

Cottrell JE. Succinylcholine and intracranial pressure. *Anesthesiology.* 2018;129(6):1159–1162.

Donnelly J, Smielewski P, Adams H, Zeiler FA, Cardim D, et al. Observations on the cerebral effects of refractory intracranial hypertension after severe traumatic brain injury. *Neurocrit Care.* 2020;32(2):437–447.

Elf K, Nilsson P, Ronne-Engstrom E, et al. Temperature disturbances in traumatic brain injury: relationship to secondary insults, barbiturate treatment and outcomes. *Neurolog Res.* 2008;30(10):1097–1105.

Farrell D, Bendo A. Perioperative management of severe traumatic brain injury: what is new? *Curr Anesthesiol Rep.* 2018;8(3): 279–289.

Meyfroidt G, Baguley IJ, Menon DK. Paroxysmal sympathetic hyperactivity: the storm after acute brain injury. *Lancet Neurol.* 2017; 16(9):721–729.

Steinberg GK, Dodd RL, Karim SA, et al. Craniotomy for trauma. In: Jaffe RA, Samuels SI, Schmiesing CA, Golianu B. eds. *Anesthesiologist's Manual of Surgical Procedures,* 5th ed. Philadelphia: Lippincott Williams and Wilkins, 2014:37–40.

Seppelt I. Intracranial hypertension after traumatic brain injury. *Indian J Crit Care Med.* 2004;8:120–126.

Tripathy S, Ahmad SR. Raised intracranial pressure syndrome: a stepwise approach. *Indian J Crit Care Med.* 2019;23(Suppl 2):S129–S135.

16

Penetrating Traumatic Injuries

KEY POINTS

- The severity of injuries that are produced by penetrating trauma vary from minor to life threatening.
- Penetrating injuries can occur from a variety of objects, including gunshot wounds (GSWs), stab wounds, or projectiles from a shotgun blast.

- Control of the airway and resuscitative interventions are the anesthetist's primary objectives when caring for a patient with a penetrating traumatic injury.

Case Synopsis

A 22-year-old man with a GSW to the abdomen is being treated in the emergency department. The entrance wound is observed in the left lower quadrant as a small hole with mild bleeding. The exit wound is present in the right upper flank on the back with moderate bleeding. He is scheduled for a diagnostic laparotomy. He is alert, talking, and states that he is having severe abdominal pain.

Preoperative Evaluation and Demographic Data

Past Medical/Surgical History

- Tonsillectomy age 5 years, no known complications

List of Medications

- Admits to smoking marijuana yesterday

Diagnostic Data

- Hemoglobin, 10.1 g/dL; hematocrit, 30.5%
- Platelets, 235,000 per microliter
- Electrolytes: sodium, 141 mEq/L; potassium, 3.9 mEq/L; chloride, 107 mEq/L; carbon dioxide, 25 mEq/L
- Blood glucose, 97 mg/dL
- Computed tomography (CT) scan reveals blood in the peritoneum

Height/Weight/Vital Signs

- 173 cm, 73 kg
- Blood pressure, 136/91; heart rate, 121 beats per minute; respiratory rate, 20 breaths per minute; room air oxygen saturation, 100% on facemask O_2 at 15 liter/min flow; temperature, 36°C

Pathophysiology

Penetrating trauma caused by a GSW has the potential to cause a tremendous amount of tissue destruction. The resulting damage is dependent on the type of instrument or projectile (e.g., knife, bullet, or fragment), the velocity of the projectile at the time of impact, and the characteristics of the tissue through which the projectile passes (e.g., fat, muscle, nervous tissue, bone, blood vessels, or organs). The amount of damage caused is a result of the amount of energy transferred to the body tissue. This phenomenon is explained by Newton's law of kinetic energy, as shown in the following equation:

$$\text{Kinetic energy} = 1/2 \ (\text{Mass} \times \text{Velocity}^2)$$

Whereas doubling the projectile's mass will double the energy, doubling the projectile's velocity will *quadruple* the energy.

When a high-velocity projectile enters body tissue, it creates a permanent and a temporary cavity, as illustrated in Fig. 16.1. High-velocity projectiles are classified as those traveling greater than 750 m/s. The permanent cavity is created by direct contact with the projectile. This is the area that experiences the greatest amount of tissue damage. Projectiles usually follow a tumbling motion, known as *yaw*, within the tissue, which can increase tissue destruction. The temporary cavity is created by the transfer of kinetic energy from the projectile to surrounding tissues (like an energy shock wave). The higher the velocity of the projectile, the more kinetic energy transferred and the greater the production of energy, which causes tissues to stretch and tear beyond the radius of the projectile, as shown in Fig. 16.1. This effect is very brief, lasting only a few milliseconds.

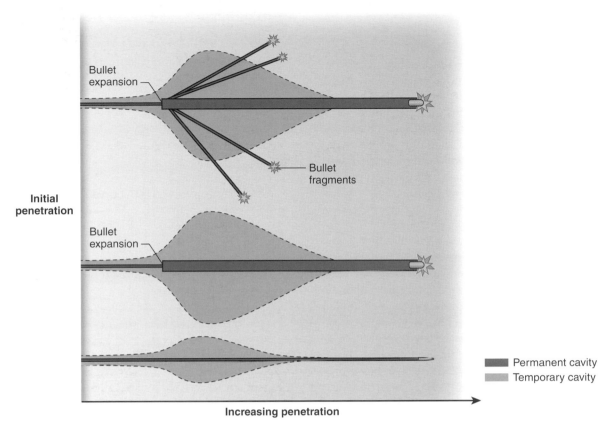

Bullet
expansion

Bullet
fragments

Initial
penetration

Bullet
expansion

Permanent cavity
Temporary cavity

Increasing penetration

• **Fig. 16.1** The cavities produced as a penetrating missile passes through tissue. (Redrawn from Caudell JN: Review of wound ballistic research and its applicability to wildlife management, *Wildlife Society Bulletin* 37[4]:824–831, 2013.)

Projectiles may fragment and ricochet within the body, damaging other structures. Solid and dense organs tend to shatter, and they are disrupted to a greater degree by high-velocity projectiles and the temporary cavity created by the transfer of kinetic energy. Elastic tissue can be directly injured or stretched and damaged by the temporary cavity. The risk of infection and sepsis is high if certain organs, such as the bowel, are ruptured or perforated. The wound can become contaminated from dirt, debris, or clothing, which is due to a vacuum effect caused by the velocity of the penetrating object. Finally, bleeding from damaged blood vessels or organs into the abdominal cavity is potentially life threatening.

Surgical Procedure

Exploratory or diagnostic laparotomy is used to visualize and examine the structures inside of the abdominal cavity to determine the extent of injury or source of pain and to perform repairs if needed. A GSW to the abdomen is an indication for an exploratory laparotomy. However, a significant number of such injuries may be managed in a non–operating room setting. The small intestine is most frequently injured, followed by the colon and liver. Sometimes a single incision extending from the xiphoid process to pubic symphysis is used, especially during trauma surgery. An upper midline incision extends from the xiphoid process to the umbilicus,

and a lower midline incision is limited by the umbilicus superiorly and by the pubic symphysis inferiorly. The midline incision allows wide access to most of the abdominal cavity. The objectives of a laparotomy are to locate and control hemorrhage, identify bowel injuries and manage fecal contamination within the peritoneum, locate and manage injuries to organs or supporting structures, and, finally, to determine whether definitive repair is needed.

Anesthetic Management and Considerations

Preoperative Period

1. *Discuss the importance of a head-to-toe physical examination for this patient.*

   A trauma assessment consisting of A (airway), B (breathing), C (circulation), D (disability), and E (exposure) allows the anesthetist to identify deficiencies in airway, breathing, or circulation, as well as to assess the possibility of tissues and/or organs damaged. Each part of the body should be inspected and palpated for pain, tenderness, crepitus, or injury, including the posterior when patients are supine. In critically ill trauma patients, assessment and treatment of traumatic injuries occur concomitantly by a trauma team.

2. *Identify the rationale for administering antibiotics during the preoperative period.*

Traumatic injuries can introduce pathogens into the body. Pathogens may enter the body via the penetrating object, the skin, the victim's clothing, any foreign material that enters or gets sucked into the wound, or by the perforation and spillage of stomach or colon contents into the peritoneum. A broad-spectrum antibiotic, which covers gram-positive and gram-negative bacteria, such as a third- or fourth-generation cephalosporin agent combined with metronidazole (Flagyl), is recommended by the American College of Surgeons to treat wound contamination and infection.

3. *Describe the types of monitoring that are required during exploratory laparotomy for a gunshot wound.*

Electrocardiograph (ECG), noninvasive blood pressure, and pulse oximetry are often initiated in prehospital treatment and continued throughout emergency treatment and the perioperative period. End tidal carbon dioxide should be monitored once the airway is controlled, and because the patient can rapidly loose heat, core temperature monitoring should be initiated. Depending on the severity of the injury and the intraoperative course, additional monitoring may include invasive blood pressure monitoring via an arterial catheter, central line placement with central venous pressure monitoring, and placement and/or intracranial pressure monitoring via an intraventricular catheter or a subarachnoid bolt.

4. *Discuss the need for intravenous (IV) access that is required for this injury.*

At least two large-bore IVs (14 to 18 gauge) should be placed during initial assessment in the upper extremities. Additional large-bore IV catheters should be placed if multiple fluid and blood product administration is anticipated. The external or internal jugular, femoral, or subclavian veins can be considered for central venous catheter placement. A level I transfusion infuser should be available for rapid administration of fluid and blood products.

5. *Discuss which laboratory values should be monitored.*

Serial laboratory evaluation should include hemoglobin, hematocrit, and platelets; serum chemical constituents, including sodium, potassium, magnesium, carbon dioxide, blood urea nitrogen, creatinine, and calcium; and serum coagulation studies consisting of prothrombin time, international normalized ratio (INR), and partial thromboplastin time. If major hemorrhaging occurs, large blood transfusions are instituted, or the patient's medication regimen dictates, these values should be repeated as long as clinically relevant. Additionally, blood glucose and arterial blood gas values should be continuously evaluated.

If a significant amount of banked blood is transfused, the patient may develop acute hypocalcemia. The preservative that is used to store blood is citrate, phosphate, dextrose, and adenine (CPDA). Citrate chelates or binds free ionized calcium, decreasing its availability for physiologic functioning. The symptoms associated with acute hypocalcemia are listed in Box 16.1. The treatment for acute hypocalcemia is to administer IV calcium chloride.

> **• BOX 16.1 Symptoms Associated With Acute Hypocalcemia**
>
> - Perioral tingling (early symptom of hypocalcemia)
> - Paresthesia (early symptom of hypocalcemia)
> - Tetany
> - Muscle spasms
> - Weakness
> - Hyperactive tendon reflexes
> - Laryngospasm
> - Bronchospasm
> - Hypotension
> - Cardiac dysrhythmias
> - ECG changes (prolonged QT interval, widened QRS complex, and/or flattened T wave)

Administration of calcium should be guided by serial blood calcium values.

6. *Compare and contrast the injuries that are caused by high-velocity missile (HVM) and low-velocity missile (LVM) wounds.*

LVMs travel at lower velocities, between 100 and 300 m/s, and exert a relatively low amount of energy, between 10 and 300 joules. LVMs crush and lacerate the surrounding tissues and structures that are in their path to form a drill hole wound, known as the permanent cavity. This cavity approximates the same diameter as the bullet. They produce a small temporary cavity, and these types of missiles may fragment or ricochet within the body, damaging other structures.

HVMs travel at greater than 750 m/s and exert a greater amount of energy, between 2000 and 3000 joules. The amount of energy transferred to surrounding tissues can create a temporary cavity 10 to 20 times the size of the permanent cavity during an HVM injury. An illustration of an HVM wound is shown in Fig. 16.1. The temporary cavity expands and collapses in a very short period, causing tissues to stretch and tear. Additionally, debris can be sucked into the wound, consequently leading to wound infection.

7. *Describe how tetrahydrocannabinol (THC) affects anesthesia during both acute and chronic use.*

The main substance that causes the drug effect in marijuana is THC. THC is extremely lipid soluble with a half-life of up to 59 hours. Acute marijuana use decreases the anesthetic requirement (decreasing minimum alveolar concentration [MAC]) due to its central nervous system depressant effects. Chronic use (this patient denies currently using) increases the anesthetic requirement (increasing MAC) due to liver enzyme induction. Similar to smoking cigarettes, chronic marijuana smoke can increase secretion production and airway hyperactivity, result in alveolar destruction, and decrease lung compliance consistent with chronic obstructive pulmonary disease.

8. *Describe how acute alcohol intoxication and chronic abuse affects anesthesia.*

Acute ingestion of alcohol decreases the anesthetic requirements (decreasing MAC) due to its depressant

TABLE 16.1	Physiologic Effects and Anesthetic Considerations Associated With Acute Substance Abuse	
	Substance Physiologic Effects	Anesthetic Considerations
CNS Stimulants		
Cocaine and amphetamines	Tachycardia, hypertension, dysrhythmias, mydriasis, hyperreflexia, euphoria, hyperpyrexia, sweating	May require increased doses of anesthetic agents; amphetamine users may have loose or rotting teeth
Phencyclidine (PCP) and lysergic acid diethylamide (LSD)	Tachycardia, hypertension, hallucinations, weak analgesic effects, psychosis in high doses	May require increased doses of anesthetic agents; PCP produces dissociative anesthesia with increased doses
CNS Depressants		
Cannabis	Tachycardia, labile blood pressure, euphoria, dysphoria, hunger	May require decreased doses of anesthetic agents; may exhibit hyperactive airway and increased secretions
Opioids	Respiratory depression, hypotension, bradycardia, constipation, euphoria, miosis	May require decreased doses of anesthetic agents; IV access may be difficult in heroin users

effects. Additionally, alcohol has an inhibitory effect on the release of antidiuretic hormone. Therefore patients who have consumed a large amount of alcohol can develop hypovolemia. This fact coupled with the vasodilation and myocardial depression associated with inhaled anesthetic agents can result in severe hypotension, especially if the situation is complicated due to hemorrhage. There is the potential for withdrawal, resulting in tremors or seizures during the postoperative course. Long-acting benzodiazepines, such as diazepam (Valium) and chlordiazepoxide (Librium), have been shown to be a safe and effective treatment for alcohol withdrawal. Chronic ingestion of alcohol increases the anesthetic requirement (increasing MAC) due to enzyme induction. Long-term abuse can result in hepatocellular degeneration and decreased production of coagulation factors.

9. *Describe how acute and chronic use of stimulants such as amphetamines or cocaine affects anesthesia.*

Acute ingestion of stimulants, such as cocaine or amphetamines, increases the anesthetic requirement (increasing MAC) due to stimulation of the sympathetic nervous system. These chemical substances are thought to increase the release or decrease the reuptake of catecholamines from postsynaptic adrenergic nerve terminals. Intense vasoconstriction occurs as a result of continuous catecholamine stimulation. When anesthesia is administered, there is a potential for severe hypotension due to vasodilation, especially in the presence of hypovolemia.

Chronic use decreases or has a minimal effect on the anesthetic requirement due to continual sympathetic nervous system stimulation and the possible depletion of catecholamines. For patients who are acutely intoxicated or chronically misusing stimulants, it is recommended that use of a direct-acting vasopressor, such as phenylephrine, be administered. A summation of the

physiologic effects and their influence on anesthetic management is presented in Table 16.1.

Intraoperative Period

10. *Describe the physiologic changes that are associated with induction of anesthesia in a hypovolemic patient.*

Anesthesia induction agents (with the exception of ketamine and, to a lesser degree, etomidate) cause direct myocardial depression and decrease systemic vascular resistance in a dose-dependent manner. Even mild decreases in systemic vascular resistance in the presence of significant hypovolemia can lead to severe hypotension. The anesthetic management for severe hypotension should be individualized to the specific patient. However, decreasing the anesthetic depth, infusing fluids or blood products, and considering administering a vasopressor should be considered.

11. *Discuss the physiologic consequences of aspiration in the trauma patient.*

Trauma patients are at risk for aspiration as a result of the possibility of a full stomach and the potential for decreased airway reflexes. Aspiration of gastric contents can lead to pulmonary aspiration, aspiration pneumonitis, airway obstruction, and hypoxemia.

12. *Construct a plan as it relates to induction of anesthesia for this patient.*

Initiating a fluid bolus of 500 mL before induction in order to decrease the severity of hypotension is prudent. A hemodynamic goal should include maintenance of systolic blood pressure greater than 90 mm Hg. Oxygen (O_2) administration at 100% should be given at least 5 minutes before induction of anesthesia to increase the hemoglobin O_2 saturation during the period of apnea after induction. The goal of preoxygenation is to achieve an SpO_2 value of greater than 90%.

Suction should be readily available. A rapid sequence induction using cricoid pressure is the standard of care in all trauma patients. Succinylcholine or rocuronium may be used for neuromuscular blockade. Propofol, in small doses, may be used if blood pressure is stable. Hypnotics, such as midazolam, may be administered to prevent recall or to provide sedation for patients who are anxious. Narcotics are frequently used because traumatic injuries can cause severe pain.

13. *Discuss the intraoperative anesthetic maintenance for this patient.*

Administration of sedative and amnesic medications should be titrated according to the patient's blood pressure. A high percentage of oxygen should be administered throughout the perioperative course due to the possibility of decreased tissue perfusion. Nondepolarizing muscle relaxation should be provided to facilitate abdominal exposure during exploratory laparotomy. Anesthetic maintenance can be achieved using inhalational agents or in combination with IV medications such as propofol, ketamine, dexmedetomidine, and opioids, and these medications should be titrated to the hemodynamic response. If the trauma patient cannot sustain an adequate blood pressure while anesthetic agents are being administered, these medications should be abandoned in favor of hemodynamic support while maintaining adequate neuromuscular blockade.

The patient with a major traumatic injury has a 10% to 43% chance of intraoperative recall. Scopolamine 0.2 to 0.4 mg administered intramuscularly (IM) or IV can help prevent recall if other hypnotic medications cannot be administered because of the patient's critical hemodynamic profile. Scopolamine crosses the blood–brain barrier, and it can cause amnesia within 10 minutes of administration for up to 2 hours.

14. *Explain the risks associated with administering nitrous oxide (N_2O) for the trauma patient.*

The use of nitrous oxide can be problematic because it is highly diffusible and has a propensity to accumulate in closed air spaces. If administered, it can worsen gas-containing conditions such as pneumothorax, pneumocephalus, air embolism, or obstructed bowel. These conditions may not occur, but over time the effects of nitrous oxide may become clinically relevant. For these reasons nitrous oxide is best avoided in the trauma patient.

15. *Examine the use of various IV fluids and blood products for a trauma patient.*

Crystalloid solutions such as lactated Ringer's and sodium chloride are used as initial volume expanders while awaiting blood for transfusion. The intravascular half-life of crystalloids is 20 to 30 minutes. Large volumes of crystalloid administration should be calculated and based on the patient's kilogram weight. Overzealous IV hydration can cause acute pulmonary edema and dilutional thrombocytopenia. Colloid solutions such as albumin are administered for intravascular fluid deficits before the arrival of blood for transfusion or for conditions associated with large protein losses (i.e., burn injuries). Blood products such as packed red blood cells (PRBCs), fresh frozen plasma (FFP), platelets, and cryoprecipitate are used to replace blood and clotting factors, which can become deficient in the trauma patient. The patient's specific blood type should be evaluated and requested from the blood bank for administration. If life-threatening hypovolemia ensues, O negative blood can be used for immediate transfusion.

The anesthetist should be aware that when administering large volumes of PRBCs (greater than 5 units), FFP and platelets should be added to avoid or treat coagulation abnormalities. Thromboelastography (TEG) can be used to assess coagulation status, and its use is indicated in this scenario. The most common cause of continuous bleeding after extreme volume resuscitation is dilutional thrombocytopenia. Patients with decreasing platelet values of less than 100,000 microliters should receive a platelet transfusion. The anesthetist should consider infusing 2 to 4 units of FFP and 4 to 6 units of platelets after infusion of 8 to 10 units of PRBCs (1 blood volume in a 70-kg person). Cryoprecipitate, which contains factor VIII, von Willebrand factor, and fibrinogen, can be used to treat thrombocytopenia and/or hypofibrinogenemia.

16. *List the signs and symptoms of intraoperative hemorrhage.*

The signs and symptoms associated with acute hemorrhage include:

- Hypotension
- Tachycardia
- Decreased urine output
- Decreased central venous pressure/pulmonary capillary wedge pressure
- Diminishing hematocrit values

Repeated surgical suctioning, use of multiple saturated lap-sponge pads, blood in the surgical field, and/or blood around the surgical field are further evidence of large amounts of blood loss. Some trauma patients can have a severe decrease in blood pressure caused by additional hemorrhage after incision because of the release of a blood clot that has been causing a tamponade effect within the abdominal vasculature.

17. *Discuss the potential adverse effects of a massive blood transfusion.*

Coagulopathies can develop from dilution of coagulation factors from massive IV fluid and blood product administration. Hypothermia can occur due to cold IV fluid and/or blood administration. A blood transfusion reaction can result if there is an incompatibility with the blood products that are administered. Anaphylaxis can develop due to antibody/antigen reactions. Hypocalcemia can arise from large amounts of banked blood being infused. Calcium is needed during myocardial contractile excitation coupling, and hypocalcemia can cause further hypotension by decreasing myocardial

TABLE 16.2	Characteristics of Stored Packed Red Blood Cells
Sodium citrate	Can lead to decreased levels of ionized calcium due to chelation of the serum ionized calcium; initially acidic, sodium citrate is converted to sodium bicarbonate in the liver and can lead to metabolic alkalosis
Deficient in platelets and clotting factors	Can lead to dilutional coagulopathy
Decreased levels of 2,3 DPG	Large replacements of 2,3 DPG–depleted blood may cause hemoglobin to have increased affinity for oxygen, leading to decreased cellular oxygenation
Increased levels of potassium	Can lead to hyperkalemia in rapid, massive blood transfusion
Microaggregates	Can cause obstruction in small capillaries (i.e., pulmonary vasculature)
Stored at 4°C	Hypothermia

contractility. Hyperkalemia may occur, though it is rare, from the high-potassium concentration contained in the banked blood preservative and from cellular breakdown. Infectious disease transmission is a potential complication. A summary of the characteristics of PRBCs is included in Table 16.2.

18. *Compare and contrast the types of vasopressor medications used to maintain blood pressure in a hypovolemic, hypotensive trauma patient.*

Ephedrine is a direct- and indirect-acting vasopressor. It may not be as efficacious as a direct-acting vasopressor due to the trauma patient's potential depletion of sympathetic neurotransmitters (catecholamines), especially for those patients using stimulants. Phenylephrine is a direct-acting vasopressor that can directly stimulate sympathetic receptors and cause increases in systemic vascular resistance. Inotropic agents such as dopamine and small intermittent boluses of epinephrine or norepinephrine can be used to positively stimulate sympathetic alpha- and beta-receptors on the heart and blood vessels, resulting in increases in blood pressure and heart rate. Additionally, epinephrine in advanced cardiac life support (ACLS) doses is used in emergency situations for resuscitative efforts.

19. *List the potential complications associated with a GSW to the abdomen.*
   - Soft tissue injury
   - Severe hemorrhage from vascular injury
   - Solid organ injury
   - Hollow organ injury
   - Diaphragm injury
   - Musculoskeletal injury
   - Infection and sepsis
   - Hypovolemia
   - Spinal cord injury
   - Death

20. *List the organs that can be injured by a GSW to the abdomen.*
   - Liver
   - Spleen
   - Small bowel
   - Large bowel
   - Stomach
   - Bladder

21. *List the organs that can be injured by a projectile in the retroperitoneal region.*
   - Kidneys
   - Pancreas
   - Aorta and/or vena cava

22. *Discuss the surgical goals during a laparotomy for a penetrating abdominal injury.*

The primary goal of a laparotomy for a penetrating abdominal injury is to stop hemorrhage. This is accomplished by initially locating injuries such as vascular damage, organ damage and/or structural injuries, and controlling hemorrhage. Other goals include controlling fecal contamination from damaged organs and determining whether temporary repair (damage control surgery) or definitive repair of an injury should occur.

23. *Explain the concept of damage control surgery (DCS).*

The decision to provide DCS is made due to life-threatening injuries that necessitate a rapid decision to move the patient to the operating room for emergency surgery. The philosophy of DCS consists of controlling hemorrhage, preventing contamination, limiting sepsis, and providing protection from further injury. It provides time to improve the physiologic state of the trauma patient until a more definitive surgical repair can be accomplished.

24. *Explain the difference between penetrating injuries that occur to solid organs compared with hollow organs.*

Solid organs such as the liver and spleen are more vascular, are denser, and are more rigid compared with hollow organs such as the stomach and intestines. A penetrating injury to a solid organ causes shattering or fracturing, which can lead to severe hemorrhage. A penetrating injury to a hollow organ leads to a perforation and spillage of contents into the peritoneum that can cause severe infections, which may lead to sepsis.

25. *Explain how a patient with a penetrating abdominal injury would be at risk for developing sepsis.*

    Intestinal perforation causes spillage of fecal matter and bacteria into the peritoneum. Sepsis can develop in as little as 2 to 4 hours after colon injury. The peritoneum may also be contaminated by bacteria from the penetrating object and/or foreign material from the skin. Thus removal of the contaminating substance, irrigation of the peritoneal cavity, and serial antibiotic administration are essential.

26. *Discuss the potential complications associated with a GSW in the thoracic region.*
    - Soft tissue damage
    - Pneumothorax
    - Hemothorax
    - Tension pneumothorax or hemothorax
    - Lung contusion
    - Cardiac tamponade
    - Cardiac contusion
    - Direct cardiac injury from projectile
    - Aorta and/or vena cava laceration or transection
    - Tracheobronchial laceration or transaction
    - Esophageal laceration or transaction
    - Diaphragmatic injury
    - Rib fracture
    - Spinal cord injury
    - Death

27. *Describe the physiologic alterations in ventilation in a patient with a penetrating abdominal injury.*

    Sympathetic nervous system stimulation in response to trauma causes the patient's heart rate and blood pressure to increase, causing an increase in myocardial oxygen demand. The compensatory mechanism includes increasing minute ventilation. A rapid shallow pattern of breathing is not uncommon as a result of pain in the abdominal region or because of a direct lung injury. Additionally, abdominal organ injuries can lead to severe hypovolemia resulting in hypotension, which can cause loss of consciousness and apnea.

28. *Describe the physiologic alterations in ventilation in a patient with a penetrating thoracic injury.*

    Pneumothorax, hemothorax, or tension pneumothorax/hemothorax can lead to hypoventilation, hypoxia, and ventilation–perfusion mismatches. Open chest injuries can lead to sucking chest wounds when air enters the thoracic cavity but is unable to leave, therefore worsening lung compression and hypoxia. Lung contusions, rib fractures, or diaphragmatic injuries can cause hypoventilation and hypoxia. Tracheobronchial disruption can cause life-threatening hypoxia and/or subcutaneous emphysema.

29. *Describe the physiologic alterations in ventilation during and after an exploratory laparotomy with a large midline incision.*

    Manipulation of abdominal organs during open laparotomy, use of general anesthesia, and administration of neuromuscular blockade can cause pressure on the diaphragm and lungs, decreasing volumes and functional residual capacity and increasing inspiratory pressures. Edema from tissue damage may lead to abdominal compartment syndrome, preventing laparotomy closure and creating pressure on the diaphragm and lungs. The increased diaphragmatic pressure increases inspiratory pressures and decreases functional residual capacity, promoting atelectasis and hypoventilation. Excessive narcotic administration can lead to bradypnea or apnea. The physiologic consequences of hypoventilation can lead to hypercarbia, decreased tissue oxygenation, acidosis, and death.

30. *Discuss the physiologic implications of hypothermia during exploratory laparotomy.*

    The trauma patient is at risk of developing hypothermia due to exposure to the environment and/or the administration of cold IV fluids. Conductive heat loss can be caused by cold beds and gurneys. Clothing is removed in order to fully assess the extent of injuries, which results in radiative heat loss. The patient is exposed to convective heat loss from cold emergency and operating rooms. Physiologic alterations caused by hypothermia include:
    - Impaired cardiorespiratory function
    - Impaired coagulation
    - Impaired hepatorenal function
    - Decreased drug clearance
    - Impaired immune response
    - Impaired wound healing

    Additionally, the oxyhemoglobin disassociation curve is shifted to the left during periods of hypothermia. The result is a greater affinity or a tighter bond between oxygen and hemoglobin that decreases oxygen delivery to the tissues.

31. *Develop a plan to minimize heat loss and prevent hypothermia in a trauma patient.*

    Preexisting hypothermia is common in the trauma patient and is attributable to environmental exposure before entering the hospital, during resuscitative efforts in the emergency department, and during the operative procedure. Interventions used to treat or minimize hypothermia include:
    - Removing wet clothing
    - Warming the operating room
    - Using forced-air warmers
    - Warming IV fluids
    - Warming/humidifying airway gases
    - Heating peritoneal or pleural lavage fluids
    - Extracorporeal rewarming (i.e., hemodialysis or cardiopulmonary bypass)

Postoperative Period

32. *Describe the risks associated with extubation after open laparotomy and repair of a penetrating injury.*

    Complications from penetrating trauma and massive blood transfusions can cause acid–base disturbances, coagulopathies, and hypothermia, which may render the patient unable to maintain adequate oxygenation and ventilation without assistance. In addition, large amounts of fluid volume and/or blood replacement may lead to third spacing and pulmonary edema; this may cause a decrease in pulmonary compliance and functional residual capacity, rendering the patient susceptible to oxygen desaturation. Finally, a large midline incision has the potential to cause intense postoperative pain, which can lead to hypoventilation, atelectasis, hypercarbia, and acidosis. The decision to extubate the patient should be individualized to each specific situation and is best guided by factors such as arterial blood gas values, the extent of the injury and surgical intervention, other associated traumatic injuries, current hemodynamic status, and amount of volume resuscitation.

33. *Explain the concerns for postoperative pain management after penetrating abdominal injury.*

Narcotic requirements may be considerable as a result of surgical trauma to the rectus abdominis muscles and the extent of the tissue damage and surgical intervention. Pain can be managed by using patient-controlled analgesia and/or parenteral narcotics. Epidural anesthesia using narcotics or low-dose local anesthetics may be considered if there is no evidence of coagulopathy. Epidural anesthesia has been shown to be beneficial for patients with rib fractures. Regional anesthesia decreases postoperative pain and narcotic requirements. Low-dose ketamine also decreases postoperative pain by antagonism of NMDA receptors.

34. *Discuss the postoperative laboratory values that would be relevant after an open laparotomy with a massive blood transfusion.*

The anesthetist should continue to monitor blood hemogram, coagulation, and chemical constituents. The following is suggested:

- Hemoglobin and hematocrit
- Platelet count
- Prothrombin time, partial thromboplastin time, INR
- Serum sodium, potassium, calcium, chloride, blood urea nitrogen, creatinine
- Blood glucose level
- Arterial blood gas values
- If disseminated intravascular coagulation is suspected or if there is evidence of unexplained bleeding, fibrin split products and a fibrinogen level should be evaluated

Review Questions

1. Which is the correct method to induce and intubate a trauma patient?
   a. Rapid sequence induction
   b. Standard induction maintaining in-line cervical stabilization
   c. Emergency cricothyrotomy
   d. Blind nasal intubation

2. Which anesthetic agent should be avoided in the acute anesthetic management of a patient with a penetrating abdominal injury?
   a. Ketamine
   b. Succinylcholine
   c. Propofol
   d. Nitrous oxide

3. Which statement regarding substance misuse is correct?
   a. Acute ingestion of alcohol increases anesthetic requirements.
   b. Acute ingestion of marijuana decreases anesthetic requirements.
   c. Acute ingestion of cocaine decreases anesthetic requirements.
   d. Acute ingestion of a narcotic has no effect on anesthetic requirements.

4. Venous air embolism can occur after trauma to which anatomic structure?
   a. Stomach
   b. Small bowel
   c. Liver
   d. Bladder

5. Which is a characteristic of a low-velocity missile wound?
   a. Produces a large temporary cavity
   b. Occurs with guns that have a high muzzle velocity
   c. Tissues are stretched and torn as a result of a large temporary cavity and a high energy shock wave
   d. Tissue destruction can be extensive

Suggested Readings

Cannon JW. Hemorrhagic shock. *N Engl J Med.* 2018;378(4):370–379.

Cherry RA, Eachempati SR, Hydo L, et al. The role of laparoscopy in penetrating abdominal stab wounds. *Surg Laparosc Endosc Percutan Tech.* 2005;15(1):14–17.

Dai W, Shi J, Carreno J, Kloner RA. Different effects of volatile and nonvolatile anesthetic agents on long-term survival in an experimental model of hemorrhagic shock. *J Cardiovasc Pharmacol Ther.* 2020:1074248420919221.

Howie WO. Trauma anesthesia. In: Nagelhout JJ, Elisha S, eds. *Nurse Anesthesia,* 6th ed. St. Louis, MO: Elsevier, 2018: 855–870.

Johnson JW, Gracias VH, Schwab CW, et al. Evolution in damage control for exsanguinating penetrating abdominal injury. *J Trauma.* 2001;51(2):261–271.

Kirkpatrick AW, Ball CG, D'Amours SK, et al. Acute resuscitation of the unstable adult trauma patient: bedside diagnosis and therapy. *Can J Surg.* 2008;51(1):57–69.

Louro J, Dudaryk R, Rodriguez Y, Dutton RP, Epstein RH. Airway management at Level 1 trauma center in the era of video laryngoscopy. *Int J Crit Illn Inj Sci.* 2020;10(1):20–24.

Morris MC, Niziolek GM, Baker JE, Huebner BR, et al. Death by decade: establishing a transfusion ceiling for futility in massive transfusion. *J Surg Res.* 2020;252:139–146.

Peng J, He F, Qin C, Que Y, Fan R, Qin B. Intraoperative dexmedetomidine versus midazolam in patients undergoing peripheral surgery with mild traumatic brain injuries: a retrospective cohort analysis. *Dose Response.* 2020;18(2):1559325820916342.

Riskin DJ, Spain DA, Jou R. Trauma surgery. In: Jaffe RA, Schmiesing RA, Golianu B, eds. *Anesthesiologist's Manual of Surgical Procedures.* Philadelphia: Lippincott Williams & Wilkins, 2014:727–747.

Stahl JL, Miller AC. What's new in critical illness and injury science? A look into trauma airway management. *Int J Crit Illn Inj Sci.* 2020;10(1):1–3.

Tobin JM, Barras WP, Bree S, Williams N, et al. Anesthesia for trauma patients. *Mil Med.* 2018;183(suppl_2):32–35.

Uchida K, Nishimura T, Hagawa N, Kaga S, et al. The impact of early administration of vasopressor agents for the resuscitation of severe hemorrhagic shock following blunt trauma. *BMC Emerg Med.* 2020;20(1):26.

17

Blunt Thoracic Injuries

KEY POINTS

- Blunt trauma to the chest is the third leading cause of traumatic injury.
- Lung injury is the most common problem resulting from thoracic trauma.
- A pneumothorax occurs in as many as 40% of all blunt thoracic injuries.

- Signs of cardiac tamponade are associated with Beck triad, which includes jugular venous distention, muffled heart sounds, and hypotension.

Case Synopsis

A 65-year-old woman arrives in the emergency department after sustaining injuries in a motor vehicle accident (MVA). She was the driver of a sport utility vehicle that was struck by another vehicle at approximately 60 mph. She was wearing her seatbelt, and the airbags deployed.

The patient arrives to the trauma center wearing a cervical collar and on a backboard. She is presently complaining of mild shortness of breath. The emergency medical technician reports that the patient has sustained an open left femur fracture. Her electrocardiogram (ECG) tracing shows normal sinus rhythm with occasional premature ventricular contractions.

Preoperative Evaluation and Demographic Data

Past Medical/Surgical History

- Osteoporosis
- Hyperlipidemia
- Caesarian section 35 years ago, spinal anesthesia administered, no problems noted

List of Medications

- Fosamax
- Lipitor

Diagnostic Data

- Initial chest X-ray was significant for multiple rib fractures to the left side of her chest
- Open left femur fracture

Height/Weight/Vital Signs

- 160 cm, 73 kg
- Blood pressure, 132/68; heart rate, 122 beats per minute; respiratory rate, 16 breaths per minute; room air

oxygen saturation, 93% on 6 liters of oxygen administered by nasal cannula

Physical Examination

The primary trauma assessment is rapidly completed upon arrival. The patient presents with an obvious orthopedic injury and complains of significant shoulder and left chest pain. She has a cervical neck collar in place and is secured to a backboard. Her breath sounds are diminished bilaterally.

Pathophysiology

Blunt trauma to the chest is the third leading cause of traumatic injury, closely following traumatic brain injury and extremity trauma. In developed nations, thoracic trauma is most often associated with motor vehicle collisions. Blunt thoracic trauma patients present a unique series of concerns for the trauma team. These patients are frequently severely injured, and multisystem involvement commonly occurs. Blunt injuries account for nearly 25% to 50% of all traumatic deaths.

Pulmonary Injuries

The most commonly reported thoracic injuries are associated with the lungs and include pulmonary contusion, pneumothorax, and hemothorax. These injuries are most consistent with high-velocity trauma and are associated with abrupt deceleration. A pulmonary contusion, which frequently develops over 24 hours, represents the most common lung injury. It is reported that as many as 70% of patients who sustain blunt thoracic traumatic injuries have some degree of pulmonary contusion. The pathologic mechanism of a pulmonary contusion includes injuries to the alveoli without disruption of the distal air sacs. The result is a *bruise* to the lung tissue resulting in the disruption of the alveolar–capillary membrane which allows protein-rich fluid to exit the pulmonary capillaries and collect within the alveolar–capillary interstitium and alveoli. Due to the widening of the pulmonary capillary membrane, pulmonary contusions result in varying degrees of reduced gas diffusion. The degree of hypoxia and hypercarbia that is induced may or may not be clinically relevant.

Pneumothoraces occur in as many as 40% of all blunt thoracic injuries. The size and location of the pneumothorax may vary throughout the lung field. It is estimated that as many as 50% of patients with a pneumothorax are not initially detected by radiographic analysis. This presents several intraoperative management issues and may alter an anesthetic plan. Like a pneumothorax, acute identification of a hemothorax is unreliable with conventional radiology. The use of early computed tomography (CT) has increased early detection, with nonoperative management via tube thoracoscopy. Despite the possibility of minimal intervention, the anesthetist needs to monitor blood loss from the chest tube and anticipate acute decomposition and massive hemorrhage (>1500 mL).

This patient has sustained multiple rib fractures to the left aspect of her chest. Rib fractures are associated with a pneumothorax, hemothorax, and/or thoracic vascular injury. Because nitrous oxide is highly diffusible and decreases the total fraction of inspired concentration, its use during this patient's anesthetic course is contraindicated.

Chest Wall Injuries

The exact incidence of blunt chest injuries (BCIs) following a traumatic event is unknown. Injuries can vary from individual rib fractures to a flail chest. The most common chest wall injury is a rib fracture. Although often clinically insignificant, this finding may serve as a sign of underlying pathology and pulmonary injury. The scapulae and thoracic musculature protects the upper thorax, and fractures that occur to three or more ribs are reflective of a high-energy trauma. This injury is associated with brachial plexus and subclavian vascular injuries. An injury that involves the lower three ribs is associated with kidney, liver, and splenic injuries.

A flail chest is defined as a series of three or more contiguous ribs that are fractured at two or more places. These fractures typically occur on the anterior or anterior lateral surface of the chest. A flail chest produces paradoxical chest wall movement during spontaneous breathing. In addition to causing respiratory compromise and extreme pain, flail chest is indicative of significant thoracic injury. It is estimated that more than 50% of patients who endure a flail chest will require surgical intervention in order to repair additional thoracic injuries.

Cardiac Injuries

The incidence of blunt cardiac trauma is between 5% and 50%, depending on the definition and the clinical criteria used to evaluate cardiac injuries. Blunt cardiac trauma, similar to pulmonary injuries, results from occult injury to the thorax, deceleration injuries, and compression of the heart against bony structures such as the sternum. Blunt cardiac trauma is categorized into those that are low- and high-energy events.

Low-energy BCIs are typically a result of a sudden strike to the precordium. Although the mechanism can vary widely, these injuries can be caused by objects such as a baseball or fist. The effect of this injury can result in ventricular fibrillation or cardiac arrest, depending on the severity of the impact time the trauma is sustained and its relation to the cardiac cycle. Advanced cardiac life support procedures will begin prior to hospital admission, and the anesthetist will assist with cardiopulmonary resuscitation. High-energy BCIs are a result of tremendous force that is transferred to the cardiac tissue resulting in significant injury. Sequelae can range from lethal arrhythmias to myocardial septal rupture and massive hemorrhage. Perioperative management is variable and depends on the extent of the injury. Clinical management can range from cardiac monitoring and assessing a cardiac enzyme profile to emergency thoracotomy and cardiac repair. Fig. 17.1 describes various treatment strategies that depict a treatment algorithm that is dependent on the severity of BCI that is sustained.

Thoracic Vascular Injuries

Injuries sustained to the thoracic aorta are caused by rapid deceleration resulting in intimal tears of the thoracic aorta and often occur near the left subclavian artery. If untreated, thoracic aortal injuries can result in vascular rupture and death. In the United States, many injuries to the thoracic aorta result from motor vehicle collisions, which account for 10% to 15% of motor vehicle fatalities.

Surgical management of thoracic aortic injuries has evolved from open vascular repair to endovascular stent grafting (EVSG). This advance in management has demonstrated a significant reduction in morbidity and mortality for these patients. Initial management for thoracic aortic injuries should focus on deliberate blood pressure control and blood replacement. Perioperative goals should include meticulous blood pressure control to reduce shear wall stress and the risk of aortic rupture. The exact "range" of blood pressure measurements that should be achieved for patients with cardiac tamponade remains unclear. Maintenance of the systolic blood pressure less than or equal to 100 mm Hg is reasonable. Pharmacologic adjuncts such as beta-blockers (esmolol) and nitrates can be used to acutely control hypertension.

Airway Injuries

Airway injuries represent a potentially lethal consequence associated with blunt thoracic trauma. The relative infrequency of airway injuries that are treatable in a trauma center is likely due to the high incidence of rapid mortality

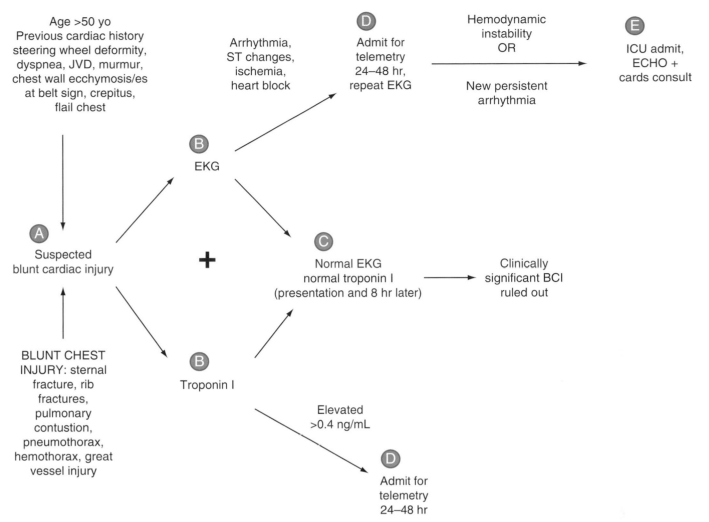

• **Fig. 17.1** Management of blunt cardiac injuries. *BCI,* Blunt chest injury; *ECHO,* echocardiography; *EKG,* electrocardiogram; *ICU,* intensive care unit; *JVD,* jugular venous distention. (From McIntyre RC, Schulick RD: *Surgical decision making,* ed 6, St. Louis, 2020, Elsevier.)

that occurs at the site of the accident and is associated with this injury. Recognition of the presence of airway injuries is often challenging. Patients with associated airway trauma that are treated at a trauma center are often unrecognized during the primary assessment despite airway management, direct laryngoscopy, and endotracheal tube (ETT) placement. This is because most thoracic airway injuries occur below the level of the carina, and definitive diagnosis is only possible during direct visual inspection by bronchoscopy or CT examination. Nevertheless, the management of a patient with a recognized or unrecognized airway injury is the same; if hypoxia, acidosis, and respiratory distress are evident, airway management and ETT intubation are mandatory.

Anesthetic Management and Considerations

1. Describe the immediate concerns regarding airway management for a patient who has sustained a high-energy blunt thoracic injury from an MVA.

Blunt thoracic trauma that is associated with a high-energy mechanism poses significant issues for both the surgical and anesthesia teams. After the advanced trauma life support (ATLS) protocol, airway assessment is the first priority of management for this patient. Acute respiratory distress or impending respiratory failure will require immediate airway intervention. A delay in airway management can result in severe hypoxemia and acidosis, which will result in cardiopulmonary decompensation.

There is a high probability of pulmonary injury as a result of high-energy blunt thoracic injuries, and the anesthetist should be prepared to manage a variety of potential complications. The anesthetist should anticipate rapid desaturation upon induction. Although all thoracic injuries are concerning, reductions in functional residual capacity (FRC) from injury or a pneumothorax may exacerbate arterial hypoxemia. Rapid desaturation should be anticipated. Simple techniques, such as prolonged and thorough preoxygenation, will be beneficial. During cricoid pressure, the anesthetist should consider bag–valve–mask ventilation using minimal peak pressures to maintain oxygenation and avoid sustained periods of desaturation. The risk of gastric aspiration exists; however, severe hypoxemia that occurs over the course of several minutes will have a negative effect on the patient's postoperative neurologic condition.

Once the ETT is in place and the location is confirmed, the patient should be closely monitored for signs of an unrecognized pneumothorax and/or tension pneumothorax. It should be remembered that the absence of a pneumothorax on radiograph does not guarantee that there is not an injury to the lung. Additionally, a tension pneumothorax is a clinical diagnosis made based on cardiovascular collapse after positive pressure ventilation ensues. Needle decompression on the affected side at the second intercostal space at the midclavicular line or chest tube thoracoscopy should be performed immediately if decompensation occurs.

2. *Describe acute respiratory distress syndrome (ARDS) and the clinical criteria to recognize this condition.*

ARDS occurs acutely within the first 24 to 48 hours after traumatic injury and can occur as a result of direct pulmonary injury (aspiration, blunt thoracic trauma) or extrapulmonary injury such as sepsis or multiple organ dysfunction syndrome. The diagnosis is based on several factors, which include a PaO_2/FiO_2 ratio of <200 mm Hg, acute onset, the presence of hypoxia, and specific cause such as thoracic trauma. The pathologic progression occurs over a 21- to 28-day span. The acute phase of ARDS occurs over the first 7 days of injury. Tissue trauma causes activation of inflammatory mediators, which causes leakage of protein-rich fluid from the capillaries that accumulates into the alveolar capillary membrane and alveoli and causes diffuse alveolar disruption and fibrosis. As a result, atelectasis occurs due to the dilution of surfactant and injury to type II pneumocytes. The thickening of the alveolar septum caused by the formation of edema leads to a reduction in gas diffusion, increased ventilation–perfusion mismatching, hypoxemia, and hypercarbia. In severe cases, arterial hypoxemia results in hypoxic pulmonary vasoconstriction and can potentially lead to acute congestive heart failure, which is a common cause of rapidly increasing pulmonary pressure. Although ARDS is a progressive disorder, the primary challenge for the anesthetist is to maintain a normal PaO_2 to provide adequate ventilation and avoid barotrauma. Decreased pulmonary compliance commonly results in increased peak airway pressures.

3. *Describe an appropriate ventilation strategy for a patient who has sustained a pulmonary contusion caused by blunt trauma. The patient's intraoperative situation during mechanical ventilation includes SpO2, 91%; arterial hypoxemia (PaO2 is 97 mm Hg with an FiO2 of 0.5); and increased ventilating pressures are required to achieve an adequate tidal volume (TV).*

Unlike elective surgery, canceling or postponing surgery for patients who have sustained major traumatic injuries is not possible, and delaying the operative procedure may result in increased morbidity and mortality. Although complex, managing pulmonary injuries is a common challenge faced by the anesthetist. Providing adequate oxygenation while minimizing excessive peak airway pressures and dead space ventilation are the ventilatory goals.

A variety of ventilation strategies have been described to best manage intraoperative ventilation for patients with an acute lung injury (ALI). Techniques vary from conventional strategies to inverse ratio ventilation (IRV). Unfortunately, a definitive protocol that outlines the "best practice" for managing ALI during the perioperative period does not currently exist. The findings of the ARDSnet study randomized patients with ALI to a low TV (6 mL/kg) group or a high TV (10 to 15 mL/kg) group. The amount of TV that was used was based on ideal body weights, and plateau and peak airway pressure were monitored over a 28-day period. A significant reduction in mortality and the number of days that patients were ventilator dependent occurred in the group that received a low TV.

Intraoperative management for this patient should be focused on maximizing oxygenation and ventilation without causing further pulmonary injury and compromise. Nitrous oxide should be avoided due to the potential expansion of an unrecognized pneumothorax. Oxygen should be diluted with air and titrated to the lowest inspired oxygen concentration to maintain an arterial oxygen saturation greater than 60 mm Hg. Inhalational anesthetics will reduce hypoxic pulmonary vasoconstriction (HPV) in a dose-dependent fashion. Although changes to HPV have been demonstrated in the laboratory, the clinical relevance has not been demonstrated.

As previously discussed, ALI/ARDS can cause noncardiogenic pulmonary edema that results in atelectasis and reduced gas diffusion, which often requires higher pressures to adequately facilitate positive pressure ventilation. Increasing the pressure during mechanical ventilation likely increases ventilation–perfusion mismatching and high-pressure alveolar trauma.

Management of these patients should focus on treating the cause of hypoxemia (i.e., atelectasis). An appropriate ventilation strategy for this patient would begin with a low TV approximately 4 to 6 mL/kg, a respiratory rate of 12 to 14 breaths per minute, and positive-end expiratory pressure (PEEP). It is recommended that plateau pressures be maintained less than 30 cm H_2O in order to reduce ventilator-associated barotrauma. The plateau phase of mechanical ventilation represents the longest period of alveolar stretch during the ventilation cycle. Peak airway pressures should be closely monitored; however, plateau pressures are more accurate in

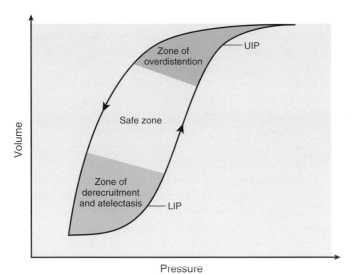

• **Fig. 17.2** Schematic of a pressure–volume curve for the lungs or total respiratory system that demonstrates hysteresis between inspiratory and expiratory limbs. The upper inflection point *(UIP)* and lower inflection point *(LIP)* are demarcated on the inspiratory limb. During mechanical ventilation, lung regions should be in the safe zone for optimal lung protection. (Redrawn from Froese AB: High-frequency oscillatory ventilation for adult respiratory distress syndrome: let's get it right this time! *Crit Care Med* 25:906–908, 1997.)

• **BOX 17.1 Perioperative Strategies Used to Manage Patients With ARDS**

- Maintain tidal volume at 6–8 mL/kg
- Minimize peak inspiratory pressure <30 cm H_2O
- PEEP
- Pressure ventilation mode
- Inverse ratio ventilation
- High-frequency jet ventilation
- Avoid aggressive fluid therapy if possible

predicting high-pressure barotrauma. Fig. 17.2 represents the zone for optimal ventilation.

The primary role of PEEP during mechanical ventilation is to maintain alveolar patency during exhalation, avoiding derecruitment or collapse. In addition, PEEP can increase the overall mean airway pressure during positive pressure ventilation, facilitating gas diffusion across the alveolar membrane. This is essential for the patient with ALI/ARDS. Although there is no consistent recommendation for the amount of PEEP that should be administered to patients with ALI/ARDS because lung compliance and opening pressures vary, many anesthetists initiate PEEP at 8 to 10 cm H_2O. Box 17.1 summarizes the strategies that can be used to help manage patients who have developed ALI/ARDS.

• **BOX 17.2 Signs Associated With Cardiac Tamponade**

- Tachycardia
- Hypoxemia
- Hypercarbia
- Myocardial ischemia
- Dysrhythmias
- Pulsus paradoxus
- Widened mediastinum
- Decreased cardiac output
- Equivalent left- and right-sided heart pressures
- Beck triad

4. *Discuss the pathophysiology, symptomatology, and treatment for cardiac tamponade.*

Cardiac tamponade is an accumulation of blood that pools within the pericardium from an intramyocardial perforation or coronary artery laceration. This type of injury is consistent with a high-speed MVA and associated rib fractures. The fibrous pericardium is extremely durable, and as little as 50 to 100 mL of acute blood accumulation in this area can cause death. If untreated, intrapericardial pressure progressively increases, which impinges on the heart and decreases cardiac performance. The pathogenesis associated with cardiac compressive shock includes decreased diastolic filling, which decreases left ventricular volume and cardiac output. A cycle resulting from systemic hypoperfusion leads to systemic acidosis, myocardial ischemia, and worsening hypotension.

The symptomatology that can be used for diagnosis of cardiac tamponade is included in Box 17.2. Objective factors that are definitively associated with this process are described by Beck triad, which includes elevated central venous pressure resulting in jugular venous distention, muffled heart sounds, and hypotension. Because the pressure exerted on the heart is equivalently distributed in each region, left- and right-sided heart pressures will become similar. Evaluation with cardiac echocardiography is a definitive method for determining the presence of blood within the pericardium.

The treatment that is used to treat cardiac tamponade is for the surgeon to create an opening in the pericardium or pericardial window or to perform a pericardiocentesis. The goals of anesthetic management are to maintain preload and to minimize myocardial depression. Bradycardia will cause acute decompensation, as the increased heart rate is the primary determinant of stroke volume in this situation. Due to its sympathomimetic effects, ketamine can be used for the induction of anesthesia. The use of etomidate is also acceptable.

Review Questions

1. The most common injury as a result of blunt thoracic trauma is:
   a. Cardiac contusion.
   b. Pneumothorax.
   c. Pulmonary contusion.
   d. Tracheal injuries below the carina.

2. Using the recommendations of the ARDSnet, which is an appropriate range of tidal volume for a male patient who is 84 kg and 72 inches tall?
   a. 350 to 500 mL
   b. 450 to 550 mL
   c. 500 to 650 mL
   d. 600 to 750 mL

3. Which factor is most predictive of the potential for barotrauma during mechanical ventilation?
   a. Plateau pressure
   b. Peak airway pressure
   c. Mean airway pressure
   d. Positive-end expiratory pressure

4. Which statement regarding blunt thoracic trauma is false?
   a. A flail chest is a continuous section of three or more rib fractures in two or more locations.
   b. ARDS is defined as a PaO_2/FiO_2 ratio less than 200 mm Hg.
   c. A chest radiograph is insensitive for detecting a pneumothorax after a blunt thoracic injury.
   d. Management of a thoracic aneurysm requires blood pressure control to decrease the heart rate and hemorrhaging.

5. Which best describes the pathologic changes that are consistent with ARDS?
   a. Ventilation–perfusion mismatching is decreased.
   b. Hypercarbia occurs due to alveolar–capillary membrane fibrosis.
   c. Right ventricular pressure is decreased.
   d. Atelectasis formation is caused by increased surfactant.

Suggested Readings

Huang FD, Yeh WB, Chen SS, et al. Early management of retained hemothorax in blunt head and chest trauma. *World J Surg.* 2018;42(7):2061–2066.

Kaewlai R, Avery LL, Asrani AV, et al. Multidetector CT of blunt thoracic trauma. *Radiographics.* 2008;28(6):1555–1570.

Ishida K, Kinoahita Y, Iwasa N, et al. Emergency room thoracotomy for acute traumatic cardiac tamponade caused by a blunt cardiac injury: a case report. *Int J Surg Case Rep.* 2017;21–24.

Lebl DR, Dicker RA, Spain DA, et al. Dramatic shift in the primary management of traumatic thoracic aortic rupture. *Arch Surg.* 2006;141:177–180.

LuoL, Shaver CM, Zhao Z, et al. Clinical predictors of hospital mortality differ between direct and indirect ARDS. *Chest.* 2017;151(4):755–763.

Manetta F, Newman J, Mattia A. Indications for Thoracic EndoVascular Aortic Repair (TEVAR): a brief review. *Int J Angiol.* 2018;27(4):177–184.

Matthay MA, Zemans RL, Zimmerman GA, et al. Acute respiratory distress syndrome. *Nat Rev Dis Primers.* 2019;5(1):18.

Miller PR, Croce MA, Kilgo PD, et al. Acute respiratory distress syndrome in blunt trauma: identification of independent risk factors. *Am Surg.* 2002;68(10):845–850.

Moloney JT, Fowler SJ, Chang W. Anesthetic management of thoracic trauma. *Curr Opin Anaesthesiol.* 2008;21(1):41–46.

Orliaguet G, Ferjani M, Riou B. The heart in blunt trauma. *Anesthesiology.* 2001;95:544–548.

Reiker M. Respiratory anatomy: thoracic surgery. In: Nagelhout JJ, Elisha S KL, eds. *Nurse Anesthesia,* 6th ed. St. Louis, MO: Elsevier, 2018:624–644.

Stafford RE, Linn J, Washington L. Incidence and management of occult hemothoraces. *Am J Surg.* 2006;192(6):722–726.

18

Pneumonectomy

KEY POINTS

- Lung cancer is the second most common cancer and the most common cause of cancer-related death in both men and women in the United States. Most pulmonary resection procedures are performed for the removal of lung cancer.
- The term *pulmonary resection* refers to a variety of procedures, including (1) segmentectomy (e.g., wedge resection), (2) lobectomy, (3) pneumonectomy (e.g., intrapericardial and extrapericardial), (4) completion pneumonectomy, (5) radical pneumonectomy, and (6) carinal pneumonectomy. Each procedure differs in terms of indication, technique, and extent of pulmonary resection.
- The anesthetist should thoroughly evaluate the degree and severity of pulmonary disease, cardiovascular disease, and comorbidities during the preoperative assessment.
- Findings from basic physical examination and preoperative testing dictate (1) the histologic type and stage of lung

cancer, (2) the need for preoperative optimization, (3) the necessity for advanced intraoperative monitoring, (4) optimal one-lung ventilation (OLV) methods, (5) periop-erative risk stratification based on the patient's ability to tolerate the proposed resection, and (6) the perioperative anesthetic plan.
- OLV allows for lung separation and provides optimal surgical visualization. It can be achieved through various methods, including (1) dual-lumen endobronchial tube (ETT), (2) bronchial blocker, or (3) endobronchial intubation with a single-lumen ETT.
- Complications of pneumonectomy include (1) cardiac herniation, (2) hemorrhage, (3) bronchial disruption, (4) arrhythmias, (5) respiratory failure, (6) right heart failure, and (7) neural injury.

Case Synopsis

A 70-year-old man is admitted to the hospital for right-sided, non–small cell lung carcinoma. He is scheduled by his thoracic surgeon to have a right extrapericardial pneumonectomy.

Preoperative Evaluation and Demographic Data

Past Medical/Surgical History

- Hypertension, chronic obstructive pulmonary disease, insulin-dependent diabetes mellitus, and gastroesophageal reflux disease
- Cigarette smoking: 50 pack-years of cigarette smoking, stopped 1 month ago
- Computed tomography (CT)–guided fine-needle biopsy: pathologic examination reveals right-sided, non–small cell lung adenocarcinoma
- Mediastinoscopy with lymph node biopsy: pathologic examination reveals no mediastinal metastases and no mediastinal lymph node involvement
- Bronchoscopy: gross visual examination reveals right bronchial involvement without carinal extension, no tracheobronchial compression

List of Medications

- Atenolol (Tenormin)
- Albuterol (ProAir)
- Regular insulin (Novolin R)
- Omeprazole (Prilosec)

Diagnostic Data

- Hemoglobin, 15.3 g/dL; hematocrit, 45.9%; platelets 300,000 mm^3
- Electrolytes: sodium, 147 mEq/L; potassium, 4.1 mEq/L; chloride, 107 mEq/L; carbon dioxide, 30 mEq/L
- Glucose, 135 mg/dL
- Blood urea nitrogen, 12 mg/dL; creatinine 1.2 mg/dL
- Chest radiograph (anterior, posterior, and lateral): Bilateral hyperinflation with increased vascular markings. Right lung: Centrally located opacity of pulmonary parenchyma, approximately 10 cm in diameter. Cardiac hypertrophy noted. No gross tracheal or bronchial deviation.
- Chest CT: Right lung, 10 cm centrally located pulmonary mass. No cardiac or tracheobronchial compression. Vascular involvement as indicated by contrast-enhanced CT.
- Chest magnetic resonance imaging (MRI): Right lung, 10 cm centrally located, high-intensity pulmonary mass. No cardiac and tracheobronchial compression.

- Pulmonary function test (pre- and post-bronchodilator therapy): FVC 70% (normal 80%); FEV_1 = 65 % of predicted (normal 80% of vital capacity); FEV_1/FVC % = 60% (normal 70% of predicted); forced expiratory flow (FEF 25% to 75%) = 3.5 L (normal 4 to 5 L or <60% of predicted)
- Arterial blood gas (21% oxygen): pH, 7.37; $PaCO_2$, 44 mm Hg; HCO_3, 25 mEq/L; PaO_2, 70 mm Hg
- Electrocardiogram (ECG), normal sinus rhythm, heart rate 67 beats per minute

Height/Weight/Vital Signs

- 170 cm, 83 kg
- Blood pressure, 135/86; heart rate, 65 beats per minute; respiratory rate, 25 breaths per minute; room air oxygen saturation, 95%; temperature, 36.9°C

Pathophysiology

Pulmonary resection procedures have been performed for a variety of etiologies, such as (1) pulmonary masses, (2) malignant mesothelioma, (3) bronchiectasis, (4) tuberculosis, (5) and thoracic trauma. Pulmonary masses may present as benign or malignant pathology. Benign pulmonary masses include carcinoid tumors, hemangiomas, bronchopulmonary sequestrations, and infection. Many pulmonary resection procedures are performed for the removal of malignant tissue (e.g., bronchogenic carcinoma).

Lung cancer is the second most common cancer (15%) and the most common cause of cancer-related deaths (29%) in both men and women in the United States. Most patients have an extensive history of smoking, and less than 10% of patients presenting with lung cancer are nonsmokers. In these cases, lung cancer can often be attributed to environmental exposure (i.e., passive smoking) or industrial exposure (i.e., asbestos or heavy metals).

Lung cancer is traditionally divided into two categories: small cell lung carcinoma (SCLC) and non–small cell lung carcinoma (NSCLC). SCLC (e.g., oat-cell carcinoma) accounts for 25% of all lung cancer. Treatment for SCLC rarely involves surgery because patients typically present with advanced staging and metastases have frequently occurred upon initial evaluation. Endocrinopathies and paraneoplastic neurologic syndromes can occur in patients with SCLC. NSCLC accounts for the remaining 75% of all lung cancer. Less than 20% of NSCLC patients present at a stage that is amendable by surgical intervention. Depending on the type and stage of lung cancer, treatment options include a combination of surgery, radiation, chemotherapy, and targeted biologic therapy.

Surgical Procedure

Extrapericardial pneumonectomy involves making a posterolateral or lateral thoracotomy incision through the fifth intercostal space, allowing exposure of the pulmonary hilum and lateral mediastinum. Partial or total rib resection may be necessary to facilitate surgical visualization. Surgical

evaluation of the thoracic cavity, mediastinum, pulmonary parenchyma, and all pleural surfaces is assessed. Instances of metastases, multistation lymph node involvement, and/or invasion of the major vascular and mediastinal structures preclude complete resection. Based on the patient's presenting pathology, the surgeon determines if a pneumonectomy is indicated or if a less dramatic pulmonary resection procedure can be performed.

Once the need for pneumonectomy is established and resection is deemed favorable, the surgeon performs a methodical biopsy of the thoracic lymph nodes. Attention is then directed to the pulmonary hilum. The surgical ligation of the hilar structures includes the (1) pulmonary artery, (2) pulmonary veins, and (3) bronchus ipsilateral to the thoracic pathology. Meticulous surgical resection is undertaken to prevent unwarranted damage to major vascular and mediastinal structures. Surgical ligation is performed using traditional sutures and/or vascular staples.

After surgical resection and hemostasis, the affected lung is extracted though the thoracotomy incision and will be examined by a pathologist. If the surgeon desires, the in vivo bronchial stump may be reinforced with synthetic material or autografted tissue/muscle. An appropriately sized chest tube is inserted, and the thoracic cavity is closed in traditional surgical fashion.

Presently, the majority of thoracic procedures performed on the lungs are accomplished via a video-assisted thoracoscopic (VATS) approach. Advances in videoscopic technology have led to the increased use of thoracoscopy to replace open thoracotomy for a variety of intrathoracic procedures. VATS usually involves general anesthesia with a double-lumen ETT. There are limited visualization and limited ability for the surgeon to manually compress the lung, and a double-lumen tube may be preferable to a bronchial blocker to facilitate lung isolation. However, the anesthetic plan should account for the potential need for rapidly obtaining arterial blood gas samples or for possible hemorrhage, which may be difficult to control in the endoscopic procedure. In cases of severe pulmonary compromise, VATS can be performed using epidural anesthesia in the spontaneous-breathing patient who is sedated with a variety of techniques. Advantages of VATS for pneumonectomy include less ventilation–perfusion mismatch and decreased postoperative pain.

Anesthetic Management and Considerations

Preoperative Period

1. *Describe the anatomy of the pulmonary hilum and lungs and its bearing on pneumonectomy.*

    The pulmonary hilum refers to the site of contact between the lung parenchyma and the mediastinum. Fig. 18.1 depicts the anatomy of the left and right pulmonary hila. The left and right pulmonary hila have four common structures: (1) the pulmonary artery, (2) superior and inferior pulmonary veins, (3) main bronchus, and (4) hilar lymph nodes. The pulmonary hila lie in intimate proximity to major vascular and mediastinal structures, including the (1) heart, (2) aorta, (3) main pulmonary artery, (4) trachea, (5) esophagus, (6) vena cava, and (7) nerves (i.e., phrenic, vagus, and recurrent laryngeal nerves). Vigilance must always be exercised by

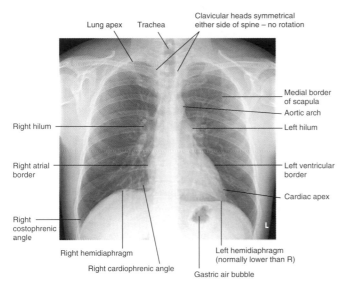

• **Fig. 18.1** Anatomy of the left and right pulmonary hila. (From Innes JA. *Davidson's essentials of medicine*, ed 3, Edinburgh, 2016, Churchill Livingstone.)

the anesthetist, because surgical damage to major vascular and mediastinal structures is a constant risk.

The major function of the lungs is for gas exchange (i.e., oxygenation and ventilation), which is dependent on the quantity and quality of functional lung tissue. The right lung represents up to 60% of the total lung volume, and the left lung represents the remaining 40%. After right-sided pneumonectomy, total lung area decreases to a greater degree than with a left-sided pneumonectomy. A right-sided pneumonectomy is therefore more physiologically taxing and is associated with a significantly higher mortality rate.

2. *Discuss an appropriate preoperative assessment for patients presenting for scheduled pneumonectomy.*

As with any disease process, the optimal anesthetic plan is based on a thorough clinical evaluation and preoperative testing that should be tailored to each patient's presenting condition and symptomatology. Preoperative symptoms exhibited by patients with bronchogenic carcinoma are listed in Table 18.1. Findings from basic physical examination and preoperative testing dictate (1) the histologic type and stage of lung cancer, (2) the need for preoperative optimization, (3) the necessity for advanced intraoperative monitoring, (4) optimal OLV methods, (5) perioperative risk stratification based on the patient's ability to tolerate the proposed resection, and (6) perioperative anesthetic plan.

TABLE 18.1	Preoperative Symptoms Exhibited by Patients Presenting With Bronchogenic Carcinoma	
Symptom Category	**Anatomy Involved**	**Symptom**
Bronchopulmonary symptoms	• Bronchial irritation • Obstruction • Infection • Ulceration	• Cough or wheezing • Dyspnea • Chest pain, rales, rhonchi, or pneumonia • Hemoptysis
Extrapulmonary intrathoracic symptoms	• Pleura • Chest wall • Esophagus • Superior vena cava • Pericardium • Brachial plexus • Recurrent laryngeal nerves (unilateral or bilateral) • Spinal cord • Cervical sympathetic nerves	• Pleural effusion • Chest pain • Dysphagia • Superior vena cava syndrome • Pericardial effusion or pericarditis • Arm pain • Coarseness or stridor • Parethesias or paralysis • Horner syndrome
Extrathoracic metastatic symptoms	Multiple sites throughout body	• Dependent on site and tumor involvement
Extrathoracic nonmetastatic symptoms	• Endocrinologic syndromes • Paraneoplastic syndromes	• Syndrome of inappropriate antidiuretic hormone hypersecretion (SIADH) • Cushing syndrome • Eaton–Lambert syndrome
Nonspecific	Variant	• Weight loss • Nocturnal diaphoresis • Anemia • Weakness • Anorexia • Lethargy • Malaise

---

• BOX 18.1   Three Tiers of Preoperative Pulmonary Function Testing and Indicators of Increased Perioperative Risk

Tier 1: Whole-lung function testing

Arterial blood gas on room air
$PaCO_2$: >45 mm Hg

Spirometry
- FEV_1: <2 L
- FEV_1/FVC: <50% predicted
- Maximum breathing capacity: <50% predicted

Lung volume
RV/TLC: >50%

Diffusing capacity CO_2
$DLCO_2$: <60% predicted

Tier 2: Split-lung function testing

Split-lung spirometry with DLT or regional lung radio-spirometry (i.e., V/Q scan)
- Predicted postoperative FEV_1: <0.85 L or <40% predicted
- Blood flow to affected lung: >70%

Tier 3: Postoperative functional capacity testing

Temporary unilateral occlusion of the right or left pulmonary artery or bronchus.
- Mean PA pressure: >40 mm Hg
- $PaCO_2$: >60 mm Hg
- PaO_2: <45 mm Hg (with supplemental oxygen)
- Signs of respiratory failure

The chest radiograph is the most common preoperative test used to evaluate intrathoracic pathology. When the patient develops symptoms consistent with bronchogenic carcinoma, a chest radiograph is frequently ordered. Anterior, posterior, and lateral chest radiographs provide information regarding tumor (1) size, (2) location, (3) density, and (4) cardiopulmonary abnormalities.

CT, MRI, and positron emission tomography (PET) studies provide more accurate information regarding tumor (1) size, (2) location, (3) density, and (4) metabolic activity. Information from these studies is used to determine the presence, type, and stage of lung cancer. Instances of metastases to distal sites or invasion of the major vascular and mediastinal structures preclude complete resection.

Preoperative bronchoscopic and mediastinoscopic examination is imperative in patients presenting with bronchogenic carcinoma. Examination allows evaluation of the patient's airway and the opportunity to obtain biopsies from tracheobronchial pathology. Gross findings and pathologic examination provide insight regarding (1) histologic typing, (2) stage of lung cancer, and (3) optimal OLV methods based on abnormalities in airway anatomy. Pulmonary function tests provide invaluable diagnostic information regarding a patient's ability to tolerate the proposed pulmonary resection (e.g., perioperative risk stratification). Pulmonary function testing should commence in a tiered approach, with each tier increasing in sensitivity, specificity, and invasiveness. Box 18.1 describes the three tiers of preoperative function testing.

The pulmonary and cardiovascular systems are physiologically intertwined. Therefore a thorough preoperative evaluation of right- and left-sided cardiac function is crucial in determining a patient's ability to tolerate pneumonectomy. Right and/or left ventricular dysfunctions (i.e., as indicated by decreased exercise capacity) indicate the need for preoperative optimization (e.g., medical management, angioplasty, or coronary artery bypass graft [CABG]) before surgery.

3. *Describe preoperative interventions that can be used to optimize high-risk patients for pneumonectomy.*

The purpose of preoperative optimization is to treat or manage conditions that predispose the patient to perioperative complications (i.e., atelectasis and pneumonia), ideally decreasing morbidity and mortality in the process. Pulmonary optimization procedures include (1) cessation of smoking, (2) bronchodilation therapy, (3) decreasing viscosity of secretions, (4) secretion mobilization, and (5) adjunct care (e.g., pharmacologic and psychologic). As discussed previously, cardiac optimization to maximize ventricular function must be instituted before surgery.

Patients that present with lung cancer typically have multiple risk factors. Preoperative interventions should be implemented with consideration of "the four Ms": (1) mass effects (e.g., bronchopulmonary and extrapulmonary intrathoracic symptoms), (2) metabolic effects (e.g., endocrinopathies and paraneoplastic neurologic syndromes), (3) metastases, and (4) medications (i.e., bleomycin and other chemotherapy drugs).

4. *Describe contraindications to performing pneumonectomy.*

The contraindications for having a pneumonectomy are due to distal metastases and/or a patient's inability to tolerate the physiologic stresses of surgery. Physical examination, preoperative testing, and preoperative optimization are aimed at determining which patients are optimal surgical candidates. Box 18.2 describes contraindications to a pneumonectomy procedure.

5. *Describe the significance of SCLC in a patient for pneumonectomy.*

Endocrinologic abnormalities and paraneoplastic neurologic syndromes are common in patients with SCLC. Table 18.2 describes common syndromes and anesthetic considerations in patients with SCLC. SCLC cells are derived from neuroendocrine tissue and commonly produce physiologically active factors. These factors clinically manifest as paraneoplastic endocrine syndromes, including syndrome of inappropriate antidiuretic hormone (SIADH) and Cushing syndrome. SIADH is present in up to 40% of patients with SCLC.

TABLE 18.2	Common Syndromes and Anesthetic Considerations in Patients With SCLC		
	SIADH	Cushing Syndrome	Myasthenic Syndrome
Signs and symptoms	• Increased urine osmolarity • Increased sodium concentration with serum hyponatremia • Decreased serum osmolarity	• Systemic hypertension • Hypokalemia • Hyperglycemia • Skeletal muscle weakness • Osteoporosis • Obesity • Poor wound healing	• Limb weakness (proximal, legs greater than arms) • Strength improved with exercise • Muscle pain common • Reflexes decreased or absent
Treatment	• Fluid restriction • Diuretics • Electrolyte replacement therapy	• Fluid and electrolyte therapy • Surgical treatment of primary cause	• Steroids • 3,4 diaminopyridine • Plasma exchange • Intravenous immunoglobulin
Anesthetic considerations	• Hyponatremia associated with altered consciousness • Diuretics may cause hypovolemia and hypotension with induction	• Blood pressure, electrolyte, and blood glucose management • Decreased doses of muscle relaxants • Need for postoperative ventilation possible	• Sensitive to succinylcholine • Sensitive to nondepolarizing muscle relaxants • Need for postoperative ventilation possible

---

• BOX 18.2 Contraindications for a Pneumonectomy Procedure

- Metastases and/or multistation lymph node involvement
- Invasion of the major vascular and/or mediastinal structures
- Inadequate pulmonary function as indicated by pulmonary function tests
- Hemodynamic instability with clamping of pulmonary artery (1–5 min) before ligation

---

Myasthenic syndrome (e.g., Eaton–Lambert syndrome) may also be present in patients with SCLC. An autoimmune reaction between tumor-related (immunoglobulin G) antibodies and presynaptic calcium channels causes a decreased presynaptic release of acetylcholine. Clinical manifestations of myasthenic syndrome frequently precede cancer identification and should be considered in patients undergoing diagnostic procedures.

Intraoperative Period

6. *Describe the different classifications of pneumonectomy.*

Pneumonectomy for lung carcinoma is typically performed for large and centrally located pulmonary masses untreatable by segmentectomy (e.g., wedge resection) or lobectomy. Several types of pneumonectomy exist. Selection of the type of pneumonectomy is dependent on the type, stage, and location of lung carcinoma. A standard pneumonectomy involves the sole removal of the affected lung. Intrapericardial and extrapericardial pneumonectomy refers to a standard pneumonectomy with the extent of surgical resection in relation to the cardiac pericardium. Completion pneumonectomy involves removing the

affected lung, after previous lung resection, that has experienced a recurrence of carcinoma. Radical pneumonectomy (e.g., extrapleural pneumonectomy) is commonly performed as treatment for malignant mesothelioma and involves removal of the entire lung, ipsilateral pleura, hemopericardium, and hemidiaphragm. Carinal pneumonectomy is the removal of the entire lung, ipsilateral mainstem bronchus, and carina. This procedure requires surgical anastomosis of the remaining mainstem bronchus and distal trachea.

7. *Describe indications for lung separation and OLV.*

OLV allows for lung separation and provides optimal surgical visualization during thoracic procedures. It can be accomplished through various methods, including (1) dual-lumen ETT (DLT), (2) bronchial blocker, or (3) endobronchial intubation with a single-lumen ETT. Absolute and relative indications for lung separation techniques and OLV are given in Table 18.3.

8. *Describe unique features of DLTs, bronchial blockers, and endobronchial intubation.*

A DLT consists of two separate channels for independent ventilation of the distal bronchus and the trachea. DLTs are designed to accommodate the left or right mainstem bronchus. The choice of a left- versus right-sided DLT is dependent on the type and side of operation. Most surgical procedures can be performed with a left-sided DLT. However, choice of a left- versus right-sided tube is not absolute. Stenosis, disruption, obstruction, or absence of a mainstem bronchus warrants placement of a DLT on the opposite side. During surgical procedures involving the mainstem bronchus (e.g., pneumonectomy), the choice of left- versus right-sided DLT must be carefully considered to avoid interference of the bronchial lumen during resection. Table 18.4 describes

TABLE 8.3   Absolute and Relative Indications for OLV and/or Lung Separation Techniques

Need	Indication	Examples
Absolute	Unilateral lung isolation	Infection and massive hemorrhage
	Unilateral ventilation control	Fistula (i.e., bronchopleural or bronchopleural cutaneous fistula), tracheobronchial surgery or disruption, large lung parenchymal mass (i.e., cyst or bulla), and unilateral lung disease causing life-threatening hypoxemia
	Unilateral pulmonary lavage	Treatment for alveolar proteinosis
Relative	Surgical exposure (high priority)	Thoracoscopy, mediastinal exposure, thoracic aortic aneurysm surgery, pneumonectomy and upper lobectomy
	Surgical exposure (low priority)	Segmentectomy, middle and lower lobectomy, esophageal surgery, minimal invasive cardiac surgery, transmyocardial revascularization, and thoracic spine surgery
	Status post-cardiopulmonary bypass	After removal of unilateral pulmonary emboli
	Unilateral lung disease	Severe hypoxemia related to lung pathology

TABLE 8.4   Advantages, Disadvantages, Complications, Relative Contraindications, and Types of DLTs

	Dual-Lumen Endobronchial Tube
Advantages	• Effective suction for secretions and lung deflation • Application of CPAP to nonventilated lung • Easy conversion between OLV and two-lung ventilation
Disadvantages	• Difficult or impossible placement with abnormal anatomy • If postoperative ventilation is required, removal may pose risk to patient
Complications	• Tracheobronchial trauma • Laryngeal trauma • Accidental suturing to mediastinal structures
Relative contraindications	• Full stomach • Difficult airway • Ventilator dependent, critically ill
Types	• Robertshaw • Carlens • White

advantages, disadvantages, complications, relative contra-indications, and types of DLTs.

When compared to the left mainstem bronchus, the right mainstem bronchus is shorter in length with variable location of the right upper lobe orifice. Right-sided DLTs have a separate opening, embedded in the endobronchial cuff, to ventilate the right upper lobe. Inadvertent obstruction of the ventilation slot has occurred. Therefore proper DLT placement should be ensured to avoid inadequate ventilation of the right upper lobe. An anomalous right upper lobe orifice that emerges above the tracheal carina is a contraindication for a right-sided DLT.

Choosing the correct size of DLT may be based on gender, height, weight, tracheal width, and/or bronchial diameter. It is important to remain cognizant that the patient's height more accurately correlates to the appropriate DLT size compared with the patient's weight. The ideal DLT size is one that (1) can safely traverse the glottis; (2) minimizes tracheobronchial trauma; (3) mini-mizes airway resistance; (4) allows the passage of the fiber-optic bronchoscope and suction catheter; and (5) requires no more than 1 to 2 mL of air to create an adequate endobronchial cuff seal. Size recommendations, placement techniques, and confirmation of placement recommendations for DLTs are given in Table 18.5. There are three methods of confirming DLT placement: (1) chest radiograph, (2) clinical signs, and (3) fiber-optic bronchoscopy. Table 18.6 describes the proper sequence of assessing DLT placement using clinical signs. Fiber-optic bronchoscopy has revealed a significant incidence of mispositioning of the DLT in cases despite proper positioning, as confirmed by relying on clinical signs. It is recommended that an appropriately sized fiber-optic bronchoscope be used in conjunction with clinical signs to confirm placement. Proper positioning of the DLT should be confirmed after (1) initial placement, (2) changes in position, and (3) instances of hypoxemia. Fig. 18.2 depicts proper placement of a left-sided DLT

TABLE 18.5	Sizing Recommendations, Placement Techniques, and Confirmation of Placement Recommendations for DLT	

	Dual-Lumen Endobronchial Tube
Sizing recommendations	Height: • 4'6" to 5'5": 35 or 37 French • 5'6" to 5'10": 37 or 39 French • 5'11" to 6'4": 39 or 41 French • Pediatrics (>8 years): 26 or 28 (only available as left-sided DLT) Gender: • Adult female: 35 or 37 French • Adult male: 39 or 41 French
Placement technique (i.e., blind technique)	• Direct laryngoscopy with appropriate laryngoscope blade to maximize visualization (i.e., Macintosh recommended) • LT passes with distal curvature concave anteriorly • After the tip passes the larynx, the DLT is rotated 90 degrees into the appropriate mainstem bronchus • Advanced to proper depth (see Fig. 18.2)
Confirmation of placement	• Chest x-ray • Clinical signs • Fiber-optic bronchoscopy

TABLE 18.6	Proper Sequence of Determining DLT Placement by Clinical Signs		

Bronchial Side Ventilated	Tracheal Side Ventilated	Situation	Action
Unilateral breath sounds on correct side	Unilateral breath sounds on correct side	DLT placed in the correct position	None required
Unilateral breath sounds	Unilateral breath sounds or no breath sounds	DLT advanced too far, tracheal lumen in mainstem bronchus	Retract DLT until properly positioned
Bilateral breath sounds	No breath sounds	DLT advanced not far enough, bronchial lumen in trachea	Advance DLT to proper positioning
Unilateral breath sounds on wrong side	No breath sounds or breath sounds on wrong side	DLT advanced into wrong mainstem bronchus	Retract DLT into trachea and rotate into appropriate mainstem bronchus
No breath sounds	No breath sounds	DLT not in trachea (e.g., esophageal placement)	Remove DLT and reattempt placement

and confirmation of placement via fiber-optic bronchoscopy. Table 18.7 describes two methods to assist in difficult placement of a DLT.

Bronchial blockers can be placed (1) in conjunction with a preexisting ETT (i.e., Fogarty catheter), (2) via a specially designed large-caliber ETT with a small integrated channel for a built-in bronchial blocker (i.e., Univent tube), (3) by wire-guided endobronchial blocker (i.e., WEB blocker), or (4) with the aid of a looped suture that can be attached to a fiber-optic bronchoscope (i.e., Arndt blocker). Advantages, disadvantages, confirmation of placement recommendations for bronchial blockers, and endobronchial intubation are given in Table 18.8. Video double-lumen tubes (VDLTs) allow for constant visualization of the trachea and bronchi throughout the intubation period and during the surgical procedure. The need for confirmation of ETT placement and checking for migration of a VDLT is only necessary if constant visualization becomes obscured (i.e., fogging, malfunction).

9. *Describe hypoxic pulmonary vasoconstriction and methods to optimize oxygenation during pneumonectomy.*

Hypoxic pulmonary vasoconstriction (HPV) is a normal physiologic response during instances of (1) primary hypoxia (i.e., low FiO_2), (2) hypoventilation, and/or (3) atelectasis to maximize oxygenation. During HPV, blood vessels perfusing nonventilated, poorly oxygenated alveoli constrict, causing a regional increase in pulmonary vascular resistance. Blood flow from these alveoli is diverted to the ventilated, well-oxygenated alveoli. This

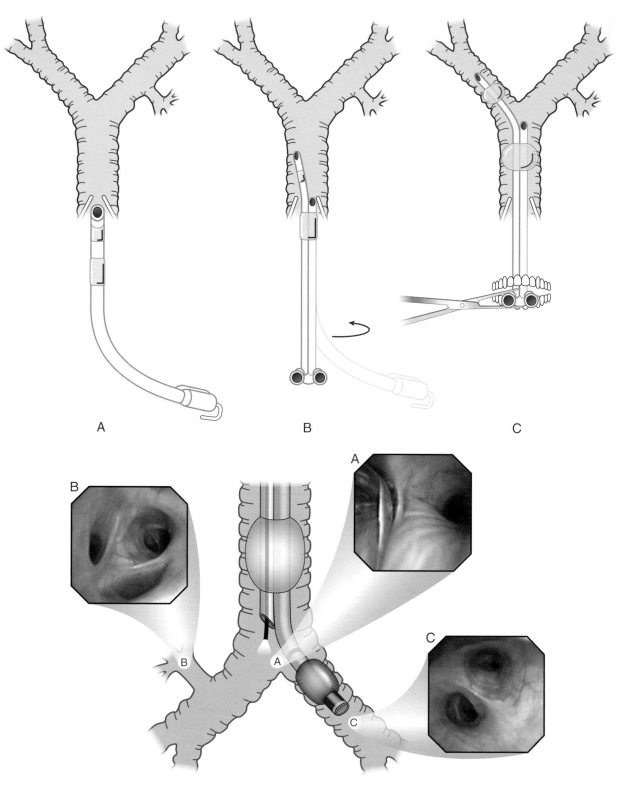

• **Fig. 18.2** *Top,* Blind method for placement of a left-sided DLT. (A) The DLT is passed with direct laryngoscopy beyond the vocal cords. (B) The DLT is rotated 90 degrees to the left (counterclockwise). (C) The DLT is advanced to an appropriate depth (in general 27–29 cm marking at the level of the teeth). *Bottom,* Fiber-optic bronchoscopic examination of a Mallinckrodt left-sided DLT. (A) The edge of the endobronchial cuff around the entrance of the left mainstem bronchus when the bronchoscope is passed through the tracheal lumen. A white line marker is seen above the tracheal carina. (B) Clear view of the right upper lobe bronchus and its three orifices: apical, anterior, and posterior segments. (C) A clear view of the bronchial bifurcation (left upper and left lower bronchi) when the left-sided DLT is in the optimal position and the fiber-optic bronchoscope is being advanced through the endobronchial lumen. (Reproduced with permission from Slinger P: *Principles and practice of anesthesia for thoracic surgery,* New York, 2011, Springer.)

TABLE 18.7 Two Methods to Assist in Difficult DLT Placement

Step 1	• DLT is positioned with both the bronchial and tracheal lumens within the trachea, the tracheal cuff is inflated
Step 2	• Bilateral lungs are ventilated, and the position is confirmed such as with a single-lumen endotracheal tube

Method 1	Method 2
Step 3 Appropriately sized fiber-optic bronchoscope is inserted into the bronchial lumen and the carina is visualized Step 4 Under direct visualization the fiber-optic bronchoscope is passed into the appropriate mainstem bronchus Step 5 The tracheal cuff is subsequently deflated and the right- or left-sided DLT may then be passed over the fiber-optic bronchoscope using it as a conduit for proper placement Step 6 The fiber-optic bronchoscope can then be inserted into the tracheal lumen to assess proper depth of insertion.	Step 3 Appropriately sized fiber-optic bronchoscope is inserted into the tracheal lumen and the carina is visualized Step 4 The tracheal cuff is deflated, and under direct visualization the right- or left-sided bronchial lumen is passed into the appropriate mainstem bronchus Step 5 Assess proper depth of insertion

TABLE 18.8 Advantages, Disadvantages, Confirmation of Placement Recommendations, and Types of Bronchial Blockers and Endobronchial Intubation

	Bronchial Blocker	Endobronchial Intubation
Advantages	• In situ endotracheal tube may be used for postoperative ventilation • May be used for pediatric patients when DLT is not possible • May be used in prone position • May be easier to place in difficult airway situations • Selective partial lung collapse possible (i.e., lobular) • Application of CPAP possible	• May be placed acutely in instances of thoracic hemorrhage or hemoptysis when visualization with a fiber-optic bronchoscope is inadequate
Disadvantages	• Small lumen of bronchial blocker may provide ineffective suction for secretions • Prolonged lung deflation and reinflation • Lumen of bronchial blocker easily occluded by secretions and blood • Bronchial blocker cuff prone to intraoperative leak or mucosal damage (e.g., improper inflation and prolonged use) • Lumen of bronchial blocker increases diameter of endotracheal tube • Malpositioning causes ineffective lung separation and impaired ventilation	• Limited in function • Allows only OLV • Inability to suction nonventilated lung • Inability to apply CPAP to nonventilated lung increases intrapulmonary shunt • Variant placement in right lung can cause ineffective ventilation of right upper lobe
Confirmation of placement	• Placed in conjunction with a self-sealing diaphragm and fiber-optic bronchoscope	• Placed blindly into mainstem bronchus in emergent situation • Self-sealing diaphragm and fiber-optic bronchoscope
Types	• Fogarty catheter • Univent • EB blockers • Arndt blocker	• Standard endotracheal tube

physiologic response to hypoxia decreases intrapulmonary shunt, while maintaining oxygenation in the process. Persistent alveolar hypoxia and pulmonary vasoconstriction may manifest as pulmonary hypertension or pulmonary vascular remodeling and may progress to cor pulmonale. The mechanism of HPV involves the activation of reduction–oxidation mitochondrial units within pulmonary artery smooth muscle cells, which regulate calcium influx and vascular tone.

In an effort to maintain patient oxygenation during instances of permissive atelectasis (e.g., OLV), it is imperative to avoid factors that inhibit HPV. Pharmacologic

TABLE 18.9	Summary of the Physiology of Positioning, Anesthesia, Ventilation, and Chest Opening		
State	**Physiology**	**Ventilation:Perfusion (V/Q) Ratio**
Upright, awake, spontaneous respiration, closed chest	• Ventilation: ↑ inferior lung regions • Perfusion: ↑ inferior lung regions	Relatively matched
Lateral, awake, spontaneous respiration, closed chest	• Ventilation: ↑ dependent lung • Perfusion: ↑ dependent lung	Relatively matched
Lateral, anesthetized, spontaneous respiration, closed chest	• Ventilation: ↑ nondependent lung • Perfusion: ↑ dependent lung	Mismatch
Lateral, anesthetized, controlled respiration, closed chest	• Ventilation: ↑ nondependent lung • Perfusion: ↑ dependent lung	Mismatch
Lateral, anesthetized, controlled respiration, open chest	• Ventilation: ↑ nondependent lung • Perfusion: ↑ dependent lung	Mismatch
Lateral, spontaneous respiration, and open chest	• Mediastinal shift • Paradoxical respiration	Mismatch

agents utilized in anesthesia have been implicated in HPV inhibition (i.e., inhalation anesthetics, calcium channel blockers, isoproterenol, nitrous oxide, and vasodilators). Dexmedetomidine does not have a significant effect on HPV and decreases the inhaled agent requirements. As such, dexmedetomidine in combination with inhaled agents may decrease the attenuation of HPV by inhaled agents. Inhibition of HPV does not preclude the use of these medications during anesthetic management. However, the degree of HPV inhibition is dependent on the amount of drug that is administered.

As with any surgical procedure, it is vital to maintain adequate patient oxygenation. Various maneuvers can be instituted during the intraoperative period, such as:

- **High FiO$_2$:** Utilization of a high fraction of inspired oxygen (up to 100%) maximizes arterial oxygenation. Utilization of 100% oxygen has been associated with absorption atelectasis and oxygen toxicity. However, the benefit of increasing PaO$_2$ in patients with marginal respiratory reserve exceeds the risks associated with hypoxia.
- **Continuous positive airway pressure (CPAP) and positive-end expiratory pressure (PEEP):** The application of 5 to 10 cm H$_2$O of CPAP to the non-ventilated lung is effective in minimizing alveolar hypoventilation, decreasing intrapulmonary shunt, and maintaining oxygenation during OLV. Furthermore, the application of PEEP to the ventilated lung has also been shown to be effective in maintaining oxygenation during OLV by preventing alveolar collapse and increasing functional residual capacity. The amount of PEEP should be maintained at less than 5 mm Hg, if possible, to avoid increasing pulmonary vascular resistance and barotrauma.
- **Tidal volume and respiratory rate:** During OLV, a tidal volume set to approximately 4 to 6 mL/kg should be used to prevent atelectasis, increases in airway

pressure, and increases in pulmonary vascular resistance. Despite the ventilation and perfusion mismatch that occurs during OLV, a 20% to 30% increase in respiratory rate is frequently adequate to maintain normal minute ventilation and physiologic PaCO$_2$.

10. *Describe physiologic differences in ventilation and perfusion comparing (1) the upright versus lateral decubitus position, (2) the awake versus anesthetized patient, (3) spontaneously breathing versus controlled ventilation patient, and (4) the closed versus open chest.*

Distribution of perfusion to the pulmonary parenchyma is affected by gravitational forces. In the upright lung, gravity causes a proportionally larger blood flow to the inferior areas when compared with the superior areas. In the lateral decubitus position, pulmonary blood flows to the dependent lung functions, much like the inferior areas of the upright lung. The increased perfusion of these areas is consistent through the physiologic states described in Table 18.9. Fig. 18.3 depicts the zones of the lung proposed by West. Note the distribution of blood flow between the upright and lateral decubitus positions.

Pulmonary compliance refers to the stiffness or mechanical compliance of lung tissue. It is defined as the change in volume for a given change in pressure. The following equation can be used to calculate pulmonary compliance (*C*):

$$C \text{ (liters/cm H}_2\text{O)} = \Delta V \text{ (change in volume) } / \Delta P \text{ (change in pressure)}$$

Regional differences in pleural pressure cause inferior areas of the upright lung to be more compliant compared with the superior portions. For a given and equal change in transpleural pressure, the inferior areas of the lung receive a larger portion of the tidal volume (e.g., increased ventilation). In the lateral decubitus position, the dependent lung functions much like the inferior regions of the upright lung.

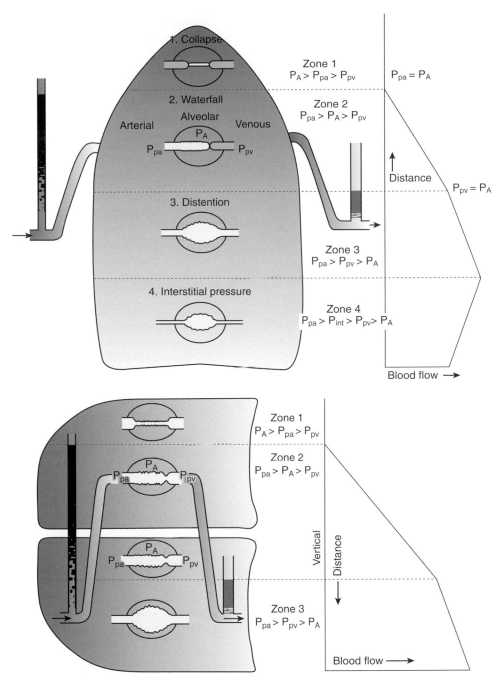

• **Fig. 18.3** The zones of the lung proposed by West. Note the distribution of blood flow in the upright and lateral decubitus positions. (*Top,* Modified from West JB, Dollery CT, Naimark A: Distribution of blood flow in isolated lung: relation to vascular and alveolar pressures, *J Appl Physiol* 19:713, 1964. *Bottom,* Modified from Triantafillou AN, et al. Physiology of the lateral decubitus position, the open chest, and one-lung ventilation. In Kaplan JA, Slinger PD, eds. *Thoracic anesthesia*, ed 3, Philadelphia, 2003, Churchill Livingstone.)

During spontaneous respiration, the increased ventilation of the inferior or dependent areas of the lung are relatively matched to the increased perfusion in these same areas. However, with the institution of (1) anesthesia, (2) controlled ventilation, and (3) thoracotomy (e.g., open chest), the dependent lung in the lateral decubitus position undergoes a decrease in pulmonary compliance, while the nondependent lung undergoes a relative increase in ventilation. Because perfusion does not change to the dependent area of the lung, a mismatch of ventilation and perfusion ensues. Table 18.9 summarizes the physiology of positioning, anesthesia, ventilation, and chest opening. Regional differences in ventilation and perfusion affect anesthetic management regarding (1) maintaining oxygenation and ventilation; (2) alterations in pulmonary resistance and compliance;

and (3) interpretation of data from invasive monitoring (i.e., pulmonary artery catheter).

Scenario: After 20 minutes of surgical resection, the following scenario occurs: blood pressure, 70/30; heart rate, 120; room air oxygen saturation, 75%; respiratory rate, 10; tidal volume, 20 mL; peak inspiratory pressure, 45 cm H$_2$O.

11. *List potential intraoperative complications that could cause this clinical scenario and the appropriate initial anesthetic interventions.*

Treatment for this patient would include immediately informing the surgeon, ventilating with 100% oxygen, and diagnosing the etiology of this scenario before instituting further treatment. A treatment plan for severe hypoxemia is given in Box 18.3. Potential intraoperative complications that can occur during pneumonectomy include:

- Pneumothorax: Treatment, emergent needle decompression, subsequent chest tube placement
- Venous air embolism: Treatment, flooding the surgical field with normal saline solution, Durant position, aspiration of the air embolus via central venous catheter, supportive measures as needed
- Hemorrhage: Treatment; surgical hemostasis; administration of crystalloids, colloids, and blood products
- Airway obstruction: Treatment, ensure airway device (e.g., lung separation and OLV method) is not occluded or surgically attached to bronchus

Postoperative Period

12. *Describe serious postoperative complications specifically related to pneumonectomy.*

A variety of postoperative complications have been reported after pneumonectomy, including (1) cardiac herniation, (2) hemorrhage, (3) bronchial disruption,

---

• BOX 18.3 Treatment Plan for Severe Hypoxemia

Prevention

1. Maintain two-lung ventilation until parietal pleura is exposed to atmosphere
2. Utilization of a high fraction of inspired oxygen (up to 100%)
3. OLV:Tv 4–6 mL/kg and adjust respiratory rate to maintain physiologic PaCO$_2$

Treatment

1. Check position of lung isolation/OLV method
2. Assess and correct hemodynamic status (e.g., mechanical or pharmacologic therapy)
3. Nondependent lung CPAP
4. Dependent lung PEEP
5. Alveolar recruitment maneuvers
6. Intermittent two-lung ventilation
7. Clamp pulmonary artery (i.e., pneumonectomy)

Alternative oxygenation methods:

1. High-frequency ventilation
2. Low-flow apneic ventilation (apneic insufflation)

---

(4) arrhythmias, (5) respiratory failure, (6) right heart failure, and (7) neural injury.

- **Cardiac herniation:** An intrapericardial approach for pneumonectomy may result in a large pericardial defect if it is unable to be closed. Herniation of the heart through this defect into the empty hemithorax causes severe impairment of cardiac function with a mortality rate of 50%. Immediate surgical exploration of the thoracic cavity is necessary.
- **Hemorrhage:** Systemic arterial bleeding, diffuse bleeding from thoracic parenchyma, failure of staples/sutures, and tracheobronchial trauma resulting from management of the airway have been reported. Uncontrolled postoperative bleeding and hypovolemia necessitate emergency thoracotomy.
- **Bronchial disruption:** The severity of a bronchopleural fistula is dependent on the size of the bronchial disruption, the accumulation of fluid within the pleural space, and the presence of a chest drain. The development of tension pneumothorax necessitates prompt resuscitation. The in vivo bronchial stump should be assessed for air leaks before closure of the thoracic cavity.
- **Arrhythmias:** Approximately 25% of patients undergoing thoracic surgery experience postoperative atrial dysrhythmias, of which atrial flutter and fibrillation are the most common. Trauma from cardiac manipulation, vagal stimulation, cardiopulmonary disease, and right atrial enlargement from increased pulmonary vascular resistance can precipitate cardiac dysrhythmias.
- **Respiratory failure:** Acute respiratory insufficiency is the most common and serious complication after pulmonary resection of bronchial carcinoma. Preexisting pulmonary pathology, pulmonary trauma, unilateral reexpansion pulmonary edema, and/or postoperative pain can precipitate inadequate respiratory effort.
- **Right heart failure:** The decrease in functional pulmonary vasculature after pulmonary resection causes an increase in pulmonary vascular resistance. The resultant increase in right ventricular afterload can precipitate acute right heart failure (e.g., cor pulmonale) and right-to-left intracardiac shunting across a patent foramen ovale.
- **Nerve injury:** During dissection, the phrenic, vagus, and recurrent laryngeal nerves may be inadvertently injured or deliberately sacrificed. Damage to the spinal branches of the intercostal arteries by dissection or diathermy may cause spinal cord ischemia. Fistula formation between the pleura and epidural space can cause spinal cord compression and ischemia from hematoma formation.

13. *Describe available pain management modalities for patients presenting for pneumonectomy.*

Intercostal nerve damage plays a significant role in the development of pain after thoracic surgery. Nerve dysfunction and muscle damage after incision, retraction, and suture placement are common. Analgesic therapies used to treat postoperative pain after pneumonectomy are included in Box 18.4. Although effective analgesic therapy reduces the prevalence and intensity of pain after thoracic surgery, up to 21% of patients still develop chronic pain. Because there are multiple pathways of nociceptive input to the central nervous system, a multimodal approach to pain management may also include a combination of nonsteroidal antiinflammatory drugs, use of patient-controlled analgesia, and narcotics.

Treating pain after pneumonectomy is important for the following reasons: (1) patient comfort and satisfaction, (2) allowing optimal respiratory effort, and (3) minimizing pulmonary complications (i.e., atelectasis and pneumonia). Lung volume may be greatly reduced after thoracic surgery, and effective analgesic therapy has been shown to improve pulmonary function.

Thoracic epidural analgesia is the current gold standard for post-thoracotomy pain and has gained increasing acceptance in providing subjectively better analgesia than any other method in thoracic surgery. Epidural anesthesia has been utilized in thoracic surgery performed in the awake patient, a testament to its versatility

---

> **• BOX 18.4 Effective Analgesic Therapies Used to Treat Postoperative Pain After Pneumonectomy**
>
> - Epidural analgesia (i.e., thoracic or upper lumbar)
> - Interpleural regional anesthesia
> - Cryoanalgesia
> - Intercostal nerve block
> - Paravertebral block
> - Local anesthetic infiltration
> - Systemic analgesia (i.e., patient-controlled analgesia)

---

as an analgesic therapy. In the absence of contraindications, patients undergoing major open thoracic surgical procedures should have a thoracic epidural catheter placed preoperatively. Typically, a thoracic epidural catheter is placed in the T6–T8 interspace. This is to be done in patients who are awake in order to assess proper placement and the presence of postprocedural complications. A clear plan must be created for the intraoperative utilization and management of a thoracic epidural catheter such as the type and volume of local anesthetic to be injected for the initial bolus and maintenance doses. The benefit of intraoperative analgesia should be weighed against the potential for sympathectomy resulting in hypotension for patients with marginal hemodynamic reserve. Postoperatively, the epidural solution used for infusion typically combines a low concentration of a long-acting local anesthetic such as bupivacaine or ropivacaine and a lipophilic opioid that includes fentanyl or hydromorphone.

Scenario: Following right-sided extrapericardial pneumonectomy, the following scenario occurs: blood pressure, 160/89; heart rate, 98; room air oxygen saturation, 88%; respiratory rate, 45; tidal volume, 150 mL; spontaneous respirations, FiO_2 100%.

14. *Describe the standard tracheal extubation criteria for patients presenting with pulmonary resections and available methods for DLT exchange.*

In patients presenting for pulmonary resection procedures, the plan for tracheal extubation should be considered within the early postoperative period to decrease the risk of pulmonary barotrauma and infection. Patients with marginal cardiopulmonary reserve may require postoperative mechanical respiratory support and should remain intubated until standard extubation criteria are met. Standard extubation criteria for patients presenting for pulmonary resection procedures are given in Box 18.5. Often, it is impossible

---

> **• BOX 18.5 Standard Extubation Criteria for Patients Presenting for Pulmonary Resection Procedures**
>
> **Global Criteria:**
> 1. Acceptable hemodynamic status
> 2. Normothermia
> 3. Ability to maintain patent airway
>   - Return of laryngeal and cough reflexes
>   - Appropriate level of consciousness
> 4. Adequate muscular strength
>   - Reversal of neuromuscular blockade as indicated by train-of-four ratio, 0.9, tetanic response to 100 Hz for 5 seconds, and double-burst stimulation without fade
>   - Head lift, 5 seconds and strong, constant hand grip
> 5. Acceptable metabolic function indicators
>   - Electrolytes
>   - Acid–base balance
> 6. Acceptable hematologic function indicators
>   - Hemoglobin level consistent with adequate oxygen delivery
> 7. Adequate analgesia for optimal respiratory effort
>
> **Respiratory Criteria:**
> 1. Adequate respiratory mechanics
>   - Vital capacity >15 mL/kg
> 2. Ability to maintain adequate oxygenation (with FiO_2, <50%)
>   - SpO_2 >90%
>   - PaO_2 >60 mm Hg
> 3. Ability to maintain adequate alveolar ventilation
>   - $PaCO_2$, <50 mm Hg
>   - Spontaneous respiratory rate (breaths/min) to tidal volume (L) ratio (e.g., rapid shallow breathing index) <100 breaths/min/L

and impractical to fulfill the criteria in its entirety. However, the anesthetist should exercise sound judgment in determining which patients are suitable for postoperative tracheal extubation.

If the decision to continue postoperative mechanical respiratory support is made and a DLT has been utilized for OLV, it should be replaced at the end of surgery with a single-lumen ETT. The DLT tube may be replaced under direct laryngoscopy or with the assistance of an airway exchange catheter depending on the preoperative history (i.e., difficult intubation). During this procedure care should be exercised by the anesthetist to minimize airway trauma, maintain adequate oxygenation, and prevent barotrauma if ventilation through the airway exchange catheter is possible.

Physical examination, preoperative testing, and preoperative optimization are aimed at determining which patients are optimal surgical candidates. Pulmonary

function tests provide invaluable diagnostic information regarding a patient's ability to tolerate the proposed pulmonary resection. Pulmonary function testing should commence in a tiered approach, with each tier increasing in sensitivity, specificity, and invasiveness. Box 18.1 describes the three tiers of preoperative function testing. Postoperative predicted (pop) FEV_1 is a method of estimating postoperative ventilatory function after pulmonary resection. It is based on the amount of functional lung tissue remaining after resection and can be calculated from ventilation and perfusion scanning of each individual lung by radioisotope. The following equation can be used to calculate the $popFEV_1$:

$$popFEV_1 = preop\ FEV_1 - (\%\ contribution$$
$$of\ diseased\ lung \times preop\ FEV_1)$$

A $popFEV_1$ of less than 0.85 l or less than 40% of predicted is associated with increased morbidity and mortality rates.

Review Questions

1. The majority of pulmonary resection procedures are performed to treat:
   a. Malignant tissue.
   b. Mesothelioma.
   c. Bronchopulmonary sequestrations.
   d. Thoracic trauma.
2. Which endocrinopathy is present in up to 40% of patients with SCLC?
   a. SIADH
   b. Cushing syndrome
   c. Myasthenic syndrome
   d. Carcinoid syndrome
3. Which accurately describes the correct placement and depth of insertion of a left-sided dual lumen tube after fiber-optic bronchoscopy?
   a. Bronchial cuff in the right mainstem bronchus, visible just below the carina
   b. Bronchial cuff in the left mainstem bronchus, not visible below the carina
   c. Bronchial cuff in the left mainstem bronchus, herniating above the level of the carina
   d. Bronchial cuff in the left mainstem bronchus, visible just below the carina

4. During which physiologic states are ventilation and perfusion most closely matched?
   a. Lateral, awake, spontaneous respiration, closed chest
   b. Lateral, anesthetized, spontaneous respiration, closed chest
   c. Lateral, anesthetized, controlled respiration, closed chest
   d. Lateral, anesthetized, controlled respiration, open chest
5. During a pneumonectomy, what surgical maneuver can be performed to decrease intrapulmonary shunt and prevent hypoxemia?
   a. Clamping of the mainstem bronchus
   b. Clamping of the superior pulmonary vein
   c. Clamping of the pulmonary artery
   d. Clamping of the inferior pulmonary vein

Suggested Readings

Asri S, Hosseinzadeh H, Eydi M, Marahem M, Dehghani A, Soleimanpour H. Effect of dexmedetomidine combined with inhalation of isoflurane on oxygenation following one-lung ventilation in thoracic surgery. *Anesth Pain Med.* 2020;10(1):e95287.

Campos JH. Current techniques for perioperative lung isolation in adults. *Anesthesiology.* 2002;97(5):1295-1301.

Campos JH, Feider A. Hypoxia during one-lung ventilation-a review and update. *Anesthesiology.* 2018;32(5):2330-2338.

Cohen E, Neustein SM, Eisenkraft JB. Anesthesia for thoracic surgery. In: Barash PG, Cullen BF, Stoelting RK, eds. *Clinical Anesthesia,* 5th ed. Philadelphia: Lippincott Williams & Wilkins, 2006:813-855.

Datta D, Lahiri B. Preoperative evaluation of patients undergoing lung resection surgery. *Chest.* 2003;123(6):2096–2103.

Divo MJ, DePietro MR, Horton JR, Maguire CA, Celli BR. Metabolic and cardiorespiratory effects of decreasing lung hyperinflation with budesonide/formoterol in COPD: a randomized, double-crossover, placebo-controlled, multicenter trial. *Respir Res.* 2020;21(1):26.

Gottschalk A, Cohen SP, Yang S, et al. Preventing and treating pain after thoracic surgery. *Anesthesiology.* 2006;104(3):594-600.

Grichnik KP, Clark JA. Pathophysiology of one-lung ventilation. *Thorac Surg Clin.* 2005;15(1):85-103.

Mineo TC. Epidural anesthesia in awake thoracic surgery. *Eur J Cardiothorac Surg.* 2007;32(1):13-19.

Pedersen CM, Green JS, Bigler DR, Andersen NE, Cromhout PF. Evaluation of time to intubation and rate of success for different healthcare professionals using a double-lumen left-sided endotracheal video tube: A prospective observational study. *J Perioper Pract.* 2020;30(12):383-388.

Reiker M. Respiratory anatomy: thoracic surgery. In: Nagelhout JJ, Elisha S, eds. *Nurse Anesthesia,* 6th ed. St. Louis, MO: Elsevier, 2018:624-644.

Tusman G, Böhm SH, Sipmann FS, Maisch S. Lung recruitment improves the efficiency of ventilation and gas exchange during one-lung ventilation anesthesia. *Anesth Analg.* 2004;98(6):1604-1609.

Mediastinoscopy

KEY POINTS

- Mediastinoscopy is a diagnostic procedure used for biopsy of mediastinal masses and staging of lung cancer.
- Compression of vital respiratory structures by a large mediastinal mass can create airway collapse or edema with severe respiratory compromise. An asymptomatic patient can develop severe respiratory compromise with anesthesia and any change in position.
- Mediastinal tumors can produce cardiac dysfunction secondary to compression of the heart and great vessels. The compression of vascular structures in the mediastinum can produce serious hemodynamic problems, including a

condition called *superior vena cava (SVC) syndrome*. Effects of SVC obstruction may worsen in the supine position and with the onset of general anesthesia.
- Mediastinal and thoracic tumors can produce abnormal hormone production, autocoids, or autoantibodies that have systemic effects and can potentially affect anesthesia management.
- Major complications of mediastinoscopy include hemorrhage, pneumothorax, compression of major blood vessels, esophageal perforation, tracheal or bronchial trauma, and recurrent laryngeal nerve injury.

Case Synopsis

A 57-year-old woman reports to her physician that she has had a recent history of respiratory distress. A chest radiograph reveals the presence of a large mediastinal mass, and the patient is subsequently scheduled for a mediastinoscopy for histologic biopsy and possible staging of tumor.

Preoperative Evaluation and Demographic Data

Past Medical/Surgical History

- Right-sided mastectomy with axillary node dissection for breast carcinoma 5 years ago
- During the past month, the patient reports increasing dyspnea, orthopnea, and a feeling of fullness in her neck.
- Smoking half a pack per day for 35 years

List of Medications

- None

Diagnostic Data

- Hemoglobin, 13.2 g/dL; hematocrit, 39.4%; glucose, 139 mg/dL; blood urea nitrogen (BUN), 15 mg/dL; creatinine, 1.1 mg/dL
- Electrolytes: sodium, 139 mEq/L; potassium, 3.9 mEq/L; chloride, 104 mEq/L; carbon dioxide, 24 mEq/L
- Chest x-ray and magnetic resonance imaging (MRI) reveal a widened mediastinum due to the suspected metastatic tumor.

Height/Weight/Vital Signs

- 160 cm, 58 kg
- Blood pressure, 152/84; heart rate, 78 beats per minute; respiratory rate, 24 breaths per minute; room air oxygen saturation, 97%; temperature, 36.8°C
- Electrocardiogram (ECG): normal sinus rhythm; heart rate, 86; ejection fraction, 60%
- Mallampati class III airway, midline trachea, clear breath sounds bilaterally

Pathophysiology

The mediastinum is the region between the two pleural cavities containing the heart, great vessels, thymus gland, esophagus, and tracheobronchial tree. The borders of the mediastinum are anterior—the sternum, posterior—the thoracic vertebrae, lateral—the pleural sacs and thoracic inlets, and inferior—the diaphragm. Evaluation of the mediastinum and its contents is often performed by mediastinoscopy, a diagnostic procedure that was first described by Carlens in 1959. The procedure is used to obtain tissue for histologic diagnosis and to help identify treatment options for various thoracic diseases.

Mediastinoscopy is an important tool for staging bronchogenic cancer to determine resectability and prognosis. Lymph fluid from the lungs drains directly into mediastinal lymph nodes, and node biopsy helps determine the extent of disease metastasis. Diseases presenting with mediastinal lymphadenopathy (e.g., sarcoidosis, lymphoma, infectious granulomatous diseases) may be diagnosed and staged with mediastinal tissue biopsy. When performed for cancerous lung tumor staging, the procedure's sensitivity is greater than 80% and specificity is 100%. Box 19.1 lists conditions that are associated with mediastinal masses.

Despite the availability of newer and less invasive imaging and diagnostic techniques (e.g., MRI, positron emission tomography [PET]), mediastinoscopy is still widely used and remains the diagnostic standard used to identify the histology of various mediastinal masses.

Surgical Procedure

Most mediastinoscopy procedures are performed under general anesthesia by way of the cervical approach through a small incision in the suprasternal notch. A tunnel created by blunt dissection through fascial layers, anterior and lateral to the trachea, allows the mediastinoscope to gain access to the subcarinal area (paratracheal, subaortic, and bronchial lymph nodes), as shown in Fig. 19.1. An alternative anterior or transthoracic approach (Chamberlain procedure) is used less frequently to inspect the lower and anterior mediastinum. The anterior approach involves entry through the second, third, or fourth left intercostal space lateral to the sternal border. Video-assisted mediastinoscopic lymph node biopsy is associated with fewer complications and greater numbers of lymph nodes dissected compared with the traditional surgical method.

The relative contraindications for cervical mediastinoscopy include factors that may distort the anatomy or interfere with the fascial plane for mediastinal dissection (scarring from a previous mediastinoscopy, radiation to the chest). Absolute contraindications to mediastinoscopy include coagulopathy, SVC obstruction, and thoracic aneurysm. Box 19.2 lists relative and absolute contraindications associated with mediastinoscopy.

Anesthesia Management Considerations

Preoperative Period

1. *Describe comorbidities often present in patients having a mediastinoscopy procedure.*

    Patients scheduled for mediastinoscopy often have significant cardiac and respiratory problems, such as coronary artery disease, peripheral vascular disease, and chronic obstructive pulmonary disease. Many of these patients are smokers, and the associated comorbidities require a thorough preoperative evaluation.

2. *Discuss preoperative evaluation of the patient scheduled for a mediastinoscopy.*

    Anesthetic management is complicated by the presence of a large mediastinal mass or enlarged mediastinal lymph nodes that compress nearby vital structures, such as the superior or inferior vena cava or the tracheobronchial tree. Preoperative evaluation should include an

---

> **• BOX 19.1 Predisposing Factors Associated With Mediastinal Masses**
>
> **Tumors**
> - Thymus gland tumors
> - Thyroid and parathyroid tumors
> - Lymphoma
> - Esophageal cancer
> - Neurogenic tumors
>
> **Benign Conditions**
> - Esophageal and bronchogenic cysts
> - Tuberculosis lymphadenopathy
> - Sarcoidosis lymphadenopathy
> - Aortic aneurysms

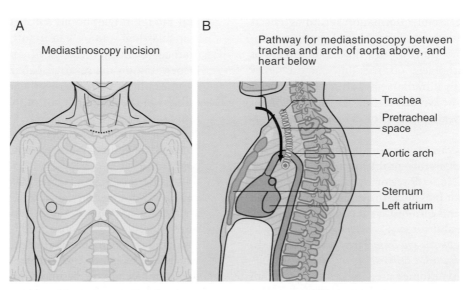

• **Fig. 19.1** Mediastinoscopy for investigation of the posterior mediastinum. (From Quick CRG, Biers SM, Arulampalam THA: *Essential surgery: problems, diagnosis and management*, ed 6, Philadelphia, 2020, Elsevier.)

• BOX 19.2 **Relative and Absolute Contraindications to Mediastinoscopy**

Relative Contraindications	Absolute Contraindications
Previous mediastinoscopy	Superior vena cava obstruction
Severe tracheal deviation	Thoracic aortic aneurysm
Cerebrovascular disease	Coagulopathy
Severe cervical spine disease that limits neck extension	
Previous chest radiotherapy	

TABLE 19.1 **Predictors of Perioperative Respiratory Insufficiency**

Preoperative cardiopulmonary clinical manifestations	Peak expiratory flow rate, 40% of predicted
Both obstructive and restrictive respiratory impairment	Tracheal diameter, 50% of predicted on CT scan

ECG, chest radiograph, and computed tomography (CT)/MRI scan to determine the size and location of the mass and any compression on adjacent vital structures. Echocardiography in the upright and supine positions may be indicated for the patient with cardiac symptoms.

Patients with tracheobronchial compression may exhibit wheezing, cyanosis, orthopnea, coughing, dyspnea, and stridor. A thorough preoperative assessment of the airway is imperative to detect distortion or obstruction. Patients should be questioned about the effect of position changes on their ventilation. Pulmonary function tests and flow-volume loops (in the upright and supine positions) provide useful information regarding effects of the tumor on pulmonary function and airway dynamics. The inspiratory limb of the flow-volume loop is blunted by extrathoracic obstruction; the expiratory limb is dampened by intrathoracic obstruction. Preoperative sedation must be avoided if clinical manifestations or laboratory tests reveal suspected or demonstrated airway obstruction.

Table 19.1 lists factors that predict an increased risk of perioperative respiratory problems in patients with a mediastinal mass. It is noteworthy that some surgical patients who do not present with symptoms may exhibit severe respiratory and cardiovascular compromise during or after anesthesia and surgery.

3. *Explore the paraneoplastic syndromes that may be associated with lung and mediastinal tumors.*

Paraneoplastic syndromes are diseases or symptoms that occur because of cytokines or hormones produced by, or in response to, a cancerous tumor. Hormones or hormone-like substances secreted from lung and mediastinal tumors can produce paraneoplastic syndromes. Disorders that may result from the liberation of abnormal humoral factors include hyperparathyroidism (parathyroid hormone secreted), Cushing syndrome (adrenal corticotropic hormone secreted), syndrome of inappropriate antidiuretic hormone (ADH secreted), and carcinoid syndrome (serotonin secreted).

Some mediastinal tumors produce humoral factors that affect muscle function. The preoperative history should include an assessment of the patient's muscle strength, as muscle weakness can be associated with thymomas or oat-cell (small cell) tumors of the lung.

Oat-cell tumors may be associated with Eaton–Lambert syndrome (myasthenic syndrome). These tumors can produce autoantibodies that inhibit calcium-dependent acetylcholine release at the presynaptic neuromuscular junction, which causes profound proximal muscle weakness. The muscle weakness associated with Eaton–Lambert syndrome typically improves with repeated movement, in contrast to the muscle weakness of myasthenia gravis, which worsens with repeated activity.

Tumors of the thymus gland (thymomas) are associated with myasthenia gravis, an autoimmune disease caused by antibodies that destroys nicotinic acetylcholine receptors on the postsynaptic neuromuscular junction. The resulting muscle weakness may be temporarily reversed by rest and anticholinesterase medications. Surgical patients with Eaton–Lambert syndrome or myasthenia gravis are at risk for aspiration and perioperative respiratory failure, and they are extremely sensitive to nondepolarizing muscle relaxants.

4. *Define the anesthetic implications associated with SVC syndrome.*

SVC compression by a mediastinal mass occurs in approximately 6% to 7% of patients with lung cancer. Masses that produce SVC compression are usually malignant and often consist of oat-cell carcinoma or non-Hodgkin lymphoma. Obstruction of the SVC by a mediastinal tumor can result in blocked venous drainage from the head, neck, and upper extremities. Depending on the severity, patients may present with dyspnea, dilated veins across the upper chest and neck, fullness in the face, or rubor of the upper body. Symptoms of SVC obstruction may be exaggerated in the supine position and may be relieved by head elevation. Steroids or diuretics are used to help control SVC congestion.

Tongue swelling and upper airway edema associated with SVC obstruction can make intubation difficult or impossible, and minor trauma during intubation can result in bleeding. SVC obstruction is considered to be a contraindication to mediastinoscopy. The surgeon may schedule radiation or chemotherapy to reduce the size of the tumor before mediastinoscopy. Compared with patients undergoing mediastinoscopy without SVC obstruction, patients with SVC syndrome have a significantly higher incidence of morbidity.

Intraoperative Period

5. *Describe the necessary equipment and monitoring modalities required for safe anesthetic management of a mediastinoscopy.*

Standard intraoperative monitors are used for most mediastinoscopy procedures. Assiduous neuromuscular blockade monitoring is particularly important for patients with mediastinal or thoracic tumors. An arterial line is optional, based on the anticipated hemodynamic stability of the patient. Preparation, a plan, and equipment for emergency thoracotomy should always be in place.

Intraoperative blood loss is usually minimal with a mediastinoscopy, but blood should be type and cross-matched because of the surgery's proximity to great vessels. The most serious complication associated with mediastinoscopy is massive hemorrhage. At least one large-bore intravenous catheter should be placed before induction of anesthesia. Should major blood loss occur through lacerated vasculature in the mediastinum, fluid and blood replacement through upper extremity cannulation sites may flow directly into the mediastinum. Under these conditions, and for the patient with SVC syndrome, fluids should be administered through lower extremity intravenous sites.

During the procedure, the rigid mediastinoscope can cause compression of major blood vessels, especially the innominate (brachiocephalic) artery (Fig. 19.2). Decreasing innominate blood flow, which perfuses the right common carotid and right subclavian arteries, increases the risk of cerebral ischemia or loss of the right radial pulse. Continuous monitoring of arterial flow in the right arm is necessary to alert the surgeon should repositioning or removal of the mediastinoscope be necessary. Intraarterial monitoring of the *right radial artery pressure or obtaining a right pulse oximetry* reading from a right finger probe may be used to monitor blood

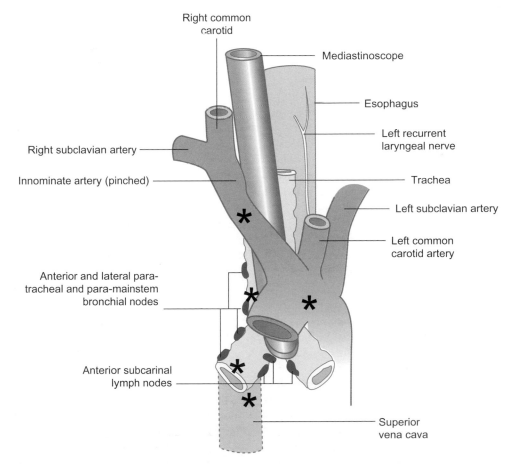

• **Fig. 19.2** Placement of a mediastinoscope into the superior mediastinum. The mediastinoscope passes anterior to the trachea but behind the thoracic aorta. This location allows for sampling of the anterior and lateral para-mainstem bronchial lymph nodes, anterior subcarinal lymph nodes, and anterior and lateral paratracheal lymph nodes. Anatomic structures that can be compressed by the mediastinoscope (see areas marked by asterisks) and result in major complications are the thoracic aorta (rupture, reflex bradycardia), innominate artery (decreased right carotid blood flow can cause cerebrovascular symptoms, and decreased right subclavian flow can cause loss of the right radial pulse), trachea (inability to ventilate, stimulus to cough), and vena cava (risk of hemorrhage with superior vena cava syndrome). (From Miller RD: *Miller's anesthesia*, ed 6, St. Louis, 2005, Elsevier.)

flow. If noninvasive blood pressure monitoring is used, the blood pressure cuff should be placed on the patient's left arm and the pulse oximeter on the right finger.

Close monitoring of breath sounds and ventilation pressures during the procedure is important to help detect the development of a pneumothorax or compression of the tracheobronchial tree by the mediastinoscope. The surgeon should be alerted immediately if any acute increase in airway pressure or change in breath sounds occurs.

6. *Describe the positioning considerations for a mediastinoscopy.*

Typically, the surgical patient is positioned supine with the shoulders elevated on a shoulder roll and the head extended and supported on a head cushion. A slight head-up position may be employed to help reduce congestion in the great veins and reduce compression on the airway. A head-up position will increase the risk of venous air embolism, especially if the patient breathes spontaneously. Changes in the patient's respiratory or cardiovascular state can occur suddenly, and plans should be in place to rapidly turn the patient if needed.

7. *Explain the key considerations for safe anesthetic management of the patient undergoing a mediastinoscopy.*

General anesthesia with mechanical ventilation is the preferred anesthetic management technique for mediastinoscopy. The ideal general anesthetic should produce profound depression of airway reflexes during instrumentation followed by rapid emergence. Due to the risk of pneumothorax with this procedure, nitrous oxide should be avoided. Cardiovascular changes during mediastinoscopy can occur suddenly, and administering vasoactive medications may be necessary for hemodynamic support. The nodes and tissue biopsies will be sent to pathology for interpretation before wound closure. The absence of surgical stimulation during this period may predispose the patient to developing profound hypotension. Titration of the inhalation agent is important, and the individual's hemodynamic response should dictate the concentration that is administered.

The patient's preoperative respiratory status is an important determinant of the type of anesthesia induction. A slow controlled induction in the sitting position is often the prudent choice for the patient with SVC syndrome. Suspected or documented obstruction of the tracheobronchial tree may necessitate an awake fiber-optic–guided intubation under local anesthesia. Case reports of cardiovascular collapse or an inability to ventilate with anesthesia induction reflect decreased thoracic muscle tone and loss of transmural distending pressure associated with the onset of anesthesia and muscle paralysis. Changing the patient's position (prone, lateral, sitting) may dramatically reverse cardiorespiratory distress by moving a mediastinal mass off of vital structures.

Equipment for emergency airway management (fiber-optic or rigid ventilating bronchoscope) should be available. A single-lumen reinforced endotracheal tube may be used to minimize the risk of kinking during the procedure.

High intrathoracic pressures associated with positive pressure ventilation and a large tidal volume decrease venous return. In a patient with venous congestion, controlled ventilation must be adjusted to provide the lowest ventilating pressure compatible with oxygenation and normal end-tidal carbon dioxide levels.

Muscle paralysis is important to prevent movement and coughing. Spontaneous ventilation with generation of negative intrathoracic pressure can increase the risk of air embolism through open venous structures. The patient should exhibit full return of reflexes and recovery of neuromuscular function before extubation. Box 19.3 outlines major complications associated with this procedure.

Postoperative Period

8. *Review the important postoperative considerations for the patient who is recovering from a mediastinoscopy.*

Routine postoperative monitoring is usually sufficient for an uncomplicated mediastinoscopy. The head of the bed should be elevated to improve respiratory function and decrease airway and surgical site edema. An uncomplicated cervical mediastinoscopy in an asymptomatic patient may be performed on an outpatient basis and the patient can return home the same day. A transthoracic mediastinoscopy generally requires at least one night of observation in the hospital before discharge.

Respiratory distress in the recovery room may be the result of inadequate reversal of muscle relaxant, airway edema, damage to the recurrent laryngeal nerve, paratracheal hematoma, compression of the tracheobronchial tree by tumor, or pneumothorax. The patient with unilateral recurrent laryngeal nerve damage will be hoarse and require close observation. Bilateral recurrent laryngeal nerve damage requires immediate reintubation. Tracheomalacia that has developed as a result of long-standing tracheal compression can cause an unexpected airway obstruction during the recovery period. A chest x-ray obtained in the postanesthesia care unit is necessary to rule out the possibility of a pneumothorax.

• BOX 19.3 Complications That Are Associated With Mediastinoscopy

Hemorrhage
Esophageal perforation
Pulmonary artery injury
Compression of major
  blood vessels
Dysrhythmias

Pneumothorax
Recurrent laryngeal nerve injury
Tracheal or bronchial trauma
Air embolism

9. *Describe future trends and developments for diagnosing and managing lung and mediastinal tumors.*

Newer, less invasive staging techniques are being developed that may redefine the need for surgical mediastinoscopy in patients with lung cancer. Video mediastinoscopy is increasingly used in selected cases and is associated with fewer complications. Endobronchial or transesophageal endoscopic ultrasound-guided fine-needle aspirations are promising, accurate, safe, and minimally invasive tools for mediastinal staging.

Review Questions

1. Eaton–Lambert syndrome (myasthenic syndrome) is associated with:
   a. Antibody-mediated depression of postsynaptic acetylcholine receptor synthesis.
   b. Oat-cell carcinoma of the lung.
   c. Profound skeletal muscle weakness that improves with rest.
   d. Derangements in calcium release from skeletal muscle sarcoplasmic reticulum.

2. Myasthenia gravis is associated with which type of mediastinal tumor?
   a. Thymoma
   b. Oat-cell carcinoma
   c. Lymphoma
   d. Adenoma

3. Which is classified as an absolute contraindication to a mediastinoscopy?
   a. Coagulopathy
   b. Myasthenic syndrome
   c. Distortion of the airway
   d. Previous chest radiotherapy

4. Anesthetists should monitor flow in the right radial artery during a mediastinoscopy to detect instrument compression on the _____.
   a. superior vena cava
   b. common carotid
   c. innominate artery
   d. right atrium

5. Near the end of a mediastinoscopy procedure, the patient becomes hypotensive and the peak inspiratory pressure increases. The trachea is noted to be deviated to the left. Which is the most likely cause of this situation?
   a. Pneumothorax
   b. Recurrent laryngeal injury
   c. Incomplete muscle relaxant reversal
   d. Bronchospasm

Suggested Readings

Bousema JE, Dijkgraaf MGW, Papen-Botterhuis NE, et al. MEDIASTinal staging of non-small cell lung cancer by endobronchial and endoscopic ultrasonography with or without additional surgical mediastinoscopy (MEDIASTrial): study protocol of a multicenter randomised controlled trial. *BMC Surg* 2018;18(1):27.

Cata JP, Lasala J, Mena GE, Mehran JR. Anesthetic considerations for mediastinal staging procedures for lung cancer. *J Cardiothorac Vasc Anesth* 2018;32(2):893-900.

Klinkenberg TJ, Bouma W, Van De Wauwer C, et al. Surgical experience and patient-related restrictions predict the adequacy of cervical mediastinoscopy in non-small cell lung carcinoma lymph node staging. *J Cardiothorac Surg* 2018;13(1):134.

Lemaire A, Nikolic I, Petersen T, et al. Nine-year single center experience with cervical mediastinoscopy: complications and false negative rate. *Ann Thorac Surg* 2006;82:1185-1189.

Leschber G, Sperling D, Klem W, et al. Does video-mediastinoscopy improve the results of conventional mediastinoscopy? *Eur J Cardiothorac Surg* 2008;33:289-293.

Madeira F, Cortesão J, Pancas R, Paiva T. Major hemorrhage during mediastinoscopy: do you panic or do you have a protocol? *Rev Port Cir Cardiotorac Vasc* 2017;24(3-4):146.

Malik R, Mullassery D, Kleine-Brueggeney M, et al. Anterior mediastinal masses - a multidisciplinary pathway for safe diagnostic procedures. *J Pediatr Surg* 2019;54(2):251-254.

Miao J, Li M, Fu Y, Hu X, Hu B, Li H. Ultrasound-guided video-assisted mediastinoscopic biopsy: a novel approach. *Ann Thorac Surg* 2016;102(5):e465-e467.

Reiker M. Respiratory anatomy: thoracic surgery. In: Nagelhout JJ, Elisha S, eds. *Nurse Anesthesia*, 6th ed. St. Louis, MO: Elsevier, 2018:624-644.

Santos Silva J, Costa AR, Calvinho P. Cervical mediastinoscopy: safety profile, feasibility and diagnostic accuracy in a decade in a single center. *Pulmonology* 2019;25(2):119-120.

Wallace MB, Pascual JM, Raimondo M, et al. Minimally invasive endoscopic staging of suspected lung cancer. *JAMA* 2008;299:540-546.

Wilson LD. Superior vena cava syndrome with malignant causes. *N Engl J Med* 2007;356:1862-1869.

20

Video-Assisted Thoracoscopic Surgery for Mediastinal Mass

KEY POINTS

- Improvements in video technology, endoscopic instruments, and surgical techniques have permitted a variety of diagnostic and therapeutic procedures to be performed using video-assisted thoracoscopic surgery (VATS).
- The advantages of VATS compared with open thoracotomy include decreased postoperative pain, reduced incidence of postoperative respiratory dysfunction, shorter postoperative course, and rapid recovery resulting in reduced duration of hospitalization and decreased cost.
- Open thoracotomy remains the gold-standard surgical approach for thoracic surgery. A VATS procedure may be emergently converted to an open thoracotomy, and this possibility must be considered during the creation of an anesthetic care plan.
- The presence of a mediastinal mass may be associated with cardiac and respiratory derangements, which include direct cardiac and great vessel compression, superior vena cava

syndrome, and tracheobronchial obstruction. Complete airway obstruction can develop perioperatively in patients, regardless of the presence of clinical symptoms associated with airway compression.
- Preoperative optimization of a patient with a mediastinal mass may include (1) a comprehensive preoperative assessment, (2) selective radiation and chemotherapy in sensitive groups, and (3) a biopsy of the mass under local anesthesia.
- Anesthetic management of high-risk patients includes (1) administration of general anesthesia without the use of muscle relaxants; (2) maintenance of spontaneous respirations; (3) remaining cognizant that cardiopulmonary bypass may be required for distal airway obstructions and hypoxemia; and (4) relieving airway obstruction by placing the patient in a lateral, prone, or semi-recumbent position.

Case Synopsis

A 26-year-old man is admitted to the hospital for a 3-cm right infrabronchial mass. He is scheduled by his thoracic surgeon to have a VATS for an excision of the mediastinal mass.

Preoperative Evaluation and Demographic Data

Past Medical/Surgical History

- The patient has had a persistent nonproductive cough for 6 months, which has been unresponsive to conventional medical treatment.

List of Medications

- Guaifenesin (Robitussin)

Diagnostic Data

- Hemoglobin, 14.1 g/dL; hematocrit, 42.3%; platelets 250,000 mm^3
- Electrolytes: sodium, 135 mEq/L; potassium, 4.1 mEq/L; chloride, 107 mEq/L; carbon dioxide, 26 mEq/L

- Blood urea nitrogen (BUN), 10 mg/dL; creatinine, 1 mg/dL
- Chest radiograph (anterior, posterior, and lateral): 3-cm right infrabronchial opacity; normal cardiac silhouette and pulmonary parenchyma; no tracheal or bronchial deviation
- Chest computed tomography (CT) scan: 3-cm right infrabronchial mass; homogeneous in nature; no cardiac and tracheobronchial compression; minimal vascular involvement as indicated by contrast-enhanced CT scan
- Magnetic resonance imaging (MRI): 3-cm right infrabronchial, high-intensity mass; no cardiac, great vessel, and tracheobronchial compression
- Pulmonary function tests (upright and supine): FVC, 4 L; FEV$_1$, 3 L; FEV$_1$/FVC 75%

Height/Weight/Vital Signs

- 170 cm, 68 kg
- Blood pressure, 120/86; heart rate, 90 beats per minute; respiratory rate, 25 breaths per minute; room air oxygen saturation, 98%; temperature, 36.9°C

Pathophysiology

Mass lesions in the mediastinum encompass a variety of pathologic etiologies and are classified as anterior, middle, or posterior based on their relationship to the heart, which occupies the middle mediastinum, as shown in Fig. 20.1. Due to the tenuous proximity to thoracic structures within a confined space, mediastinal masses may be associated with cardiac and respiratory derangements, including (1) direct cardiac and great vessel compression, (2) superior vena cava syndrome, and (3) tracheobronchial obstruction.

The incidence of mediastinal masses varies according to the age of the patient and location of the lesion. In adults, most mediastinal tumors occur in the anterior mediastinum. The two most common neoplasms of the anterior mediastinum are thymomas and lymphomas, which account for 30% of the pathology. In children, most mediastinal tumors occur in the posterior mediastinum. Tumors of the posterior mediastinum are typically neurogenic in nature and comprise 12% to 21% of all mediastinal masses.

Surgical Procedure

Improvements in video technology, endoscopic instruments, and surgical techniques have permitted surgeons to perform a variety of diagnostic and therapeutic procedures using the VATS technique. The indications for VATS procedures are listed in Table 20.1. VATS involves making three or more small incisions through which access ports are inserted into the chest wall. This allows the introduction of a high-resolution video camera and endoscopic surgical instruments into the thoracic cavity for surgical resection.

Typically, the sixth or seventh intercostal space in the midaxillary line is ideal for initial access to the pleural cavity. This allows for the introduction of a high-resolution video camera and a clear view of the mediastinum, all pleural surfaces, and the pulmonary parenchyma. Under direct thoracoscopic vision additional intercostal access ports are created, allowing the introduction of various surgical instruments into the thoracic cavity. The positioning of the patient, operating team, video monitor, camera, and surgical access ports are determined by the location within the thoracic cavity of the area of surgical concern. Positioning varies, and it is dependent on the individual surgeon's needs, but the principle of triangulation used for laparoscopic surgery is applicable to the thoracic cavity for VATS, as shown in Fig. 20.2. The thoracoscopic camera and endoscopic instruments should be oriented to face the target pathology from the same direction and triangulate the lesion.

After meticulous surgical resection of the mediastinal mass and hemostasis, a retrieval device is used for extraction of the mass. The tissue that is removed will be examined by a pathologist to determine if the specimen is cancerous. The adequacy of pulmonary reexpansion is observed under direct visualization. An appropriately sized chest tube is then inserted, and the thoracic cavity is closed in traditional surgical fashion.

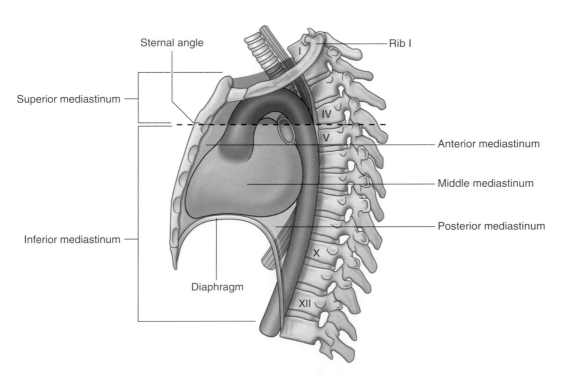

• **Fig. 20.1** Anatomic representation of the mediastinum with associated mediastinal pathologic abnormalities. (From Drake RL, Vogl AW, Mitchell AWM: *Gray's anatomy for students*, ed 4, Philadelphia, 2020, Elsevier.)

TABLE 20.1	Indications for Diagnostic and Therapeutic VATS
Pulmonary disease	• Biopsy and staging of cancer • Identification of disease (i.e., tuberculosis, mesothelioma, pulmonary interstitial fibrosis, and solitary nodules) • Lung resection or lobectomy • Lung volume reduction surgery • Drainage and treatment of pleural effusions (e.g., pleurodesis by talc, thermal, chemical, or mechanical means) • Traumatic thoracic injury evaluation • Diaphragmatic disease • Tissue resection (i.e., decortication, empyemectomy, bullae, blebs, and granulomas)
Esophageal disease	• Biopsy and staging of cancer • Tissue resection (i.e., vagotomy, Heller myotomy, Zenker diverticulum, and esophagectomy) • Gastroesophageal reflux treatment (e.g., Nissen fundoplication)
Mediastinal disease	• Biopsy and staging of cancer • Surgical resection of tumors of the anterior, middle, and posterior mediastinum
Cardiac and vascular procedures	• Patent ductus arteriosus ligation • Internal mammary artery dissection • Pericardial window and stripping • Minimally invasive direct coronary artery bypass
Miscellaneous	• Sympathectomy (i.e., treatment of hyperhidrosis or chronic reflex pain syndrome) • Thoracic anterior vertebral surgery • Removal of intrathoracic foreign bodies (i.e., sheared catheters)

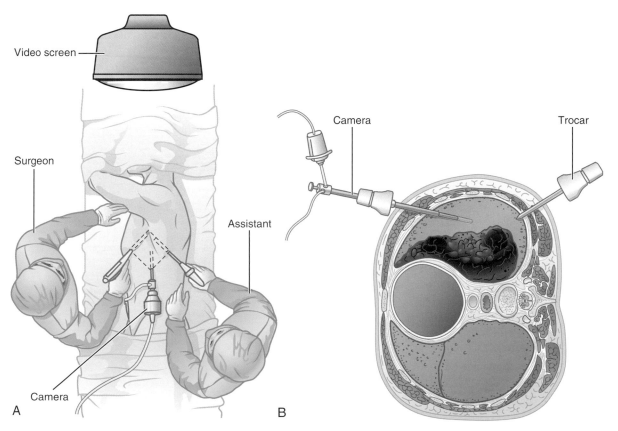

• **Fig. 20.2** Schematic representation of VATS. (A) Patient is positioned in a 30-degree semi-supine position. Note the triangular fashion in which the high-resolution video camera and surgical instruments are placed to promote adequate surgical visualization and resection. (B) Transverse plane view. (From Good VS, Kirkwood PL: *Advanced critical care nursing*, ed 2, St. Louis, 2018, Elsevier.)

Anesthetic Management and Considerations

Preoperative Period

1. *Describe the anatomy of the mediastinum and its bearing on mediastinal masses.*

The mediastinum extends superiorly to the thoracic inlet and inferiorly to the diaphragm and is bound laterally by the mediastinal parietal pleura. The mediastinum is separated into the superior and inferior mediastinum by an imaginary plane that extends from the sternal angle to the lower body of the fourth thoracic vertebra. The inferior mediastinum is further separated into the anterior, middle, and posterior mediastinum based on their relationship to the heart, which occupies the middle mediastinum.

At the convergence of the superior, anterior, and middle mediastinum are (1) the middle portion of the superior vena cava, (2) the tracheal bifurcation, (3) the main pulmonary artery, (4) the aortic arch, and (5) the cephalad surface of the heart. Mediastinal masses are associated with direct cardiac and great vessel compression, superior vena cava syndrome, and tracheobronchial obstruction. Each of these complications is potentially life-threatening, resulting in acute cardiac and respiratory deterioration and death during anesthesia if not appropriately managed.

2. *Discuss an appropriate preoperative assessment for patients presenting with mediastinal masses.*

As with any disease process, the optimal anesthetic plan is based on a thorough clinical evaluation and preoperative testing that should be tailored to each patient's presenting condition and symptomatology. Preoperative symptoms exhibited by patients presenting with mediastinal masses are listed in Table 20.2.

This is of utmost importance in patients with mediastinal masses due to the possibility of cardiac, great vessel,

TABLE 20.2 Preoperative Symptoms Exhibited by Patients Presenting With Mediastinal Masses

Symptom Category	Anatomy Involved	Symptom
Bronchopulmonary symptoms	• Bronchial irritation • Obstruction • Infection • Ulceration	• Cough or wheezing • Dyspnea • Chest pain, rales, rhonchi, or pneumonia • Hemoptysis
Extrapulmonary intrathoracic symptoms	• Pleura • Chest wall • Esophagus • Superior vena cava • Pericardium • Brachial plexus • Recurrent laryngeal nerves (unilateral or bilateral) • Spinal cord • Cervical sympathetic nerves	• Pleural effusion • Chest pain • Dysphagia • Superior vena cava syndrome • Pericardial effusion or pericarditis • Arm pain • Hoarseness or stridor • Paresthesia or paralysis • Horner syndrome
Extrathoracic metastatic symptoms	• Brain • Skeleton • Liver • Kidneys • Adrenal glands • Gastrointestinal tract • Pancreas	• Dependent on site and tumor involvement • Detection of metastases precludes curative surgery
Extrathoracic nonmetastatic symptoms	• Endocrinologic syndromes • Paraneoplastic syndromes	• Myasthenia gravis • Syndrome of inappropriate secretions of antidiuretic hormone (SIADH) • Cushing syndrome • Carcinoid syndrome • Eaton–Lambert syndrome • Pheochromocytoma
Nonspecific	• Variant	• Weight loss • Nocturnal diaphoresis • Anemia • Weakness • Anorexia • Lethargy • Malaise

and tracheobronchial compression. Findings from basic physical examination and preoperative testing dictate (1) the severity of the mediastinal mass, (2) the necessity for advanced intraoperative monitoring, and (3) the perioperative anesthetic plan.

The chest radiograph is the most common preoperative test used to evaluate intrathoracic pathology. When the patient develops symptoms consistent with a mediastinal mass, the chest radiograph is frequently ordered. Anterior, posterior, and lateral chest radiographs provide information regarding mediastinal mass (1) size, (2) location, (3) density, and (4) cardiopulmonary compression.

CT with contrast enhancement and MRI studies provide more accurate information regarding the location and density (i.e., solid, cystic, soft tissue, or vascular) of a mediastinal mass. The degree of cardiac and airway compression, which is not always obvious on chest radiograph, can be quantified. Perioperative risk of airway obstruction increases in patients with tracheal compression greater than 50% of predicted cross-sectional area. Box 20.1 lists indicators of patients who are at high risk for perioperative complications from a mediastinal mass.

Pulmonary function tests performed in the upright and supine positions can be useful in differentiating between obstructive versus restrictive mediastinal pathology. In addition, variable intrathoracic, variable extrathoracic, and fixed airway obstructions can be determined. This makes it a valuable diagnostic tool for evaluating the dynamic nature of the mediastinal mass and its compression of tracheobronchial structures throughout the respiratory cycle.

When constructing the anesthetic plan, additional tests may be advantageous for staging, planning operative therapy, and deciding on the method for one-lung ventilation (OLV). These tests should only be performed when the condition and age of the patient allow. These preoperative tests include (1) transthoracic echocardiography, (2) ultrasonography, (3) venography, (4) angiography, (5) radionucleotide scan, (6) biochemical marker testing, and (7) awake fiber-optic bronchoscopy.

3. *Evaluate the significance of superior vena cava syndrome.*

Mediastinal masses may cause compression of the superior vena cava or major tributaries, causing obstruction to venous drainage from the upper thorax. The two most common causes of superior vena cava obstruction are bronchial carcinoma and malignant lymphoma. The inherent low pressure of the venous circulatory system, including the pulmonary artery, predisposes it to extrinsic compression. The resultant increase in central venous pressure causes a myriad of symptoms, which can create physiologic instability. Patients who present with superior vena syndrome are at high risk for developing perioperative cardiopulmonary collapse. Box 20.2 lists the signs, symptoms, and anesthetic considerations for patients who present with superior vena cava syndrome.

4. *Describe the preoperative interventions that can be used to optimize high-risk patients with a mediastinal mass.*

The mediastinal mass is a foreign structure within the small confines of the thoracic cavity, and further compression occurs when the patient lies in a supine position. Therefore mediastinal masses pose a dilemma for the anesthetist due to the possibility of cardiac, great vessel, and tracheobronchial compression. These situations can result in hypotension, hypoxia, and cardiac arrest. Procedures such as tumor debulking, cystic aspiration, and tracheobronchial stenting have been cited in the literature and have successfully alleviated extrinsic compression.

Most anterior mediastinal masses that cause airway obstruction are lymphomatous in origin and are usually responsive to radiation and chemotherapy. Preoperative radiotherapy and chemotherapy have been used to reduce mediastinal mass size and compression. Significant diminution in mediastinal mass size and an improvement in symptoms after a single dose of chemotherapy have been reported.

• BOX 20.1 Indicators of Patients Who Are at High Risk of Perioperative Complications

- Cardiopulmonary signs and symptoms at presentation (i.e., dyspnea or orthopnea)
- Combined obstructive and restrictive pattern on pulmonary function tests
- Tracheal compression greater than 50% of predicted cross-sectional area
- Pericardial effusion at presentation

• BOX 20.2 Signs, Symptoms, and Anesthetic Considerations Associated With Superior Vena Cava Syndrome

Signs and Symptoms

- Dilation of jugular veins and collateral veins of the neck and upper thorax
- Edema of the face, neck, and upper thorax
- Cyanosis
- Papilledema or edema of the conjunctiva
- Central nervous system symptoms (i.e., headache, visual disturbances, or altered mental status)

Anesthetic Considerations

- Placement of central or peripheral venous catheter below the level of obstruction (i.e., femoral vein or lower extremity)
- Drug distributions from upper extremity intravenous injections are unpredictable and are therefore less desirable
- The presence of facial and neck edema correlates with edema of the mouth, oropharynx, and hypopharynx; a careful airway assessment is imperative
- Increased venous bleeding is possible due to high venous pressures (e.g., as high as 40 mm Hg)
- Increased arterial bleeding is possible due to vessel compression and/or difficult mass dissection

Determination of a mediastinal mass's sensitivity to radiation and chemotherapy can be determined only after biopsy. However, the induction of general anesthesia in symptomatic patients with mediastinal masses is associated with increased perioperative risk. Therefore it is prudent to perform diagnostic procedures such as fine needle or cervical node biopsy by administering local anesthesia and minimal sedation in cooperative and age-appropriate patients.

5. Describe contraindications to performing VATS.

The contraindications for having a VATS procedure are often due to a tenuous patient condition and/or inadequate surgical exposure. The specific contraindications for VATS are listed in Box 20.3. An open thoracotomy remains the gold-standard approach to thoracic procedures. Conversion of a VATS procedure to an open thoracotomy always exists and should be considered when formulating the anesthetic plan. Conversion to a limited thoracotomy or a standard open thoracotomy is justified if the patient's diagnostic and therapeutic condition is severely compromised.

Intraoperative Period

6. Describe the effects of general anesthesia on airway compression in a patient with a mediastinal mass.

Surgery and general anesthesia are associated with a variety of physiologic changes that can precipitate acute airway compression in a patient with a mediastinal mass. These physiologic effects include:

- Placement of the patient in the supine position causes a decrease in the anteroposterior diameter of the chest wall and cephalic displacement of the diaphragm. These actions increase the risk of airway compression by reducing the anatomic dimensions of the thoracic cavity and total lung capacity.
- Placement of the patient in the supine position causes an increase in central blood volume. In highly vascular mediastinal masses, this phenomenon can cause an increase in tumor blood volume and size, which exacerbates external compression of the tracheobronchial tree.

• BOX 20.3 Contraindications for VATS

- Hemodynamic instability and indication(s) for emergent open thoracotomy
- Bleeding diathesis (i.e., coagulopathy or grossly abnormal coagulation studies)
- Visceral and parietal pleural adhesions secondary to empyema, granulomatous infection, pleurodesis, or previous thoracotomy
- Inability to tolerate OLV or lateral decubitus position, as manifested by acute or chronic respiratory insufficiency and/or dependency on mechanical ventilation
- Pulmonary resection due to inaccessible location or size

- Induction of anesthesia and institution of inhalation anesthetics cause a decrease in tracheobronchial smooth muscle tone. This increases the extrinsic compressibility of the trachea and bronchi.
- Institution of positive-pressure ventilation eliminates the normal transpleural pressure gradient. This decreases airway diameter and increases the risk of extrinsic compression. Even in the absence of extrinsic tracheal compression, the presence of tracheomalacia and weakening of tracheal structures can cause complete tracheal collapse.

7. Describe the effects of muscle relaxants and positive pressure ventilation on airway compression in a patient with a mediastinal mass.

Under normal circumstances, inspiratory muscle contraction during spontaneous ventilation causes caudal movement of the diaphragm and an increase in the anteroposterior diameter of the chest wall. The opposing interaction between the expanding chest wall and the elastic recoil of the lungs creates a negative intrathoracic pressure (23 to 25 cm H_2O). In addition, a transpleural pressure gradient develops within the thoracic cavity. These distending forces that result from spontaneous respiration increase airway diameter and minimize airway compression.

The use of muscle relaxants and/or the institution of positive-pressure ventilation inhibit spontaneous respiration and effectively eliminate the normal transpleural pressure gradient. The resulting decrease in the caliber of the airways increases the risk of partial or complete airway obstruction.

8. Describe three methods of induction of general anesthesia that preserve spontaneous respiration.

Preanesthetic optimization is imperative to minimizing risks associated with induction of general anesthesia. Before induction of anesthesia, patients who exhibit signs and symptoms of respiratory difficulty should be placed in the semi-recumbent position to relieve preexisting airway obstruction. In high-risk patients, cannulation of the femoral vein and arteries, in anticipation of the need for cardiopulmonary bypass, has been suggested. Cardiopulmonary bypass may be required for distal airway obstructions and hypoxemia that are untreatable by conventional emergency airway methods. Emergency tracheotomy or placement of a rigid ventilating bronchoscope may prove futile if the airway compression occurs in the distal trachea or bronchial segments.

The following methods preserve spontaneous respiration and are used to minimize the risks associated with induction of general anesthesia:

- Awake intubation, followed by a gradual intravenous or inhalation induction
- Inhalation induction with a volatile anesthetic, followed by intubation
- Intravenous induction with ketamine, followed by intubation

9. Describe methods to optimize visualization and maintain oxygenation during VATS.

As with any surgical procedure, it is of utmost importance to provide adequate surgical visualization and maintain adequate patient oxygenation. Various maneuvers can be instituted during the intraoperative period, such as:

Visualization

- **Position:** The positioning of the patient (i.e., supine, prone, or lateral decubitus) is determined by the location of the mass within the thoracic cavity. The lateral decubitus position allows for intercostal surgical access and visualization of mediastinal structures. The affected side is typically placed in a nondependent position. The operating room table can then be rotated and manipulated (i.e., Trendelenburg, reverse Trendelenburg, or flexed positioned), utilizing gravity to increase surgical visualization.
- **OLV:** A dual-lumen endobronchial tube (DLT), bronchial blocker, or endobronchial intubation with a single-lumen endotracheal tube allows (1) ventilatory control, (2) selective lung separation, (3) deflation of the lung ipsilateral to the area of surgical concern, and (4) improved surgical exposure. Suction that is applied to the DLT can facilitate rapid lung deflation. Due to the relatively small diameter of the bronchial blocker, it may take up to 30 minutes for complete lung collapse to occur. Allowing adequate time for lung deflation is imperative in order to provide adequate surgical exposure.
- **Carbon dioxide insufflation:** In rare circumstances, carbon dioxide can be insufflated into the pleural cavity to facilitate visualization. It may be used at the beginning of the procedure to facilitate expeditious and complete ipsilateral lung collapse. Insufflation pressure should be maintained as low as possible (less than 5 mm Hg) and the CO_2 inflow rate kept less than 2 L/min. Higher pressures and/or a rapid insufflation rate can cause mediastinal shift and hemodynamic compromise, as occurs in a tension pneumothorax.

Oxygenation

- **High FiO_2:** Utilization of a high fraction of inspired oxygen (up to 100%) maximizes arterial oxygenation. It is important to note that the utilization of 100% oxygen has been associated with absorption atelectasis and oxygen toxicity. However, the benefits of increasing PaO_2 in patients with marginal respiratory reserve exceed the risks.
- **Continuous positive airway pressure (CPAP) and positive-end expiratory pressure (PEEP):** By minimizing the intrapulmonary shunt, the application of 5 to 10 cm H_2O of CPAP to the nonventilated lung is effective in maximizing oxygenation during OLV. Furthermore, the application of PEEP to the ventilated lung has also been shown to be effective in maintaining oxygenation during OLV by preventing alveolar collapse and increasing

functional residual capacity. PEEP should be maintained at less than 5 mm Hg to avoid adversely increasing pulmonary vascular resistance.
- **Tidal volume and respiratory rate:** During OLV, a tidal volume set to approximately 4 to 6 mL/kg should be used to prevent (1) atelectasis, (2) increases in airway pressure, and (3) increases in pulmonary vascular resistance. Despite the ventilation and perfusion mismatch that occurs during OLV, a 20% to 30% increase in respiratory rate is frequently adequate to maintain normal minute ventilation and physiologic $PaCO_2$.

Scenario: After 20 minutes of surgical resection, the following scenario occurs: blood pressure, 70/30; heart rate, 110; room air oxygen saturation, 87%; respiratory rate, 10; tidal volume, 20 mL; peak inspiratory pressure, 40 cm H_2O.

10. List potential intraoperative complications and appropriate initial interventions during VATS for mediastinal mass that could cause this clinical scenario.

Treatment for this patient would include immediately informing the surgeon, ventilating with 100% oxygen, and diagnosing the etiology of this scenario before instituting further treatment. Potential intraoperative complications that can occur during VATS for mediastinal mass include:

- Pneumothorax: Treatment, emergent needle decompression, subsequent chest tube placement
- Embolism: Treatment, left lateral decubitus positioning (Durant position), aspiration of embolus via central venous catheter, supportive measures as needed
- Hemorrhage: Treatment, surgical hemostasis, administration of crystalloids, colloids, and blood products
- Cardiac, great vessel, and tracheobronchial compression: A treatment plan is included in Box 20.4

• BOX 20.4 Treatment Plan for Cardiac, Great Vessel, and Tracheobronchial Compression

- Stop surgery
- Minimize or reverse the deleterious effects of (1) general anesthesia, (2) muscle relaxants, and (3) positive-pressure ventilation
- Change patient position to lateral, prone, or semi-recumbent to decrease compression
- Place rigid ventilating bronchoscope to apply tension to weakened tracheobronchial tree
- Place rigid ventilating bronchoscope to bypass distal obstructions
- Helium–oxygen mixture to reduce the resistance to airflow through compressed airway
- Emergency thoracotomy, median sternotomy, and tumor debulking to decrease extrinsic compression
- Utilize advanced cardiac life support protocol as needed
- Cardiopulmonary bypass to restore oxygenation

Postoperative Period

11. Describe serious postoperative complications specifically related to VATS.

A variety of postoperative complications have been reported after VATS, and constant vigilance is necessary during the postoperative period.

- **Airway obstruction:** Despite adequate surgical resection of a mediastinal mass, the presence of tracheomalacia and inadequate cartilaginous tracheal support can cause tracheal collapse and necessitate postoperative intubation and ventilatory support.
- **Hemorrhage:** Systemic arterial bleeding, diffuse bleeding from thoracic parenchyma, failure of endoscopic staples/sutures, and tracheal lacerations resulting from management of the airway have been reported. Uncontrolled postoperative bleeding and hypovolemia necessitate emergency thoracotomy.
- **Dysrhythmias:** Trauma from cardiac manipulation, vagal stimulation, and cardiopulmonary disease can precipitate cardiac dysrhythmias. Approximately 25% of patients undergoing thoracic surgery experience postoperative atrial dysrhythmias, of which atrial flutter and fibrillation are the most common.
- **Respiratory insufficiency:** Acute respiratory insufficiency is the most common and serious complication after pulmonary resection, which occurs in nearly 15% of patients after resection of bronchial carcinoma. Preexisting pulmonary pathology, pulmonary transudate, pulmonary trauma, and/or postoperative pain can precipitate inadequate respiratory effort.
- **Neural injury:** During dissection of mediastinal masses, the phrenic, vagus, and recurrent laryngeal nerves may be inadvertently injured or deliberately sacrificed. Damage to the spinal branches of the intercostal arteries by dissection or diathermy may cause spinal cord ischemia. In addition, after dissection in the posterior mediastinum, a fistula can

form between the pleura and epidural space in which blood can enter and cause spinal cord compression and ischemia.

12. Describe available pain management modalities for patients presenting for VATS.

The advantages of VATS over open thoracotomy include decreased postoperative pain, reduction in the incidence of postoperative respiratory dysfunction, shorter postoperative course, and promotion of a rapid recovery. These benefits result in a reduced length of hospital stay and decreased costs. Analgesic interventions that are used to treat postoperative pain after VATS are included in Box 20.5.

Despite this minimally invasive approach to thoracic surgery, there is the potential for chronic pain in patients after VATS. Intercostal nerve damage resulting from chest wall trauma and muscle damage from instrumentation can result in intercostal neuritis, postoperative neuralgia, and chronic pain.

Treating pain after VATS is important for the following reasons: (1) patient comfort and satisfaction; (2) allowing optimal respiratory effort; and (3) minimizing pulmonary complications (i.e., retention of secretions, airway closure, and atelectasis). Because there are multiple pathways of nociceptive input to the central nervous system, a multimodal approach to pain management may also include a combination of nonsteroidal antiinflammatory drugs, acetaminophen, dexmedetomidine, ketamine, regional anesthesia with liposomal bupivacaine, patient-controlled analgesia, epidural analgesia, and narcotics.

> **• BOX 20.5   Effective Analgesic Therapies Used to Treat Postoperative Pain After VATS**
>
> - Regional anesthesia (paravertebral block, serratus plane block, intercostal nerve block)
> - Epidural analgesia (i.e., thoracic or upper lumbar)
> - Cryoanalgesia
> - Local anesthetic infiltration
> - Systemic analgesia (i.e., patient-controlled analgesia)

Review Questions

1. The two most common neoplasms present in the anterior mediastinum are:
   a. Thymoma and lymphoma.
   b. Lymphoma and teratoma.
   c. Teratoma and bronchogenic cyst.
   d. Bronchogenic cyst and neurogenic tumor.
2. Which is not associated with a mediastinal mass?
   a. Cardiac compression
   b. Pulmonary artery dilation
   c. Superior vena cava syndrome
   d. Tracheobronchial obstruction
3. Which can precipitate tracheobronchial collapse?
   a. Maintaining spontaneous ventilation
   b. Local anesthesia and minimal sedation
   c. Tracheomalacia
   d. Intravenous induction with ketamine

4. Which statement is false regarding VATS?
   a. Diagnostic and therapeutic procedures can be performed using VATS.
   b. The principle of surgical triangulation is applicable to VATS.
   c. VATS is associated with more pain than an open thoracotomy.
   d. Conversion from a VATS procedure to open thoracotomy may be necessary.

5. Which is the most common postoperative complication after VATS for bronchial carcinoma?
   a. Respiratory insufficiency
   b. Airway obstruction
   c. Neural injury
   d. Hemorrhage

Suggested Readings

Allain PA, Carella M, Agrafiotis AC, Burey J, et al. Comparison of several methods for pain management after video-assisted thoracic surgery for pneumothorax: an observational study. *BMC Anesthesiol* 2019;19(1):120.

Béchard P, Létourneau L, Lacasse Y, et al. Perioperative cardiopulmonary complications in adults with mediastinal mass. *Anesthesiology* 2004;100(4):826-834.

Chu L, Zhang X, Lu Y, Xie G, Song S, Fang X, Cheng B. Improved analgesic effect of paravertebral blocks before and after video-assisted thoracic surgery: a prospective, double-blinded, randomized controlled trial. *Pain Res Manag* 2019;2019:9158653.

Cirino LM, Campos JR, Fernandez A, et al. Diagnosis and treatment of mediastinal mass by thoracoscopy. *Chest* 2000;117(6):1787-1792.

Cohen E, Neustein SM, Eisenkraft JB. Anesthesia for thoracic surgery. In: Barash PG, Cullen BF, Stoelting RK, eds. *Clinical Anesthesia,* 5th ed. Philadelphia: Lippincott Williams & Wilkins, 2006:813-855.

Duwe BV, Sterman DH, Musani AI. Tumors of the mediastinum. *Chest* 2005;128(4):2893-2909.

Gottschalk A, Cohen SP, Yang S, et al. Preventing and treating pain after thoracic surgery. *Anesthesiology* 2006;104(3):594-600.

Lederman D, Easwar J, Feldman J, Shapiro V. Anesthetic considerations for lung resection: preoperative assessment, intraoperative challenges and postoperative analgesia. *Ann Transl Med* 2019; 7(15):356.

Massone PBG, Lequaglie C, Magnani B, et al. The real impact and usefulness of video-assisted thoracoscopic surgery in the diagnosis and therapy of clinical lymphadenopathies of the mediastinum. *Ann Surg Oncol* 2003;10(10):1197-1202.

NeMoyer RE, Pantin E, Aisner J, Jongco R, et al. Paravertebral nerve block with liposomal bupivacaine for pain control following video-assisted thoracoscopic surgery and thoracotomy. *J Surg Res* 2020;246:19-25.

Reiker M. Respiratory anatomy: thoracic surgery. In: Nagelhout JJ, Elisha S KL, eds. *Nurse Anesthesia,* 6th ed. St. Louis, MO: Elsevier, 2018:624-644.

Sun K, Liu D, Chen J, Yu S, Bai Y, Chen C, et al. Moderate-severe postoperative pain in patients undergoing video-assisted thoracoscopic surgery: a retrospective study. *Sci Rep* 2020;10(1):795.

Tseng WC, Lin WL, Lai HC, Huang TW, et al. Fentanyl-based intravenous patient-controlled analgesia with low dose of ketamine is not inferior to thoracic epidural analgesia for acute post-thoracotomy pain following video-assisted thoracic surgery: a randomized controlled study. *Medicine (Baltimore)* 2019;98(28):e16403.

Viti A, Bertoglio P, Zamperini M, Tubaro A, et al. Serratus plane block for video-assisted thoracoscopic surgery major lung resection: a randomized controlled trial. *Interact Cardiovasc Thorac Surg* 2020;30(3):366-372.

Yang H, Dong Q, Liang L, Liu J, Jiang L, Liang H, Xu S. The comparison of ultrasound-guided thoracic paravertebral blockade and internal intercostal nerve block for non-intubated video-assisted thoracic surgery. *J Thorac Dis* 2019;11(8):3476-3481.

21

Anesthesia Management for Thymectomy

KEY POINTS

- The thymus is responsible for the production of T lymphocytes that are involved in cell-mediated immunity.
- Thymomas are frequently associated with paraneoplastic syndromes, which include hypogammaglobulinemia, pure red cell aplasia, Cushing syndrome, Graves disease, pernicious anemia, and several autoimmune diseases, especially myasthenia gravis (MG).

- Symptoms that are associated with a thymoma are primarily due to the impingement of mediastinal structures, or they are related to MG.
- MG and Lambert–Eaton myasthenic syndrome (LEMS) are two different physiologic disease processes that are associated with implications for anesthetic management.
- Anticholinesterase medications are the primary treatment for symptoms associated with MG.

Case Synopsis

A 52-year-old woman with a history of Class III MG and a stage III thymoma is admitted for a thymectomy. Before admission, she received a 3-month course of chemotherapy with doxorubicin, cisplatin, vincristine, and cyclophosphamide. She is scheduled for a postoperative course of mediastinal radiation.

Preoperative Evaluation and Demographic Data

Past Medical/Surgical History

- MG Class III for 14 years
- Stage III thymoma
- Thyroidectomy for Graves disease 4 years ago
- Laparoscopic cholecystectomy 10 years ago

List of Medications

- Pyridostigmine 600 mg daily
- Prednisolone 100 mg every second day
- Synthroid 0.15 mg daily

Diagnostic Data

- Hemoglobin, 11.9 mg/dL; hematocrit, 35%
- Glucose, 88 mg/dL
- Electrolytes: sodium, 139 mEq/L; potassium, 3.8 mEq/L; chloride, 106 mEq/L; carbon dioxide, 22 mEq/L
- Electrocardiogram (ECG): Normal sinus rhythm, heart rate 88

Height/Weight/Vital Signs

- 163 cm, 63 kg
- Blood pressure, 130/84; heart rate, 80 beats per minute; respiratory rate, 16 breaths per minute; temperature, 37°C; room air oxygen saturation, 98%

Pathophysiology

Named for its resemblance to the bud of the thyme herb, the thymus is embryonically derived from the third, and occasionally the fourth, pair of pharyngeal pouches. As seen in Fig. 21.1, it is composed of two fused different-sized lobes, enclosed by a dense capsule. The thymus is located in the upper thorax, at the level of the fourth costal cartilage, right beneath the sternum. It can extend upward into the neck as high as the lower border of the thyroid gland. Each thymic lobe is made up of numerous lobules of varying size. The cortical portion of the lobules is mainly composed of lymphoid cells, and the medulla is primarily epithelial cells. Blood supply to the thymus is derived from the internal mammary and superior and inferior thyroid arteries. Venous blood drains into the innominate veins and the thyroid sinus. The organ receives both sympathetic and parasympathetic innervation (vagus). The thymus gland weighs 10 to 30 mg at birth. It increases in size throughout childhood until puberty, at which time it starts to atrophy in response to increased levels of sex hormones; over time it is gradually replaced by adipose tissue.

There are two main types of immune system cells: B lymphocytes (B cells) and T lymphocytes (T cells). B cells are

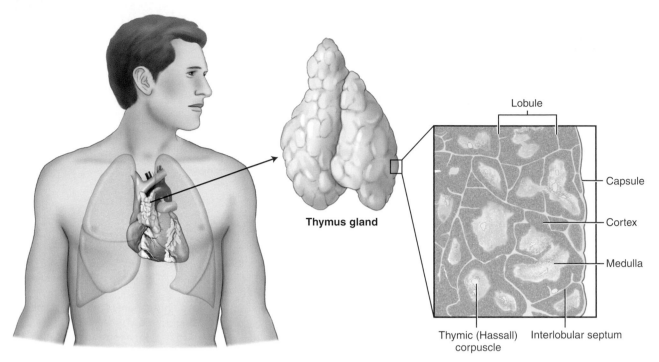

• **Fig. 21.1** Anatomy of the thymus gland. (From VanMeter KC, Huber RJ: *Microbiology for the healthcare professional*, ed 2, St. Louis, 2016, Elsevier.)

produced by bone marrow stem cells and are responsible for humoral immunity that is mediated by antibody production and complement activation. T cells, bone marrow stem cells that mature in the thymus, are involved in cell-mediated immunity and include helper T cells (effector T cells or T_h cells), cytotoxic T cells (T_C cells), memory T cells (regulatory T cells, T_{reg} cells, formerly known as *suppressor T cells*), natural killer T cells (NKT), and gamma/delta T cells (gd T cells). In addition to their role in fighting infection and cancer, T cells are responsible for rejection of transplanted organs, autoimmune diseases, and allergies.

The main function of the thymus is the development of immunocompetent T cells. Bone marrow stem cells migrate to the thymus and enter the cortex of the thymic lobules, where they mature into T cells in response to the thymic hormones thymopoietin and thymosin. Each stem cell has T-cell receptor (TCR) genes, which undergo genetic rearrangement during thymocyte maturation. The resultant T cells have a unique TCR that can recognize specific cell-bound antigens in lymphoid organs. T cells account for approximately 65% of blood lymphocytes; they are also found in lymphoid organs.

Surgical Procedure

Three cell types cause thymic cancers. Epithelial cells give rise to thymic carcinoma and thymomas; lymphocytes are associated with Hodgkin disease or non-Hodgkin lymphomas; Kulchitsky cells (neuroendocrine cells) give rise to thymic carcinoid tumors. Thymolipoma is composed of thymic tissue and fatty tissue. Thymomas are the most common type of thymic tumor. Although the overall incidence is low—0.15 cases per 100,000 and 0.5% of all cancers—they account for 20% of all mediastinal tumors and 50% of anterior mediastinal tumors. Surgery is the mainstay of treatment; despite their indolent nature, thymomas have the potential for local spread, especially into the pleural space. Chemotherapy may be instituted preoperatively to shrink large, malignant tumors; postoperative chemotherapy and radiation may be indicated for large invasive tumors. Thymomas are frequently associated with several autoimmune diseases, especially MG, which is found in 30% to 65% of patients with a thymoma. Approximately 10% to 15% of patients with MG have a thymoma, and myasthenic patients are routinely screened for thymic tumors.

Surgical thymectomy is also indicated for patients with generalized MG to induce remission or sufficiently reduce symptoms to allow a reduction in immunosuppressive medication. Due to the role of the thymus in development of the immune system, it is preferable to delay thymectomy until puberty. After the age of 60, there is a questionable amount of viable thymic tissue, which reduces the probability of a positive response to thymectomy in older patients who have MG. Of the paraneoplastic syndromes associated with thymomas, only MG, pure red cell aplasia, and hypogammaglobulinemia have a positive response to thymectomy.

Anesthetic Management and Considerations

Preoperative Period

1. Describe the symptoms that are commonly associated with thymomas.

Thymomas are capable of local invasion, and the majority of symptoms are due to impingement of mediastinal structures or associated myasthenic symptoms. Patients may present with a chronic cough from phrenic nerve encroachment, superior vena cava syndrome, dysphagia, and shortness of breath (SOB) as a result of a paralyzed hemidiaphragm, hoarseness, chest pain, hemoptysis, and pleural effusion. However, 30% to 50% of patients have no symptoms and the mass is discovered incidentally during chest x-ray (CXR) or computed tomography (CT) scan for an unrelated problem. Thymomas are rare in children and adults older than 40 years; they affect females and males equally.

In addition to MG, thymomas are associated with other paraneoplastic syndromes. These rare disorders are due to an immune system response to a neoplasm. The symptoms occur remotely from the tumor and can affect multiple systems, including the endocrine, neuromuscular or musculoskeletal, cardiovascular, cutaneous, hematologic, renal, or gastrointestinal systems. Symptoms of a paraneoplastic syndrome are due to humoral factors emanating from the tumor or an immune response to the tumor; they are frequently present before the neoplasm is recognized. Paraneoplastic syndromes that are associated with thymomas and thymic carcinoma include pure red cell aplasia, Graves disease, acquired hypogammaglobulinemia, Cushing syndrome, and pernicious anemia.

2. Compare the impact of thymic dysfunction in adults and children.

After puberty, the thymus gradually decreases in size and thymic tissue is replaced by adipose tissue. The majority of T cells are produced early in life, and thymic dysfunction or a thymectomy has no significant impact on immune function in the adult. In contrast, congenital athymia, or loss of thymus gland function in childhood, is associated with a lack of functional T cells, resulting in severe immunodeficiency and increased susceptibility to infection. DiGeorge syndrome, a congenital disorder due to deletion of genes from chromosome 22, causes developmental abnormalities in the third and fourth pharyngeal pouches. Characteristics of DiGeorge syndrome include facial abnormality; congenital heart defects; absence or hypoplasia of the thymus; hypoparathyroidism; conotruncal abnormalities; cognitive, behavioral, and psychiatric problems; and increased susceptibility to infections. Immune deficiency is seen with partial DiGeorge syndrome but improves over time. Patients with athymia are categorized

as having complete DiGeorge syndrome, have few detectable peripheral T cells, and usually die within the first 2 years of life unless they undergo thymus transplantation.

3. Discuss the relationship between the thymus gland and MG.

MG is an antibody-mediated autoimmune disease of the neuromuscular junction (NMJ), specifically the postsynaptic membrane. Immunoglobulin G antibodies (IgG) to the alpha subunit of the postsynaptic nicotinic acetylcholine receptor (nAChR) are present in approximately 80% of patients with the disease. The antibodies mechanically block the acetylcholine (ACh) binding sites on the nAChR and ultimately destroy them. Over time, the architecture of the postsynaptic membrane is degraded and it takes on a simplified appearance, with a decreased number of nAChR and junctional folds on the postsynaptic membrane; the resultant widening of the postsynaptic cleft increases the chance of ACh escaping before it can reach the postsynaptic membrane (Fig. 21.2). Symptoms of MG are present when the number of functional nAChRs is <30% normal. The thymus contains myeloid (muscle-like) cells, which expose the T cells to the nAChR; this may help to explain the relationship between MG and the thymus. The nicotinic cholinergic receptors of the autonomic nervous system (ANS) and the central nervous system (CNS) have a different antigenicity, accounting for the lack of ANS and CNS symptoms in MG patients. Thymectomy improves the symptoms of MG but does not cure the disease, supporting the theory that nAChR antibodies are also produced in organs other than the thymus.

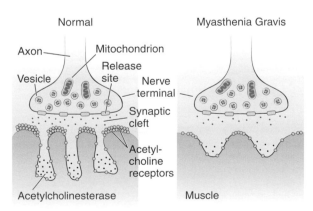

• **Fig. 21.2** Neuromuscular junctions. Acetylcholine is released from presynaptic vesicles and diffuses across the synaptic cleft to the postsynaptic receptors. Acetylcholinesterase, located deep within the synaptic folds, hydrolyzes acetylcholine. In myasthenia gravis there are a reduced number of postsynaptic acetylcholine receptors, which can lead to failed neuromuscular transmission and weakness. (From Roberts JR: *Roberts and Hedges' clinical procedures in emergency medicine and acute care*, ed 7, St. Louis, 2019, Elsevier.)

4. Review the diagnosis and treatment for MG.

Muscle weakness is a common symptom associated with many neuromuscular disorders, and it is not uncommon for a delayed diagnosis in the myasthenic patient. Weakness of the skeletal muscles is characteristic, but symptoms can vary in type and severity. Muscular weakness increases with activity and improves after periods of rest, frequently affecting muscles that control eye and eyelid movements, facial expression, chewing, talking, and swallowing. In some patients, muscle weakness is limited to the eye muscles (ocular myasthenia). In 20% of patients, MG will initially affect the bulbar muscles, but the majority of patients present with generalized weakness involving the limbs. Respiratory involvement occurs late in the disease and is associated with numerous other symptoms. Common symptoms of generalized MG include ptosis, diplopia, facial muscle weakness, dysphagia, dysarthria, dysphonia, limb weakness, and SOB. The highest incidence of MG occurs in females <40 years and males >60 years. Classifications of MG are listed in Box 21.1.

Standard electromyography (EMG), single-fiber electromyography (SFEMG), and repetitive nerve stimulation (RNS) are used for diagnosis of the disease. Diagnostic specificity for MG is close to 100% when nAChR antibodies are present: they are detected in >80% of patients with MG but may be absent in patients with ocular myasthenia. The edrophonium or Tensilon challenge test is also used for diagnosis of MG; improvement in muscle strength within 5 minutes after administration of edrophonium 10 mg intravenously (IV) is confirmatory for the disease. A positive response is not completely specific for MG and can be seen with other conditions such as amyotrophic lateral sclerosis (ALS). The sensitivity of both RNS and the edrophonium challenge is dependent on the type and severity of symptoms. SFEMG is the most sensitive test for ocular and generalized muscle involvement. CT can identify an abnormal thymus gland or thymoma.

• BOX 21.1 Osserman Classification System for Myasthenia Gravis

Class I: Eye muscle weakness (ocular myasthenia)
Class II: Eye muscle weakness, mild weakness of other muscles
Class IIa: Predominantly limb or axial muscle weakness
Class IIb: Predominantly bulbar and/or respiratory muscle weakness
Class III: Eye muscle weakness, moderate weakness of other muscles
Class IIIa: Predominantly limb or axial muscle weakness
Class IIIb: Predominantly bulbar and/or respiratory muscle weakness
Class IV: Eye muscle weakness, severe weakness of other muscles
Class IVa: Predominantly limb or axial muscle weakness
Class IVb: Predominantly bulbar and/or respiratory muscle weakness
Class V: Myasthenic crisis

Pregnancy can cause exacerbation or remission of the disease; it is also associated with a transient neonatal myasthenia in response to placental transfer of maternal antibodies. Normally, alpha-fetoprotein inhibits binding of maternal nAChR antibodies to fetal ACh receptors, and <20% of neonates born to myasthenic mothers have transient myasthenia. Alpha-fetoprotein may also contribute to the remission that often occurs during the second and third trimesters of pregnancy. Signs of neonatal myasthenia are usually present at birth and include difficulty in sucking, swallowing, and breathing; ptosis; and facial weakness. In severe cases, the infant is treated with oral neostigmine. Maternal antibodies are present in breast milk and may accentuate neonatal myasthenia. Spontaneous remission of symptoms usually occurs within 2 to 4 weeks with no risk of relapse.

Treatment of MG includes administration of anticholinesterase medication, immune suppression, and thymectomy. Anticholinesterase agents are the first line of treatment, and pyridostigmine (Mestinon) is the most widely used anticholinesterase. It has a half-life of 4 hours, and effects are seen within 30 minutes. Dosage is patient dependent; the average dose is 600 mg daily, spaced to provide maximum effects during periods of intense muscle activity. Higher doses are associated with increased muscle weakness. A sustained-release preparation is available for night administration for treatment of nighttime or early morning weakness.

Immunosuppression can attenuate the destruction of the nAChR. High-dose steroid treatment includes prednisolone (Prednisone) 100 mg per day for 2 to 4 weeks and then 100 mg every other day; improvement of symptoms is typically seen within 2 to 3 weeks. High-dose steroids are associated with a transient deterioration of NMJ function during the first weeks of treatment. For less severe cases, prednisolone 10 to 20 mg/day is initiated and increased by 5 mg every 3 to 5 days. The target daily dose of 100 mg is reached within 6 to 8 weeks, at which time the patient is switched to alternate-day dosing. This approach minimizes the negative effects on the NMJ, but the onset of improvement will be significantly prolonged.

Administration of the antimetabolite azathioprine (Imuran) is associated with inhibition of T cells and decreased plasma levels of nAChR antibodies. It is beneficial for patients who relapse on prednisolone or as a steroid-sparing precaution in patients with a history of long-time steroid use. The response to azathioprine is much slower than steroids and can take 3 to 12 months; consequently, a combination of corticosteroids and azathioprine may be used for the initial treatment of myasthenic patients. Another immunosuppressant, cyclosporine (Sandimmune, Neoral), is also used for management of myasthenic symptoms. It inhibits helper T cells, facilitates suppressor T cells, and blocks the production and secretion of interleukin-2. Long-term use of both azathioprine and cyclosporine is associated with an increased risk for malignancy. With similar efficacy and significantly reduced toxicity, mycophenolate mofetil (MyM, CellCept), an immunosuppressive agent used in organ transplantation, is an effective alternative to azathioprine and cyclosporine.

Plasmapheresis involves exchanges of 3 to 5 liters of plasma; four to six exchanges effectively remove nAChR antibodies from the circulation and allow recovery of the nAChR. Improvement of symptoms is seen within days and can last for several weeks. Plasmapheresis is especially effective for treatment of myasthenic crisis, and it is frequently used to improve muscle strength before thymectomy. Chronic, intermittent plasmapheresis may be indicated for patients refractory to other treatment modalities. Approximately 65% of myasthenic patients show improvement within days to weeks after receiving intravenous immunoglobulin (IVIg). Its exact mechanism of action is unknown, and IVIg has no consistent effect on plasma nAChR antibody levels. The incidence of side effects is low, and IVIg is used for the treatment of MG patients who are refractory to other immunosuppressive agents. Cost of the drug is a significant limitation to its use. Thymectomy, with or without the presence of thymoma, is an effective treatment for MG, especially if performed within 1 year of the onset of symptoms. The remission response to thymectomy is not immediate, and only 25% achieve remission within the first year.

5. *Contrast MG and LEMS.*

In contrast to MG, which is associated with postsynaptic nAChR antibodies, LEMS is associated with autoantibodies that antagonize the function of the presynaptic ACh voltage-gated Ca^{2+} channels. The antibodies interfere with the opening of the calcium channels and restrict the release of ACh. Decreased ACh release, characteristic of LEMS, is associated with muscle weakness in the proximal limbs; depressed tendon reflexes; posttetanic potentiation; and ANS abnormalities, including gastroparesis, orthostatic hypotension, and urinary retention. Presynaptic ACh stores and the postsynaptic response to ACh remain intact; consequently, rapid repetitive stimulation or voluntary activation will increase ACh release and improve muscle strength. Symptoms of LEMS include progressive muscle weakness, but it does not usually involve the facial or respiratory muscles. Muscle weakness is worse in the morning and improves with exercise or nerve stimulation. Autonomic symptoms are frequently present. The presence of calcium-channel antibodies and improved muscle strength with RNS is confirmatory for the disease. Guanidine hydrochloride enhances the release of ACh and is used to improve muscle strength; 3,4-diaminopyridine increases the action potential duration by blocking the potassium channel efflux. This allows the Ca^{2+} channels to remain open and release a larger amount of ACh. Patients with LEMS may also be treated with steroids. Plasmapheresis and IVIg are associated with transient improvement in muscle strength; anticholinesterases have little effect. Similar to other paraneoplastic syndromes, the majority of patients with LEMS have an identifiable cancer, most notably small cell, which is also known as oat-cell carcinoma of the lung.

6. *Design a preoperative assessment plan for a patient with MG.*

Optimizing the patient's preoperative condition can markedly improve the surgical outcome for myasthenic patients. Onset, duration, and severity of the disease should be determined, and close attention should be paid to a history of related autoimmune diseases. Preoperative evaluation must include assessment of voluntary muscle strength. The ability to cough, clear secretions, and maintain a patent airway should be assessed, especially in patients with bulbar involvement. Pulmonary function testing (PFT) is mandatory in patients with generalized MG; serial forced vital capacity (FVC) measurements are a good indicator of respiratory reserve and can help identify the patients who may need postoperative mechanical ventilation. Pulmonary flow-volume loops in the supine and sitting position can identify fixed or dynamic respiratory impairments in patients with a thymoma. Patients who have a dynamic impairment are at risk for an intrathoracic airway obstruction during induction of general anesthesia. All myasthenic patients should be informed of the possibility of postoperative intubation and mechanical ventilation. Patients undergoing thymectomy for a thymoma may present with undiagnosed MG; complaints of generalized weakness and reduced exercise tolerance that improves with rest should alert the anesthetist to the possibility of the disease. It may be prudent to order preoperative PFT on these individuals.

Patients with advanced stages of MG should receive their full morning dose of pyridostigmine; patients with mild disease may take half or skip their morning dose. Before induction, hydrocortisone 100 mg IV should be administered to patients on steroid therapy; the dose can be repeated twice within 24 hours. To allow time for restoration of coagulation factors, plasma cholinesterase levels, and immunoglobulins, plasmapheresis should not be performed within 24 hours of surgery. Careful attention should be paid to the drug history of the myasthenic patient, as many medications may provoke acute exacerbations. A list of these drugs is provided in Box 21.2. Premedication is best avoided, especially in patients with limited respiratory reserve and bulbar symptoms. Aspiration prophylaxis is mandatory in patients with bulbar symptoms.

> **• BOX 21.2 Medications Associated With Acute Exacerbations of Myasthenia Gravis**
>
> - **Antibiotics:** macrolides, fluoroquinolones, aminoglycosides, tetracycline, and chloroquine
> - **Antidysrhythmics:** beta-blockers, calcium-channel blockers, quinidine, lidocaine, procainamide
> - **Miscellaneous:** diphenylhydantoin, lithium, chlorpromazine, muscle relaxants, levothyroxine, adrenocorticotropic hormone (ACTH), trimetaphan, and, paradoxically, corticosteroids

Intraoperative Period

7. *Differentiate between a myasthenic crisis and a cholinergic crisis.*

Myasthenic crisis is an acute exacerbation of symptoms associated with MG that requires immediate intubation and mechanical ventilation. Increasing generalized weakness may precede the crisis. Failure of the respiratory muscle to maintain adequate ventilation will trigger acute hypoxemia, hypercarbia, and acidosis; inability to clear bronchial secretions can result in pneumonia. Severe bulbar weakness is associated with a poor or absent gag reflex and an increased risk for aspiration. Myasthenic crisis can be precipitated by fever, infection, stress, menstruation, radiographic contrast dyes, certain medications, and insufficient treatment with anticholinesterase and/or immunosuppressant medications.

Cholinergic crisis is due to a large amount of ACh at the NMJ, the consequence of overadministration of an anticholinesterase medication. The excess ACh causes increased stimulation of striated muscle, producing a flaccid muscle paralysis that is clinically indistinguishable from the weakness seen during a myasthenic crisis. However, deep tendon reflexes are preserved during a cholinergic crisis. Bradycardia, bronchospasm, miosis, increased lacrimation and salivation, urinary incontinence, and diarrhea are usually present.

There are no laboratory tests to differentiate between a myasthenic crisis and cholinergic crisis, but the presence of muscarinic symptoms supports the suspicion of a cholinergic crisis. The edrophonium challenge test is useful for distinguishing between the two occurrences. After tracheal intubation and initiation of mechanical ventilation, an initial IV test dose of edrophonium 1 mg is administered, followed by varying increments to a maximum of 10 mg. During myasthenic crisis, the patient will demonstrate an immediate and dramatic improvement in muscle strength, respiratory function, and facial expression. If cholinergic crisis is the problem, the patient will respond to edrophonium with increased salivation, bronchopulmonary secretions, diaphoresis, and possibly bradycardia caused by further increases in ACh, but improvement in muscle strength will not occur.

Although the half-life of edrophonium is short, approximately 10 minutes, the patient must be monitored carefully during the test because serious side effects, including significant bradycardia, heart block, and asystole, can occur. Patients with myasthenic crisis will require additional doses of an anticholinesterase; pyridostigmine 1 mg intramuscularly (IM) or IV is equivalent to 30 mg orally. Other treatments of myasthenic crisis include plasmapheresis and IVIg administration. Steroids should be used cautiously, as they may worsen the degree of muscle weakness. Management of cholinergic crisis includes discontinuation of all cholinergic medications and IV administration of atropine sulfate 1 to 2 mg. Continued intubation and mechanical ventilation may also be necessary in these patients.

8. *Discuss the surgical resection of a thymoma or the thymus.*

Surgical resection is the preferred treatment of patients with a thymoma. To rule out a lymphoma, which is not treated surgically, an initial biopsy is indicated for large masses with indistinct margins. The World Health Organization (WHO) uses a histologic classification system to classify thymomas. The Masaoka system (Box 21.3) is the most frequently used classification system. It allows diagnosis and staging at the time of surgical intervention and appears to have the greatest correlation with mortality.

Thymectomy with resection of surrounding tissue is indicated for stage I thymomas. Postoperative adjunctive therapy is not necessary in the absence of capsular invasion, and these patients have a 100% 5-year survival rate and a 0.9% risk of recurrence. Surgery is also indicated for stage II and III lesions. A preoperative course of chemotherapy may be indicated for patients with stage III lesions. Postoperative radiotherapy after complete resection reduces the recurrence rate from 28% to 36% to 0% to 5% for stage II and from 53% to 28% for stage III thymomas. Surgery for an invasive stage IVa thymoma involves resection of invaded local structures and may require major vascular resections, including removal and reconstruction of the superior vena cava, innominate vein, aortic arch, and pulmonary artery. Unilateral resection of the phrenic nerve, pericardial resection, and pleuropneumonectomy may also be indicated. Preoperative chemoradiation may be indicated to reduce tumor volume. Incomplete resection or debulking of a stage IVa thymoma combined with postoperative chemoradiation can improve survival rates in these patients. Treatment of stage IVb thymoma is limited to chemotherapy.

An anterior approach, utilizing a parasternal approach at the second or third intercostal space (ICS), is used for mediastinoscopic biopsies of the thymus. Surgical approach for a thymectomy is controversial and dependent on the degree of involvement of local tissues. For myasthenic patients, a video-assisted thoracoscopic surgery (VATS) or robotics-assisted thoracoscopic surgery (RATS) will allow a simple thymectomy. A complete resection of the thymus and surrounding tissues is necessary. An upper sternal split with division only of the manubrium or a transcervical approach similar to that used for a thyroidectomy will provide good surgical access for an early-stage

---

• **BOX 21.3** Thymoma Staging System (Masaoka)

   I. Macroscopically, completely encapsulated; microscopically, no capsular invasion
  II. Macroscopic invasion into surrounding fatty tissue or mediastinal pleura; microscopic invasion into capsule
 III. Macroscopic invasion into neighboring organs (pericardium, lung, and great vessels)
IVa. Pleural or pericardial dissemination
IVb. Lymphogenous or hematogenous metastases

thymoma. With advanced stages of thymoma, a complete sternotomy is necessary for removal of all anterior mediastinal tissue that may have thymic metastasis.

Postsurgical complications associated with thymectomy include:

- Unilateral phrenic nerve injury with short-term dyspnea upon exertion
- Pleural effusion
- Hemorrhage
- Respiratory insufficiency
- Postoperative thrombosis after dissection near the innominate vein
- Left recurrent nerve injury
- Vocal cord paralysis after dissection near the aortopulmonary window

Surgical mortality is <2% and is frequently related to diseases such as MG and other autoimmune diseases. Thymectomy in adults does not influence the immune system; in young children, it is associated with severe immunodeficiency and increased susceptibility to infection.

9. *Analyze the major anesthetic considerations for an MG patient undergoing a thymectomy.*

General endotracheal anesthesia (GETA) is required for a thymectomy. A double-lumen tube and one-lung ventilation are required for a VATS or RATS technique. Patients with advanced stages of the disease or isolated bulbar involvement are at risk for aspiration, and an awake fiber-optic intubation (FOI) is the safest technique for securing the airway.

With a 70% reduction in the number of nAChRs, myasthenic patients are generally resistant to the neuromuscular blocking effects associated with succinylcholine, and higher doses are required for intubation. However, responses can be unpredictable, and myasthenic patients are more likely to develop a phase II block, especially with repeat doses of succinylcholine. Preoperative anticholinesterase therapy or plasmapheresis may prolong the duration of succinylcholine. Myasthenic patients are extremely sensitive to nondepolarizing neuromuscular blockers (NDMRs) and it is best to avoid them. Even a small defasciculating dose before succinylcholine administration can result in respiratory distress and loss of airway protection. Sevoflurane or propofol and remifentanil can be used for induction and tracheal intubation. If muscle relaxants are required for intubation, succinylcholine is the best choice. Surgical muscle relaxation can be accomplished with a volatile anesthesia. Small doses of intermediate-acting relaxants (10% to 25% of the ED_{95}) such as cisatracurium have been used successfully in myasthenic patients. Due to the unique manner of degradation associated with cisatracurium, a combination of Hoffman elimination and ester hydrolysis, reversal may not be necessary. Use of a peripheral nerve stimulator (PNS) is mandatory; a control twitch should be assessed before the administration of an NDMR, and a single twitch should be maintained during surgery. Use of an electromyogram (EMG) or a mechanomyogram (MMG) is preferable for monitoring the neuromuscular function.

If an NDMR is used, the decision to reverse residual neuromuscular blockade at the end of surgery is controversial. Administration of an anticholinesterase and antimuscarinic will confound the differential diagnosis of a myasthenic crisis versus a cholinergic crisis. In addition, reversal of an NDMR block with an anticholinesterase agent may be ineffective due to chronic pyridostigmine administration. Therefore reversal of neuromuscular blockade is best accomplished by administering sugammadex. Extubation after spontaneous recovery of neuromuscular function and consistent demonstration of acceptable respiratory parameters may be preferable to pharmacologic reversal of the neuromuscular blockade. A prolonged recovery from anesthesia should be anticipated if high concentrations of an inhalation agent were administered to provide muscle relaxation.

Inhibition of plasma cholinesterase activity can result in decreased metabolism of ester local anesthetics and succinylcholine. Azathioprine can inhibit phosphodiesterase and antagonize neuromuscular blockade, and cyclosporine is associated with prolonged neuromuscular blockade.

10. *Identify the major side effect of radiation therapy.*

Thymomas are highly radiosensitive, and postoperative radiation therapy is frequently indicated after surgical resection of a large or invasive thymoma. Radiation is also synergistic with concurrent induction chemotherapy. Short-term side effects of radiotherapy include loss of hair and reddening, swelling, and blistering of the skin over the irradiated area. Effects on the skin resemble sunburn, and the skin may become dry, flaky, or peel with resolution of the changes within a few weeks of finishing treatment. A dry cough and SOB, lasting for a few days or weeks, are not uncommon.

Long-term side effects of radiation therapy include radiation pneumonitis, an inflammatory response of the lungs that can occur 1 to 6 months after radiotherapy. It occurs in approximately 10% of chest-irradiated patients. Symptoms include a fever, cough, SOB, and CXR changes. It may be treated with a short course of steroids and usually resolves over time. Pulmonary fibrosis is also a risk of chest radiotherapy, with a reduction in the number and efficiency of functioning lung units within the irradiated region. CT scans of irradiated lungs reveal increased lung densities, decreased lung volume, pleural thickening, and severe vascular damage within the radiation beam boundaries. Bronchiolitis obliterans, pneumothorax, mesothelioma, and lung cancer may also occur with radiotherapy.

Irradiation of the mediastinum and left side of the chest can have serious side effects on the cardiovascular system, including cardiomyopathy, premature coronary artery stenosis, ascending aortic calcification, pericardial disease, valvular injury, and conduction abnormalities. Radiation-induced heart disease is directly correlated with previous chemotherapy and duration of radiation exposure. Formation of thymic cysts, calcified lymph nodes, esophageal damage, radiation-induced sarcomas, osteochondroma, and rib or clavicle fractures are also recognized risks of radiation therapy. A patient with a history of chest radiotherapy should be assessed for loss of skin integrity, pulmonary fibrosis, pericardial or pleural effusion, myocardial fibrosis, valvular disorders, and fistula formation.

11. *Discuss the anesthetic concerns for patients who have had preoperative chemotherapy.*

A preoperative course of chemotherapy may be indicated for patients with stage III and IVa thymomas. Commonly used agents include bleomycin (Blenoxane), cisplatin (Platinol), cyclophosphamide (Cytoxan), doxorubicin (Adriamycin), lomustine (CeeNU), vincristine (Oncovin), and ifosfamide (Mitoxana). In varying degrees of severity, all chemotherapeutic agents have a depressant effect on all rapid turnover cells, resulting in hair loss; gastrointestinal distress, including nausea, vomiting, anorexia, ulceration, and ileus; sensory loss and paresthesias; muscle wasting; neuritic pain; and myelosuppression, as evidenced by leucopenia, thrombocytopenia, and anemia. In general, these effects are dose dependent and reversible. Reactivation of hepatitis B virus (HBV) may also occur during systemic chemotherapy. Several antimetabolites have the potential to enhance radiation injury to tissues (radiation recall reactions), and recurrent injury to a previously radiated site can occur weeks to months after radiotherapy.

Several of the antimetabolites used in the treatment of thymic carcinoma present additional concerns for the anesthetist. Cisplatin is associated with renal toxicity, especially in the elderly population. Renal damage is greatest with high doses and repeated courses of the drug. Electrolyte abnormalities may be present, a function of the depressed renal function. Peripheral neuropathies are also reported with the use of cisplatin. A dose-dependent cardiomyopathy is associated with doxorubicin, and potentially fatal congestive heart failure (CHF) may occur months to years after treatment.

Approximately 10% of patients treated with bleomycin develop pneumonitis that can progress to pulmonary fibrosis. Symptoms include a dry, hacking cough; dyspnea; tachypnea; fever; and cyanosis; 20% of patients will have abnormal PFT results. Symptoms can appear in 1 to 3 months after treatment, and death occurs in 1% of patients with bleomycin pneumonitis. Risk factors include age >70 years, preexisting pulmonary disease, coexisting renal failure, prior or concomitant thoracic radiation therapy, subsequent high-dose oxygen exposure, smoking, or previous exposure to bleomycin. Corticosteroids are used to treat bleomycin pneumonitis but are of questionable value once interstitial fibrosis has occurred.

Preoperative testing of patients with a history of chemotherapy should include a complete blood count

(CBC), electrolytes, and renal and liver function tests. Patients with a history of doxorubicin treatment should also have an ECG and echocardiography (ECHO). A CXR and PFTs are indicated in patients who have received bleomycin. To decrease possible superoxide and free radical damage, the inspired oxygen concentration (FiO_2) should not exceed 28% during anesthesia. Blood and third-space losses should be replaced with colloids to prevent the development of pulmonary interstitial edema. Due to the possibility of persistent immunosuppression in patients who have a recent history of chemotherapy, strict attention must be paid to infection control, and the use of aseptic technique is mandatory during insertion of intravenous lines, arterial lines, airways, and nasogastric tubes during the perioperative period.

Postoperative Period

12. *Discuss the implication of damage to the phrenic nerve during a thymectomy.*

Injury to the phrenic nerve can occur during thymectomy, resulting in a temporary or permanent diaphragmatic paralysis. Phrenic nerve damage must be considered in any patient presenting with unexplained respiratory difficulty in the postoperative period. Symptoms of unilateral damage include dyspnea and atelectasis, and a CXR will reveal elevation of the ipsilateral hemidiaphragm and pulmonary infiltrates on the affected side. Bilateral injury of the phrenic nerve causes paralysis of both hemidiaphragms resulting in a reduced vital capacity (VC), residual volume (RV), and total lung capacity (TLC). The resultant hypoxemia and hypercapnia mandate continuation of mechanical ventilation during the postoperative period. The transient neurapraxia that is seen with phrenic nerve injury usually resolves spontaneously within 7 to 10 days.

13. *Review the postoperative management concerns for a patient with MG.*

Patients who have MG have an increased risk of developing postoperative respiratory failure, and approximately 50% will require prolonged postoperative ventilation after a transsternal thymectomy. Sustained respiratory muscle strength and resumption of spontaneous ventilation must be confirmed before extubation, especially in patients with bulbar and/or respiratory muscle weakness. Postoperative mechanical ventilation should be anticipated for patients presenting with:

- Long history (>6 years) of MG
- Significant bulbar weakness
- History of other chronic respiratory disease
- Grades III and IV MG
- Preoperative vital capacity <2.9 L

Arterial blood gases (ABGs) should be used to guide respiratory management; a CXR is indicated if aspiration is suspected. Myasthenic patients should be closely monitored for muscular weakness in the postoperative period. Differential diagnosis of residual weakness includes myasthenic crisis, cholinergic crisis, and residual effects of anesthetics; or nonanesthetic drugs that interfere with neuromuscular transmission; and a myasthenic or cholinergic crisis. Hypothermia and hypokalemia may also increase muscle weakness in the postoperative period.

Postoperative pain management can be challenging in the myasthenic patient, as there is a significant risk of respiratory depression if potent opioids are administered. Postoperative pain can be successfully managed with a thoracic or lumbar epidural, especially for patients undergoing a transsternal thymectomy. If inserted preoperatively, an epidural offers the additional advantage of intraoperative analgesia. Amide local anesthetics are preferable, as metabolism of ester local anesthetics may be prolonged by maintenance anticholinesterase therapy. The need for anticholinesterase medication is decreased in the postoperative period; approximately 75% of the preoperative dose is required for the first few postoperative days. The benefits of thymectomy are usually delayed for months to years after surgery.

14. *Discuss the long-term prognosis for patients with thymomas.*

The majority of thymomas are associated with autoimmune disorders, and metastasis is usually limited to the pleura. Advanced-stage thymomas are associated with pleura, kidney, bone, liver, and brain metastasis. Invasive thymomas are prone to recurrence and can recur 5 to 10 years after surgery; recurrence rates are significantly reduced with postoperative radiation therapy. Prognosis of this relatively indolent disease is good: the 10-year survival is 80% to 100% for stage I, 60% to 95% for stage II, 45% to 47% for stage III, and 30% to 47% for stage IV. Approximately 15% of patients with a thymoma will develop a second cancer. Patients with MG have a near-normal life expectancy.

Review Questions

1. Thymic epithelial cells are associated with the development of:
   a. Thymomas.
   b. Non-Hodgkin lymphomas.
   c. Hodgkin disease.
   d. Deficient humoral immunity.

2. Which symptoms are associated with myasthenic crisis? (Choose three.)
   a. Myosis
   b. Increased lacrimation
   c. Increased salivation
   d. Flaccid paralysis

3. The most effective treatment for myasthenic crisis includes:
   a. Prednisolone.
   b. Plasmapheresis.
   c. Atropine.
   d. Thymectomy.

4. Thymomas are most often associated with which of the following conditions?
   a. Hyperthyroidism
   b. Anemia
   c. Small cell carcinoma
   d. Myasthenia gravis

5. In the pediatric patient, thymic dysfunction is associated with:
   a. DiGeorge syndrome.
   b. Small cell carcinoma.
   c. Myasthenia gravis.
   d. Cushing syndrome.

Suggested Readings

Béchard P, Letourneau L, Lacasse Y, et al. Perioperative cardiorespiratory complications in adult with mediastinal masses: incidence and risk factors. *Anesthesiology* 2004;100:826-834.

Dontukurthy S, Wisler C, Raman V, Tobias JD. Myasthenia gravis and sugammadex: a case report and review of the literature. *Saudi J Anaesth* 2020;14(2):244-248.

Fok M, Bashir M, Harky A, Sladden D, DiMartino M, et al. Video-assisted thoracoscopic versus robotic-assisted thoracoscopic thymectomy: systematic review and meta-analysis. *Innovations (Phila)* 2017;12(4):259-264.

Gothard JWW. Anesthetic considerations for patients with anterior mediastinal masses. *Anesthesiol Clin* 2008;26:305-314.

Hu B, Niu L, Jiang Z, Xu S, Hu Y, Cao K. LncRNA XLOC_003810 promotes T cell activation and inhibits PD-1/PD-L1 expression in patients with myasthenia gravis-related thymoma. *Scand J Immunol* 2020;92(1):e12886.

Karlet MC. Musculoskeletal system anatomy, physiology, pathophysiology, and anesthesia management. In: Nagelhout JJ, Elisha S, eds. *Nurse Anesthesia*, 6th ed. St. Louis, MO: Elsevier, 2018:760-781.

Markert ML, Alexieff MJ, Li J, et al. Postnatal thymus transplantation with immunosuppression as treatment for DiGeorge syndrome. *Blood* 2004;104:2574-2581.

Muckler VC, O'Brien JM, Matson SE, Rice AN. Perianesthetic implications and considerations for myasthenia gravis. *J Perianesth Nurs* 2019;34(1):4-15.

Schoser B, Eymard B, Datt J, Mantegazza R. Lambert-Eaton myasthenic syndrome (LEMS): a rare autoimmune presynaptic disorder often associated with cancer. *J Neurol* 2017;264(9):1854-1863.

Tian W, Li X, Tong H, Weng W, Yang F, Jiang G, Wang J. Surgical effect and prognostic factors of myasthenia gravis with thymomas. *Thorac Cancer* 2020;11(5):1288-1296.

Tormoehlen LM, Pascuzzi RM. Thymoma, myasthenia gravis, and other paraneoplastic syndromes. *Hematol Oncol Clin North Am* 2008;22:509-526.

Wang A, Zhang X, Yi J, Zhu M, Zhang Y. Successful treatment of advanced lung adenocarcinoma complicated with Lambert-Eaton myasthenic syndrome: a case report and literature review. *Thorac Cancer* 2020;11(5):1334-1338.

Zhao J, Bhatnagar V, Ding L, Atay SM, et al. A systematic review of paraneoplastic syndromes associated with thymoma: treatment modalities, recurrence, and outcomes in resected cases. *J Thorac Cardiovasc Surg* 2020;160(1):306-314.e14.

22

Multiorgan Procurement

KEY POINTS

- An individual's signature on a driver's license or donor card attesting to their desire to be an organ/tissue donor is legally binding and does not require family permission.
- Absolute contraindications for organ donation include age >80 years, human immunodeficiency virus (HIV) infection, active metastatic cancer, prolonged hypotension or hypothermia, active infection, disseminated intravascular coagulation (DIC), sickle cell anemia, or other hemoglobinopathy.

- Aggressive donor management increases the number and quality of retrieved organs and improves both the number and outcome of subsequent transplantations.
- The most frequently transplanted organ is the kidney; the lung is the least transplanted organ.
- Anesthesia services are required for organ donation after brain death (DBD) but not for donation after cardiac death (DCD).

Case Synopsis

A 35-year-old man is admitted, unresponsive, to the emergency department after a gunshot injury to the head. The patient is intubated and mechanically ventilated. His Glasgow Coma Scale (GCS) score is 4, and a computed tomography (CT) scan reveals a large subdural hematoma and extensive cerebral edema with a midline shift.

Preoperative Evaluation and Demographic Data

Past Medical/Surgical History

- Healthy male
- Nonsmoker, no recreational drug use, no alcohol intake
- Appendectomy at age 22

List of Medications

- Ibuprofen

Diagnostic Data

- Hemoglobin, 11.4 mg/dL; hematocrit, 37%
- Glucose, 250 mg/dL
- Electrolytes: sodium, 158 mEq/L; potassium, 3.2 mEq/L; chloride, 106 mEq/L; carbon dioxide, 22 mEq/L
- Electrocardiogram (ECG): Sinus tachycardia, heart rate 154, with T inversion in multiple leads

Height/Weight/Vital Signs

- 180 cm, 86 kg
- Blood pressure, 100/60; heart rate, 154 beats per minute; room air oxygen saturation, 95%

- No spontaneous respirations; mechanical ventilation; tidal volume, 800; respiratory rate, 12 breaths per minute; inspired oxygen concentration, 40%

Pathophysiology

The first solid organ transplant involved a kidney transplant between identical twins in 1954 followed by liver, lung, heart, and pancreas transplants in the 1960s. Cyclosporine, introduced in 1978, had a major impact on the growth and success of transplant surgery by decreasing the incidence of host rejection. Organs and tissues that can be transplanted include the heart, kidneys, lungs, pancreas, liver, intestines, corneas, skin, tendons, bone, and heart valves. Kidney and liver (whole organ or segmental) are the most frequently transplanted organs. The federally supported United Network for Organ Sharing (UNOS) links all organ procurement and transplant centers in the United States. When a donor is identified, individuals on waiting lists are matched and ranked via computer against the donor's characteristics. Ranking is based on blood type, tissue match, length of time on list, immune status, and geographical distance between donor and potential recipient. Other factors considered include pediatric patients in specific age categories, reciprocal-sharing arrangements or payback agreements, dual-organ recipient, and acute failure of a recently transplanted organ. Medical urgency is considered for heart, liver, and intestinal transplantation.

Absolute contraindications to organ donation include age >80 years, HIV infection, active metastatic cancer, prolonged hypotension or hypothermia, active infection, DIC, and hemoglobinopathy. Relative contraindications include malignancy other than in the central nervous system (CNS) or skin that is in remission, hypertension, diabetes mellitus, age >70 years, hepatitis B or C, and a history of smoking.

The medical condition of the donor at the time of death determines the viability of retrieved organs. After a cardiac arrest, the viability of the vital organs deteriorates quickly, whereas other tissues, such as bone, skin, heart valves, and corneas, can be donated within 24 hours after death. Minimizing the time interval (warm ischemic time) between cardiac death and perfusion of donor organs with cold preservation solutions increases the viability of the organs. The length of time is organ specific; the heart and liver must be retrieved within 30 minutes, and kidneys and pancreas can be retrieved up to 60 minutes after cardiac death.

Classifications of Organ Donors

Living Organ Donors

A healthy individual who is between 18 and 60 years of age and free from hypertension, diabetes, cancer, kidney disease, and heart disease can be considered for a living organ donation. Kidney donation is the most frequent type of living organ donation; individuals can also donate a lung or segments of the liver or pancreas. Some heart–lung recipients can donate their heart (domino transplant) if they have lung but not heart pathology. Living donors account for 44% of all donors and are frequently related to the recipients.

Deceased Organ Donors

The U.S. Uniform Determination of Death Act (1980) defines death as the irreversible cessation of circulatory and respiratory functions or of all functions of the entire brain, including the brainstem. Deceased organ donors include DBD and DCD. For DBD, causes of brain death include severe head trauma, cerebral ischemia, infarction or hemorrhage, prolonged cardiopulmonary arrest, and intracranial tumors. Diagnosis of brain death is primarily based on clinical examination, but diagnostic tests are often used for confirmation. The patient is considered legally dead at the time that a physician determines that brain death has occurred.

In the event of cardiac death, also known as *non-heartbeating cadaver donation (NHBCD)*, the removal of transplantable organs occurs immediately after the patient has been declared dead using specific cardiac criteria. These patients are typically ventilator dependent, have a severe neurologic injury after a cerebrovascular accident (CVA) or cerebral anoxia, have a high spinal cord injury, or have an end-stage neuromuscular disease. They do not meet brain death criteria but are not expected to recover, and the physician and family have decided to withdraw life support. The patient is considered legally dead at the time of asystole. In controlled DCD, organ procurement occurs immediately after withdrawal of life support and declaration of cardiac death, allowing retrieval of kidneys, liver, lungs, and pancreas. Hearts are rarely retrieved due to concerns about sustained ischemic injury after cardiac arrest. In uncontrolled DCD, the cardiac death is not anticipated, and there may be a considerable time for warm ischemia to occur that limits retrieval to kidneys and nonvital tissues. DCD currently accounts for approximately 8% of all deceased donors and has significant potential for increasing the number of available organs.

Surgical Procedure

State organ procurement organizations (OPOs) are subject to regulations set forth by UNOS. Once a patient has been declared brain dead or a cardiac death is imminent, an OPO coordinator is sent to evaluate the patient and coordinate the organ procurement process. Surgical transplant teams are not involved until the donor is declared dead by the attending physician. Initially, the organs are allocated locally and then offered to other regional or state OPOs.

During organ procurement, surgical access is provided via a midline incision from the suprasternal notch to the pubis and a median sternotomy. The aortic arch, inferior vena cava (IVC), abdominal aorta, and portal vein or tributaries are cannulated for infusion of a cold preservative solution, and the heart, lung, liver, kidneys, and pancreas are dissected from supporting structures. After administration of heparin 300 units/kg, the abdominal aorta is crossclamped; a cold preservative solution is infused through the inferior aortic, portal, and cardiac cannulae; and the thoracic and abdominal cavities are packed with ice. The warm ischemic time must be minimized, and organs are removed in order of susceptibility to warm ischemic damage; the heart is removed first, followed by the lungs, liver, pancreas, small intestines, and kidneys. An en bloc resection of organs may be utilized in which the organs are removed together and dissected in vitro either in the operating room or at the site of transplantation. Before transport, organs are flushed with a cold preservative solution, packed in wet ice, and stored at 48°C. Recipients are required to be at the transplant center within 4 to 6 hours of notification; for a heart or lung recipient, this time may be shortened.

Anesthetic Management and Considerations

Preoperative Period

1. *Identify the sources of consent for organ donation.*

   An individual's desire to be an organ donor can be documented on a driver's license, a donor card, a living will or durable power of attorney, or through verbal communication with family. Historically, family consent was required for organ donation, even in the presence of a signed driver's license or donor card. In states with first-person consent laws, an individual's signature is legally binding and does not require family permission. In the absence of a signed consent, the family, legal guardian, or medical coroner can agree to organ donation. Knowledge of the donor's wishes or families who had previous discussion regarding donation are more likely to agree to donate in the face of an unexpected terminal condition of a family member. To increase the number of donated organs, the Uniform Anatomical Gift Act (UAGA) was revised, granting new authority to OPOs over individuals with a signed driver's license or donor card. The OPO must be notified when a donor or potential donor is dead or near death; if necessary, the OPO will seek consent from family or authorized persons. The OPO can direct life-sustaining interventions before death to increase the viability of organs unless an advance directive specifically forbids them from doing so. The act empowers a minor, eligible under other law to apply for a driver's license, to be a donor without family consent. The National Organ Transplant Act (1984) prohibits the sale of organs for transplantation.

2. *Discuss the physiologic responses associated with brain death.*

Brain death is a result of severe rostral caudal ischemia. Intense sympathetic activity, an attempt to maintain cerebral perfusion pressure, is the initial response to cerebral ischemia and increased intracranial pressure (ICP). A mixed vagal and sympathetic response is seen with ischemia of the pons, and Cushing response, hypertension, bradycardia, and altered respirations are present. Medullary ischemia causes an intense sympathetic response, loss of thermoregulatory control, and endocrinopathy due to hypothalamic and pituitary impairment. Catecholamine release causes a significant increase in systemic vascular resistance (SVR), increasing myocardial work and compromising cardiac function. Hypothermia can lead to myocardial depression, coagulopathy, and decreased oxygen (O_2) delivery to tissues. Disruption of the hypothalamic–pituitary axis results in adrenal insufficiency, loss of glycemic control, reduced antidiuretic hormone (ADH) secretion, and hypothyroidism. Brainstem herniation is associated with bradycardia, decreased SVR, low cardiac output (CO), pulmonary edema and dysfunction, and cardiopulmonary arrest. DIC may occur as the coagulation cascade is activated in response to the release of necrotic brain tissue. A systemic inflammatory response is associated with brain death; inflammatory mediators decrease SVR, increase lung injury, and may increase immune sensitivity after transplantation.

3. *Discuss the preoperative management of an organ donor.*

Hemodynamic instability can seriously compromise organ function; >80% of organ donors require hemodynamic support, and approximately 20% of potential donors are lost because of hemodynamic instability. Initial management includes aggressive fluid resuscitation with crystalloids and colloids; colloids are more effective than crystalloids in preventing pulmonary edema and congestion of other organs. Packed red blood cells (PRBCs) may be required to maintain a hemoglobin of >10 mg/dL, and fresh frozen plasma (FFP) is administered if the prothrombin time (PT) and partial thromboplastin time (PTT) are 1.5 times greater than control values.

Central venous pressure (CVP) is used to guide fluid management. The infusion of inotropic medications is frequently indicated; dopamine 2 to 10 mcg/kg/min is the initial drug of choice. Dobutamine 3 to 15 mcg/kg/min, norepinephrine 0.5 to 5 mcg/min, or epinephrine 0.1 to 1 mcg/kg/min may also be required to maintain effective perfusion pressures. The goals of anesthetic management include mean arterial pressure (MAP) >60 mm Hg, CVP 12 mm Hg, SVR 800 to 1200 dynes/cm^5, systolic blood pressure (SBP) >100 mm Hg, and cardiac index (CI) >2.5. Because the cardiac center is located within the medulla oblongata, when brain death occurs, functional myocardial denervation occurs, and as a result atropine has a limited effect on increasing heart rate. Bradycardia is most effectively treated with isoproterenol, epinephrine, or cardiac pacing. Electrolytes are monitored frequently to maintain plasma sodium ≤150 mEq/dL and potassium ≥4.0 mEq/dL.

Brain death has a profound impact on lung function, and lung recovery occurs in only 20% of actual donors. Neurogenic pulmonary edema occurs in response to the early elevation of SVR and left atrial and pulmonary capillary pressures. The inflammatory response and release of proteases, cytokines, and leukotrienes are associated with lung damage and decreased pulmonary function. The development of a coagulopathy may produce pulmonary microemboli. With brainstem death, the fall in SVR will increase ventilation/perfusion mismatch. In addition, aspiration, pulmonary contusion, excessive fluid resuscitation, atelectasis, and barotrauma negatively affect pulmonary function. Pulmonary management includes delivery of large tidal volumes (12 to 15 mg/kg); low peak inspiratory pressure (PIP), ideally <30 cm H_2O; positive-end expiratory pressure (PEEP) ≤7.5 cm H_2O; and an FiO_2 ≤40% in order to maintain arterial saturation (SaO_2) of >90%, arterial oxygen pressure (PaO_2) >60 mm Hg, arterial carbon dioxide pressure ($PaCO_2$) 30 to 35 mm Hg, and arterial pH 7.35 to 7.45. Careful fluid management, chest physiotherapy, frequent suctioning, and administration of antibiotics (cefazolin or equivalent) are also indicated to minimize lung trauma.

4. *Discuss the common physiologic complications associated with brain death.*

Donors are vulnerable to a variety of complications, especially endocrine dysfunction. Diabetes insipidus (DI) is caused by a lack of ADH production and/or release as a result of damage to the hypothalamus and/or pituitary gland. This syndrome is treated with vasopressin or desmopressin acetate (DDAVP [1-deamino-D-arginine vasopressin]), and the associated hypovolemia is corrected with hypotonic saline or dextrose and water and electrolyte replacement as indicated. Thyroid dysfunction is characterized by low triiodothyronine (T_3), a result of decreased thyroid-stimulating hormone (TSH) secretion and reduced conversion of thyroxine (T_4) to T_3. Anaerobic glycolysis and mitochondrial dysfunction are seen with T_3 deficiency, resulting in widespread acidosis. Sympathetically mediated hyperglycemia and depletion of insulin stores can contribute to hypovolemia (osmotic diuresis) and are best managed with an insulin infusion. A protocol for hormonal replacement for patients undergoing organ procurement is included in Box 22.1.

The profound hypothermia that occurs with loss of thermoregulatory control is associated with cardiac depression, cold diuresis, coagulopathy, and reduced tissue oxygenation. Warming blankets, fluid warmers, and heated humidifiers are indicated to maintain core temperature greater than 34.8°C. Coagulation abnormalities are common due to release of thromboplastin, tissue plasminogen, and fibrinogen from necrotic brain tissue and reduced platelet aggregation secondary to hypothermia. A dilutional coagulopathy may occur if large amounts of crystalloids are used for resuscitation. Blood products, including FFP, platelets, and cryoprecipitate, are indicated to correct coagulation abnormalities. Immediate organ retrieval is indicated for severe fibrinolysis resistant to therapy.

Hypovolemia can result from fluid restriction for treatment of cerebral edema, DI, hemorrhage, hyperglycemic osmotic diuresis, cold diuresis, and decreased SVR. Crystalloids, colloids, and red blood cells are administered to maintain SBP >100 mm Hg, urine output >1 mL/kg/hr, and hematocrit >30%. Cardiopulmonary management for organ procurement utilizing the rule of 100 is listed in Box 22.2.

5. *List the criteria used to confirm brain death.*

Diagnosis of brain death is primarily based on the absence of brainstem reflexes and respiratory effort. Optional confirmatory tests include an electroencephalogram (EEG), cerebral blood flow studies, and brainstem auditory-evoked responses (BAER). Potentially

reversible causes of coma (hypothermia, metabolic disturbances, medications, hypoxia, or hypocarbia) must be corrected before brain death can be confirmed. The GCS provides an objective and reliable method of assessing the status of the CNS, and the criteria are listed in Table 22.1. A fully awake patient will have a score of 15; a score ≤8 is indicative of a severe coma, 9 to 2 a moderate coma, and ≥13 a minor coma. The Pediatric GCS has a modified verbal response for assessment of young children.

- **Cerebral motor responses to pain:** Cerebrally modulated motor responses of extremities to painful stimulation are abnormal with brain death. Eye opening, facial grimacing, and purposeful withdrawal of limbs from a noxious stimulus are an indication that consciousness is not greatly impaired. Asymmetric motor responses to pain or deep tendon reflexes may indicate a focal hemispheric lesion. Decorticate posturing is associated with damage to the cerebral hemispheres, internal capsule, and thalamus. A decerebrate response to pain indicates damage to the brainstem, midbrain, and cerebellum. Minor flexion of an extremity in response to painful stimulation of the same limb represents spinal cord reflexes and not cortical activity. Spinal automatism (Lazarus sign), limb flexion, gasping motions, and head turning also occur at the spinal cord level. It is more common in young adults and can occur spontaneously during apnea testing in the presence of hypoxia or hypotension or brisk neck flexion.
- **Brainstem reflexes**
  - **Pupillary response to light:** Pupils may be round, oval, or irregularly shaped, and midsize (4 to 6 mm), but pupillary light reflex (constriction) is absent in brain death. Drugs such as atropine can influence pupillary size but not the response to light.
  - **Oculocephalic reflex (doll's eyes):** When the head is rapidly turned from side to side, the eyes normally rotate to the opposite side. With brainstem death, there is no movement of the eyes and they remain fixed.
  - **Oculovestibular reflex (caloric reflex):** Irrigation of both ear canals with iced saline or water will result in nystagmus and deviation of the eyes toward the side of irrigation. This reflex is absent in brain death. Several drugs can inhibit this reflex, including sedatives, tricyclic antidepressants, aminoglycosides, anticholinergics, and antiseizure agents.
  - **Corneal reflex (blink reflex):** Normal closing of the eyelid in response to corneal stimulation is absent with brainstem death.
- **Apnea test:** After ventilation with 100% O_2 to normocapnia, the patient is disconnected from the ventilator but continues to receive O_2 by continuous positive airway pressure. The patient is observed for up to 10 minutes for signs of spontaneous breathing; arterial blood gases (ABGs) are drawn at the end of

---

• BOX 22.1   Hormonal Replacement Protocol

- Methylprednisolone: 15 mg/kg bolus every 24 hours
- Triiodothyronine (T_3): 4 mcg bolus followed by 3 mcg/hr infusion
- Thyroxin (T_4): 20 mcg bolus, followed by 10 mcg/hr infusion
- Arginine vasopressin: 1-unit bolus followed by 0.5–4 units/hr titrated to SVR of 800–1200 dynes/cm^5 and urine output >200 mL/hr or desmopressin 8 ng/kg, followed by 4 ng/kg/hr
- Insulin infusion: 1 unit/hr titrated to maintain blood glucose 120–180 mg/dL

• BOX 22.2   Anesthetic Management for Organ Procurement: Rule of 100

- Systolic blood pressure >100 mm Hg
- Heart rate <100 beats per minute
- Urine output >100 mL/hr
- PaO_2 >100 mm Hg

TABLE 22.1 Glasgow Coma Scale

	Score 1	Score 3	Score 3	Score 4	Score 5	Score 6
Response of Eyes	Does not open eyes	Opens eyes in response to painful stimuli	Opens eyes in response to voice	Opens eyes spontaneously	N/A	N/A
Verbal Response	Makes no sounds	Incomprehensible sounds	Utters inappropriate words	Confused, disoriented	Oriented, converses normally	N/A
Motor Response	Makes no movements	Decerebrate posturing	Decorticate posturing	Flexion/ withdrawal to painful stimuli	Localizes painful stimuli	Obeys commands

the observation period. A lack of spontaneous respirations and $PaCO_2$ >55 to 60 mm Hg are indicative of brain death.

6. *Discuss the laboratory evaluation for potential organ donors.*

A variety of tests are required for the evaluation of potential DBD and DCD organ donors. These include a complete blood count (CBC); glucose; electrolytes; blood urea nitrogen (BUN); creatinine; ABG; ABO and human leukocyte antigen (HLA) typing; blood, sputum, and urine cultures; and Venereal Disease Research Laboratory (VDRL), HIV, Epstein–Barr virus (EBV), cytomegalovirus (CMV), human T-cell leukemia virus type 1 (HTLV-1), and hepatitis B and C virus serologies. An ECG, chest x-ray (CXR), echocardiogram, creatine kinase (CK) and muscle and brain subunits (CK-MB), and troponin levels are required for heart donors; serial ABGs, CXR, and bronchoscopy for lung donors; serial blood glucoses and amylase and lipase levels for pancreas donors; and liver function tests (LFTs), PTT, and PT for liver donors.

7. *Discuss the signs and management of DI.*

ADH (vasopressin) is produced by the hypothalamus and stored and released from the posterior pituitary gland. It increases water permeability in the renal collecting ducts and distal convoluted tubule, where reabsorption of water maintains normovolemia. Central DI is caused by a deficiency of ADH secondary to autoimmune disease, malignancy, head trauma, intracranial tumor, infection, renal disease, and vascular disease. Signs of DI include polyuria (urine output ≥25 mL/kg/hr) with a specific gravity of ≤1.005, lethargy, excessive thirst, hypernatremia, tachycardia, hypotension, fatigue, vomiting, and seizures. DI that occurs from neurologic dysfunction is caused by damage of the hypothalamus and/or pituitary gland. In nephrogenic DI, the kidney fails to respond to ADH. Certain drugs such as lithium, amphotericin B, and demeclocycline and hypercalcemia can cause nephrogenic DI.

Diagnosis of DI is accomplished by restricting fluid and then monitoring the plasma and urine sodium and urine specific gravity. When ADH levels and kidney function are within normal limits, the urine output and

plasma sodium levels will decrease, and urine specific gravity will increase. With DI, there is no change, and the diagnosis of central DI is confirmed if the urine output decreases and specific gravity increases in response to ADH administration. Mild cases of central DI are treated with drugs that are used to stimulate ADH production such as chlorpropamide, carbamazepine, and clofibrate. Nephrogenic DI is treated with indomethacin, hydrochlorothiazide, or amiloride.

DI occurs in approximately 70% to 80% of DBD donors. If the donor is hemodynamically unstable, vasopressin is the preferred treatment; desmopressin can be used if the donor is hemodynamically stable. Electrolytes are monitored frequently, and after correction of hypovolemia, the plasma sodium should return to normal without any additional intervention.

8. *Discuss the role of steroids in the preoperative management of organ donors.*

Steroids increase tissue oxygenation and attenuate the effects of proinflammatory cytokines that are released in response to brain death. They improve donor organ function, increase the number of organs transplanted from each donor, and improve graft survival, especially in heart and lung recipients. Methylprednisolone 15 to 30 mg/kg is administered every 24 hours. To protect the heart and lungs from ischemia, an additional 30 mg/kg may be administered 1 to 2 hours before actual organ procurement.

Intraoperative Period

9. *Describe the requirements for declaring death in a DCD donor.*

A variety of tools, such as the University of Wisconsin DCD Evaluation Tool, is used to predict DCD donors who will expire within 60 minutes after extubation. The DCD donor is transported to the operating room with O_2 and manual ventilation. Heparin is administered to prevent thrombi formation; vasodilators and antioxidants such as steroids, vitamin E, or N-acetylcysteine are also frequently administered. Large arteries and veins are cannulated to facilitate the rapid infusion of organ-preservation solutions, and the donor is surgically prepped and draped. Analgesics and sedatives may be administered by the treating physician to prevent or relieve suffering during termination of life support but not with the intention of hastening death. The donor is extubated and all medications discontinued. The Institute of Medicine (IOM) recommends an observation period of 5 minutes to ensure lack of cardiac reanimation (flat ECG tracing, flat pressure arterial line tracing, absence of carotid pulse). The National Conference of Donation after Cardiac Death recommends >2 minutes but <5 minutes of observation. Once the patient is pronounced dead, a cold preservative solution is infused, and organ procurement is instituted immediately to limit the time of warm ischemia and increase organ viability. If death does not occur within 60 minutes after termination of life support, the procedure is canceled and palliative care/life support is resumed for the patient; this occurs in approximately 20% of cases. Anesthesia services are not required for treatment of DCD donors.

10. *Discuss the anesthetic requirements of a DBD donor during organ retrieval.*

There is no perception of pain in the higher brain centers because of neuronal death, and providing anesthesia with the intent of inhibition of cerebral function is not required for DBD donors. However, anesthesia services are required to manage the physiologic responses to surgical trauma, spinal cord reflexes, catecholamine release, and release of inflammatory mediators that can damage the vital organs before procurement. The American Society of Anesthesiologists Physical Status Category VI is used for DBD donors who require anesthesia care. In addition to standard monitors, an arterial line and CVP/PA catheter are used for pressure monitoring; warming blankets, fluid warmers, and heated humidifiers are necessary to prevent intraoperative hypothermia. The donor is mechanically ventilated with 100% O_2 unless lung retrieval is planned, in which case a $FiO_2 \leq 0.4$ is indicated. Dopamine, norepinephrine, epinephrine, dobutamine, or vasopressin infusions are continued to support hemodynamics and organ perfusion during organ procurement. Hemodynamic responses to surgical stimulation occur at the spinal cord level and can be managed with alpha- and beta-blockers and/or volatile anesthetics. A long-acting muscle relaxant is administered to provide maximal intrathoracic and intraabdominal surgical exposure and to prevent donor movements that are also initiated by spinal reflexes. Heparin 20,000 to 30,000 units is administered to prevent postmortem clotting. Other drugs that may be required include mannitol, furosemide, allopurinol, methylprednisolone, and PGE_1. After aortic cross-clamping, vasodilators, such as phentolamine, may be required to treat an increased SVR. Significant third-space losses occur during multiple organ procurement, and glucose-free crystalloids, colloids, and PRBCs are used to maintain normovolemia, SBP >100 mm Hg, and hematocrit >30%. Colloids are preferable for lung and pancreas donors to increase viability of these organs. Serial evaluation of electrolytes, glucose, hemoglobin, hematocrit, and ABGs are monitored, especially for heart and lung donors. For liver and pancreas retrieval, a Betadine and amphotericin B solution is inserted via a nasogastric tube to decontaminate the intestinal tract (not gastrointestinal system).

Several surgical teams are involved in the organ procurement. Organs are removed in order of their susceptibility to ischemia, with the heart first and the kidneys last. Anesthesia care is terminated when the aorta is cross-clamped and the heart removed (at that time mechanical ventilation and monitors are turned off and all medications discontinued). If lung retrieval is planned, mechanical ventilation is continued until the surgeon is ready to remove the lungs, at which time the endotracheal tube is suctioned and removed. In the event of a premature cardiac arrest, cardiopulmonary resuscitation (CPR) is instituted to preserve viability of the organs; unsuccessful CPR will eliminate the heart and lungs for donation, but rapid aortic cross-clamping and infusion of a cold preservative solution allow retrieval of liver, pancreas, and kidneys. The maximum time before organ transplantation must occur varies according to the different vital organs, ranging from 5 hours for the heart to 3 days for kidneys, and this information is included in Table 22.2.

Postoperative Period

11. *Discuss the long-term survival of transplant recipients.*

In the United States, there are over 163,000 individuals living with a functioning transplanted organ. One-year survival rates are highest for kidney and pancreas recipients (95% to 98%). One-year survival for liver, intestine, lung, and heart recipients is 81% to 91%. The lowest survival rate (75%) is seen with heart–lung recipients. Long-term graft survival of a DCD kidney is similar to a DBD kidney, but the DCD liver graft survival is significantly less than a DBD liver.

TABLE 22.2	Organ Preservation Times
Heart	≤5 hours
Lung	≤5 hours
Intestines	≤8 hours
Liver	≤18 hours
Pancreas	≤20 hours
Kidney	≤72 hours
Corneas	≤10 days
Skin	≥5 years
Bone	≥5 years
Heart valves	≥5 years

12. *Discuss the professional conflicts health care providers en-*
counter with organ donation.

The majority of health care providers are supportive of organ donation, but some providers may feel conflicted when required to transfer the emphasis of care from the donor to the recipient. The family may question the ability of the providers to continue with quality end-of-life care for their family member. Physicians and nurses must continue to provide quality end-of-life care for the donor and should not be involved with the care of the recipient or with the organ procurement or transplantation process. It is never appropriate for them to discuss organ donation or obtain a consent from the family. The OPO is responsible for evaluating the donor, verifying or obtaining consent, coordinating the procurement and transplantation procedures, and assisting the family with the bereavement process. The treating physician is responsible for declaring death using brain or cardiac criteria; the transplant team cannot participate in end-of-life care or the declaration of death. Anesthetists, who provide anesthesia care for organ procurement, are required to withdraw life support in the operating room, an action that may appear contrary to their professional standards of practice.

13. *Compare a signed driver's license or organ donor card with*
a surgical consent.

An informed surgical consent advises the patient of what the procedure entails, the risks and benefits to be expected, and alternative options for care. A signed driver's license or donor card is a limited informed consent, as the risks and benefits are not explained and the donor agrees to a procedure without knowing specific details. Most donors do not know that their end-of-life care may be significantly altered and that a third party, the OPO, and not their treating physician, may direct their care. Under the UAGA, the OPO can decide what premortem medications and procedures (heparin, CVP and PA catheter, femoral cannulae) are implemented and when mechanical ventilation is discontinued. To restrict their end-of-life care solely to their personal physician, a voluntary donor must specify this directive in a living will.

Review Questions

1. Which parameter is representative of the rule of 100 during organ procurement?
   a. Systolic blood pressure <100 mm Hg
   b. Urine output <100 mL/hr
   c. PaO_2 ≥100 mm Hg
   d. Heart rate >100 mm Hg
2. Which is true regarding diabetes insipidus?
   a. Rarely seen in donors who have sustained brain death
   b. Associated with hypovolemia, hypernatremia, and hypokalemia
   c. Causes hypertonic diuresis
   d. Best treated with intramuscular Pitressin
3. Viability of harvested organs is primarily dependent on the:
   a. Length of warm ischemic time.
   b. Age of the patient.
   c. Early administration of steroids.
   d. Corrections of fluid deficits.

4. Anesthesia is required for DBD donors to prevent:
   a. Recall.
   b. Spinal reflexes.
   c. Pain.
   d. Parasympathetic activation.
5. An organ procurement organization can only direct end-of-life care and implement donor management protocols without family consent if the patient:
   a. Has a signed driver's license or donor card.
   b. Is ≥12 years old.
   c. Has a living will that restricts end-of-life care to their treating physician.
   d. Has signed a refusal that bars others from making a gift of their organs after death.

Suggested Readings

Anderson MJ, Willhite CJ. Anesthesia for organ transplantation. In: Nagelhout JJ, Elisha S KL, eds. *Nurse Anesthesia*, 6th ed. St. Louis, MO: Elsevier, 2018:871-888.

Anderson TA, Bekker P, Vagefi PA. Anesthetic considerations in organ procurement surgery: a narrative review. *Can J Anaesth* 2015; 62(5):529-39.

Jawoniyi O, Gormley K, McGleenan E, Noble HR. Organ donation and transplantation: awareness and roles of healthcare professionals-a systematic literature review. *J Clin Nurs* 2018; 27(5-6):e726-e738.

Mascia L, Bosma K, Pasero D, et al. Ventilatory and hemodynamic management of potential organ donors: an observational survey. *Crit Care Med* 2006;34(2): 321–327.

McKeown DW, Bonser RS, Kellum JA. Management of the heart beating brain-dead organ donor. *Br J Anaesth* 2012;108 Suppl 1:i96-107.

Milan Z, Cortes M, Sarma N. Anaesthetic management of organ transplant patients. *Injury* 2019;50 Suppl 5:S126-S130.

Mittel AM, Wagener G. Anesthesia for kidney and pancreas transplantation. *Anesthesiol Clin* 2017;35(3):439-452.

Robba C, Fossi F, Citerio G. Organ donation: from diagnosis to transplant. *Curr Opin Anaesthesiol* 2020;33(2):146-155.

Rosendale JD, Kauffman HM, McBride MA, et al. Aggressive pharmacological donor management results in more transplanted organs. *Transplantation* 2003;75:482-487.

Steinbrook R. Donation after cardiac death. *N Engl J Med* 2007; 357(3):209-213.

Wilson L, Carter A. Organ donation. *Br J Hosp Med (Lond)* 2018; 79(1):C8-C12.

23
Carotid Endarterectomy

KEY POINTS

- Cerebrovascular accidents (CVAs) are the third leading cause of death in the United States per year.
- Patients presenting with a recent hemispheric transient ischemic attack (TIA) and high-grade stenosis (70% to 99%) have a 65% risk reduction for the development of an ipsilateral stroke within 2 years of carotid endarterectomy (CEA).
- Chronic essential hypertension is present in most patients undergoing CEA and is associated with an increased incidence of postoperative stroke or death.
- Monitoring neurologic function under general anesthesia is necessary to detect episodes of cerebral ischemia, hypoperfusion, and cerebral embolization.

- Regional anesthesia allows for the continuous monitoring of the patient's neurologic status but requires patient cooperation throughout the procedure.
- Hemodynamic instability occurs regardless of the anesthetic technique employed and requires prompt management to decrease the incidence of postoperative complications.
- Postoperative complications of CEA include hypertension, hypotension, myocardial ischemia/infarction, stroke, cerebral hyperperfusion syndrome, recurrent laryngeal nerve damage, hematoma, tension pneumothorax, and respiratory failure.

Case Synopsis

A 78-year-old woman presents with a recent history of a TIA with complete resolution of symptoms. Carotid angiography shows a 90% stenosis of the right carotid artery and 50% stenosis of the left carotid artery. She is scheduled for a right-sided CEA.

Preoperative Evaluation and Demographic Data

Past Medical/Surgical History

- Hypertension
- Stable angina
- Percutaneous transluminal coronary angioplasty 1 year ago
- Smoker with 40-pack/year history
- History of TIA, no residual deficits

List of Medications

- Plavix
- Metoprolol
- Lisinopril

Diagnostic Data

- Hemoglobin, 12.1 g/dL; hematocrit, 36.2%
- International normalized ratio, 1.08

- Electrolytes: sodium, 140 mEq/L; potassium, 3.7; chloride, 104 mEq/L; carbon dioxide (CO_2), 23 mEq/L
- Glucose, 108 mg/dL

Height/Weight/Vital Signs

- 157 cm, 60 kg
- Blood pressure, 156/88; heart rate, 64 beats per minute; respiratory rate, 18 breaths per minute; room air oxygen saturation, 97%; temperature, 36.8°C
- Electrocardiogram (ECG): normal sinus rhythm, first-degree atrioventricular (AV) block, nonspecific ST-T wave changes, evidence of old inferior-wall myocardial infarction
- Dobutamine stress test: normal left ventricular function, no evidence of ischemia, normal study

Pathophysiology

Each year in the United States over 700,000 individuals experience an adverse cerebrovascular event. Stroke is the third leading cause of death and the number one cause of major morbidity. Atherosclerotic disease accounts for approximately 30% of all of these strokes. It is estimated that 0.5% of individuals over the age of 60 and 10% of people over the age of 80 have carotid artery stenosis, accounting for the increased prevalence of stroke in the elderly population. CEA is therefore a prophylactic treatment, performed for individuals who are at increased risk of decreased cerebral perfusion.

Blood is supplied to the brain via the right and left internal carotid arteries and the vertebral arteries. The two internal carotid arteries are responsible for 80% to 90% of the blood supply, and the remainder comes from the vertebrobasilar system. These vessels join to form the circle of Willis and the major intracranial vessels, including the anterior cerebral arteries, the middle cerebral arteries, and the posterior cerebral arteries, as is shown in Fig. 23.1. Occlusion of a major cerebral vessel results in a predictable pattern of neurologic symptoms specific to the area of the brain supplied by the vessel.

Cerebral blood flow (CBF) is dependent on several factors, which are summarized in Box 23.1. CBF is normally autoregulated over a range of mean arterial pressures (MAPs) from 60 to 150 mm Hg. Cerebral perfusion pressure (CPP) is calculated using the following equation. The normal range for CPP is 80 to 100 mm Hg. In the absence of increased intracranial pressure (ICP) or an elevated central venous pressure, the major determinant of CPP is MAP.

$$CPP = MAP - ICP \text{ or } CVP$$

Note: The value that is higher, ICP or CVP, is used. *CPP*, Cerebral perfusion pressure; *CVP*, central venous pressure; *ICP*, intracranial pressure; *MAP*, mean arterial pressure.

In patients who have hypertension, the autoregulation curve is shifted to the right such that higher perfusion pressures are required to maintain consistent CBF. Normal cerebral metabolic requirements for oxygen ($CMRO_2$) range from 3.0 to 3.8 mL O_2/100 g brain tissue/minute. These requirements can be decreased by hypothermia, barbiturates, benzodiazepines, and volatile anesthetics. However, hyperthermia, seizure disorders, and ketamine all increase $CMRO_2$. Finally, CO_2 is a potent cerebral vasodilator such that CBF is increased 1 mL/100 g/minute for each 1 mm Hg increase in $PaCO_2$. Therefore dramatic increases in CBF will occur in the presence of hypercarbia.

Carotid artery stenosis most frequently occurs where the common carotid artery bifurcates into the internal and external carotid arteries. This results in turbulent blood flow, which leads to endothelial cell damage and plaque formation. Carotid plaques usually take one of two forms: homogeneous or heterogeneous. *Homogeneous plaques* are stable deposits of fatty streaks and fibrous tissues that rarely rupture, and therefore patients may be asymptomatic. However, over time, the plaque becomes covered by a fibrous cap, which can rupture, releasing the underlying debris into the cerebral circulation. Restabilization of the ruptured cap results in the development of *heterogeneous plaques,* which are unstable and can rupture. Patients who are symptomatic

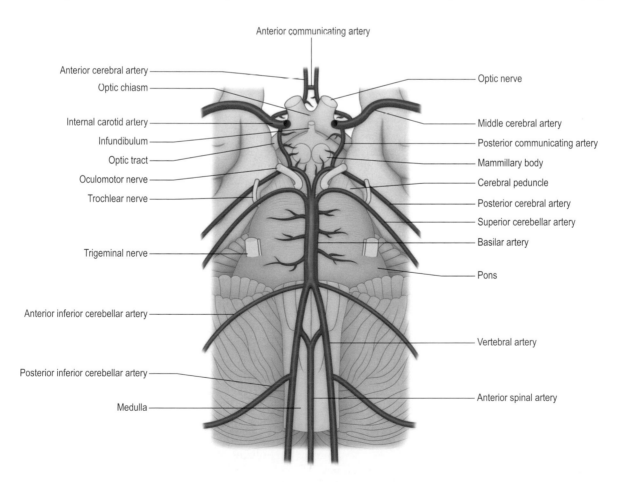

• **Fig. 23.1** The blood supply to the brain (circle of Willis). (From Crossman AR, Neary D: *Neuroanatomy: an illustrated colour text*, ed 6, London, 2020, Elsevier.)

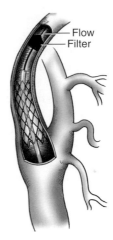

• **Fig. 23.2** Carotid artery stenting. (From Pellerito JS, Polak JF: *Introduction to vascular ultrasonography*, ed 7, St. Louis, 2020, Elsevier.)

are most likely to have heterogeneous plaques that are prone to acute disruption and spontaneous embolization, which is the cause of most strokes resulting from carotid artery stenosis. Carotid endarterectomy is recommended for symptomatic patients with greater than 70% carotid stenosis in the associated carotid artery.

Surgical Procedure

CEA involves careful exposure of the common carotid artery, including its bifurcation into the internal and external carotid arteries. Once exposure is complete, the external, internal, and common carotid arteries are cross-clamped so that the carotid bifurcation can be isolated from the circulation. The artery is then opened through a longitudinal incision and the plaque is removed, extending as far cephalad into the internal carotid as feasible. A synthetic patch graft is then utilized to close the vessel in order to increase the diameter of the artery and prevent restenosis. Several surgeons utilize an eversion CEA technique in which the carotid artery is completely transected and turned inside out in order to remove the plaque. A shunt may or may not be utilized. Regardless of the technique that is performed, it is essential that the surgeon remove all debris from the vessel intima in order to prevent embolization and postoperative neurologic sequelae.

Anesthetic Management and Considerations

Preoperative Period

1. *Discuss the indications for CEA, including criteria for patient selection.*

    The American Academy of Neurology reviewed the indications for CEA, and they have identified two groups of patients that are candidates for surgical treatment: symptomatic and asymptomatic patients. Symptomatic patients are considered when rupture of the plaque releases emboli into the cerebral circulation causing TIAs that produce reversible neurologic effects. Asymptomatic patients have carotid artery stenosis but there is no history of a neurologic event that is attributable to the carotid lesion.

    Several large studies have compared patient outcomes after surgery and medical treatment. They found that for symptomatic patients with greater than 70% stenosis, there was an absolute risk reduction of 16% for perioperative death and subsequent stroke over the next 5 years. A reduction in the patients' risk was not observed in symptomatic patients with less than 70% stenosis, and no benefits were demonstrated in patients with 30% to 49% stenosis or total occlusion. CEA was shown to be harmful in patients who had less than 30% carotid artery stenosis. CEA is therefore recommended for symptomatic patients with greater than 70% carotid artery stenosis.

2. *Discuss a minimally invasive surgical procedure used to treat carotid artery stenosis.*

    Carotid artery angioplasty and stent placement (CAS) is a nonsurgical alternative to CEA that has recently become available for the primary and secondary prevention of a CVA as a result of carotid artery stenosis, as shown in Fig. 23.2. Hemodynamic changes are similar to those seen with CEA, including reperfusion hypotension due to baroreceptor dysfunction. Anesthesia services may be provided for sedation and hemodynamic monitoring for CAS. Complications associated with CAS are related to anticoagulation, balloon angioplasty, and the stent placement and are presented in Box 23.2.

3. *Discuss the common coexisting disease states, preoperative medications, and factors that contribute to morbidity and mortality in patients undergoing CEA.*

    The majority of patients presenting for CEA suffer from significant atherosclerotic disease in both the coronary and peripheral vasculature and are at risk for developing myocardial ischemia and/or infarction. Most of these patients will be medically managed preoperatively, utilizing a combination of beta-blockers, calcium channel blockers, antiarrhythmics, nitrates, diuretics, angiotensin-converting enzyme (ACE) inhibitors, and other

• **BOX 23.2** **Complications Associated With Carotid Artery Angioplasty and Stenting**

- Stroke
- Myocardial infarction/ischemia
- Death
- Bradycardia and hypotension from stimulation baroreceptor reflex
- Stent thrombosis and embolization
- Carotid artery dissection from stent placement
- Cerebral hyperperfusion syndrome
- Horner syndrome
- Hemorrhage

• **BOX 23.3** **Preoperative Risk Factors Associated With Perioperative Events During CEA**

- Chronic essential hypertension
- Coronary artery disease (CAD)
- Peripheral vascular disease
- Preexisting renal disease
- Symptomatic carotid artery stenosis in combination with severe CAD

antihypertensive drugs. In addition, some patients may be receiving antiplatelet therapy with aspirin (ASA) and/or clopidogrel (Plavix). Current recommendations are that all patients with carotid artery disease be on low-dose aspirin therapy on a regular basis and it should be continued through the perioperative period. There is no evidence to support the continued use of other antiplatelet medications, and these should be discontinued a week before surgery to ensure that platelet function has normalized.

The incidence of perioperative myocardial infarction has been reported to range from 0% to 4%, and this complication is the leading cause of mortality after CEA. Patients presenting with both significant coronary artery disease and carotid artery disease requiring surgical intervention present a specific problem because it is unclear which surgical procedure to undertake first. Patients undergoing CEA before coronary revascularization are at significant risk for cardiac events. However, coronary revascularization has improved, and distal embolic protection devices have been developed. The risk of adverse neurologic events appears to be higher with CAS, particularly during catheterization and ballooning, but restenosis rates appear to be comparable to the traditional CEA technique.

Chronic essential hypertension is highly associated with carotid artery stenosis and increases the morbidity and mortality for patients undergoing CEA.

- There is a significant association between postoperative stroke or death and a *preoperative* systolic blood pressure >180 mm Hg.
- A *postoperative* systolic blood pressure >220 mm Hg is associated with an increased risk of stroke or death after CEA.
- A preoperative systolic blood pressure of >160 mm Hg is a risk factor for postoperative hypertension.
- It is recommended that blood pressure control be achieved preoperatively in patients with a systolic blood pressure >180 mm Hg, who do not have severe bilateral carotid artery disease, and who are not having frequent adverse neurologic events.

The anesthetist must consider that cerebral autoregulation is shifted to the right, requiring a higher MAP in patients with hypertension, and it is unknown how long it takes for the mechanism to reset. The concern is that patients with severe hypertension will be at increased risk for impaired cerebral perfusion during surgical correction. The preoperative risk factors associated with perioperative events during CEA are presented in Box 23.3.

4. *Discuss the preoperative evaluation of the patient undergoing CEA, including cardiac risk assessment.*

Preoperative evaluation of the patient undergoing CEA should include the conduct of a comprehensive history and physical examination. All preexisting neurologic deficits should be documented in the patient's record. A careful cardiovascular assessment should be carried out because the possibility of cardiovascular disease is high. This should include a preoperative ECG, echocardiogram, or cardiac stress test, as dictated by the patient's history and presentation. A careful assessment of preoperative blood pressure is also necessary because the risk of preoperative neurologic events is high in the patient with hypertension. All patients undergoing CEA should be evaluated by a cardiologist before surgery.

In addition to the cardiac assessment, the patient's preoperative respiratory function should be assessed to determine their pulmonary reserve. Information regarding the patient's smoking history is also essential, as cigarette smoking is associated with an increase in the risk of a stroke. Other preoperative factors associated with an increased risk of stroke include preexisting renal disease, diabetes mellitus, hyperlipidemia, and excessive alcohol consumption.

Intraoperative Period

5. *Describe the various anesthetic techniques utilized for CEA.*

Anesthesia for CEA can be provided utilizing either regional or general anesthesia. The choice of technique is dependent on the patient's, surgeon's, and anesthetist's preference, as well as familiarity with a particular technique and the patient's status. The advantages comparing regional and general anesthesia for CEA are listed in Box 23.4. Regardless of anesthetic technique, it is necessary to provide cerebral and cardiac protection,

---

• BOX 23.4 Advantages of Regional Versus General Anesthesia for CEA

Regional Anesthesia
- Superior perioperative neurologic assessment
- Improved postoperative analgesia
- Maintenance cerebral blood flow
- Decreased rate of elective shunting
- Decreased length of stay

General Anesthesia
- Does not require patient cooperation
- Anesthetic-induced decrease in $CMRO_2$ may provide cerebral protection

---

• BOX 23.5 Methods of Monitoring for Cerebral Ischemia During CEA

- **EEG:** Monitors cortical events but does not disclose ischemia in deeper structures
- **SSEP:** Assesses the integrity of sensory pathways in both cortical and deep structures of the brain
- **NIRS (cerebral oximetry):** Measures regional cerebral oxygenation
- **Transcranial Doppler:** Allows ultrasonic measurement of blood flow through the middle cerebral artery; can be used to monitor both cerebral hemodynamics and the occurrence of emboli

---

as well as control of blood pressure, heart rate, and the stress response to surgery. Standard monitoring includes an intraarterial catheter for continuous beat-to-beat blood pressure monitoring, noninvasive blood pressure monitoring, ECG, pulse oximetry, and capnography. Patients with poor left ventricular function may benefit from a pulmonary artery catheter, but the benefits must be weighed against the risks of accidental carotid puncture. When general anesthesia is employed, transesophageal echocardiography can be used.

General Anesthesia—General anesthesia for CEA can be safely administered utilizing a variety of anesthetic agents. Comparisons of inhalation versus narcotic-based techniques have shown no difference in outcome because both volatile anesthetics and narcotics decrease $CMRO_2$. Dexmedetomidine can improve the hemodynamic stability intraoperatively and postoperatively. If somatosensory evoked potentials (SSEPs) are to be monitored intraoperatively, inhalation anesthetics may have to be avoided because they have been shown to depress the amplitude and increase the latency of SSEP transmission. However, regardless of the anesthetic agents utilized, it is essential that hemodynamic stability be maintained and that emergence occurs promptly so that immediate assessment of postoperative neurologic functioning can occur in the operating room.

Regional Anesthesia—Regional anesthesia for CEA can be accomplished using either local infiltration or superficial and/or deep cervical plexus block. The greatest advantage of this technique is the ability to assess the patient's neurologic functioning. Signs of impaired neurologic function include:
- Dizziness
- Slurred speech
- Weakness
- Dysphasia
- Altered level of consciousness

It has not been conclusively determined that regional anesthesia performed for CEA improves long-term outcomes. Because the patient is awake for the duration of the procedure, preoperative patient education is essential. Anxiety and fear can stimulate the stress response and create hemodynamic instability unrelated to the underlying surgical intervention. Mild sedation can be utilized, but deep sedation can impair neurologic assessment and produce hypoventilation, which increases CO_2. It is also difficult to convert to a general anesthetic because access to the patient's airway is limited. It is therefore essential to determine those candidates who are appropriate for regional anesthesia.

6. *Discuss the rationale and methods for monitoring neurologic status during CEA.*

Monitoring neurologic function under general anesthesia is necessary in order to detect episodes of cerebral ischemia, hypoperfusion, and cerebral embolization. These monitors are employed to identify patients who would benefit from the use of a carotid artery shunt during carotid artery cross-clamping. A number of methods of monitoring are currently available and are outlined in Box 23.5:
- **Electroencephalogram (EEG)** can be used to monitor neurologic functioning under general anesthesia for CEA. Although the technique is sensitive when detecting cerebral ischemia, the signal only reflects cortical events and does not detect ischemia in deeper structures of the brain.
- **SSEPs** have many advantages compared with the EEG to detect cerebral ischemia. The information determined from SSEPs examines both cortical and deep brain structures because they assess transmission along the entire sensory nerve pathway. However, like the EEG, they are sensitive to the effect of global ischemia rather than regional ischemia. In addition, volatile anesthetics suppress the SSEP, and if they are used, the agent concentration should be ≤0.5 minimum alveolar concentration (MAC).
- **Near infrared spectroscopy (NIRS)**, also known as *cerebral oximetry*, provides information regarding regional cerebral oxygenation (rSO_2), which is

a composite measure of arterial, venous, and capillary oxygenation. The predominant influence on the value comes from the venous blood. Carotid cross-clamping is associated with decreases in rSO_2 but there are no well-defined parameters for the "normal" range of values. In addition, changes in rSO_2 can be related to changes in the regional distribution of blood flow as a result of anesthesia rather than as a result of ischemia. This monitoring modality has been associated with a high false-positive rate.

- **Transcranial Doppler** measures velocity of flow through the middle cerebral artery by way of a probe placed on the thin petrous temporal bone. A marked reduction in velocity during carotid artery cross-clamping is an indication for the use of a carotid shunt. Studies assessing the efficacy of this technique are conflicting. Unlike other monitors utilized, the transcranial Doppler is capable of detecting the presence of emboli. Because the majority of untoward neurologic events during CEA are embolic in nature, this technique provides advantages over those previously discussed.

7. *Describe the methods available for providing cerebral protection and reducing the risk of neurologic injury during CEA.*

Stump Pressure Measurement—Before the introduction of more sophisticated forms of cerebral monitoring, stump pressures have been traditionally used to determine the need for shunt placement during carotid cross-clamping. Once the common carotid and external carotid arteries are clamped, the pressure measured within the internal carotid artery reflects the perfusion pressure within the circle of Willis, and thus the adequacy of collateral blood flow. A wide range of pressures (25 to 70 mm Hg) have been proposed as acceptable during carotid artery cross-clamping, and it has been determined that stump pressures tend to be specific (ability to detect true negatives) but not sensitive (ability to detect true positives) for the development of cerebral ischemia.

Carotid Shunting—Frequently shunts are utilized during carotid cross-clamping to ensure the adequacy of CBF during CEA. A shunt is inserted in the proximal and distal aspects of the carotid artery. The surgeons dissect the plaque within the carotid artery as blood flows from the common carotid artery through the shunt, bypasses the surgical field, and enters the circle of Willis. Although this technique would appear to be extremely useful to prevent postoperative neurologic sequelae, it is associated with risks. Complications of shunt insertion include air embolization, plaque embolization, tears of the vessel intima, and carotid dissection. In addition, there is an increased risk of local complications, including the development of hematomas, infection, nerve injury, and carotid restenosis. Because up to 95% of postoperative neurologic deficits are the result of embolic events, many surgeons do not routinely shunt but place shunts selectively based on evidence of cerebral hypoperfusion in response to cross-clamping. Determining factors include measuring of stump pressures and assessing changes in neurologic monitoring parameters. Patients undergoing CEA with intraoperative EEG and SSEP monitoring who have selective shunting demonstrate a significantly reduced rate of developing a stroke. Patients who received selective shunting are thought to be more than seven times less likely to experience a perioperative stroke.

8. *Discuss the rationale for anticoagulation during carotid cross-clamping.*

Heparin is administered intraoperatively, before carotid artery cross-clamping, to reduce the risk of thromboembolic complications. Several different methods are employed by anesthetists to guide the dosing for heparin, but 50 to 100 units/kg is commonly administered. Inadequate heparinization is associated with a higher incidence of neurologic deficits in patients who have not been adequately anticoagulated, as determined by the activated clotting time (ACT). Heparin administration on a units/kg basis is associated with more consistent plasma levels and a lower risk for the development of postoperative hematoma. Redosing is determined based on the duration of anticoagulation needed and the amount of drug left in the body. The elimination half-time of heparin is 1.5 hours with a range of 1 to 2 hours. Despite the improved control achieved with weight-based dosing, no statistically significant advantage has been demonstrated in clinical studies to advocate for weight-based versus fixed dosing.

The decision to reverse the anticoagulation effects of heparin with protamine is made on an individual basis and depends on the presence of bleeding. There is an increased incidence of stroke associated with protamine administration but a decreased risk for postoperative hematoma requiring surgical decompression. The dose of protamine administered assumes that 1 mg/100 units of heparin are left in the blood at the time of reversal. Therefore, 25 mg of protamine should be sufficient to reverse the effects of 5000 units of heparin of heparin administered an hour before reversal. Protamine administration can result in hypotension and anaphylaxis.

9. *Explain the importance of controlling the patient's blood pressure during CEA.*

As previously stated, hypertension is present in many patients presenting for CEA. In general, hypertensive patients suffer from profound blood pressure lability during the perioperative period, especially when general anesthesia is utilized. Cardiovascular instability is even more pronounced when these patients undergo CEA. Hypotension and/or hypertension can occur as a result of carotid sinus baroreceptor stimulation and manipulation. In addition, carotid artery cross-clamping is associated with marked increases in arterial pressure regardless of the anesthetic technique. The cardiovascular changes produced as a result of the combined effect of anesthesia and carotid sinus manipulation place the patients undergoing CEA at risk for negative perioperative cardiac and cerebrovascular events. It is recommended to maintain the patient's MAP ≥20% of the preoperative MAP throughout the cross-clamp time.

10. *Describe the methods utilized for control of blood pressure during CEA.*

Intraoperative blood pressure control begins during the preoperative period, as outlined previously. The patient's cardiovascular and neurologic conditions should be optimized before surgical intervention. All antihypertensive medications should be continued throughout the perioperative period. Because multiple intraoperative events can result in sympathetic stimulation, including induction of anesthesia, incision, carotid cross-clamping, and emergence, short-acting beta-adrenergic blocking agents should be readily available. If hypertension is sustained, nitroglycerin and nitroprusside can be utilized for titratable control of blood pressure. Bradycardia associated with manipulation of the carotid sinus can be blocked with local infiltration of local anesthetic by the surgeon. The initial treatment for bradycardia that is caused by the baroreceptor reflex and results in severe hypotension is to notify the surgeon to release pressure on the carotid sinus. Sustained hypotension can be treated by administering intravenous fluids and vasopressors. Bradycardia that is unresponsive to local infiltration may require the administration of atropine sulfate.

Postoperative Period

11. *Discuss the pathophysiology and treatment of commonly occurring postoperative complications associated with CEA.*

The most frequently occurring postoperative complications associated with CEA are summarized in Box 23.6. Both hypertension and hypotension are common after CEA. It has been estimated that hypertension is seen in approximately 25% of patients, and hypotension occurs in approximately 10% of

patients; however, the specific causes have not been completely explained. Unrecognized bleeding and/or inadequate intraoperative fluid replacement may cause postoperative hypotension. It has been hypothesized that postoperative hypertension results from a decreased baroreceptor reflex responsiveness as a result of mechanical injury during surgical manipulation. In addition, patients with bilateral carotid artery disease have been shown to exhibit more severe deterioration in baroreceptor function after surgery. Sustained systolic blood pressures >180 mm Hg are associated with an increased risk of TIA, stroke, and myocardial infarction in the postoperative period. The intervention should be determined by the individual anesthetist, but nitrates may be useful in this setting because they are more likely to maintain CBF.

Cerebral hyperperfusion syndrome occurs in 1% to 3% of patients undergoing CEA. These patients develop profound increases in CBF and often demonstrate an increased flow velocity in the middle cerebral artery estimated to be 100% greater than the values measured preoperatively. These patients develop an ipsilateral (operative side) headache, severe arterial hypertension, seizures, and, often, focal neurologic deficits. If left untreated, cerebral hyperperfusion syndrome can progress to cerebral edema, intracranial hemorrhage, and death. Preoperative risk factors for the development of cerebral hyperperfusion syndrome include decreased cerebrovascular reserve, preoperative hypertension, previous CVA, or surgery for >90% carotid artery stenosis. Therefore it is essential that blood pressure control be achieved before the day of surgery and throughout the perioperative period. Box 23.7 summarizes the risk factors associated with the development of cerebral hyperperfusion syndrome.

The development of a postoperative stroke is most commonly attributed to thrombus formation and embolization of plaque debris during the insertion of shunts and removal of the intimal plaque. Neurologic assessment is conducted within the operating room immediately after emergence in order to identify the presence of neurologic deficits.

• BOX 23.6   Postoperative Complications After CEA

- Hemodynamic instability (hypotension and hypertension)
- Myocardial ischemia/infarction
- Carotid sinus dysfunction
- Stroke
- Cerebral hyperperfusion syndrome
- Recurrent/superior laryngeal nerve damage
- Hematoma
- Tension pneumothorax
- Respiratory failure

• BOX 23.7   Risk Factors for Developing Cerebral Hyperperfusion Syndrome

- Diminished cerebrovascular reserve
- Preoperative uncontrolled hypertension
- Recent ipsilateral nonhemorrhagic stroke
- Previous ischemic cerebral infarction
- Surgery for >90% ipsilateral carotid stenosis
- Intraoperative ischemia/embolization
- Postoperative hypertension
- Hyperperfusion lasting longer than several hours after CEA

Postoperative bleeding is infrequent but can occur after a CEA. When bleeding is significant, it can cause the development of an incisional hematoma that may be large enough to cause airway compromise. The initial intervention after a hematoma is discovered is to immediately notify the surgeon to evacuate the hematoma, followed by airway management. This seems counterintuitive; however, the definitive treatment is to relieve the pressure on the structures of the neck. Normally viewed anatomic structures that are identifiable during direct laryngoscopy may not be visualized during subsequent attempts. It may also become difficult or impossible to ventilate the patient. Immediate re-exploration of the surgical site is mandatory. Tension pneumothorax can also occur in the postoperative period because the apices of the lungs extend above the clavicles and the pleural cavity may be inadvertently entered during surgical dissection of the neck. This will require immediate decompression.

12. *Describe the neurologic cranial nerve assessment for a patient having a CEA.*

During dissection and retraction of neck structures, it is possible for damage to occur to the underlying cranial nerves as they pass through the surrounding tissues. The postoperative evaluation of the patient's neurologic and cognitive function should include an assessment of the integrity of cranial nerves VII (facial), IX (glossopharyngeal), X (vagus), XI (spinal accessory), and XII (hypoglossal).

The facial nerve is a mixed sensory and motor nerve responsible for motor control to the muscles of the face and for the secretion of saliva. Damage to the facial nerve results in an asymmetric ipsilateral smile. Contralateral asymmetry may be indicative of a possible intraoperative CVA.

The glossopharyngeal nerve controls the pharyngeal muscles and the ability to swallow. Damage to this nerve will result in difficulty swallowing and ipsilateral Horner syndrome. Horner syndrome is associated with miosis, ptosis, and anhidrosis.

Branches of the vagus nerve divide to form the superior and recurrent laryngeal nerves, which control the intrinsic muscles of the larynx. Unilateral damage to the internal branch of the superior laryngeal nerve,

TABLE 23.1	Assessment of Cranial Nerve Function After CEA
Cranial Nerve	**Abnormal Assessment**
• Facial nerve (VII)	• Ipsilateral smile asymmetry
• Glossopharyngeal nerve (IX)	• Difficulty swallowing • Ipsilateral Horner syndrome
• Vagus nerve (X) (recurrent and superior laryngeal nerves)	• Unilateral vocal cord paralysis • Hoarseness • Impairment of the gag reflex • Voice fatigue
• Spinal accessory nerve (XI)	• Ipsilateral weakness of the trapezius and sternocleidomastoid muscles • Ipsilateral weakness of the neck and shoulder against resistance
• Hypoglossal nerve (XII)	• Ipsilateral tongue drift • Difficulty with speech • Difficulty with chewing

which innervates the cricothyroid muscle, will result in hoarseness. Unilateral damage to the recurrent laryngeal nerve, which innervates the posterior and lateral cricoarytenoid muscles, can cause vocal cord paralysis on the operative side, hoarseness, impairment of the gag reflex, difficult vocalization, and respiratory difficulty, especially in those patients with preoperative respiratory insufficiency.

The spinal accessory nerve controls the sternocleidomastoid and the trapezius muscles. Damage to this nerve during CEA will result in ipsilateral weakness in the neck and shoulder. Patients will have difficulty turning their head or shrugging against resistance.

Finally, the hypoglossal nerve is responsible for control of the muscles of the tongue. Damage to this structure will result in ipsilateral drift of the tongue when patients are asked to stick out their tongue. In addition, patients may have difficulties with speech and chewing. A summary of the cranial nerves that should be assessed is included in Table 23.1.

Review Questions

1. Which is a disadvantage of regional anesthesia administered for carotid endarterectomy?
   a. Results in an increased length of stay
   b. Associated with increased morbidity and mortality
   c. Requires patient cooperation
   d. Increases hemodynamic instability

2. Monitoring carotid artery stump pressures is:
   a. Reflective of perfusion pressure in the internal carotid artery.
   b. Highly sensitive for the development of cerebral ischemia.
   c. Measured before the application of the carotid cross-clamp.
   d. A specific indicator of cerebral hypoperfusion.

3. One hour after a dose of heparin, 7000 units have been administered. The appropriate initial dose of protamine for this patient who weighs 60 kg is:
   a. 70 mg.
   b. 50 mg.
   c. 35 mg.
   d. 15 mg.

4. Which is not caused by cranial nerve injury during carotid endarterectomy?
   a. Contralateral facial asymmetry
   b. Unilateral vocal cord paralysis
   c. Horner syndrome
   d. Ipsilateral tongue drift

5. The majority of postoperative neurologic deficits occur as a result of:
   a. Perioperative hypertensive episodes.
   b. Thromboembolic events.
   c. Carotid dissection.
   d. Cranial nerve injury.

Suggested Readings

Ahmed N, Kelleher D, Madan M, et al. Carotid endarterectomy following thrombolysis for acute ischaemic stroke. *Vasa* 2017; 46(2):116-120.

Borghese O, Pisani A, Lapergue B, Di Centa I. Early carotid endarterectomy for symptomatic stenosis of internal carotid artery in patients affected by transient ischemic attack or minor-to-moderate ischemic acute stroke: a single-center experience. *Ann Vasc Surg* 2020;65:232-239.

Cao P, De Rango P, Verzini F, et al. Outcome of carotid stenting versus endarterectomy: a case-control study. *Stroke* 2006;37(5): 1221-1226.

Chaturvedi S, Bruno A, Feasby T, et al. Carotid endarterectomy—an evidence-based review: report of the Therapeutics and Technology Assessment Subcommittee of the American Academy of Neurology. *Neurology* 2005;65(6):794-801.

Elisha S. Anesthesia for vascular surgery. In: Nagelhout JJ, Elisha S, eds. *Nurse Anesthesia*, 6th ed. St. Louis, MO: Elsevier, 2018:535-563.

Grecu L, Nikhil C. Vascular disease. In: Hines RL, Marschall KE, eds. *Stoelting's Anesthesia and Coexisting Disease,* 7th ed. Philadelphia: Churchill Livingstone, 2018:237–263.

Kim JW, Huh U, Song S, et al. Outcomes of carotid endarterectomy according to the anesthetic method: general versus regional anesthesia. *Korean J Thorac Cardiovasc Surg* 2019;52(6):392-399.

Kuzkov VV, Obraztsov MY, et al. Total intravenous versus volatile induction and maintenance of anesthesia in elective carotid endarterectomy: effects on cerebral oxygenation and cognitive functions. *J Cardiothorac Vasc Anesth* 2018;32(4):1701-1708.

Martín-Morales E, Jiménez-Román R, et al. Results and complications of carotid endarterectomy in a hospital from Madrid, Spain. *Cir Cir* 2019;87(5):501-507.

Macfarlane AJR, Vlassakov K, Elkassabany N. Regional anesthesia for vascular surgery: does the anesthetic choice influence outcome? *Curr Opin Anaesthesiol* 2019;32(5):690-696.

Newman JE, Bown MJ, Sayers RD, Thompson JP, et al. Post-carotid endarterectomy hypertension. Part 2: association with perioperative clinical, anaesthetic, and transcranial doppler derived parameters. *Eur J Vasc Endovasc Surg* 2017;54(5):564-572.

Nouraei SA, Al-Rawi PG, Sigaudo-Roussel D, et al. Carotid endarterectomy impairs blood pressure homeostasis by reducing the physiologic baroreflex reserve. *J Vasc Surg* 2005;41(4):631–S637.

Otite FO, Khandelwal P, Malik AM, Chaturvedi S. National patterns of carotid revascularization before and after the Carotid Revascularization Endarterectomy vs Stenting Trial (CREST). *JAMA Neurol* 2018;75(1):51-57.

Rasheed AS, White RS, Tangel V, et al. Carotid revascularization procedures and perioperative outcomes: a multistate analysis, 2007-2014. *J Cardiothorac Vasc Anesth* 2019;33(7):1963-1972.

Rots ML, Fassaert LMM, Kappelle LJ, et al. Intra-operative hypotension is a risk factor for post-operative silent brain ischaemia in patients with pre-operative hypertension undergoing carotid endarterectomy. *Eur J Vasc Endovasc Surg* 2020;59(4):526-534.

Tsujikawa S, Ikeshita K. Low-dose dexmedetomidine provides hemodynamics stabilization during emergence and recovery from general anesthesia in patients undergoing carotid endarterectomy: a randomized double-blind, placebo-controlled trial. *J Anesth* 2019; 33(2):266-272.

24

Acute Aortic Dissection and Repair

KEY POINTS

- The incidence of acute aortic dissection is rare and is estimated to be 5 to 30 cases per 1 million people per year in the United States.
- Aortic dissection is associated with a tear in the intimal layer of the aorta.
- An acute aortic dissection may involve the ascending and/or the descending aorta.

- The incidence of acute aortic dissection occurs more frequently in men than in women.
- The morbidity and mortality rate associated with acute aortic dissection even when treatment occurs is 90% within a 3-month period.

Case Synopsis

A 65-year-old man presents to the emergency room (ER) with severe sharp chest pain that radiates to his upper back. A transesophageal echocardiogram (TEE) reveals an acute ascending aortic dissection.

Preoperative Evaluation and Demographic Data

Past Medical/Surgical History

- Hypertension
- Coronary artery disease
- Coronary artery bypass grafting 1 year ago
- Right inguinal hernia repair 20 years ago

List of Medications

- Zestril (Lisinopril)
- Atorvastatin (Lipitor)
- Aspirin (80 mg)

Diagnostic Data

- Hemoglobin, 12.8 g/dL; hematocrit, 38.2%
- Electrolytes: sodium, 141 mEq/L; potassium, 3.7 mEq/L; chloride, 101 mEq/L; carbon dioxide, 19 mEq/L
- Electrocardiogram (ECG): normal sinus rhythm; heart rate, 95 beats per minute
- Chest x-ray: widening mediastinum, otherwise normal

Height/Weight/Vital Signs

- 183 cm, 85 kg
- Blood pressure, 165/100; heart rate, 95 beats per minute; respiratory rate, 18 breaths per minute; room air oxygen saturation, 96%; temperature, 37°C

Pathophysiology

Acute aortic dissection is an uncommon yet life-threatening condition that involves a disruption of the intimal layer of the aorta. The aorta is exposed to constantly high pressure, which creates shear stress on the intimal layer. The high degree of wall tension within the aorta can be described by the law of Laplace. When patients have long-term untreated hypertension and plaque formation within the aorta, there is an increased incidence of dissection. Once the intimal layer is damaged, blood flows through the disruption between the intima and media, creating a false lumen that separates the middle and outer layers of the aorta. The false lumen may eventually rupture.

Numerous classification systems exist to describe the location of the aortic dissection (Box 24.1). The Stanford classification system is the most commonly used to differentiate between the regions of the aortic defect. This system divides aortic dissection into a type A and a type B, as shown in Fig. 24.1. The type A dissection involves the ascending thoracic aorta with or without the involvement of the descending thoracic aorta. The Stanford type B dissection involves the descending thoracic aorta. Aortic dissections can extend to the aortic root and produce aortic valve insufficiency. Untreated aortic dissections have a 50% mortality rate in the first 48 hours and a 90% mortality rate within 3 months. The most common anatomic positions for an aortic dissection to occur include the aortic arch, distal to the left subclavian artery and immediately superior to the aortic root.

A Stanford type A acute aortic dissection requires immediate medical treatment and surgical intervention. The Stanford type B acute aortic dissection is most often treated with medical management unless the patient has uncontrolled hypertension, poor perfusion to the gastrointestinal

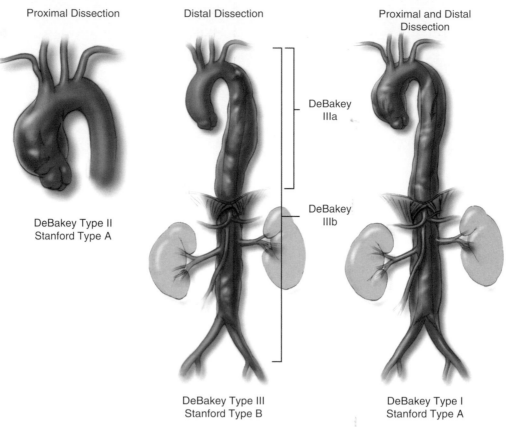

Proximal Dissection

DeBakey Type II
Stanford Type A

Distal Dissection

DeBakey
IIIa

DeBakey
IIIb

DeBakey Type III
Stanford Type B

Proximal and Distal
Dissection

DeBakey Type I
Stanford Type A

• **Fig. 24.1** This simplified, descriptive classification scheme categorizes aortic dissection based on involvement of the proximal aorta, distal aorta, or both segments. Corresponding DeBakey classifications are included for comparison. The primary limitation of the Stanford classification is that it is based solely on the presence (type A) or absence (type B) of ascending aortic involvement; it does not provide information about distal aortic involvement, a factor that has important management and prognostic implications. (From Creager MA, Beckman JA, Loscalzo J: *Vascular medicine: a companion to Braunwald's heart disease*, ed 3, Philadelphia, 2020, Elsevier.)

• BOX 24.1 Stanford and DeBakey Classification Systems for Aortic Dissection

Stanford Classification

- Type A dissection involves the ascending aorta.
- Type B dissection involves the descending aorta.

DeBakey Classification

- Type I dissection involves both the ascending and descending aorta.
- Type II dissection involves only the ascending aorta.
- Type III dissection involves only the descending aorta.
  - Type IIIA dissection involves the descending aorta between the left subclavian artery and the diaphragm.
  - Type IIIB dissection involves the descending aorta below the level of the diaphragm.

---

tract or lower extremities, and rupture of the aorta. Surgical treatment is warranted in these cases.

Open surgical repair of the aorta is the usual procedure used to correct the Stanford type B aortic dissection. Endovascular aortic repair (EVAR) is being explored as a treatment option for aortic aneurysms, and recent evidence supports the effectiveness of this technique. It is estimated that 70% of patients who develop an aortic dissection have hypertension. Aneurysms of the aorta may or may not be present before aortic dissection. TEE is a first-line diagnostic tool used to identify the presence of an acute aortic dissection. The TEE can reveal the extent of the dissection into the aortic root, as well as the condition of the aortic valve. Computed tomography (CT) and magnetic resonance imaging (MRI) techniques provide definitive data as to the presence, location, and size of the aortic dissections. A repair of a dissection of the ascending aorta is illustrated in Fig. 24.2.

Medical Management

The Stanford type B aortic dissection is routinely medically treated by administering beta-adrenergic blocking drugs. If the use of beta-adrenergic blocking drugs is contraindicated, then calcium channel blocking agents and sodium nitroprusside may be used. The goal of medical management is to avoid aortic rupture. Antihypertensive therapy is titrated to maintain the systolic blood pressure between 100 and 120 mm Hg, which decreases the mechanical stress exerted on the aortic wall. Careful monitoring for aortic

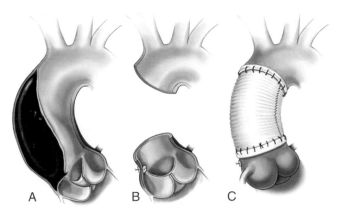

• **Fig. 24.2** Ascending aortic dissection repair. (A) The dissecting hematoma is seen and usually extends all the way to the iliac arteries. (B) The compromised commissure of the valve is resuspended by a full-thickness pledgeted suture. (C) The ascending aorta is replaced with a vascular graft, usually using strips of felt to reinforce the delicate adventitial tissues. (From Otto CM, Bonow RO: *Valvular heart disease: a companion to Braunwald's heart disease,* ed 3, Philadelphia, 2009, Elsevier.)

rupture is necessary. Obtaining data from serial TEE, CT scans, or MRI can be utilized to monitor for progressive increases or decreases in the size of the aortic dissection and aortic rupture.

Surgical Management

The Stanford type A aortic dissection requires immediate surgery to resect the ascending aorta. It is necessary to use cardiopulmonary bypass, hypothermia, and potentially circulatory arrest. If the dissection involves the aortic root and aortic valve, replacement with a prosthetic valve is usually performed due to the likelihood of developing aortic valvular pathology in the future. EVAR using endovascular stenting techniques is also used for elective and acute treatment of Stanford type B aortic aneurysms. There is a decrease in the 30-day mortality rate associated with EVAR compared with an open approach; however, the 1-year postoperative mortality rates are similar for both surgical approaches.

Anesthetic Management and Consideration

Preoperative Period

1. *Describe the usual signs and symptoms associated with acute aortic dissection.*

    It is estimated that up to 50% of patients who develop an acute aortic dissection are initially misdiagnosed because the symptoms can be easily mistaken for other medical problems. The typical symptoms include sharp, tearing, or ripping chest pain and hypertension or hypotension, which is less common. The hypertension that ensues is thought to be caused by the release

---

Neurologic
- Altered level of consciousness
- Syncope
- Cerebrovascular accident
- Paraplegia

Cardiovascular
- Hypertension and bounding peripheral pulses
- Hypotension and decreased peripheral pulses
- Congestive heart failure
- Acute aortic regurgitation
- Cardiac tamponade
- Sudden onset of severe chest pain (anterior and/or posterior)
- Jugular venous distention
- Widening pulse pressure
- Dysrhythmias
- Superior vena cava syndrome

Respiratory
- Shortness of breath
- Bilateral rales
- Hemothorax
- Hoarseness caused by impingement on the left recurrent laryngeal nerve

---

of catecholamines resulting from sympathetic nervous system predominance from decreased peripheral perfusion. Hypotension is suggestive of cardiac tamponade or hypovolemia resulting for partial or complete rupture of the aorta. Some patients have presented with epigastric pain or paraplegia. At times, only after an autopsy is the diagnosis of aortic dissection confirmed.

   This patient has severe chest pain that radiates to his back, which is symptomatic of an acute aortic dissection. His chest x-ray revealed a widening of the mediastinum, which may be indicative of an aortic dissection. A finding of a widening mediastinum should prompt further testing such as a CT scan, angiography, or TEE to confirm aortic dissection. A widening mediastinum can also be found with an aortic aneurysm, esophageal rupture, pericardial effusion, and other pathologies. A complete list of signs and symptoms associated with acute aortic dissection is listed in Box 24.2.

2. *Examine the various coexisting disease processes that may be associated with patients presenting with an acute aortic dissection.*

   The most common comorbidities that are associated with aortic dissection in the order of frequency include hypertension, atherosclerosis, aortic aneurysm, and Marfan syndrome. Males are more likely to have acute aortic dissections. Chronic hypertension can cause thickening of arteries, atherosclerosis, and arterial aneurysms. Constant high blood pressure in thickened, atherosclerotic, or aneurismal arteries can predispose the patient to aortic dissection. Atherosclerosis causes decreased compliance of the arterial walls. This alteration will increase the patient's susceptibility to aortic dissection. Weakness in the aortic wall can lead to an aneurysm, which is a "bulging" or "ballooning" of the vessel wall, and with constant pressure the aneurysm may rupture. Inherited connective tissue disorders such as Marfan syndrome alter the normal physiology of arterial vessels and increase the probability of aortic dissection. A complete list of coexisting disease factors that are related to acute aortic dissection is given in Box 24.3.

3. *Discuss the preoperative preparation and monitoring considerations for this patient.*
   - If the patient is hemodynamically unstable, then the time available for a thorough preoperative history and physical may be limited.
   - Control hemodynamic variability with vasopressors and vasodilators.
     - Treatment for hypertension: beta-adrenergic antagonists, calcium channel blockers, nitrovasodilators
     - Treatment for hypotension: phenylephrine, dopamine, dobutamine, epinephrine, norepinephrine
   - Large-bore intravenous (IV) lines.
   - Right-side radial arterial line. The left subclavian artery provides perfusion to the left radial artery. During aortic cross-clamp application, impingement of the left subclavian artery will decrease the effectiveness of arterial monitoring if the left radial artery is cannulated. Insertion of femoral arterial lines may be used, but the femoral arteries should be spared for the arterial cannulation associated with cardiopulmonary bypass.
   - Central venous catheter to infuse fluid/blood and monitor central venous pressure.
   - Pulmonary artery catheter if a specific indication exists.
   - Cell saver and rapid transfusion devices.
   - TEE.
   - Packed red blood cells, fresh frozen plasma, and platelets.

• BOX 24.3 **Coexisting Diseases That Are Associated With Acute Aortic Dissection**

- Pain
- Abdominal distention
- Bloating
- Constipation
- Nausea and vomiting
- Fever
- Leukocytosis
- Hemodynamic variability
- Intraluminal gas fluid within the lumen of segments proximal to the obstruction
- Free air present within the peritoneum (suggestive of bowel perforation)

Intraoperative Period

4. *Describe common surgical corrections of acute aortic dissection.*

   The most common procedure used to correct acute aortic dissection is the Stanford type A, and this is accomplished by performing a sternotomy utilizing cardiopulmonary bypass, deep hypothermia, and circulatory arrest. If aortic cannulation for cardiopulmonary bypass is unable to be achieved due to the dissection, the right axillary artery and the right femoral artery can be used. Intraoperative electroencephalography (EEG) or cerebral oximetry and TEE are commonly used to evaluate neurologic function and cardiac function, respectively. Preservation of neurologic function is accomplished by administering barbiturates, utilizing cerebral perfusion via the cardiopulmonary bypass machine, and instituting deep hypothermic circulatory arrest (DHCA). These measures decrease the cerebral metabolic rate of oxygen consumption and protect the brain during periods of decreased perfusion. Repair of the acute aortic dissection may include replacement of the aortic root (with reimplantation of coronary arteries), replacement of aortic root and aortic valve (with reimplantation of coronary arteries), replacement of the aortic root keeping the native valve, ascending aortic graft, and ascending aortic graft with aortic valve replacement.

5. *Identify the key components of anesthetic management for the patient with an acute aortic dissection.*
   - The induction of anesthesia should provide cardiovascular stability while ensuring loss of consciousness.
   - It is vital that all attempts be made to keep the patient hemodynamically stable.
   - The systolic blood pressure should remain between 100 and 120 mm Hg.
   - Maintenance of anesthesia can be accomplished by administering narcotics, dexmedetomidine, inhaled anesthetic agents, and neuromuscular blocking agents.
   - The information gained from the TEE will guide vasodilator and vasopressor therapy.
   - Ideally a baseline EEG tracing or cerebral oximetry measurement will be established before the induction of anesthesia. The EEG will be continuously monitored throughout the case. Burst suppression should be achieved during DHCA.
   - Initiation of cardiopulmonary bypass and cooling to between 188°C and 258°C.
   - Propofol administration can occur before DHCA; however, there is a lack of definitive clinical evidence that this intervention offers additional cerebral protection.
   - Steroid administration is warranted before DHCA for brain and multiorgan protection.
   - Mannitol may be given to preserve renal function and to decrease cerebral edema. DHCA is initiated when the surgeon is ready to repair the aorta. There is a lack

of scientific evidence that proves that mannitol and furosemide decrease postoperative renal failure.
- Selective cerebral perfusion may be used during aortic dissection repair to protect the brain and to prolong circulatory arrest time to 45 minutes while decreasing the potential for neurologic damage. Infusion of cold, oxygenated blood can be achieved by antegrade and/or retrograde cannulation. Antegrade cannulation is commonly accomplished via the innominate and left carotid arteries. Retrograde cannulation usually occurs in the superior vena cava.

6. *Discuss DHCA.*

DHCA has been utilized since the 1970s to protect the brain during surgery when cerebral perfusion is compromised. Cardiopulmonary bypass is initiated, and the patient is cooled. Once hypothermia is achieved and the surgeon is ready to repair the aorta, circulatory arrest is initiated. The method by which circulatory arrest occurs is by turning the cardiopulmonary bypass machine off and thereby stopping perfusion to the entire body. Circulatory arrest should only be employed for 30 minutes or less because increased time can result in organ ischemia. Retrograde and/or antegrade perfusion is continued during circulatory arrest to provide additional cerebral protection. The head may be packed in ice to provide additional cooling. Care must be taken to protect exposed skin surfaces to the ice and to avoid the development of frostbite. Once the aorta has been repaired or replaced, cardiopulmonary bypass is reinitiated and incremental warning begins. The glucose level should be monitored to avoid global cerebral ischemia. Allowing the blood pH to be more alkaline as hypothermia is accomplished helps preserve cerebral autoregulation. The rewarming process should be slow because cerebral hyperthermia results in increased metabolic demands and may result in cerebral injury.

7. *List the physiologic alterations associated with deep hypothermia.*
- Decreased cerebral metabolic rate of oxygen consumption
- Decreased organ metabolic rate of oxygen consumption
- Increased blood viscosity
- Coagulopathy
- Hemorrhage
- Thrombocytopenia
- Peripheral vasoconstriction
- Impaired renal and liver function

Postoperative Period

8. *Identify the postoperative anesthetic concerns after acute aortic dissection repair.*

After the surgical procedure, patients remain intubated and are transferred to the intensive care unit. Careful monitoring of the blood pressure, urine output, and bleeding is required. The patient should also be assessed for other potential complications related to the surgery such as stroke, ventricular dysrhythmias, myocardial infarction, and renal failure. If the patient remains hemodynamically stable, they should be extubated as soon as possible in order to assess for adequate neurologic integrity. Decreasing the amount of vasoactive medication should be accomplished as expeditiously as possible.

Review Questions

1. Which intervention is used to prolong the amount of time that deep hypothermic circulatory arrest can be used?
a. Administration of propofol
b. Administration of steroids
c. Retrograde cerebral perfusion
d. Selective antegrade perfusion
2. A TEE reveals that a patient has an aortic dissection that extends to the aortic root and the aortic arch. Which Stanford classification type is consistent with these findings?
a. Type A
b. Type B
c. Type C
d. Type D
3. Retrograde cerebral perfusion is accomplished by cannulating the:
a. Right axillary artery.
b. Right carotid artery.
c. Internal jugular vein.
d. Left subclavian vein.
4. The most common comorbid factor that is associated with an acute aortic dissection is:
a. Diabetes.
b. Hypertension.
c. Atherosclerosis.
d. Deep vein thrombosis.
5. Which complication is associated with deep hypothermia circulatory arrest?
a. Hyperoxia
b. Thrombocytopenia
c. Deep vein thrombosis
d. Atherosclerosis

Suggested Readings

Chen Y, Zhang S, Liu L, et al. Retrograde type A aortic dissection after thoracic endovascular aortic repair: a systematic review and meta-analysis. *J Am Heart Assoc* 2017;6(9):e004649.

Elisha S. Vascular surgery. In: Nagelhout JJ, Elisha S, eds. *Nurse Anesthesia,* 6th ed. St Louis, MO: Elsevier, 2018:535-562.

Elsayed RS, Cohen RG, Fleischman F, et al. Acute type a aortic dissection. *Cardiol Clin* 2017;35(3):331-345.

Grecu L, Nikhil C. Vascular disease. In: Hines RL, Marschall KE, eds. *Stoelting's Anesthesia and Coexisting Disease,* 7th ed. Philadelphia: Churchill Livingstone, 2018:237–263.

Guo MH, Appoo JJ, Saczkowski R, et al. Association of mortality and acute aortic events with ascending aortic aneurysm: a systematic review and meta-analysis. *JAMA Netw Open* 2018;1(4):e181281.

Henly WS. Acute aortic dissection and visceral ischemia. *JMDHVC* 2008;4:12-13.

Kazimi M, Deo SV, Altarabsheh SE, et al. Acute aortic dissection in patients presenting to US emergency department, 2006-2014. *Am J Emerg Med* 2020;38(12):2745-2747.

Kocher AA, Bonaros N, Nagiller J, et al. Acute aortic dissection mimicking cholecystitis. *Eur Surg* 2007;39:203-205.

Lee SJ, Kang WC, Ko YG, Woo Y, et al. Aortic remodeling and clinical outcomes in type B aortic dissection according to the timing of thoracic endovascular aortic repair. *Ann Vasc Surg* 2020; 67:322-331.

López Espada C, Linares Palomino JP, et al. Endovascular treatment of descending thoracic aortic pathology: results of the Regis-TEVAR Study. *Ann Vasc Surg* 2020;67:306-315.

Patel PD, Arora RR. Pathophysiology, diagnosis, and management of aortic dissection. *Ther Adv Cardiovasc Dis* 2008;2:439-468.

Reser D, Morjan M, Savic V, et al. Outcomes of patients operated for acute type A aortic dissection requiring preoperative cardiopulmonary resuscitation. *J Card Surg* 2020;35(7):1425-1430.

Thomas RP, Amin SS, Eldergash O, Kowald T, et al. Urgent endovascular treatment for non-traumatic descending thoracic aortic rupture. *Cardiovasc Intervent Radiol* 2018;41(9):1318-1323.

25
Thoracic Aneurysm Repair

KEY POINTS

- Significant comorbidities are prevalent in patients with atherosclerotic lesions of the thoracic aorta. These include hypertension, coronary artery disease, chronic obstructive pulmonary disease (COPD), renal insufficiency, and cerebrovascular disease.
- Mortality rates for open repairs of thoracic aortic aneurysms (TAAs) are approximately 8% in centers with concentrated experience and may approach 20% for all cases in the United States.
- One-lung anesthesia is typically required to facilitate surgical access to the descending thoracic aorta.

- Monitoring and regulation of proximal and distal perfusion during aortic cross-clamping of the thoracic aorta are central to the anesthetic management of patients undergoing aneurysm repair.
- Aortic reconstruction that is performed superior to the level of the renal arteries poses an increased risk of temporary or permanent spinal cord injury. The incidence of paraplegia associated with thoracic aortic surgery ranges from 2% to 16%.
- Aneurysmal leakage, rupture, and aortic dissection increase the risk for intraoperative hemorrhage and massive transfusion.

Case Synopsis

A 67-year-old man has been diagnosed with a descending TAA that was discovered on a recent history and physical examination for a chronic cough and mild interscapular back pain. He is scheduled for an open repair of the aneurysm under general anesthesia.

Preoperative Evaluation and Demographic Data

Past Medical/Surgical History

- Hypertension, COPD, cigarette smoking
- Inguinal hernia repair under local/monitored anesthesia care

List of Medications

- Atenolol, lisinopril, atorvastatin (Lipitor), budesonide and formoterol (Symbicort), albuterol

Diagnostic Data

- Complete blood count: white blood cells, 4.31 K/mcL; red blood cells, 5.28 K/mcL; hemoglobin, 14.1 g/dL; hematocrit, 42.3%; platelets, 285 K/mcL
- Coagulation: prothrombin time, 11.2 s; international normalized ratio, 1.1; partial thromboplastin time, 29.2 s
- Electrolytes: sodium, 139 mmol/L; potassium, 4.1 mmol/L; chloride, 105 mmol/L; carbon dioxide, 38 mmol/L
- Glucose, 98 mg/dL
- Blood urea nitrogen, 28 mg/dL; creatinine, 1.4 mg/dL

- Electrocardiogram: sinus rhythm, nonspecific ST abnormalities
- Chest x-ray: widened mediastinum consistent with a TAA; no infiltrates
- Pulmonary function testing: moderate COPD; FEV_1/FVC = 68% predicted
- Echocardiogram: no wall motion abnormalities; ejection fraction, 61%
- Computed tomography (CT) scan: 5.2 cm TAA just distal to the left subclavian artery

Height/Weight/Vital Signs

- 185 cm, 87 kg
- Blood pressure, 147/82; heart rate, 76 beats per minute; respiratory rate, 18 breaths per minute; room air oxygen saturation, 94%

Pathophysiology

A TAA is defined as a permanent dilation in any area of the aorta above the diaphragm that measures at least 1.5 times the expected normal diameter, as shown in Fig. 25.1. The majority of TAAs are caused by atherosclerotic degenerative disease, but the aneurysm may also develop from chronic aortic dissection, connective tissue disease, infection, trauma, or after surgical procedures that require aortic cannulation or cross-clamping. Aortic aneurysms are also seen in congenital disorders of metabolism, such as Marfan syndrome and Ehlers–Danlos syndrome. Regardless of etiology, a TAA arises from a weakening of the aortic wall, which

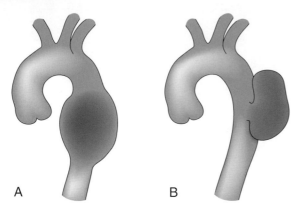

• **Fig. 25.1** Thoracic aortic aneurysm. (A) Tubular. (B) Saccular. (From Garden OJ, Parks RW: *Principles and practice of surgery*, ed 7, Philadelphia, 2018, Elsevier.)

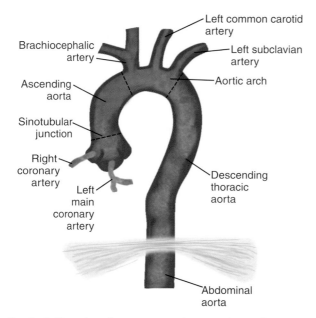

• **Fig. 25.2** Normal aortic anatomy and nomenclature. The thoracic aorta can be partitioned into three segments: the ascending aorta, the aortic arch, and the descending thoracic aorta. (From Taylor AJ: *Atlas of cardiovascular computed tomography: an imaging companion to Braunwald's heart disease*, Philadelphia, 2010, Elsevier.)

results in a progressive dilation of all three structural layers of the vessel (*intima, media,* and *adventitia*). The increased diameter of the aortic lumen compromises aortic blood flow, compresses surrounding structures, and increases arterial wall tension, placing the patient at risk for aortic rupture, exsanguination, and death.

TAAs constitute 30% to 40% of all aortic aneurysms and may develop in one or more anatomic segments along the course of the aorta within the thorax. The thoracic aorta originates from the aortic root and encompasses the ascending aorta, the aortic arch, and the descending thoracic aorta. The descending aorta originates distal to the left subclavian artery and terminates at the diaphragm, as shown in Fig. 25.2. Thoracic lesions can also extend below the level of the diaphragm into the abdominal aorta in the form of thoracoabdominal

aneurysm, as is illustrated in Fig. 25.3. The majority of all TAAs involve the aortic root and/or the ascending aorta. Approximately 40% of all TAAs involve areas of the descending aorta. Dissections of the thoracic aorta are also classified with reference to their anatomic location. Dissections occur when a tear in the intima allows blood to enter the medial layer, creating an extraluminal channel (false lumen) that can course along the length of the aorta.

The clinical presentation varies with the location of the TAA and the mechanism of vessel dilation. Many patients are asymptomatic; however, the aneurysm may be discovered as an incidental finding while investigating an unrelated problem. Degenerative lesions are less likely to cause symptoms than those caused by dissection, from which up to 85% of patients may be symptomatic. A common symptom is back pain, often interscapular. Pain may also be felt in the neck and jaw, the precordium, or the left thoracic region. The aneurysm can often be localized by symptoms that result from its expansion at the expense of surrounding structures. Compression of the left mainstem bronchus can cause dyspnea, coughing, wheezing, and stridor, as well as tracheal deviation. Aneurysm expansion near the esophagus produces dysphagia and even weight loss. The left recurrent laryngeal nerve is situated around the aortic arch, and impingement from the aneurysm manifests as hoarseness and unilateral left-sided vocal cord paralysis. Horner syndrome can be precipitated by encroachment in the area of the stellate ganglia. Compression of the vena cava can produce facial edema and may occasion dyspnea and other symptoms consistent with a superior vena cava syndrome. Aortic root and ascending thoracic aneurysms may give rise to symptoms of congestive heart failure produced by aortic valve dilation and regurgitation. A local mass effect in the aortic root may provoke myocardial ischemia due to compression or dissection of the coronary arteries. Finally, patients with a ruptured TAA may present with profound hypovolemia and hemorrhagic shock, as well as the signs and symptoms of hemothorax or hemopericardium.

Surgical Procedure

Repair of the descending thoracic aorta is usually performed with the patient positioned in right lateral decubitus. Rotation of the hips up to 45 degrees is necessary to facilitate access to the descending aorta and the femoral vessels. Once the lesion is isolated, the repair is often accomplished with a tube graft. The aneurysm may be either excised or oversewn around the completed aortic graft. The repair requires clamping of the thoracic aorta, normally above and below the area of the lesion. The proximal clamp is most commonly placed just distal to the left subclavian artery, as is shown in Fig. 25.4. The distal clamp may be placed sequentially along the aorta with the goal of minimizing visceral ischemia.

In addition to the aortic cross-clamp, procedures that are performed on the descending thoracic aorta may require the placement of shunts or extracorporeal support

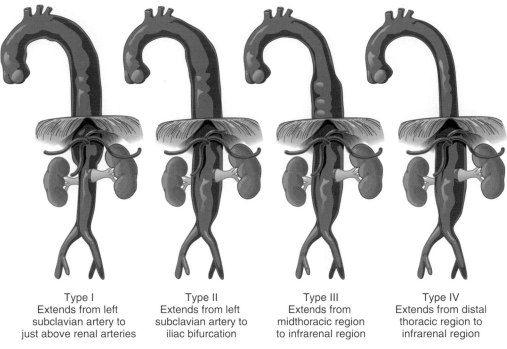

Type I	Type II	Type III	Type IV
Extends from left subclavian artery to just above renal arteries	Extends from left subclavian artery to iliac bifurcation	Extends from midthoracic region to infrarenal region	Extends from distal thoracic region to infrarenal region

• **Fig. 25.3** Types of thoracoabdominal aneurysms. (From Good VS, Kirkwood PL: *Advanced critical care nursing*, ed 2, St. Louis, 2018, Elsevier.)

with partial cardiopulmonary bypass (CPB) in order to maintain lower body perfusion and to provide adequate spinal cord and visceral blood supply distal to the clamp. Complete CPB is indicated for ascending aorta aneurysms that involve the aortic arch. For descending aorta aneurysms, aortic clamping techniques with or without shunts or partial distal bypass are most commonly employed. The intercostal or segmental spinal arteries may be incorporated into the graft or reimplanted into the descending aorta to prevent ischemic spinal cord injury after excision of the aneurysm. Visceral branches (celiac, mesentery, renal arteries) must be preserved, and these arteries are incorporated into the aortic graft.

Anesthetic Management and Considerations

Preoperative Period

1. Describe the comorbidities associated with atherosclerotic lesions of the thoracic aorta and the measures to evaluate the extent of coexisting disease in the preoperative period.

   Most patients with atherosclerotic lesions of the thoracic aorta are of advanced age and have significant comorbidities. The scope of the preoperative evaluation will depend on the urgency of the surgical procedure. TAAs that are leaking or dissecting or have ruptured should be repaired immediately, and the limited preoperative time allows for a rapid assessment of the patient's condition. For elective surgery, a complete health history and thorough assessment of all systems are warranted in order to reveal the extent of coexisting disease, to optimize the patient's preoperative condition, and to help reduce the risk of perioperative complications.

   Atherosclerosis is a systemic disease that can cause degenerative changes in the entire arterial system, which may cause coronary artery disease, cerebrovascular disease, and renal dysfunction. Chronic hypertension is another key risk factor for aneurysm formation and is usually evident preoperatively. Patients often have a long history of cigarette habituation; significant COPD is a common finding. Preoperative renal dysfunction may be present in up to 30% of patients, particularly with descending aortic aneurysms when the lesion extends to the renal arteries.

   Cardiac status is evaluated by electrocardiography (ECG) to detect myocardial ischemia and/or infarction, conduction abnormalities, and ventricular hypertrophy and by echocardiography to evaluate the size and location of the TAA, ventricular function, and valvular competence. Angiography is performed to assess the dimensions and location of the TAA, the coronary vascular anatomy, and cardiac function. Pulmonary status may be assessed with arterial blood gas analysis, chest radiography, and pulmonary function testing. Airway obstruction caused by the aneurysm can be detected by pulmonary function testing. A thorough neurologic history may be supplemented in some patients by carotid artery angiography or carotid duplex studies, as well as a neuropsychological consultation to establish a baseline for postoperative assessment. Routine preoperative measurement of blood urea nitrogen (BUN) and creatinine will help identify the presence of renal dysfunction.

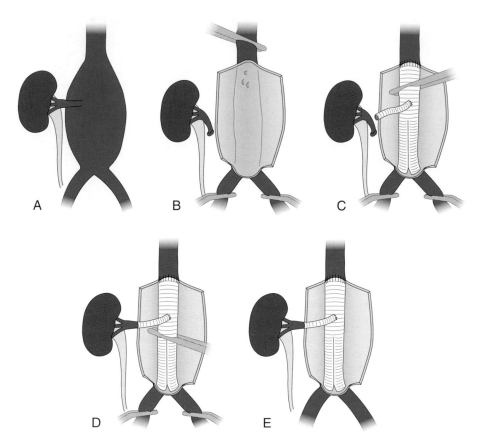

• **Fig. 25.4** Mobilization of aortic cross-clamp during open abdominal aortic aneurysm repair. To minimize unnecessary ischemic time on visceral organs, the aortic cross-clamp is moved sequentially lower on the graft as each anastomosis is completed. Each cross-clamp release will result in metabolic washout to the previously ischemic organs, although the subsequent quick replacement of the cross-clamp lower on the graft will mitigate some of the hemodynamic alterations. (A) Native aneurysm with right renal artery. (B) The aortal and iliac arteries are clamped. The aneurysm sack is opened, and the right renal artery is dissected. (C) Aortobifemoral graft with a separate arterial graft sewn in. The aortic clamp is moved from the native aorta to the proximal graft. (D) The right renal artery is anastomosed, with perfusion to the right kidney achieved by moving the aortic cross-clamp distal. (E) Reperfusion of the legs: all arterial clamps are removed. Aortic cross-clamp placement and tube graft repair. (Modified from Woo EY, Damrauer SM: Abdominal aortic aneurysms: open surgical treatment. In Cronenwett JL, Johnston KW, eds: *Rutherford's vascular surgery*, ed 8, Philadelphia, 2014, Elsevier.)

2. *Discuss the natural history and strategies used to treat thoracic aortic aneurysms.*

Atherosclerotic TAAs generally develop over time, and the destruction of the supporting matrix of the aorta causes vessel dilation at a rate of 0.5 cm or less per year. Patients who are asymptomatic and have TAAs whose anteroposterior diameter is less than 5 to 6 cm may be managed medically. As the risk of rupture increases with elevations in diastolic blood pressure and obstructive lung disease, medical management focuses on risk factor modification, including the strict control of blood pressure, low-sodium diet, and cessation of smoking. A TAA that is >6 cm in diameter increases the potential for rupture by fivefold. The natural course of luminal expansion results in aortic rupture or dissection and death. Surgical intervention is warranted in large aneurysms, as well as in acutely symptomatic patients, in rapidly expanding lesions, and in type B dissections. The risk of death with descending TAA surgery is about 8% in centers with concentrated experience and may reach 20% nationally.

3. *Explain the mechanism for airway compromise for patients who have a thoracic aneurysm.*

Expansion of a TAA may distort the airway due to the proximity of anatomic structures along the course of the thoracic aorta. Ascending TAAs may compress the right mainstem bronchus, whereas descending TAAs may cause tracheal deviation and compression of the left mainstem bronchus. Airway compression may cause dyspnea or stridor. Larger ascending thoracic aneurysms can create a mediastinal mass effect and complicate induction and intubation. These patients may not be able to breathe if they are placed supine. Prolonged compression of airway structures can lead to tracheomalacia.

Aneurysms may also leak into the airways precipitating hemoptysis.

4. *Discuss spinal cord vascular anatomy and perfusion in the context of thoracic aneurysm surgery.*

The spinal cord receives its blood supply from three principal sources: the anterior spinal artery (75%) and two posterior spinal arteries (25%). The anterior spinal cord receives supplementation of blood flow by way of the spinal branches of the intercostal arteries in the thorax and the lumbar arteries in the abdomen. These collateral vessels originate in the posterior aorta, the most important of which is the artery of Adamkiewicz (greater radicular artery). This artery's origin is positioned on the left in 80% of the population and joins the anterior spinal artery in 60% of patients at the T9–T12 vertebral segments, at the T5–T8 vertebral segments in 15%, and at the L1–L2 vertebral segments in 25% of the population. As the anterior spinal artery tapers in the thorax, the artery of Adamkiewicz provides most of the blood supply to the anterior, lower two-thirds of the spinal cord. Thus spinal cord ischemia can occur to the anterior portion of the spinal cord, which is involved in motor function, from hypotension, aortic cross-clamping, and interruption of segmental arteries. The incidence of paraplegia has been estimated to be approximately 20% after elective surgery and as high as 40% during aortic reconstruction for dissecting or ruptured TAAs. Dexmedetomidine is associated with decreased spinal cord ischemic reperfusion injury due to inhibition of mast cell degranulation.

5. *Describe the potential for blood loss and list techniques for venous access in patients undergoing repair of the descending thoracic aorta.*

The risk of major hemorrhage is substantial during repair of a TAA. The estimated blood loss ranges from 5000 to 8000 mL. This is particularly true if only proximal clamping of the aorta is used, which causes retrograde blood flow and bleeding from visceral vessels. Sudden and catastrophic blood loss from aortic rupture is also possible throughout the surgical procedure. Insertion of one or two large-bore (14 to 16 gauge) peripheral intravenous catheters is routine, along with the placement of central introducer cannulae (7 to 9 French) in the internal jugular, subclavian, or femoral veins.

6. *Describe the requirements for fluid, blood, and blood product requirements necessary for thoracic aortic surgery.*

The incision for thoracic aorta surgery is extensive and exposes both the thoracic and abdominal cavities to the extracorporeal environment. As a result, insensible fluid losses from evaporation are large. Due to the potential for major hemorrhage, the availability of sufficient blood products and systems for their infusion is imperative. Eight to fifteen units of packed red blood cells (PRBCs) should be readily accessible in the operative suite. The administration of fresh frozen plasma (FFP) and platelets should also be anticipated, as massive fluid resuscitation and the development of an intraoperative coagulopathy are common. A rapid infusion or cell salvage system and fluid warming capabilities should be primed and in place before the beginning of surgery. Intraoperative assessment of hematologic and coagulation laboratory values and thromboelastography is imperative.

Intraoperative Period

7. *Describe the cardiovascular and hemodynamic monitoring modalities for thoracic aorta surgery.*

The dynamic nature of patient responses during TAA and the risk of complications due to existing comorbidities and intraoperative events make hemodynamic monitoring a complex and critical process. Standard ECG with ST-segment analysis in leads II and V5 is indicated for the detection of myocardial ischemia, injury, and dysrhythmias. The risk of a myocardial infarction is considerable, and it is the major cause of perioperative mortality.

Dramatic and precipitous changes in hemodynamics during thoracic aorta repairs are common due to aortic cross-clamping/unclamping and ongoing major blood loss. These changes necessitate placement of an arterial catheter for beat-to-beat monitoring of blood pressure. Serial sampling of blood for laboratory analysis is likewise facilitated. The *right radial artery* is the preferred site for blood pressure assessment during a descending aorta repair. This is due to the fact that aortic cross-clamping is occasionally required proximal to the left subclavian artery, making the left upper extremity unsuitable for arterial pressure monitoring. A right brachial arterial line is considered a safe alternative. Pulse oximetry and plethysmography should be avoided in the left upper extremity for the same reason. Femoral artery blood pressures may be monitored in order to determine the adequacy of distal perfusion during the aortic cross-clamping. The assessment of femoral arterial pressures allows timely interventions to be made for low distal perfusion, which may reduce overall spinal and renal ischemia.

In contrast to the descending aorta, repairs of the ascending aorta require monitoring of arterial blood pressure in the *left upper extremity*, as the innominate (brachiocephalic) artery may be clamped. Noninvasive blood pressure cuffs can also be placed on both arms to document differences in upper extremity perfusion. Pulmonary artery (PA) catheter placement has been frequently advocated for use in thoracic aorta surgery to assess cardiac function, volume status, and mixed venous oxygen saturation. The insertion of PA catheters is associated with complications such as pneumothorax, intrathoracic bleeding, inadvertent carotid artery puncture, dysrhythmias, pulmonary artery ischemia, and infection. Pulmonary artery occlusion pressures

(PAOPs) may substantially overestimate the left ventricular end-diastolic pressures (LVEDPs) during one-lung anesthesia (OLA). Moreover, the usefulness of mixed venous oxygen saturation as an indicator of cardiac output during cross-clamping of the aorta has been questioned. Noninvasive hemodynamic monitoring is an alternative to the use of PA catheterization.

Transesophageal echocardiography (TEE) has become a routine modality for intraoperative monitoring during thoracic aorta surgery. It is a minimally invasive technique used to assess biventricular function, volume status, and the development of myocardial ischemia. The information obtained from the TEE assessment has been found to be more accurate in estimating preload than PA catheters and more effective in detecting early myocardial ischemia than ECG monitoring. The TEE is an important tool in the diagnosis of acute aortic dissection and can confirm proper placement of central access devices. Passage of the TEE probe may cause injury to the oropharynx and esophagus and precipitate rupture of the aneurysm, and compression can make placement difficult.

8. *Explain induction techniques for thoracic aorta surgery that serve to minimize the hypertensive response and the risk of aneurysm rupture.*

The goals for the induction of anesthesia in thoracic aorta surgery focus primarily on myocardial preservation and the prevention of hemodynamic stress on the aortic lesion. Tachycardia and hypertension are the principal concerns, especially during laryngoscopy and endotracheal intubation. Tight control of heart rate and blood pressure during induction helps decrease the potential for myocardial ischemia or infarction. Tachycardia and hypertension may also trigger the rupture of an aneurysm or may extend an aortic dissection by increasing the shearing forces present within the aorta. Adequate anesthesia depth is essential.

The hemodynamic stability that is associated with etomidate is desirable for induction agent prior to TAA repair. High-dose narcotic techniques have been advocated but must be used with caution before the establishment of mask ventilation due to the risk of chest wall rigidity and consequent sympathetic stimulation. Careful titration of narcotics, such as fentanyl or sufentanil, is preferred and is considered a safe and effective method to blunt the hemodynamic effects of airway manipulation. Dexmedetomidine provides intraoperative hemodynamic stability and enhances postoperative analgesia. Beta-adrenergic antagonists, particularly short-acting agents such as esmolol, are useful adjuncts in treating tachycardia and hypertension during induction. Treatment of hypertension may require the administration of vasoactive agents; nitroglycerin or sodium nitroprusside may be helpful in reducing blood pressure in the context of a normal heart rate.

9. *Discuss the potential problems during management of OLA for repair of descending thoracic aneurysms.*

The use of a double-lumen endotracheal tube (DLT) is a standard practice for surgeries of the descending thoracic aorta that are performed through a left thoracotomy incision. Lung separation and the subsequent collapse of the left lung facilitate exposure of the thoracic aorta and reduce iatrogenic trauma to the left lung from surgical retraction. OLA for thoracotomy typically makes use of a left-sided DLT, although airway distortion of the left bronchus from a large descending lesion may make placement difficult. Fiber-optic examination of the left bronchus may facilitate proper left endobronchial intubation; findings of pulsatile compression or frank erosion within the left bronchus warrant the use of a right-sided DLT in order to avoid complications. Proper positioning of the right-sided DLT should be confirmed with fiber-optic evaluation to ensure adequate right upper lobe ventilation with OLA. After surgery, DLTs are generally changed to single-lumen devices for postoperative ventilatory support. An alternative to using a DLT for OLA is a single-lumen tube with a retractable bronchial blocking device. If the patient requires postoperative ventilation, then the DLT should be replaced by a standard endotracheal tube.

Patients undergoing OLA during thoracic aorta surgery are at substantial risk for developing hypoxemia. Collapse of the nondependent lung creates a significant right-to-left shunt, which may be further exacerbated in those with preexisting lung disease. Maintenance of 100% oxygen may lower the incidence of hypoxemia with OLA, as hypoxic pulmonary vasoconstriction (HPV), which shunts blood from the nonventilated left lung to the ventilated right lung, is inhibited. The effectiveness of HPV may be diminished by the administration of potent vasodilators, such as inhalation of anesthetic agents, nitroglycerin, and sodium nitroprusside. Effective measures in addressing hypoxemia during OLA include use of 100% oxygen, application of 5 to 10 cm H_2O continuous positive airway pressure (CPAP) to the collapsed left lung, positive end-expiratory pressure (PEEP) to the ventilated right lung, intermittent reinflation and ventilation of both lungs, and ligation of the pulmonary artery to the collapsed lung. High peak airway pressures (greater than 30 cm H_2O) may also counteract the beneficial effects of HPV and can be managed with slight reductions in tidal volume (5 to 7 mL/kg) and increases in respiratory rate in order to maintain minute ventilation at a lower pressure.

10. *Describe the physiologic and hemodynamic impact of aortic clamping/unclamping during repair of a TAA.*

Application of a cross clamp to the descending aorta causes significant hemodynamic alteration. Acute occlusion of the aorta increases afterload, resulting in a reduction of ventricular ejection and a rise in LVEDP. Preload is augmented by a redistribution of blood from vessels below the clamp. Ventricular contractility may be enhanced by increased filling and by catecholamine release in response to clamping. These changes may precipitate acute left ventricular failure or myocardial ischemia, especially in patients with preexisting cardiac disease. Proximal to the clamp, arterial blood pressure dramatically increases and often requires active intervention when bypass techniques are not utilized. Vasodilators, such as sodium nitroprusside and nitroglycerin, may be used. Higher concentrations of inhalation anesthetics may be helpful in lowering proximal blood pressure in patients with normal ventricular function. Esmolol may be administered to control proximal hypertension without compromising spinal cord perfusion. Peripheral perfusion is significantly decreased distal to the aortic clamp, causing severe reductions in end-organ blood flow and autoregulation, notably to the kidneys, the abdominal viscera, and the distal spinal cord. Impaired perfusion to organs and tissues results in anaerobic metabolism with lactic acid production and metabolic acidosis. Reduced hepatic blood flow impairs lactate clearance and exacerbates acidosis.

Unclamping of the aorta causes profound hemodynamic instability. Systemic vascular resistance and blood pressure may be reduced by 50%, creating a "declamping shock" state. Arterial hypotension is most likely caused by massive peripheral vasodilation, made worse by the redistribution of blood from the upper to lower body. Myocardial depression, central hypovolemia, and the systemic effects of ischemic metabolites exacerbate the reduction in blood pressure. Reperfusion of ischemic tissues causes inflammatory mediators, and oxygen free radicals, which cause cellular damage, are produced and released. In anticipation of this profound hypotension, aggressive volume loading may be instituted, along with decreasing the anesthetic depth and stopping the infusion of vasodilators. A staged or slow removal of the aortic clamp by the surgeon may reduce the intensity of the response, but hypotension is usually unavoidable. The minute ventilation may be increased and sodium bicarbonate administered to counter the acidosis. Once the clamp is removed, the administration of vasopressors, such as phenylephrine, may be necessary to stabilize the blood pressure, as well as calcium chloride to correct hypocalcemia if present. Hypertension should be avoided, as it may place stress on the suture lines of the graft and cause bleeding.

11. *List methods to improve lower body perfusion during repair of the descending thoracic aorta.*

Distal perfusion techniques are generally indicated for complex repairs of the descending aorta that may require prolonged aortic cross-clamping. They are designed to maintain lower body perfusion, to reduce ischemic injury, and to decrease the incidence of paraplegia and renal failure. Distal perfusion techniques can also attenuate the proximal hypertension associated with the placement of the clamp, the development of metabolic acidosis during clamping, and the profound hypotension that occurs with unclamping.

The least complex technique for lower body perfusion utilizes a conduit that diverts blood flow from the proximal descending aorta or the left ventricle to the distal aorta. Blood flows through the shunt passively using the pressure in the proximal source as its driving force. The Gott shunt is heparin coated, which eliminates the need for systemic heparinization. The most common technique for distal aortic perfusion is partial bypass or left-heart bypass, which uses a centrifugal pump to direct blood from the left atrium to the left femoral artery. Other proximal sites with partial bypass include the aortic arch, the proximal descending aorta, or the pulmonary vein. The bypass circuits are also coated with heparin, so a reduced dose of systemic heparin may be given (100 units/kg). The pump allows for adjustments in blood flow to be made during aortic cross-clamping to correct alterations in preload or afterload and to control proximal hypertension. Both radial and femoral blood pressure monitoring are indicated with partial bypass techniques in order to assess pressures above and below the aortic cross-clamp. Finally, extracorporeal support for lower body perfusion can also be achieved with a femoral vein–femoral artery bypass, which provides retrograde perfusion below the clamp. This approach requires an oxygenator, a roller clamp, and systemic heparinization.

Distal perfusion techniques reduce visceral and renal ischemia and may decrease the risk of paraplegia during descending aortic surgery. The provision of perfusion to the lower body prevents metabolic acidosis and the accumulation of hypoxia-induced metabolites. Bypass techniques provide an effective means for controlling proximal hypertension during aortic cross-clamping and for preventing post-clamp hypotension. Their large cannulae supply access for rapid volume infusion; their flexible configuration allows for extracorporeal oxygenation and temperature manipulation. The disadvantages of distal perfusion techniques include bleeding, dislodgement, increased operative time, and injury to anatomic structures. As with all extracorporeal support, there is an increased risk of air emboli and embolic stroke. The anticoagulation required for many techniques increases the risk of hemorrhage and adverse medication reactions from heparin and protamine.

12. *Compare and contrast modalities used to monitor the integrity of the spinal cord during thoracic aortic surgery.*

The integrity of the spinal cord may be assessed by neurophysiologic monitoring using evoked potentials. Evoked potentials refer to the electrical activity of the nervous system that is elicited in response to a stimulus. With this form of monitoring, a stimulus is generated and the evoked waveform is measured in terms of amplitude (strength) and latency (delay). The pathways between the brain and the peripheral nervous system or vice versa, including the spinal cord, may be continually evaluated in this manner. Decreases in amplitude and increases in latency may indicate an alteration in neuronal function, which is most likely caused by hypotension, hypothermia, or spinal cord ischemia. Somatosensory evoked potential (SSEP) monitoring involves the initiation of a signal in the periphery, usually at the posterior tibial or peroneal nerves, and the measurement of the cortical response in the brain by means of scalp electrodes. SSEP monitoring reflects the integrity of ascending sensory pathways in the lateral and posterior tracts of the spinal cord. Motor evoked potential (MEP) monitoring is achieved by stimulation of the motor cortex of the brain and measurement of the motor neuron response in the periphery or at the level of the spinal cord itself. MEP reflects the integrity of the descending motor pathways in the anterior tracts of the spinal cord.

Both SSEPs and MEPs have been used to monitor spinal cord integrity during thoracic aortic surgery. SSEPs reliably deteriorate from impaired perfusion to the cord during aortic cross-clamping or hypotension, but this deterioration may not predict permanent spinal cord injury with any degree of certainty. There does appear to be a strong correlation between the aortic cross-clamp time and the loss of SSEPs. Although the preservation of evoked potentials during surgery presumes adequate spinal cord perfusion, postoperative paraplegia has been observed despite normal intraoperative SSEPs. This suggests that monitoring of the posterior sensory tracts may be of less clinical significance than that of the anterior motor tracts, given the nature of thoracic spinal perfusion and the vulnerability of the distal anterior cord during thoracic aortic surgery. MEPs may be better suited to detect clinically relevant spinal cord ischemia with greater sensitivity and specificity. Aortic cross-clamp placement and spinal cord protective measures can be directed, in part, by neurophysiologic monitoring. Identification of collateral vessels that may be critical to the perfusion of a specific segment of the spinal cord can also be facilitated by evoked potential data, allowing the surgeon to revascularize the area by reimplantation of segmental arteries or by endarterectomy.

Evoked potential monitoring may be affected by a number of factors. The type and depth of anesthesia can alter both SSEP and MEP monitoring. All volatile anesthetic agents interfere with evoked potential monitoring, causing dose-related reductions in amplitude and increases in latency. Avoidance of these agents or reduction of delivered concentrations is necessary; the use of isoflurane at 0.5 MAC with 60% nitrous oxide, for example, is felt to be compatible with effective SSEP monitoring. Intravenous anesthetic agents depress the SSEP waveform, although ketamine and etomidate may increase the amplitudes of both SSEP and MEP by reducing inhibitory mechanisms. Opioids have a minimal effect on both SSEP and MEP. Muscle relaxants profoundly inhibit MEPs; complete blockade renders the modality useless as a monitor of ventral tract integrity. It is recommended that muscle twitches in response to neuromuscular blockade monitor be maintained at a minimum of 30% of baseline to avoid interference with MEP. Patient parameters, such as temperature, hematocrit, and oxygen saturation, can also adversely affect evoked potential monitoring.

13. *Outline intraoperative methods that may be used to protect the spinal cord from ischemic injury during the repair of the descending thoracic aorta.*

Aortic cross-clamping of the descending thoracic aorta poses a risk for spinal cord ischemia and injury due to the resultant hypoperfusion. Paraparesis and paraplegia are the most devastating consequences of this iatrogenic impairment of spinal perfusion. The reported incidences of postoperative neurologic deficits in thoracic aortic surgery vary widely; rates for paraplegia average 2% to 16%. Risk factors for spinal cord injury include advanced patient age, the urgency of the procedure, the presence of rupture or dissection, and the level and the duration of aortic cross-clamping. A history of preoperative renal dysfunction is also an important risk factor for the development of spinal cord ischemia during thoracic aortic surgery. Spinal cord integrity may also be impaired by perioperative hypotension and hypoxemia, elevations in cerebrospinal fluid (CSF) pressure, and surgical transection of spinal arteries.

The management of perfusion distal to the aortic clamp is a key element in spinal cord protection. Foremost, the limitation of clamp time may help reduce the overall risk of spinal deficits by reducing the total ischemic time, although cases of paraplegia have been reported when the aortic clamp time is less than 20 minutes. The provision of distal perfusion during aortic cross-clamping by means of shunts or bypass techniques attempts to prevent end-organ ischemia, including the spinal cord. No one surgical intervention, however, has proven to be totally protective. The modulation of acute changes in CSF pressure after cross-clamping has been advocated, as spinal cord perfusion pressure (SCPP) is a function of the difference between MAP and CSF shown in the following equation.

$$SCPP = MAP - CSF$$

CSF, Cerebrospinal fluid; *MAP*, mean arterial pressure; *SCPP*, spinal cord perfusion pressure.

Attenuation of CSF pressure increases may be achieved with the placement of a lumbar catheter and the drainage of CSF fluid, which serves to increase SCPP by lowering CSF pressure. Risks of lumbar drainage include cerebral herniation, spinal headache, meningitis, and epidural hematoma.

Hypothermia provides a reliable method of neuronal protection and prolongs cross-clamp time even with the use of mild hypothermia (34°C). It can be achieved systemically before clamping with passive cooling or partial bypass, or regionally by means of local spinal cord cooling through epidural or spinal catheters. A number of pharmacologic interventions have been studied, including systemic administration of corticosteroids, mannitol, magnesium, and naloxone, with varying degrees of spinal cord protection. Intrathecal papaverine has been used to improve the perfusion through spinal arteries by vasodilation. Dexmedetomidine may decrease spinal cord injury by decreasing the degranulation of mast cell and inflammation.

14. *Discuss strategies to monitor and maintain renal perfusion during repair of thoracic aneurysm surgery.*

Urinary output is measured with a Foley catheter, which provides an indirect, albeit inconsistent, means of assessing volume status and renal perfusion. Renal dysfunction after repairs of the descending thoracic aorta can be as high as 14% and is associated with a substantially increased mortality rate. Advanced age, preoperative renal dysfunction, operative complexity, and prolonged aortic cross-clamp times predispose patients to perioperative renal failure. The mechanism of renal injury is most commonly ischemia caused by reduced renal perfusion due to aortic cross-clamping or hemodynamic instability. Oxygen free radicals and other inflammatory compounds affect the renal vasculature and may play an important role as well.

Renal protective strategies begin with the minimization of aortic cross-clamp time. Adequate renal perfusion should likewise be assured through the maintenance of intravascular volume and the avoidance of arterial hypotension during the perioperative period. Distal hypoperfusion during cross-clamping should be avoided and may be obviated by the use of shunts or bypass. Hypothermia, either systemic or regional, reduces renal oxygen requirements and metabolism and can protect the kidneys during ischemia. Pharmacologic interventions are varied and a matter of considerable debate. Mannitol may improve renal blood flow and glomerular filtration during ischemia and diminish the impact of reperfusion injuries through its capacity for oxygen free radical scavenging. Low-dose dopamine (3 mcg/kg/min) acts as a vasodilator on the renal vasculature to improve blood flow and exerts a natriuretic effect by inhibiting sodium transport. There is no evidence that dopamine decreases renal failure during ischemia. Other drugs that increase renal blood flow and natriuresis include furosemide, prostaglandin E1, and fenoldopam, a dopamine-1 selective agonist.

15. *Describe sources of altered coagulation function in descending thoracic aortic surgery and outline methods of treatment.*

The development of coagulopathies is common during thoracic aortic surgery, especially when extreme intraoperative blood loss and massive fluid resuscitation occur. Patients may require replacement of several blood volumes during repair of descending thoracic aneurysms. Alterations in normal coagulation function can occur from hypothermia, heparinization, acidemia, and dilutional thrombocytopenia. Profound hypoperfusion may cause disseminated intravascular coagulation (DIC). Visceral ischemia may initiate fibrinolysis; liver ischemia may result in reduced production of coagulation factors. In addition to monitoring the patient's hematocrit and hemoglobin, frequent assessment of the prothrombin time (PT), partial thromboplastin time (PTT), fibrinogen, and platelets is warranted during massive transfusions. Early administration of FFP and platelets may be effective in preventing severe derangements in coagulation. Cryoprecipitate may be necessary to correct coagulopathies that occur in the context of volume overload from massive fluid resuscitation. The use of antifibrinolytics, such as tranexamic acid, is associated with decreased perioperative bleeding during thoracic aortic surgery. Aprotinin, another fibrinolytic, is no longer used because of adverse renal, cardiac, and neurologic outcomes.

Postoperative Period

16. *List the potential complications after thoracic aortic surgery.*
    - Myocardial infarction
    - Respiratory failure
    - Renal failure
    - Hemorrhage
    - Paraplegia
    - Cerebrovascular accident

Spinal cord injury in the immediate postoperative period presents with paraparesis or flaccid paralysis. An anterior spinal artery syndrome may be present with a loss of motor function and pinprick sensation but sparing of vibratory sensation and proprioception. The delayed onset of neurologic deficits is most likely caused by postoperative hypotension in patients with severe atherosclerotic disease.

17. *Explain strategies for postoperative pain management in patients undergoing TAA.*

The large incision required for descending thoracic aortic surgery creates significant postoperative pain. Both the thoracic and abdominal components of the incision require transection of major muscle groups. The posterolateral thoracotomy may entail removal of one or more ribs. Pleural chest tube sites are another source of patient pain and discomfort. The use of thoracic epidural analgesia after descending TAA repair is common but has a number of associated concerns, including intraoperative hypotension.

The potential benefits of pain relief and the reduction of pulmonary and cardiac morbidity must be weighed against the risks of hypotension and epidural hematoma formation after anticoagulation. Early recognition of an anterior spinal artery syndrome may be delayed by the use of neuraxial local anesthetics. Parenteral narcotics administered by intermittent bolus, continuous infusion, or patient-controlled analgesia may also be used for pain management but must be titrated carefully to prevent excessive respiratory depression. Coughing and deep breathing are essential to avoid developing postoperative pneumonia, which requires adequate analgesia.

18. *Discuss emerging evidence for the advantages and disadvantages of endovascular techniques for repair of thoracic aneurysms.*

EVAR has become an alternative to open techniques for the repair of aneurysms of the thoracic aorta. Endovascular stenting avoids the extensive surgical exposure required for an open repair and the protracted cross-clamping of the thoracic aorta. Preliminary data suggest that endovascular repairs have a lower incidence of neurologic complications in patients with descending TAAs and a significantly reduced perioperative mortality rate. A reduction in hospital and critical care stay may be an additional benefit of endovascular techniques. Endovascular stenting may be unsuitable for anatomically complex lesions, and endograft longevity has not been fully established.

Review Questions

1. The inability of a patient to tolerate the supine position during a preoperative evaluation before thoracic aortic surgery is suggestive of aneurysmal compression of the:
   a. Stellate ganglia.
   b. Superior vena cava.
   c. Left mainstem bronchus.
   d. Esophagus.

2. The anterior spinal artery is most commonly supplemented in the thoracic region by which blood vessel?
   a. Vertebral artery
   b. Artery of Adamkiewicz
   c. Basilar artery
   d. Celiac artery

3. The preferred site for placement of an arterial cannula to monitor blood pressure in surgery on the descending thoracic aorta is the:
   a. Right radial artery.
   b. Left radial artery.
   c. Left femoral artery.
   d. Right femoral artery.

4. Evoked potential monitoring during surgery on the descending thoracic aorta would be least affected by:
   a. Isoflurane.
   b. Hypothermia.
   c. Hypotension.
   d. Fentanyl.

5. Spinal cord perfusion pressure (SCPP) is defined as the difference between the mean arterial blood pressure and which of the following measures?
   a. Central venous pressure
   b. Diastolic blood pressure
   c. Cerebrospinal fluid pressure
   d. Thoracic pleural pressure

Suggested Readings

Kumar A, Duttas V, Negi S, Puri GD. Vascular airway compression management in a case of aortic arch and descending thoracic aortic aneurysm. *Ann Card Anaesth* 2016;19(3):568-571.

Awad H, Ramadan ME, et al. Spinal cord injury after thoracic endovascular aortic aneurysm repair. *Can J Anaesth* 2017;64(12):1218-1235.

Elisha S. Vascular surgery. In: Nagelhout JJ, Elisha S, eds. *Nurse Anesthesia*, 6th ed. St Louis, MO: Elsevier, 2018:535-562.

Grecu L, Nikhil C. Vascular disease. In: Hines RL, Marschall KE, eds. *Stoelting's Anesthesia and Coexisting Disease*, 7th ed. Philadelphia: Churchill Livingstone, 2018;237–263.

Ma J, Zhang L, Wang C, et al. Dexmedetomidine alleviates the spinal cord ischemia-reperfusion injury through blocking mast cell degranulation. *Int J Clin Exp Med* 2015;8(9):14741-14749.

Kahn RA, Stone ME, Moskowitz DM. Anesthetic considerations for descending thoracic aortic aneurysm repair. *Semin Cardiovasc Vasc Anesth* 2007;11:205-223.

Makkad B, Pilling S. Management of thoracic aneurysm. *Semin Cardiovasc Vasc Anesth* 2005;9:227-240.

Goel N, Jain D, Savlania A, Bansal A. Thoracoabdominal aortic aneurysm repair: what should the anaesthetist know? *Turk J Anaesthesiol Reanim* 2019;47(1):1-11.

Silvay G, Stone ME. Repair of thoracic aneurysms, with special emphasis on the preoperative work-up. *Semin Cardiovasc Vasc Anesth* 2006;10:11-15.

Soliman R, Zohry G. The myocardial protective effect of dexmedetomidine in high-risk patients undergoing aortic vascular surgery. *Ann Card Anaesth* 2016;19(4):606-613.

Taterra D, Skinningsrud B, Pękala PA, et al. Artery of Adamkiewicz: a meta-analysis of anatomical characteristics. *Neuroradiology* 2019;61(8):869-880.

26

Abdominal Aortic Aneurysm Repair

KEY POINTS

- Risk factors for developing an abdominal aortic aneurysm (AAA) include male gender, increasing age, smoking, elevated plasma cholesterol levels, hypertension, and a family history of AAAs.
- A thorough preoperative evaluation is essential in this patient population due to the presence of multiple underlying comorbidities.
- Coronary artery disease is the single most significant risk factor that influences long-term outcomes, and a definitive cardiac evaluation is vital before an elective repair.

- Surgical repair utilizing an open or endovascular technique remains the only definitive treatment.
- Hemodynamic changes from the application and removal of the abdominal aortic cross-clamp are one of the most challenging aspects of patient management for the anesthetist.
- Myocardial dysfunction is the single most likely cause of morbidity after vascular surgery.

Case Synopsis

A 65-year-old man presents for surgical repair of a 6.5-cm AAA. He is scheduled for an open abdominal repair procedure.

Preoperative Evaluation and Demographic Data

Past Medical/Surgical History

- 42-pack/year smoking history
- Hypertension
- Hypercholesteremia

List of Medications

- Lovastatin
- Atenolol
- Hydrochlorothiazide

Diagnostic Data

- Hemoglobin, 14 g/dL; hematocrit, 42%
- Glucose, 107 mg/dL
- Blood urea nitrogen, 10 mg/dL; creatinine, 0.8 mg/dL
- Electrolytes: sodium, 142 mEq/L; potassium, 3.6 mEq/L; chloride, 104 mEq/L; carbon dioxide, 26 mEq/L
- Coagulation studies: prothrombin time, 12 s; international normalized ratio, 1.0; partial thromboplastin time, 28 s

Height/Weight/Vital Signs

- 183 cm, 80 kg
- Blood pressure,142/84; heart rate, 61 beats per minute; respiratory rate, 18 breaths per minute; room air oxygen saturation, 98%; temperature, 36.8°C

- Electrocardiogram (ECG): normal sinus rhythm; heart rate, 61
- Cardiac Doppler ultrasound: mild left ventricular hypertrophy; estimated ejection fraction, 50%
- Chest x-ray: within normal limits

Pathophysiology

The proposed pathophysiology associated with the development of an AAA is complex and multifaceted. AAA is defined as a weakening of the aortic wall that results in progressive dilatation that can eventually rupture. The most common site of an AAA is infrarenal (>90%), as shown in Fig. 26.1; however, the aneurysm may occur in a juxtarenal or suprarenal position. AAAs affect approximately 5% of elderly men and are estimated to account for about 2% of all deaths within the United States. However, it is believed that the incidence is an underestimation due to sudden death that is caused by cardiac disease compared with an undiagnosed AAA. Even though the reason has not been elucidated, the incidence of AAA is increasing. Potential causes may include increased incidence of obesity and atherosclerosis or improved detection and diagnostic screening modalities. The pathophysiologic process associated with AAA remains unclear, but it is believed that they develop from the combination of lipid deposition within that aortic adventitia. Cytokines and proteolytic enzymes degrade the elastin and collagen causing inflammation and atherosclerosis.

Surgical Procedure

Surgical repair of an AAA is recommended once the aneurysm expands to >5 cm in cross-section dimension, if the

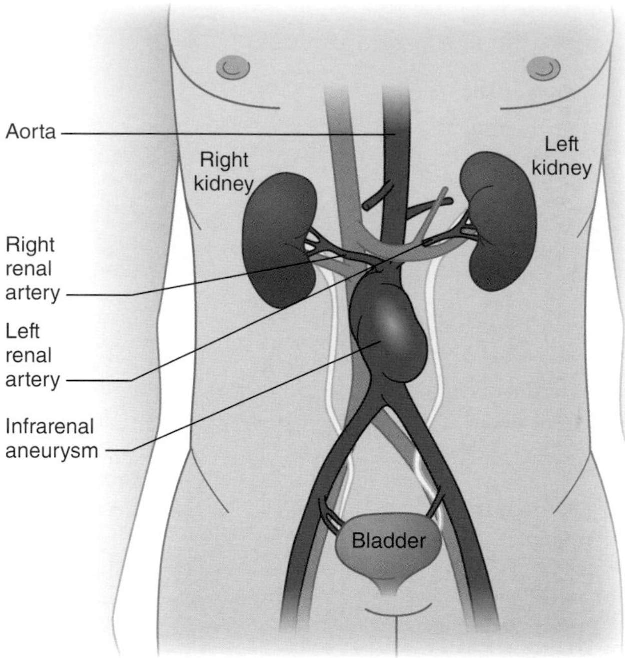

• **Fig. 26.1** Anatomic representation of infrarenal aneurysm.

AAA is between 4.0 and 5.0 cm with expansion of >0.5 cm within 6 months, if the patient is exhibiting signs and symptoms associated with AAA, or if the aneurysm is dissecting or has ruptured. Traditionally, the procedure is done via open abdominal incision and the patient is placed in the supine position. The operation may also be performed via a retroperitoneal approach. Once the aorta is exposed, the aortic cross-clamp is applied above the aneurysm and the aneurysm is dissected and removed. A Dacron graft replaces the diseased portion of the aorta. It is sewn into the normal proximal and distal aorta.

Advances in endovascular procedures have now made AAA repair less invasive. An endograft is placed inside the lumen of the aorta at the level of the aneurysm. The deployment device is advanced via the femoral arteries. The position of the endograft is assessed under fluoroscopy before final placement. Because the surgeon does not have to cross-clamp the aorta, the dramatic cardiac and metabolic manifestations associated with this process do not occur. Endovascular aortic repair (EVAR) is associated with a decreased incidence of cardiovascular, pulmonary, and renal complications compared with a traditional open approach. However, there is no significant difference in the long-term survivability when comparing these two surgical techniques to AAA repair. A complication that is specific to EVAR is endoleak. Blood from the proximal aorta leaks around the graft into the aneurysm sac and can cause aortic aneurysm rupture. Several interventions can be performed if this circumstance occurs, such as placement of a graft extension, use of a coil or fibrin glue to seal the entrance to the aneurysm sac, or removal of the graft and direct aortic repair via

an open approach. A comparison of these surgical techniques is represented in Fig. 26.2.

Anesthetic Management and Considerations

Preoperative Period

1. *Discuss the risk factors associated with the development of an AAA.*

   The occurrence of AAAs is greater in men than in women, at an incidence of approximately 9:1. AAAs are more frequently diagnosed in men over the age of 55 and women at age 65. Ethnicity may play a role in the development of an AAA, and this disease has been reported to be more common in whites than in blacks. In patients that develop an AAA, 90% have a history of current or previous smoking. Smoking is the strongest independent risk factor for the development of an AAA. Hypertension is present in 60% of patients with AAA; other risk factors are listed in Box 26.1.

2. *Describe the components of a comprehensive preoperative evaluation for a patient with an AAA.*

   Three-fourths of patients are asymptomatic when they are diagnosed with an AAA. Typically, the diagnosis is made either on a radiologic examination or physical examination, which reveals a pulsatile epigastric mass. Patients that do experience symptoms usually complain of vague abdominal pain, back pain, or, rarely, gastrointestinal or ureteral obstruction. Symptoms associated with a ruptured AAA include persistent, severe pain that

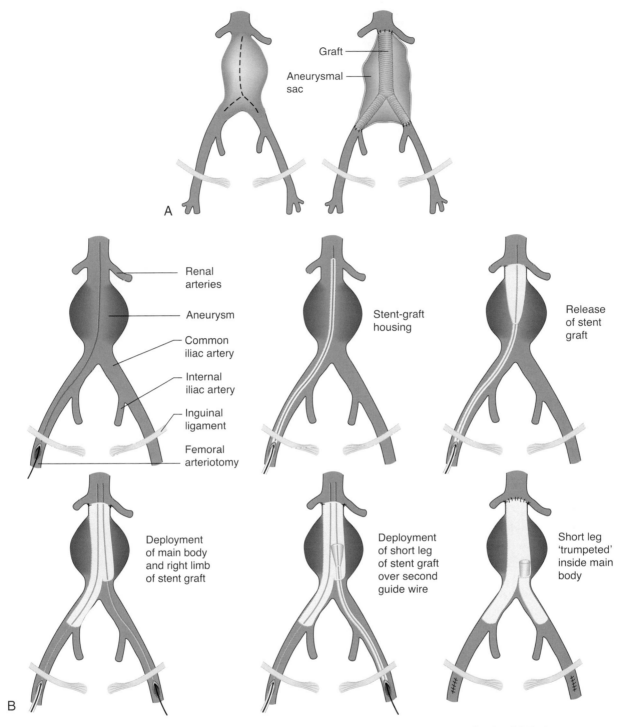

• **Fig. 26.2** Comparison of an open (A) versus EVAR (B) technique for AAA repair. (From Garden OJ, Parks RW: *Principles and practice of surgery*, ed 7, Edinburgh, 2018, Elsevier.)

radiates to the back and groin. Coronary artery disease (CAD) is present in 30% to 40% of patients who have AAA. Aortoiliac or peripheral arterial occlusive disease manifests as tissue ischemia, such as claudication of the lower extremities.

For elective repair of an AAA, the most common imaging studies performed, ultrasound and computed tomography (CT), reveal the location and size of the aneurysm.

The size of the aortic aneurysm is the most important determining factor for rupture. Further imaging studies completed before elective repair include chest radiograph and ECG. If a patient is identified as having symptomatic CAD, further cardiac evaluation is recommended. The most dependable diagnostic tool in determining the extent of CAD is coronary angiography. A thorough preoperative evaluation and an appreciation of the anticipated

- Family history
- Coronary artery disease
- History of myocardial infarction
- Hypertension
- Hyperlipidemia
- Peripheral vascular disease
- Obesity
- Smoking
- Chronic obstructive pulmonary disease
- History of stroke
- Renal insufficiency
- Gender (male > female)
- Elevated C-reactive protein

postoperative outcomes are essential when providing anesthetic care for patients with an AAA.

3. *Differentiate between a suprarenal, juxtarenal, and infrarenal AAA and the associated anesthetic management concerns.*

Approximately 90% of AAAs are infrarenal. Juxtarenal aneurysms are found at the level of the renal arteries but do not extend into the orifice of the renal arteries. Suprarenal aneurysms are located above the renal arteries and may involve some of the visceral vessels. Thus renal failure, though possible with aortic cross-clamping at any level, occurs more frequently with suprarenal aortic occlusion due to decreased renal perfusion. Anesthetic management aimed to counter this effect would include maintaining adequate intravascular volume, administration of osmotic diuretics before clamp application (mannitol), and a loop diuretic (Lasix). A low-dose dopamine infusion (2 to 5 mcg/kg/min) may also help preserve renal perfusion. There is a lack of scientific evidence showing a decreased incidence of renal failure from either mannitol administration or from renal dose dopamine infusion. The most significant predictor of postoperative renal failure after AAA repair is determined by the presence or absence of preoperative renal impairment. Ultimately, the effects of aortic cross-clamping are similar for all types of abdominal aneurysms, but the cardiovascular and hemodynamic alterations are more dramatic, as the clamp is placed more proximally.

4. *Contrast the advantages and disadvantages of open AAA repair versus EVAR.*

The first successful elective open repair of an AAA occurred in 1952. Since then, great advances have been made in improving outcomes and decreasing morbidity and mortality. However, the elective open repair is a highly invasive procedure that is costly to not only the patient's physical well-being but also to the health care system. The average intensive care stay for a patient undergoing an open repair is 2.58 days and an overall hospital stay of 19 days. The physiologic stress that the patient must endure is immense. On average, a patient will lose 2000 to 5000 mL of blood. The list of potential adverse complications associated with the traditional AAA repair is presented in Box 26.2. However, the durability of AAA repair is superior compared with EVAR. In addition, patients must meet specific anatomic requirements such as the size and distance from the aneurysm to the renal arteries in order to be an acceptable candidate for the EVAR procedure.

In 1991, the introduction of EVAR for AAA repair drastically changed the way this disease can be surgically managed. It has been demonstrated that EVAR reduces the time spent in the intensive care unit to 0.33 days, hospital stays to 6 days, and blood loss to 200 to 500 mL. However, EVAR is also associated with unique complications such as endoleak, stent graft migration and collapse, and endograft limb occlusions. As a result, contrast-enhanced CT scans must be performed frequently in order to monitor the stent graft. Therefore decreased renal function from graft migration and renal artery occlusion are risks associated with EVAR. Presently, EVAR is most commonly performed for AAA repair for patients with appropriate vascular access and anatomy.

5. *Distinguish between the transperitoneal versus retroperitoneal approach for surgical repair of the AAA.*

Most commonly, open repair of AAAs is carried out via the transperitoneal approach. This technique involves a large midabdominal incision with the patient in the supine position. The retroperitoneal approach involves the patient being in the right lateral decubitus position. The skin is then incised from the lateral edge of the left rectus muscle to the bottom of the twelfth rib. The benefits of the retroperitoneal position include decreased postoperative ileus, reduced pulmonary complications, and minimized postoperative incision pain.

6. *Identify the contraindications to elective repair of AAA.*

Patients in which the aneurysm diameter measures <5 cm are medically managed, as the benefit of repair is outweighed by the risks of the procedure. Contradictions to elective repair of AAAs include recent myocardial infarction, pulmonary insufficiency/disorders, unstable angina pectoris, and chronic renal insufficiency.

- Hemorrhage
- Myocardial ischemia/infarction
- Cerebral ischemia/infarction
- Thrombus/embolization
- Mesenteric traction syndrome
- Organ ischemia
- Wound infection
- Renal failure
- Graft failure/thrombosis/infection
- Respiratory insufficiency
- Lower extremity ischemia

7. *Describe the nonsurgical management of AAA.*

In patients in which repair of the AAA is contradicted or deferred, the nonsurgical management is similar to that of a patient with CAD. These interventions help reduce the rate of aneurysm expansion. Modifiable lifestyle changes are among the most important treatment modalities. Smoking cessation is crucial, as nicotine abuse is not only a factor in developing an AAA but it also increases the expansion, risk for rupture, and worsens the prognosis of an AAA. Medically, research demonstrates that the control of hypercholesteremia with statin drugs, combined with angiotensin II inhibitors, macrolides, and antiinflammatory agents, reduce the production of proteolytic enzymes and cytokines. Treatment of hypertension and sodium restriction is also vital.

Intraoperative Period

8. *Identify appropriate intraoperative anesthetic monitoring techniques for open repair of an AAA.*

Appropriate intraoperative monitoring for patients undergoing AAA repair is crucial in order to detect changes in hemodynamic status. Cardiac morbidity is of the utmost concern during this procedure. ECG monitoring of leads II and V5 will detect approximately 80% of ischemic events. Arterial monitoring is essential for continuous assessment of the blood pressure, fluctuations in hemodynamics due to aortic cross-clamping, and access for blood sampling. Central line placement and central venous pressure assessment can help guide fluid resuscitation. Due to the wide fluctuations in systemic vascular resistance that result from the aortic cross-clamp, pulmonary artery catheters may also be utilized to monitor left-heart filling pressures. Transesophageal echocardiography (TEE) can also be used to monitor cardiac function.

9. *List other pharmacologic agents that are utilized during anesthetic management of open AAA.*

Heparin 50 to 100 units/kg is administered approximately 5 minutes before the application of the cross-clamp to inhibit thrombus formation. If the clamp time is prolonged, additional doses may be needed. Decisions regarding anticoagulation are guided by activated clotting time (ACT) measurements. After the clamp is removed, protamine can be given to inhibit the anticoagulant effects of heparin. Protamine should not be administered faster than 50 mg/min to avoid hypotension.

10. *Discuss acceptable anesthetic techniques for induction and maintenance for this patient.*

It is most important when formulating an anesthetic plan to tailor the plan individually to each patient. However, most patients presenting for abdominal aortic reconstruction are elderly with coexisting morbidities. Titration is essential because not every patient will require the same amount of medications. Premedication is used if the patient is hemodynamically stable. An epidural catheter placed before induction can provide adequate analgesia during the intraoperative and postoperative periods. It also allows for a combined epidural and general technique, which lowers the level of volatile agents consumed, decreases spinal cord sensitization, and causes vasodilation, which decreases the blood pressure during aortic cross-clamping. The disadvantage of infusing local anesthesia into the epidural catheter during the intraoperative period is that if severe hypotension occurs from hemorrhage or myocardial dysfunction, then treating the hypotension may be more difficult. Also, concerns regarding the development of an epidural hematoma are warranted due to systemic anticoagulation.

Induction should be accomplished to maintain hemodynamic stability (mean arterial pressure [MAP] within 20% of preoperative values). Hypertension and tachycardia should be avoided. For maintenance of general anesthesia, patients who have poor myocardial performance may develop hypotension due to the myocardial depressant effects of the inhaled agents. In this instance, it may be prudent to administer lower concentrations of inhalation agents (<1 MAC) and narcotics and dexmedetomidine. Overall, constant vigilance combined with accurate interpretations and interventions are the keys to a successful anesthetic, regardless of the anesthetic technique that is employed.

11. *Describe the hemodynamic changes that occur with the application and removal of the aortic cross-clamp.*

The initial response to aortic cross-clamp application is arterial hypertension that results from an increased systemic vascular resistance and increased impedance to aortic flow. In the majority of patients who undergo aortic reconstruction, the cross-clamp is placed below the level of the renal arteries due to the high prevalence of infrarenal aneurysms. The organs above the clamp experience a redistribution of blood volume, and blood flow to the pelvis and lower extremities will cease. With infrarenal cross-clamping, the arterial blood pressure can increase 7% to 10% above the clamp. In general, patients with normal cardiac reserve can tolerate this increase. However, in patients with significant cardiac dysfunction, even the slightest change in pressure will precipitate heart failure and ischemia. Table 26.1 outlines the hemodynamic

TABLE 26.1	Hemodynamic Changes That Occur in Response to Aortic Cross-Clamping	
Cardiovascular Variable	**Response to Aortic Cross-Clamp**
Mean arterial pressure	Increases
Systemic vascular resistance	Increases
Cardiac output	No change or decreases
Pulmonary artery occlusion pressure	Increases

changes that occur in response to aortic cross-clamp application.

The removal of the aortic cross-clamp is not a benign process, and constant communication between the surgeon and anesthetist is vitally important. The clamp should be removed incrementally in order to avoid drastic reductions in blood pressure due to the abrupt decrease in systemic vascular resistance combined with the release of metabolites such as lactate, which is created due to reperfusion of the ischemic lower extremities. Adequate fluid administration combined with vasopressor administration helps minimize severe hypotension.

These metabolites cause vasodilation and myocardial depression. Hypotension can be treated by infusing a fluid bolus, decreasing the depth of anesthesia, and administering medications that cause vasoconstriction such as phenylephrine or norepinephrine. The surgeon should also reapply the cross-clamp as needed in case of severe and persistent hypotension. Interestingly, patients who have occlusive disease develop collateral circulation, which can continue to perfuse the patient's lower extremities during cross-clamping. Thus these patients may experience less dramatic hemodynamic changes during the procedure.

12. *Discuss appropriate pharmacologic responses to the changes in hemodynamic parameters that occur during AAA repair.*

The appropriate pharmacologic therapies utilized in the management of the patient undergoing aortic aneurysm reconstruction require a comprehensive understanding by the anesthetist. In anticipation of the application of the aortic cross-clamp, the anesthetist should have the patient at a deep level of anesthesia. Once the clamp is applied, the main goal is to decrease afterload with arterial dilators (nitroprusside) and to maintain preload with venodilators (nitroglycerin). There is increased incidence of acute renal dysfunction when the MAP is >60 mm Hg for longer than 15 minutes.

Postoperative Period

The total resection time for this surgery was 270 minutes. In the postanesthesia care unit, the patient exhibits the following acute symptoms: restlessness, pain, shivering, blood pressure of 178/86, respiratory rate 28/min, sinus tachycardia rate 102, oxygen saturation 98%, temperature 35.4°C, lungs clear to auscultation, and decreased urine output.

13. *Examine the patient's vital signs. What would be an appropriate treatment?*

Administration of a fluid bolus would be appropriate at this time. Aggressive volume administration to allow for third-space loss in the first 12 hours postoperatively is recommended. However, in the patient with limited cardiac reserve, careful fluid resuscitation is warranted in order to prevent heart failure. Shivering dramatically increases myocardial oxygen consumption, and meperidine (Demerol) can be administered

to decrease this response. If the patient has an epidural catheter in place, a test dose may be given to assess proper placement, then local anesthesia can be administered in order to provide pain relief. Blood should be drawn to assess the hemoglobin value, electrolyte, and coagulation status, and an arterial blood gas to determine the adequacy of ventilation.

14. *Identify the potential postoperative complications after AAA repair.*

The mortality rate for an elective repair of an AAA is approximately 2% to 5%; for emergent repair this rate dramatically increases to 50%. Multiple complications can occur postoperatively. These complication rates are increased parallel to the number of comorbidities that may already exist in each patient. The most common postoperative morbidity is myocardial infarction, with a reported rate of 10% to 15%. Continuous cardiac monitoring is recommended for at least 48 hours after surgery to monitor for ischemic events. Respiratory and renal complications may also occur postoperatively. Adequate pain relief should be ensured, but not at the expense of adequate ventilation. Postoperative atelectasis commonly leads to pneumonia in this patient population. Urine output should be maintained at 1 mL/kg/hr. The administration of fluid and diuretics may be necessary. Other less common complications include bleeding, leg ischemia, and stroke.

15. *Discuss the development and treatment associated with acute renal insufficiency.*

Reports of acute renal injury in patients undergoing abdominal aneurysm repair vary with estimates between 2% and 22%. Most patients that experience acute renal dysfunction have preoperative elevated plasma creatinine levels. Intrarenal aortic cross-clamp placement can decrease renal blood flow by as much as 40%. Also, in response to the cross-clamp, it is believed that the kidneys respond by activating the renin–angiotensin system. These combined factors can exacerbate renal insufficiency postoperatively. Fortunately, the reported incidence of renal failure requiring dialysis postoperatively is 0.6%. Mannitol may be given 20 to 30 minutes before the application of the cross-clamp to preserve renal function. However, adequate fluid replacement is the best prophylaxis for avoiding acute renal failure.

Furosemide (Lasix), a loop diuretic, may be given postoperatively, but an adequate fluid and electrolyte status must be maintained. Low-dose dopamine (1 to 4 mcg/kg/min) may be instituted in order to increase renal blood flow and glomerular filtration rate. However, research has shown limited evidence that these interventions prevent acute renal failure. The most predictive factor determining acute renal failure after AAA repair is the degree of preoperative renal compromise.

16. *Discuss the anesthetic management of a ruptured AAA.*

Ruptured abdominal aneurysms are associated with a mortality rate as high as 94% and are the tenth leading cause of mortality in white men over the age of 65. Patients typically present with abdominal discomfort, pulsatile abdominal mass, decreased distal pulses, back pain, and hypotension.

A patient who has a ruptured AAA is taken to the operating room for immediate surgical exploration. A brief preoperative examination is conducted, and venous access as well as arterial line and central line placement are rapidly accomplished. Etomidate is the drug of choice for induction for these patients.

Fluid resuscitation should be carried out with crystalloid and colloid solutions until blood and blood products are available. The patient's hemodynamic response to the application and removal of the aortic cross-clamp is frequently more extreme. Postoperative mechanical ventilation postoperatively due to the large volumes of fluid and blood replacement is required throughout the procedure. Endovascular grafting techniques have been used to treat dissecting and ruptured AAAs.

Review Questions

1. Which independent risk factor is most highly correlated with the development of an AAA?
   a. Hypertension
   b. Smoking
   c. Coronary artery disease
   d. Diabetes
2. Which is the initial hemodynamic consequence that occurs in response to application of the aortic cross-clamp?
   a. Hypotension
   b. Hypertension
   c. Increased cardiac output
   d. Decreased pulmonary artery occlusion pressure
3. Which statement best describes reactive hyperemia?
   a. Elevation in body temperature
   b. Chemical reaction involving the kidneys
   c. Transient vasodilation secondary to the restoration of blood flow to ischemic tissue
   d. Muscle spasms that occur in response to application of the aortic cross-clamp

4. Which postoperative complication is associated with the highest morbidity rate after AAA repair?
   a. Renal failure
   b. Graft rupture
   c. Myocardial infarction
   d. Deep vein thrombosis
5. Which is an advantage to the EVAR compared with the open approach for AAA repair?
   a. Absence of aortic cross-clamping
   b. Increased postoperative pain
   c. Potential for endoleak
   d. Higher incidence of renal insufficiency

Suggested Readings

Barakat HM, Shahin Y, Din W, et al. Perioperative, postoperative, and long-term outcomes following open surgical repair of ruptured abdominal aortic aneurysm. Angiology 2020;71(7):626-632.

Bardia A, Sood A, Mahmood F, et al. Combined epidural-general anesthesia vs general anesthesia alone for elective abdominal aortic aneurysm repair. *JAMA Surg* 2016;151(12):1116-1123.

Elisha S. Vascular surgery. In: Nagelhout JJ, Elisha S, eds. *Nurse Anesthesia,* 6th ed. St Louis, MO: Elsevier, 2018:535-562.

Golledge J. Abdominal aortic aneurysm: update on pathogenesis and medical treatments. *Nat Rev Cardiol* 2019;16(4):225-242.

Grecu L, Nikhil C. Vascular disease. In: Hines RL, Marschall KE, eds. *Stoelting's Anesthesia and Coexisting Disease,* 7th ed. Philadelphia: Churchill Livingstone, 2018;237–263.

Guessous I, Periard D, Lorenzetti D, et al. The efficacy of pharmacotherapy for decreasing the expansion rate of abdominal aortic aneurysms: a systematic review and meta-analysis. *Plos ONE* 2008;3(3):1-10.

Latz CA, Boitano L, Schwartz S, Schermerhorn M, et al. Contemporary mortality following emergent open repair of complex abdominal aortic aneurysms. *J Vasc Surg* 2021;73(1):39-47.e1.

Ulug P, Hinchliffe RJ, Sweeting MJ, Gomes M, et al. Strategy of endovascular versus open repair for patients with clinical diagnosis of ruptured abdominal aortic aneurysm: the IMPROVE RCT. *Health Technol Assess* 2018;22(31):1-122.

Yokoyama Y, Kuno T, Takagi H, et al. Meta-analysis of phase-specific survival after elective endovascular versus surgical repair of abdominal aortic aneurysm from randomized control and propensity-score matched studies. *J Vasc Surg* 2020;72(4):1464-1472.e6.

Zankl AR, Schumacher H, Krumsdorf U, et al. Pathology, natural history and treatment of abdominal aortic aneurysms. *Clin Res Cardiol* 2007;96:140-151.

27

Minimally Invasive Coronary Artery Bypass Graft

KEY POINTS

- Extracardiac procedures, such as coronary artery bypass grafting (CABG), are often performed while the heart is beating.
- Intracardiac CABG is accomplished while using cardiopulmonary bypass.
- The surgery is performed via a mini-thoracotomy or a mini-sternotomy.
- Thoracoscopic video-assisted surgery, often with robotic assistance, necessitates prolonged one-lung ventilation to optimize exposure.
- Adequate flow during cardiopulmonary bypass may increase the risk of air emboli.

- Limited exposure of the heart during surgery poses surgical and anesthetic challenges, which include arrhythmias, hemostasis, myocardial protection, and de-airing at the end of surgery.
- Patient selection is important to avoid intraoperative and postoperative complications. Prolonged one-lung ventilation, incomplete revascularization in hybrid procedures, and limited access for rapid intervention pose challenges with patient management.
- Conversion to sternotomy may be required, and extension of the laparoscopic portals extended over several dermatome segments mandate the need for postoperative analgesia.

Case Synopsis

A 53-year-old man with diabetes and new-onset chest pain undergoes cardiac catheterization, after a positive cardiac stress test study. He is scheduled for a minimally invasive direct CABG (MIDCABG).

Preoperative Evaluation and Demographic Data

Past Medical/Surgical History

- Hypertension
- Obesity
- Diabetes
- Hyperlipidemia
- Peripheral neuropathy
- Anterior cruciate ligament reconstruction on right knee; no anesthetic complications

List of Medications

- Atenolol
- Simvastatin
- Insulin regular
- Aspirin
- Lisinopril

Laboratory and Diagnostic Data

- Chest x-ray: cardiomegaly is stable; prominent pulmonary vasculature centrally without interstitial edema
- Electrocardiogram (ECG): normal sinus rhythm with first-degree atrioventricular (AV) block; heart rate, 74 beats per minute; possible left atrial enlargement (LAE)
- Cardiac catheterization: proximal left anterior descending (LAD) artery occlusion; mild proximal occlusion of the circumflex artery; proximal right coronary artery occlusion; ejection fraction 65%; biatrial enlargement is present; right ventricle, left ventricle, and aortic root are of normal size; the tricuspid and mitral valves are of normal appearance; right ventricular systolic function is normal
- Adenosine myocardial perfusion study: overall, moderately abnormal myocardial perfusion study; consistent with prior infarct involving the inferior wall with moderate peri-infarct ischemia; consistent with mild stress-induced myocardial ischemia involving the mid-to-distal anterior/anterolateral wall
- Hemoglobin, 14.7 g/dL; hematocrit, 41.5%; white blood cells, 5.8×10^9/L; platelets, 176/mm³; hemoglobin A1C, 6.0%
- Cholesterol, 141 mg/dL; high-density lipoproteins, 34 mg/dL; triglycerides, 143 mg/dL; alanine aminotransferase (ALT) 30 units/mL

- Blood urea nitrogen (BUN), 14 mg/dL; creatinine, 0.9 mg/dL
- Electrolytes: sodium, 139 mEq/L; potassium, 3.8 mEq/L; serum bicarbonate, 24 mEq/L; chloride, 103 mEq/L; international normalized ratio, 1.1
- Glucose, 121 mg/dL; fasting glucose, 105 mg/dL

Height/Weight/Vital Signs

- 183 cm, 152.862 kg
- Blood pressure, 176/68; heart rate, 68 beats per minute; respiratory rate, 18 breaths per minute; room air oxygen saturation, 99%; temperature, 37°C
- Denies tobacco and alcohol use

Pathophysiology

Coronary artery disease (CAD) is the narrowing of the coronary arteries (the blood vessels that supply oxygen and nutrients to the heart muscle), caused by accumulation of fatty material within the walls of the arteries. This buildup causes the inside of the arteries to become rough and narrowed, limiting the supply of oxygen-rich blood to the heart muscle, as is shown in Fig. 27.1.

One method used to treat the blocked or narrowed coronary arteries is to bypass the blocked portion of the coronary artery with another piece of blood vessel. Blood vessels, or grafts, used for the bypass procedure may be pieces of a vein taken from the legs, the internal mammary artery, or the radial artery. One end of the graft is attached above the blockage and the other end is attached below the blockage.

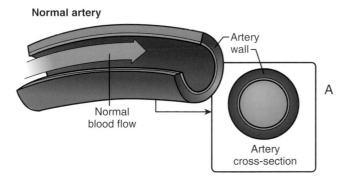

Normal artery

Artery wall

Normal blood flow

Artery cross-section

A

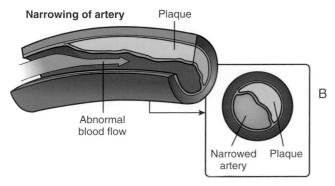

Narrowing of artery

Plaque

Abnormal blood flow

Narrowed artery

Plaque

B

• **Fig. 27.1** (A) Normal artery. (B) Plaque on the artery wall in atherosclerosis. (From Sorrentino SA, Remmert LN: *Mosby's textbook for nursing assistants*, ed 10, St. Louis, 2021, Elsevier.)

Thus the blood is rerouted around, or bypasses, the blockage through the new graft to reach the heart muscle. This bypass of the blocked coronary artery can be done by performing CABG surgery.

Traditionally, in order to bypass the blocked coronary artery in this manner, the chest is opened via sternotomy and the heart is stopped so that the surgeon can perform the bypass. To open the chest, the breastbone (sternum) is cut in half and spread apart. Once the heart is exposed, tubes are inserted into the heart so that the blood can be pumped through the body during the surgery by a cardiopulmonary bypass machine (heart–lung machine). The bypass machine is necessary to pump blood while the heart is stopped and kept still for the surgeon to perform the bypass operation.

Although the traditional "open heart" procedure is still performed and often preferred in many situations, newer, less invasive techniques have been developed to bypass blocked coronary arteries. "Off-pump" procedures, in which the heart does not have to be stopped, were developed in the 1990s. Other minimally invasive procedures, such as keyhole surgery (performed through very small incisions) and robotic procedures (performed with the aid of a moving mechanical device), are also in development.

Surgical Procedure

MIDCABG surgery is an option for patients who require a left internal mammary artery bypass graft to the LAD artery. A small, 2- to 3-inch incision is made in the chest wall between the ribs, whereas the incision made during traditional CABG surgery is about 6 to 8 inches long and is made down the center of the sternum (breastbone). Keyhole approaches or port-access techniques are also available for some types of surgery.

The patient is intubated with a double-lumen endotracheal tube, and transesophageal echocardiography is used to position coronary sinus cardioplegia and pulmonary artery vent catheters. This procedure can be performed either without cardiopulmonary bypass while the heart remains beating or with cardiopulmonary bypass. After the patient has been positioned in the supine position with the right side of the chest elevated, the femoral vessels are exposed. The right lung is then deflated, and the endoscope of the da Vinci Robotic Surgical System is inserted through a 12-mm port placed in the fourth or fifth intercostal space at or just medial to the right anterior axillary line. The 30 degrees up endoscope with the "wide angle" da Vinci camera is moved manually to confirm access to the mediastinum. The handle of the atrial septal retractor is then inserted through a 16 French introducer set in the same intercostal space as the endoscope just lateral to the right internal thoracic artery. The endoscope is removed and a 37-mm service port incision is made in the same intercostal space 20 to 30 mm lateral to the endoscope port. With the surgeon's finger in this service port to protect intrathoracic structures, trocars for the robotic instrument arms, 14-gauge angiocatheters for traction sutures and infusion of carbon dioxide, and a 20 French DLP cardiac sump for left atrial suction are inserted, as shown in Fig. 27.2. Heparin is administered and the femoral vessels are cannulated for port access. A 20-mm flexible port is temporarily placed in the service port incision.

Cardiopulmonary bypass is initiated, endoaortic balloon occlusion is achieved, and cardioplegic solution is administered. All knot tying is performed extracorporeally by the assistant using a shafted knot pusher. Approaching the mediastinum from the more lateral chest allows more working space for pericardiotomy and placement of traction sutures before initiating cardiopulmonary bypass. Because the surgical approach is endoscopic, the surgical field can be enhanced by pressurizing the right pleural space by insufflation of carbon dioxide. This technique also has the advantage of creating high carbon dioxide levels in the left cardiac chambers, potentially reducing the risk of air embolism. Cutting and suturing can be performed by the console surgeon, who has three-dimensional vision and intracorporeal robotic wrists, while suctioning of blood, retraction, and suture retrieval can be simultaneously performed by the patient-side assistant. This technique uses retrograde femoral artery perfusion and is contraindicated for *patients with advanced atherosclerosis or marked tortuosity of the aorta.*

To avoid a median sternotomy scar, an arterial inflow cannula is placed in a femoral artery and the venous outflow cannula is placed through a femoral vein. A catheter with a balloon is advanced up the aorta and the balloon is inflated in the ascending aortic arch. Cardioplegia is then delivered antegrade to the coronary arteries, which have been separated from the systemic circulation by the ascending aortic arch balloon. A catheter is advanced from the internal jugular vein into the pulmonary artery for venting the left ventricle. The patient is placed on fem-fem bypass and cardioplegia established. A single-vessel CABG is then performed either through a mini-thoracotomy or thoracoscopically. Complications associated with CABG surgery are postoperative neuropsychiatric disorders and strokes caused by extracorporeal circulation.

A mini-thoracotomy without using bypass can be accomplished by stabilizing the heart by placing latex sutures under the LAD artery proximal and distal to the site of the anastomosis. Blood flow is stopped in the target vessel by the stabilizing sutures. The technique requires improved technical skill on the part of the surgeon in that the heart is moving (contraction as well as movement of the chest wall during ventilation). It also requires increased technical skill on the part of the anesthetist because an area of the myocardium is ischemic, nonfunctional, and prone to reperfusion arrhythmias. The advantage of the operation includes reduced cost (no extracorporeal circulation, reduced hospitalization time) and reduced risk of stroke (no extracorporeal circulation).

Anesthetic Management and Considerations

Preoperative Period

1. *Identify the major obstacles that are experienced during anesthetic management for minimally invasive CABG.*
   - Preservation of ventricular function and systemic perfusion
   - Detection and treatment of myocardial ischemia
   - Prevention of hypothermia in CABG on the beating heart
   - Intermittent selective ventilation of the collapsed lung using continuous positive airway pressure (CPAP) in case of limited thoracotomy (to prevent hypoxemia)
2. *Discuss the type and frequency of comorbidities associated with CAD.*
   See Table 27.1.
3. *Identify the cardiovascular risk associated with diabetes.*
   Cardiovascular disease is the primary cause of morbidity and mortality among patients with diabetes. Although microvascular pathologies, including retinopathy and

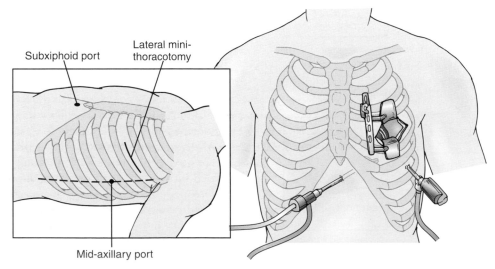

• **Fig. 27.2** Position of instruments used for MIDCABG. (From Antman EM, Sabatine MS: *Cardiovascular therapeutics: A companion to Braunwald's Heart Disease*, ed 4, St. Louis, 2013, Elsevier.)

TABLE 27.1	Type and Frequency of Comorbidities Associated With CAD	
• Hypertension	75%	
• >65 years of age	57%	
• Obesity	66%	
• Smoker	25%	
• Diabetes mellitus	24%	
• Coronary artery disease	29%	
• Chronic kidney disease	25%	
• Congestive heart failure	17%	
• Peripheral arterial disease	11%	

nephropathy, have been shown to be strongly associated with glycemic control, macrovascular complications, including heart disease and cerebrovascular disease, appear to be less responsive to glycemic control. Strategies to reduce the risks associated with diabetes are focused on controlling other risk factors such as hypertension, hyperlipidemia, smoking, and obesity.

It is estimated that over three-quarters of diabetic patients are diagnosed with hypertension. Patients with type 2 diabetes develop subclinical left ventricular (LV) dysfunction characterized by reduced myocardial functional reserve. This influence becomes quantitatively more pronounced in the presence of coexistent CAD and hypertension. The coexistence of type 2 diabetes and hypertension appears to have additive negative effects on both systolic and diastolic LV function, even in the absence of CAD.

4. *Identify the comorbidities that are associated with obesity.*

Numerous comorbidities are associated with obesity that present specific anesthetic challenges, and these factors are listed in Box 27.1.

5. *Discuss how gender, race, and age affect cardiovascular health.*

Increasing age is positively associated with all cardiovascular comorbidities. Male sex is associated with a higher incidence and prevalence of all comorbidities except hypertension. Disparities associated with race/

ethnicity vary categorically. Non-Hispanic whites have lower rates of hypertension than African Americans but higher rates of heart disease, especially myocardial infarctions. Asians and Hispanics had more favorable outcomes on several measures.

6. *Discuss the link between hypertension and concentric LV hypertrophy in this patient.*

Compared with normotensive patients, prehypertensive and hypertensive patients have hypertrophic interventricular septal and LV wall thickness. The LV internal dimension and relative wall thickness are increased, and as a result, LV mass was greater in patients with prehypertension and hypertension. The prevalence of LV hypertrophy was twofold higher in the prehypertensive group and threefold higher in the hypertensive group compared with the normotensive group. Concentric LV hypertrophy, which was rare in this age population, showed a slightly higher prevalence in the prehypertensive and hypertensive groups, but the prevalence of eccentric LV hypertrophy was twofold and threefold higher in the prehypertensive and hypertensive groups, respectively.

7. *Explain the mechanism of action and the side effects associated with this patient's medication regimen.*

- **Atenolol** (Tenormin) can be used to treat cardiovascular diseases and conditions such as *hypertension, CAD, arrhythmias, and angina* and reduces the risk of heart complications after myocardial infarction. Beta-blocking medications have cardioprotective properties because they increase myocardial oxygen supply by decreasing heart rate, which increases diastolic filling time and decreases demand by inhibiting heart rate, contractility, and cardiac conduction. Atenolol is a B_1-selective (cardioselective) drug that exerts greater inhibitory effect on myocardial B_1-adrenergic receptors compared with B_2-adrenergic receptors, which, among other places in the body, are in the lungs. B blockade can result in bronchospasm and for this reason caution should be exerted if atenolol is administered to patients with asthma. Unlike most other beta-blockers, atenolol is excreted almost exclusively by the kidneys.

- **Simvastatin** decreases lipid concentrations, and this medication can decrease low-density lipoprotein (LDL) levels by up to 50%. It has become apparent that simvastatin and other statin medications inhibit the progression of atherosclerosis beyond their effects on LDL. Many explanations have been proposed such as an inhibitory effect on macrophages that are present within the atherosclerotic plaque lesions. All statins act by inhibiting 3-hydroxy-3-methylglutaryl coenzyme A (HMG-CoA) reductase, the rate-limiting enzyme of the HMG-CoA reductase pathway. This metabolic pathway is responsible for the endogenous production of cholesterol. However, statins reduce cardiovascular disease events and total mortality irrespective of the initial cholesterol concentration. A rare but serious side effect associated with simvastatin is rhabdomyolysis, and this complication is enhanced if amiodarone is

• BOX 27.1 Comorbidities Associated With Obesity

- Cancer (kidney, colorectal, prostate, ovarian, uterine/endometrial, esophageal, pancreatic, breast)
- Type 2 diabetes
- Cardiovascular disease (hypertension, coronary artery disease, congestive heart failure, pulmonary embolism, stroke, dyslipidemia)
- Gallbladder disease
- Chronic back pain
- Osteoarthritis
- Asthma
- Obstructive sleep apnea

concomitantly administered. More common side effects may include abdominal pain, diarrhea, indigestion, and a general feeling of weakness. Rare side effects include joint pain, memory loss, and muscle cramps.

- **Insulin** is a hormone that has extensive effects on metabolism and other body functions, such as vascular compliance. Insulin causes cells in the liver, muscle, and fat tissue to absorb glucose from the blood and store it as glycogen in the liver and muscle. When insulin is absent (or low), glucose is not transported into body cells and the body begins to use fat as an energy source, for example, by transfer of lipids from adipose tissue to the liver for mobilization as an energy source. Patients with type 1 diabetes mellitus depend on external insulin (most commonly injected subcutaneously) to survive because the hormone is no longer produced by the islets of Langerhans within the pancreas. Patients with type 2 diabetes mellitus are insulin resistant, and because of such resistance, may suffer from a *relative* insulin deficiency. Some patients with type 2 diabetes may eventually require insulin when other medications fail to control blood glucose levels adequately.

- **Aspirin (acetylsalicylic acid)** is a salicylate drug often used as an analgesic to relieve minor aches and pains, as an antipyretic to reduce fever, and as an antiinflammatory medication. Additionally, aspirin causes anticoagulation due to the drug's antiplatelet effects by inhibiting thromboxane and decreasing prostaglandin synthesis. As a result, aspirin is administered for long periods in low dosages to prevent heart attacks, strokes, and thromboembolism. Low-dose aspirin may be given immediately after myocardial infarction to reduce the risk of another heart attack or of the death of cardiac tissue. The main side effects associated with aspirin are gastrointestinal ulcers, stomach bleeding, and tinnitus, which is more likely to occur if high dosages are given.

- **Lisinopril** is an angiotensin-converting enzyme (ACE) inhibitor that is primarily used in the treatment of hypertension, congestive heart failure, and heart attacks and in preventing renal and retinal complications associated with diabetes. This drug has a long half-life that allows for once-a-day dosing, which aids patient compliance. Lisinopril causes the kidneys to reabsorb potassium, which may lead to hyperkalemia. A severe and rare allergic reaction can occur that rarely can affect the internal lumen of the bowel causing abdominal pain. It has been known to cause vasoplegic syndrome leading to refractory hypotension.

8. *Explain the presence of cardiomegaly on this patient's chest x-ray and the association with obesity.*

   The cardiomyopathy associated with morbid obesity is characterized by:
   - Cardiomegaly
   - LV dilatation
   - Myocyte hypertrophy without interstitial fibrosis

Cardiomyopathy is the most common cause of sudden cardiac death in these patients. Dilated cardiomyopathy is the most frequent cause of sudden cardiac death, followed by severe coronary atherosclerosis, concentric LV hypertrophy without LV dilatation, pulmonary embolism, and hypoplastic coronary arteries.

9. *Explain why an adenosine perfusion study was chosen instead of a stress treadmill in order to assess his cardiac function.*

   The dobutamine stress echocardiography has been the gold standard for myocardial stress procedures. Now the use of tissue velocity echocardiography (TVE) is associated with superior quantification of the longitudinal LV wall motion, with improved sensitivity and specificity to diagnose CAD. There has been continued interest in this technique for assessing subclinical myocardial systolic and diastolic function for patients who have diabetes, hypertension, and chronic kidney disease.

Intraoperative Period

10. *Discuss the concerns regarding gastroesophageal reflux disease (GERD) and transesophageal echocardiography.*

    GERD, which is defined as acid regurgitation that occurs more often than twice per week, can cause inflammation of the esophagus. This condition can also exacerbate asthma, chronic cough, insomnia, and pulmonary fibrosis. If left untreated, GERD is considered a relative contraindication to the use of transesophageal echocardiography, because the probe is inserted into the esophagus. There is a risk of esophageal perforation, which can lead to leakage of acids from the esophagus into the chest, sepsis, and death.

11. *Is the need for a three-vessel bypass a contraindication to performing MIDCABG?*

    A three-vessel bypass can be performed using a MIDCABG technique. However, aortic atherosclerotic disease is a definite contraindication for this operation. An arterial inflow cannula is placed in a femoral artery, and the venous outflow is placed through a femoral vein. A catheter with a balloon is advanced up the aorta and the balloon inflated in the ascending aortic arch. Therefore aortic atherosclerotic disease is an absolute contraindication for this operation.

12. *Describe the advantages of placing a thoracic epidural as an adjunct to general anesthesia.*

    See Box 27.2.

13. *Explain the major advantages associated with avoiding cardiopulmonary bypass.*

    Patients who undergo MIDCABG have a significant reduction in the systemic inflammatory response, postoperative morbidity, and hospital stay compared with patients who undergo conventional CABG with cardiopulmonary bypass.

- Inhibition of sympathetic nervous system hyperactivity
- Cardiac sympathectomy
- Inhibition of inflammatory mediator release
- Postoperative analgesia without causing respiratory or gastrointestinal depression
- Improved respiratory function

14. *Explain the major advantages and disadvantages associated with MIDCABG.*

The advantages associated with minimally invasive cardiac surgery include:
- Reduced surgical trauma
- Decreased morbidity
- Lower procedural costs
- Increased patient satisfaction
- Decreased infusion of blood and blood products
- If cardiopulmonary bypass is not used, the absence of complications associated with extracorporeal circulation
- Shortened hospitalization and quicker return to activities of daily living
- The disadvantages associated with minimally invasive cardiac surgery include:
- Technically challenging
- Increased risk of graft occlusion
- Limited to vessels on the anterior aspect of the heart
- Inability for vessel bypass on the posterior aspect of the heart
- Learning curve before proficiency

Postoperative Period

15. *List the most significant postoperative complications for a patient with diabetes and obesity after median sternotomy.*
- Wound infection
- Pain control
- Prolonged intubation
- Prolonged hospitalization period

16. *List emerging innovative surgical methods for performing CABG.*

The technological advancements improve the equipment and the operating conditions that are used for MIDCABG. However, the physical limitations by which access to the heart is minimized remain problematic. One of the first problems to address is to formulate an intervention if and when ventricular fibrillation occurs. If the surgical plan consists of a small thoracotomy, what will occur when ischemia caused by the stabilizing sutures or reperfusion arrhythmias caused by releasing the sutures progresses to ventricular fibrillation?

If the surgical and anesthesia teams can continue to develop strategies to overcome the technical challenges (motion, bleeding, arrhythmias, hemodynamic variability, decreased cardiac exposure), this technique could continue to emerge as a viable option for patients who need coronary artery revascularization.

Review Questions

1. Which is an advantage of minimally invasive cardiac surgery for CABG?
   a. Larger surgical incision
   b. Increased postoperative pain
   c. Improved wound healing
   d. Higher incidence of cerebrovascular accident
2. Which factor increases the risk of cardiovascular disease?
   a. Diabetes
   b. Osteoarthritis
   c. Gastroesophageal reflux disease
   d. Asthma
3. Which condition is an absolute contraindication for having a MIDCABG?
   a. Ejection fraction of 42%
   b. Triple-vessel disease
   c. Aortic atherosclerotic disease
   d. History of myocardial infarction
4. Which condition disqualifies the use of transesophageal echocardiography?
   a. Carotid artery stenosis
   b. Esophageal varices
   c. Chronic renal insufficiency
   d. Obstructive sleep apnea
5. Which is true regarding the physiologic effects associated with atenolol (Tenormin)?
   a. Decreases myocardial oxygen supply
   b. Causes bronchodilation
   c. Enhances the effects of angiotensin-converting enzyme
   d. Inhibits myocardial contractility

Suggested Readings

Cao C, Harris C, Croce B, et al. Robotic mitral valve surgery. *Ann Cardiothorac Surg* 2017 Jan;6(1):73.

Casselman FP, Slycke SV, Helge D, et al. Endoscopic mitral valve repair: feasible, reproducible, and durable. *J Thorac Cardiovasc Surg* 2003;125:273-282.

Hemli JM, Patel NC. Robotic cardiac surgery. *Surg Clin North Am* 2020;100(2):219-236.

Ishikawa N, Watanabe G. Ultra-minimally invasive cardiac surgery: robotic surgery and awake CABG. *Surg Today* 2015;45(1): 1-7.

Moscarelli M, Fattouch K, Gaudino M, et al. Minimal access versus sternotomy for complex mitral valve repair: a meta-analysis. *Ann Thorac Surg* 2020;109(3):737-744.

Nifong LW, Chu VF, Bailey M, et al. Robotic mitral valve repair: experience with the da Vinci system. *Ann Thorac Surg* 2003; 75:438-443.

Paparella D, Fattouch K, Moscarelli M, et al. Current trends in mitral valve surgery: a multicenter national comparison between full-sternotomy and minimally-invasive approach. *Int J Cardiol* 2020;306:147-151.

Repossini A, Di Bacco L, Nicoli F, et al. Minimally invasive coronary artery bypass: twenty-year experience. *J Thorac Cardiovasc Surg* 2019;158(1):127-138.

Sidler M, Wong ZH, Eaton S, et al. Insufflation in minimally invasive surgery: is there any advantage in staying low? *J Pediatr Surg* 2020; 55(7):1356-1362.

Torregrossa G, Balkhy HH. The role of robotic totally endoscopic coronary artery bypass in the future of coronary artery revascularization. *Eur J Cardiothorac Surg* 2020;58(2):217-220.

Vandewiele K, De Somer F, et al. The impact of cardiopulmonary bypass management on outcome: a propensity matched comparison between minimally invasive and conventional valve surgery. *Interact Cardiovasc Thorac Surg* 2020;31(1):48-55.

Wahl S. Cardiac surgery: beyond conventional sternotomy with cardiopulmonary bypass. *Crit Care Nurse* 2020;40(1):66-73.

28

Intracranial Tumor Debulking

KEY POINTS

- The composition of the cranial vault is composed of three components: brain tissue (80%), blood (12%), and cerebrospinal fluid (CSF) (8%), which together determine intracranial pressure (ICP).
  - Brain: 1300 grams (3 lb or 2% of total body weight)
  - Blood: 15% to 20% of cardiac output, 750 mL/min
  - CSF: 150 mL total in cranium and spinal cord, 75 mL in cranium at any given time
- Normal ICP is ≤10 mm Hg.
- CSF production by choroid plexuses in lateral ventricles makes approximately 400 mL/day.
- The circle of Willis allows bilateral communication of internal carotid and vertebral artery blood flow.
- Tumor locations are generally described as supratentorial or infratentorial.

Case Synopsis

A 50-year-old woman with a 1-year history of fatigue, depression, memory loss, and headaches presents with an acute-onset severe headache, syncope, nausea, and vomiting, followed by a seizure. Computed tomography (CT) scan reveals hydrocephalus with displacement of the lateral and third ventricles by a large intracranial mass. Stereotactic biopsy confirms a diagnosis of glioblastoma. A ventriculostomy drain was placed and drained clear CSF.

Preoperative Evaluation and Demographic Data

Social History

- Smoker 1 pack/day for 25 years
- Drinks alcohol socially (2 glasses wine/week)
- Denies drug misuse

Past Medical/Surgical History

- Controlled hypertension
- Migraine headaches
- Severe gastroesophageal reflux disease (GERD)
- Appendectomy at age 19, splenectomy at age 40, no anesthetic complications

List of Medications

- Phenytoin (Dilantin)
- Propranolol (Inderal)
- Esomeprazole magnesium (Nexium)
- Oxycodone (Percocet)
- Zolpidem tartrate (Ambien)

Diagnostic Data

- Hemoglobin, 13.5 g/dL; hematocrit, 40.1%
- Glucose, 110 mg/dL; blood urea nitrogen, 11 mg/dL; creatinine, 0.9 mg/dL
- Electrolytes: sodium, 142 mEq/L; potassium, 4.0 mEq/L; chloride, 100 mEq/L; carbon dioxide, 26 mEq/L
- Chest x-ray: normal chest x-ray, normal heart size, no evidence of infiltrates or consolidations
- CT scan: Hydrocephalus with displacement of the lateral and third ventricles by an intracranial mass measuring 5 × 4 cm. Diffuse edematous tissues surrounding mass with suspected patchy necrotic infiltrates.

Height/Weight/Vital Signs

- 165 cm, 67 kg
- Blood pressure, 133/78; heart rate, 62 beats per minute; respiratory rate, 18 breaths per minute; room air oxygen saturation, 97%; temperature, 36.6°C
- Electrocardiogram (ECG): sinus bradycardia; heart rate, 58 beats per minute

Cerebral Physiology

CSF Flow Through the Brain

Cerebrospinal fluid produced by the choroid plexus located in the two lateral ventricles, flows through the interventricular foramen of Monro and into the third ventricle. The CSF flow then proceeds from the third ventricle through the aqueduct of Sylvius and into the fourth ventricle. From the fourth ventricle, CSF moves through the foramen of Magendie and two foramina of Luschka into the cerebellomedullary cistern (cistern magna) and then into the subarachnoid space and spinal column. The CSF is absorbed in the subarachnoid space by arachnoid villi of the venous system. Fig. 28.1 illustrates the structures and flow of CSF through the brain.

Cerebral Blood Flow (CBF)

- Average: 50 mL/100 g/min (total 750 mL/min) (range: 10 to 300 mL/100 g/min)
- Gray matter (neuronal bodies): 80 mL/100 g/min
- White matter (axons): 20 mL/100 g/min

Alterations in CBF may be detrimental by decreasing blood flow to ischemic areas or beneficial by providing more blood, and hence oxygen, to ischemic areas. Box 28.1 lists factors that can affect CBF. CBF occurs through the circle of Willis, which is included in Fig. 28.2.

Determinants of CBF

- **$PaCO_2$:** Linear relationship, 1 mm Hg ↑ $PaCO_2$ = ↑ 1 to 2 mL/100 g/min CBF
- **PaO_2:** Profound increase in CBF only at PaO_2 <50 mm Hg
- **Cerebral perfusion pressure:** Cerebral perfusion pressure (CPP) = mean arterial pressure (MAP) − ICP (or central venous pressure [CVP])
  - Normal CPP = 100 mm Hg
  - CPP <50 mm Hg = electroencephalogram (EEG) slowing
  - CPP = 25 to 40 mm Hg = EEG flat
  - CPP <25 mm Hg = permanent neurologic damage
- **Autoregulation:** Cerebrovascular autoregulation occurs by vasoconstriction or vasodilation that occurs between a MAP of 60 and 160 mm Hg, as shown in Fig. 28.3. If the MAP is less than 60 mm Hg or exceeds 160 mm Hg, additional vasoconstriction or vasodilation in order to maintain constant CBF will not occur. Blood flow becomes solely dependent on pressure, as the vasculature

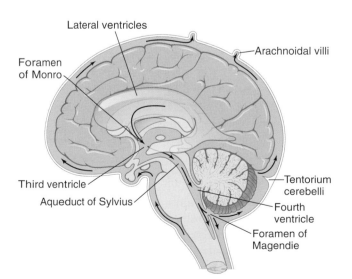

Lateral ventricles

Foramen of Monro

Arachnoidal villi

Third ventricle

Aqueduct of Sylvius

Tentorium cerebelli

Fourth ventricle

Foramen of Magendie

• **Fig. 28.1** The *arrows* show the pathway of cerebrospinal fluid flow from the choroid plexuses in the lateral ventricles to the arachnoidal villi protruding into the dural sinuses. (From Hall JE, Hall ME: *Guyton and Hall textbook of medical physiology*, ed 14, St. Louis, 2021, Elsevier.)

• BOX 28.1 Alterations in Cerebral Blood Flow

1. **Luxury perfusion:** Perfusion in excess of metabolic needs. Luxury perfusion may be beneficial in healthy brains, but may cause a "steal phenomenon" in brains that have ischemic areas. Examples include:
   a. Tumor metabolites that cause vasodilatation in surrounding tissues.
   b. Inhalation anesthetic agents decrease $CMRO_2$ and increase CBF.
2. **Steal phenomenon:** Detrimental. Increased PCO_2 or VAA globally "steals" blood flow from ischemic areas of the brain by causing vasodilatation in healthy areas of the brain. Ischemic brain tissue, which already has maximally dilated vessels due to released vasodilator substances, loses the luxury perfusion benefit due to global shunting of blood flow.
3. **Inverse steal or Robin Hood phenomenon:** Decreased PCO_2 constricts normal vessels but not necessarily in ischemic areas due to vasomotor paralysis. This is one rationale for hyperventilating patients with intracranial tumors associated with increased ICP, especially when administering VAAs, which cause vasodilatation.

VAA, Volatile anesthetic agent.

---

cannot further constrict or dilate to maintain CBF. The autoregulation curve is shifted to the right for patients with chronic hypertension. Therefore these patients require a higher MAP to maintain CBF.

- **Volatile anesthetic agents (VAAs):** All VAAs increase CBF in a dose-dependent manner.

Cerebral Metabolic Rate of Oxygen Consumption ($CMRO_2$)

- Cerebral metabolic rate is expressed as milliliters of oxygen consumed per 100 g of brain tissue per minute.
- $CMRO_2$ = 3 to 3.8 mL O_2/100 g/min
- Coupling is the direct linear relationship of $CMRO_2$ to CPP. As $CMRO_2$ increases (or decreases), CPP will correspondingly increase (or decrease).
- The direct linear relationship between $CMRO_2$ and CBF can be modified and altered by anesthetics and anesthetic management.
- All VAAs, propofol, and benzodiazepines decrease $CMRO_2$.
- VAAs decrease $CMRO_2$ while increasing CPP, disrupting the relationship of $CMRO_2$ to CPP.
- Glucose is the main energy substrate used by the brain. Glucose consumption averages 5 mg/100 g/min.

Determinants of $CMRO_2$

- Coupling: As metabolic demands increase, so does CBF and vice versa.
- Temperature: For each 1°C decrease in temperature, there is approximately a 7% decrease in $CMRO_2$. At 20°C body temperature, an EEG is flat, showing no brain activity.
- Seizures increase $CMRO_2$.

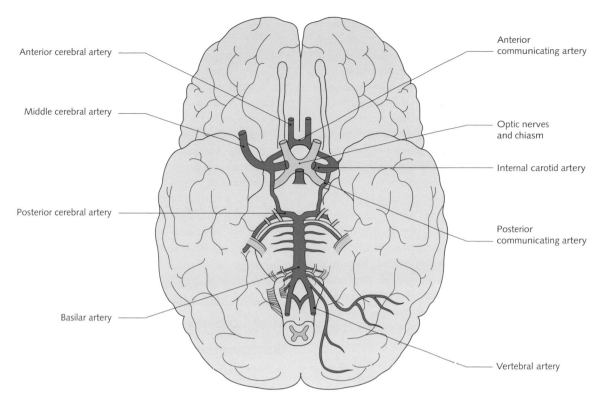

• **Fig. 28.2** Circle of Willis. (From Vivekananda U: *Crash course: Neurology*, ed 5, Philadelphia, 2019, Elsevier.)

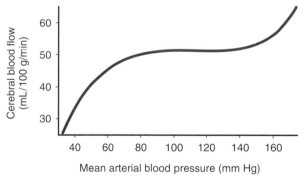

• **Fig. 28.3** The influence of autoregulation on cerebral blood flow. (From Vanderah TW, Gould DJ: *Nolte's the human brain*, ed 8, St. Louis, 2021, Elsevier.)

ICP

- Normal ICP is ≤10 mm Hg. Temporary elevation of ICP occurs during coughing, Valsalva maneuver, and hypertensive episodes.
- Sustained elevated ICP >15 mm Hg decreases CPP and increases the risk of cerebral ischemia. Severely increased ICP may lead to brainstem herniation through the foramen magnum.
- Intracranial tumors are space-occupying lesions and, depending on their size and location, may increase ICP.
- Preventing increases in ICP is a primary anesthetic concern.
- Hyperventilation decreases CBF by causing cerebral vascular vasoconstriction, which decreases CBF.

- Decreasing cerebral blood volume (CBV) decreases ICP.
- Diuretics decrease brain tissue water content, thereby decreasing ICP.
- Ventriculostomy and intrathecal catheters allow CSF to drain, which decreases ICP.

Pathophysiology

Glioblastomas are tumors that rapidly expand and arise from white or gray matter usually in the frontal or temporal regions of the brain. Often these tumors are surrounded by inflammatory and necrotic tissue. Glioblastomas can become large rapidly before the patient developing significant symptoms. Tumors that infiltrate or displace the ventricles may cause obstructive hydrocephalus. Treatment includes tumor debulking, CSF diversion, chemotherapy, and radiation to the affected site. Despite these treatments, survival remains low.

Intracranial tumors may not cause serious symptoms initially because of compensatory physiologic mechanisms that help maintain normal ICP. Glioblastomas often develop rapidly and cause increases in ICP. When CPP requirements exceed the arterial pressure, hypothalamic sympathetic reflex increases blood pressure to restore CBF. The increased blood pressure stimulates carotid bodies, which lowers the heart rate by initiating the Cushing reflex. The Cushing reflex is one of the body's most potent physiologic responses that, when stimulated, dramatically increases sympathetic nervous system predominance. The cardiovascular response includes *hypertension* and *bradycardia*. Bradycardia is the result of baroreceptor stimulation in response to increased systemic vascular resistance. If ICP continues to increase, for which the Cushing reflex cannot adequately compensate, pressure on the brainstem causes irregular respiration. The Cushing triad, which includes *hypertension*, *bradycardia*, and *irregular respirations*, reflects severe increases in ICP and severe cerebral ischemia, and impending herniation of the brainstem down through the foramen magnum can occur. It is estimated that up to 33% of patients with elevated ICP display all three components of the Cushing triad.

Surgical Procedure

The planned surgical procedure is an open craniotomy for tumor debulking utilizing a parietal approach with the patient in the lateral position. An intraoperative biopsy for tumor confirmation and identification will be performed. Before surgical closure, tumor boundaries (margins) will be biopsied to assess the absence of tumor tissues. Complete removal of the tumor is desired because tumor remnants may regrow.

Differences Between Supratentorial and Infratentorial Tumors

- Supratentorial tumors occupy the area of the midbrain and cerebral cortex.
- Infratentorial tumors occupy the area of the vital centers of the cerebellum and brainstem.

The location of the tentorium is illustrated in Fig. 28.4.
- The location of an intracranial tumor necessitates specific positioning for neurosurgical access. Unique neurosurgical positioning requirements are sometimes associated with increased risks. It is important to note that complications such as venous air emboli (VAE), nerve injuries, and postoperative vision loss (POVL) can occur when the patient is placed in any position.
- Sitting position: Increased VAE risk.
- Lateral oblique position: Brachial plexus injury.
- Prone position: POVL risk associated with lengthy prone position cases and intraoperative hypotension, especially in diabetic patients.
- Supine position: May have head and neck rotation or extension; may have cranial pinning/fixation in head tongs.

Anesthetic Management and Considerations

Preoperative Period

1. *Discuss the goals associated with anesthetic management that is associated with intracranial tumor debulking.*

    The preoperative goals include maintaining, or achieving, normal ICP and maintaining CPP (minimum 70 mm Hg) to optimize cerebral circulation and oxygenation. Maintenance of adequate CPP limits ischemia around the tumor and during intraoperative brain

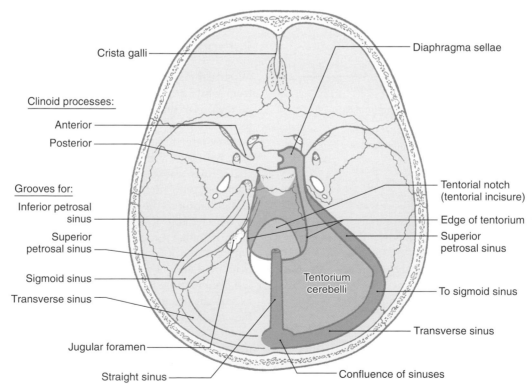

• **Fig. 28.4** Location of tentorium. (From Haines DE, Mihailoff GA: *Fundamental neuroscience for basic and clinical applications*, ed 5, St. Louis, 2018, Elsevier.)

retraction. If there are no changes in mental status, midazolam 0.025 to 0.05 mg/kg IV may be given to attenuate increases in blood pressure and ICP related to anxiety. Other preoperative interventions include:

- Place at least one large-bore intravenous (IV) access preoperatively and another after induction.
- Avoid narcotics preoperatively, as these agents depress respiratory function and raise PCO_2 causing cerebral vessel dilation and corresponding increases in ICP.
- Administer antibiotics and corticosteroids (dexamethasone 4 to 10 mg IV) per surgeon preference before induction. Dexamethasone given before induction has an antiemetic effect in addition to attenuating inflammatory responses intraoperatively and postoperatively.

2. *List the signs and symptoms of elevated ICP.*

The signs and symptoms that are associated with elevated ICP progress on a continuum from mild to severe. Symptoms may include headache, difficulty concentrating, memory disturbances, vision disturbances, vertigo, syncope, nausea, vomiting, severe headache, the Cushing reflex, Cushing's triad, seizures, or coma.

3. *Do all intracranial tumors cause increases in ICP?*

No. Small tumors and larger, slow-growing tumors associated with cerebral physiologic compensation may present with delayed increases in ICP. The compensation that occurs includes the nonlinear compliance of cerebral tissues with CSF and CBV displacement out of the cranial vault. Once ICP is increased due to a tumor, small increases in MAP can result in profound elevations of ICP. Intracranial tumors are often identified after compensatory mechanisms can no longer maintain normal ICP. Additionally, any tumor that obstructs the flow of CSF from the cranial vault to spinal canal (obstructive hydrocephalus) will raise ICP. Pituitary tumors are usually small and rarely associated with increased ICP.

4. *Discuss the most prevalent location of intracranial tumors, infratentorial or supratentorial.*

The location of most neurosurgical procedures for tumor resection is supratentorial and involves the cerebral hemispheres. The cerebral hemispheres are divided by the medial longitudinal fissure. The right and left hemispheres are connected by a bundle of nerve fibers called the corpus callosum. The cerebral cortex is composed of the frontal, parietal, temporal, and occipital lobes. Infratentorial refers to the location of the brainstem consisting of the midbrain, medulla, cerebellum, and pons; it contains major motor and sensory pathways and the cranial nerve nuclei.

5. *Explain how the location of an intracranial tumor influences patient positioning.*

Infratentorial tumors usually require a prone or lateral position for surgical access. Supratentorial tumors are often resected while the patient is positioned supine or lateral. Lateral or semi-lateral positions may use foam supports or a bean bag vacuum mattresses to support the patient. The sitting position is associated with the increased risk of VAE and excessive neck flexion. Venous drainage from the head is impeded by neck flexion. Mild head elevation (reverse Trendelenburg) may be done with any surgical position. The patient's head may be held by a horseshoe-shaped support, a foam support, or pinned in tongs, which fixes the skull to a support frame. Discussion of the patient and operating room table position should be discussed preoperatively in order to plan for intraoperative airway and invasive line access.

Intraoperative Period

6. *Discuss the anesthetic concerns during induction for a patient with elevated ICP.*

Hypoxia, hypercarbia, hypertension, and hypotension are the primary concerns during induction. A smooth induction is appropriate with hyperventilation by proper mask ventilation; however, because this patient has severe GERD, a rapid sequence induction is indicated. Continuous blood pressure monitoring is important, and placement of an arterial line at this time may be beneficial in order to assess an accurate MAP. Arterial blood pressure monitoring before induction should be considered.

Induction agents may depress cardiac function and cause hypotension, and conversely, laryngoscopy may cause sympathetic stimulation and hypertension. Hypotension decreases CBF and risks further ischemic injury to brain tissue. Hypertension can increase ICP and impede adequate cerebral circulation. Inducing an adequate depth of anesthesia before direct laryngoscopy should be assured to prevent sympathetic stimulation and the associated increases in blood pressure.

7. *What are the primary intraoperative goals of anesthesia care for the patient with elevated ICP?*

- Decreasing intracranial volume to prevent increases in ICP
- Maintaining adequate CPP by manipulating the blood pressure
- Decreasing $CMRO_2$

8. *Describe various methods that can be used to decrease $CMRO_2$.*

- **IV agents:** IV agents such as propofol, etomidate, and midazolam all lower $CMRO_2$ and CBF. The modulation of gamma-aminobutyric acid (GABA) receptors by these agents lowers neuronal activity, which corresponds with lower cerebral oxygen consumption. "Barbiturate coma" is a neuroprotective measure sometimes used to maximally suppress $CMRO_2$ and is reflected by an isoelectric EEG.
- **VAAs:** VAAs decrease $CMRO_2$ and increase CBF. VAAs decrease neuronal activity, which lowers oxygen and glucose consumption by brain tissue. The vasodilatory effects of VAAs may provide additional oxygen to brain tissue.

- **Temperature:** Some anesthetists allow a mild decrease in body temperature to help lower $CMRO_2$. Each 1°C decrease in body temperature corresponds to a 7% decrease in $CMRO_2$. The rationale for hypothermia is to lower $CMRO_2$ and metabolite formation in order to protect brain tissue, but this practice remains controversial. Although hypothermia may or may not provide benefit, hyperthermia should be avoided because it has been found to be detrimental.

9. *Explain the term "coupling" in the relationship of $CMRO_2$ to CBF.*

Coupling is the direct relationship of $CMRO_2$ to CBF. An increase in one corresponds to an increase in the other. During normal functioning, increases in cerebral metabolic activity will correlate with an increase in CBF. Decreases in cerebral metabolic activity require less oxygen and glucose, and CBF decreases accordingly. Benzodiazepines, etomidate, and propofol all decrease $CMRO_2$ and allow normal regulatory decreases in CBF (coupling). VAAs disrupt, or "uncouple," this relationship by decreasing $CMRO_2$ while increasing CBF. The term *uncoupling* is controversial in its definition. VAAs change the direct relationship of $CMRO_2$ and CBF to an inverse relationship. Some refer to this as uncoupling. Others assume a more stringent definition of uncoupling that requires a proportionally inverse relationship. All VAAs to varying degrees, and in a dose-dependent manner, decrease $CMRO_2$ while increasing CBF due to their vasodilating effects.

A decrease in $CMRO_2$ is beneficial to ischemic brain tissue, but increases in CBF may cause detrimental increases in ICP and possibly divert blood flow away from ischemic areas to nonischemic areas. This is known as the *steal phenomenon*, and this physiologic effect is listed in Box 28.1.

10. *Describe the methods used to lower ICP.*

Methods used to lower ICP address the need to decrease one or more of the three components of the cranial vault producing ICP: brain, blood, and CSF. Decreasing the volume of these components reduces ICP. Specific interventions used to decrease ICP are reviewed in Table 28.1.

11. *Describe the rationale for each method that decreases intracranial volume.*

Brain: Diuretics are administered to decrease blood and brain volume. These agents "shrink" the brain size and therefore lower ICP.

- Furosemide is a loop diuretic and lowers blood volume.
- Mannitol is specifically used for its osmotic diuretic effect, which extracts fluid from brain tissues thereby decreasing its volume. Unfortunately, mannitol also increases renal excretion of water causing hypovolemia, which contributes to hypotension.

TABLE 28.1	Methods to Lower Intracranial Volume and ICP
Component	**Intervention to Intracranial Volume and ICP**
Brain	Diuretics: loop (furosemide 10–100 mg) and osmotic (mannitol 12.5–50 g) Hypertonic saline (3%) at 20 mL/hr or 20-mL bolus (23.2%) Corticosteroids (dexamethasone 10–20 mg; methylprednisolone [Solu-Medrol] 11 g)
Blood	Hyperventilation (PCO_2 25–30 mm Hg) Limit intravenous fluids (<1 L) Elevate head of bed (30 degrees)
CSF	Ventriculostomy Subdural drain Lumbar drain (rarely)

- Hypertonic saline administration osmotically decreases brain water content without causing hypovolemia. Hypertonic saline causes water to be held intravascularly with minimal renal effects compared with mannitol. This improves maintenance of MAP intraoperatively. Hypertonic saline administration is guided by serum sodium (target 155 to 157 mEq/L) and serum osmolality (target 310 to 315 mOsm/L).
- Corticosteroids block inflammatory responses and may prevent further brain edema. The effectiveness of high-dose steroids has come under question; no definitive studies have shown improved outcomes with their use.

Blood: An effective method used to decrease intracranial blood volume is hyperventilation; it decreases PCO_2 causing cerebral vasoconstriction.

- Hyperventilation ($PaCO_2$ <30 mm Hg) causes cerebral vasoconstriction, thereby lowering the amount of blood (CBV) within the cranial vault at any given moment. Lowering the PCO_2 to 25 to 30 mm Hg is effective for lowering the ICP, but this action occurs for approximately 24 hours. Prolonged hypocarbia is associated with increased mortality in patients with increased ICP due to vasoconstriction-mediated hypoperfusion.
- Limiting IV fluid prevents increases in intravascular volume and increases in hydrostatic pressure. Intraoperative fluid administration is often limited to 1 to 1.5 L or less until the intracranial tumor is removed. This may make it difficult to maintain adequate blood pressure. Hypotension caused by hypovolemia can be attenuated by the

administration of hypertonic saline, which increases intravascular volume by establishing an osmotic gradient. Elevating the head of the bed and maintaining a neutral head position facilitates venous drainage.

CSF: Cerebrospinal fluid drainage removes volume from the cranial vault and aids in lowering ICP. A ventriculostomy or lumbar drain may be placed preoperatively or intraoperatively to drain CSF. The level of the CSF drain and amount of CSF drained should be discussed with the surgeon and closely monitored throughout the perioperative period.

12. *Describe how hyperventilation is beneficial for patients with increased ICP.*

Hyperventilation is a universal treatment for acute increases in ICP because hypocarbia causes cerebral vessel constriction, which decreases the amount of blood within the cranial vault. Vasoconstriction is thought to occur in areas of the brain that are not ischemic. Injured areas of brain tissue contain ischemic-mediated vasodilator substances and are not likely to respond to hyperventilation with vasoconstriction. Theoretically, this mechanism inhibits the benefits of the inverse steal, or Robin Hood phenomenon, in which CBF is diverted toward ischemic areas of brain and away from adequately oxygenated areas. A growing body of evidence suggests that hyperventilation may indeed worsen existing ischemia in acutely injured brain tissues. Therefore the use of hyperventilation should be thoroughly assessed and discussed with the surgeon. No conclusive evidence exists regarding the benefit or detriment of hyperventilation and ischemic tissue perfusion. Hyperventilation decreases CBF with resultant decrease in overall intracranial volume. This effect lowers ICP, improving global CBF, and improves surgical exposure and visualization. An ICP of greater than 20 mm Hg impedes CBF to such a great extent that the potential risks of hyperventilation are outweighed by the benefits. Hyperventilation starts to lose its effectiveness to cause cerebral vasoconstriction after 6 to 8 hours.

13. *Analyze the need for neuromuscular blockade (NMB) during tumor debulking procedures.*

Adequate NMB is important for immobility. Neurologic patients are often taking medications such as phenytoin, which induces the hepatic enzymes causing increased metabolism of certain drugs such as neuromuscular blocking agents such as vecuronium and rocuronium (amino–steroid compounds). Increased doses of NMBs may be required for motor function suppression. Neuromuscular monitoring by peripheral twitch monitor or accelerometry is prudent. Patient movement during intracranial procedures may have devastating consequences. Coughing or "bucking" against positive pressure ventilation also risks cervical injury when the head is fixed in tongs. NMB also prevents shivering, which may occur. Shivering increases metabolic requirements of oxygen and interferes with surgical visualization, especially during cases using visual magnification. Maintaining one out of four twitches on train of four (TOF) monitoring often provides adequate NMB with the ability to reverse the paralysis with a cholinesterase inhibitor. Sugammadex can also be administered to reverse neuromuscular blockade, and the dose given will be determined by the degree of blockade.

14. *Discuss intraoperative monitoring for a patient undergoing intracranial tumor debulking.*

Standard American Association of Nurse Anesthetists (AANA) monitoring should be used, as with all general anesthetic procedures. An arterial line for continuous blood pressure monitoring and serial arterial blood gases should be placed before or immediately after induction. Note the correlation of arterial carbon dioxide ($PaCO_2$) to end tidal carbon dioxide ($ETCO_2$) ($PaCO_2$ 5 to 10 mm Hg higher than $ETCO_2$).

EEG, evoked potentials (EPs), brain tissue oxygen ($PtiO_2$), and transcranial perfusion monitoring may also be used. These neurologic monitoring modalities, though used more often before and after surgery, may be used intraoperatively. An EEG reflects an increase or decrease in brain activity, whereas EP monitoring provides more specific data regarding sensory and motor functions. Stimulation of a peripheral nerve and measuring the time (latency) and degree (amplitude) of brain response are the basis of EP monitoring. In general, increases in latency and decreases in amplitude reflect impaired neurologic function. VAAs increase latency and decrease amplitude in a dose-dependent manner. A minimum alveolar concentration (MAC) of 0.5% is often acceptable; above this concentration significant suppression may occur. Monitoring brain tissue oxygenation is specific to the area of the brain that surrounds a sensor probe. The probe uses a polarographic sensor that measures the diffused oxygen from local brain tissues. Ongoing studies are exploring the specific interpretations that may be made regarding the correlation of $PtiO_2$ to CBF and $CMRO_2$. It appears that $PtiO_2$ increases with regional increases of CBF, although $PtiO_2$ will also increase with increased inspired oxygen (FiO_2).

15. *Analyze the IV fluids that are acceptable for use in patients with elevated ICP.*

Normal saline and lactated Ringer's solution are superior to other fluids that contain higher percentages of free water. Infusion of free water must be avoided, as it lowers the osmotic pressure and promotes increased extravascular volume resulting in swelling. Dextrose-containing solutions are also avoided because metabolism of the glucose will lower the osmotic pressure of the fluid. Dextrose-containing solutions also oppose the goal of decreasing cerebral metabolism. Glucose is the main energy substrate used by the brain and increases cerebral metabolism, which risks further ischemic insult.

16. *Cite the specific concerns associated with positioning for intracranial tumor resection.*
    - **Head fixation:** Movement or coughing while in head pins risks catastrophic injury. Assure adequate anesthetic depth and neuromuscular blockade unless the surgeon requires intact motor function for neurophysiologic monitoring. The risks associated with placement of the patient's head in pins include excessive neck flexion, airway swelling, cervical cord compression, and decreased venous outflow. The cranial nerves IX, X, XI, and XII, which control airway patency, respiration, and hemodynamics, are at particular risk with excessive neck flexion and during posterior fossa surgery. A list of these cranial nerves and their function is included in Table 28.2. The potential of injury to these cranial nerves and swelling of the brainstem requires thorough discussion and assessment with the surgeon before the decision to extubate the patient.
    - **VAE:** VAE can occur due to the entrainment of air into the open venous system, which is above the level of heart in the sitting position. As the air enters the venous system, it travels to the right atria and ventricle, entering the pulmonary arterioles. A right ventricular airlock is created and can cause hypoxemia, CO_2 retention, decreased $ETCO_2$, and heart failure. Additionally, reflex pulmonary and bronchial constriction due to the release of endothelial mediators causes pulmonary hypertension and increased peak inspiratory pressures. Venous bleeding decreases the risk for VAE, as the venous pressure likely exceeds atmospheric pressure and air will not be entrained into the venous system.

17. *Evaluate the methods used to detect VAE.*

    The most sensitive to least sensitive monitoring modalities that are used to determine if a VAE has occurred include transesophageal echocardiography, precordial Doppler, $ETCO_2$, pulmonary artery catheter, cardiac output, central venous pressure, ECG changes, blood pressure changes, and a precordial stethoscope. When air is present in the right atrium, the sound is described as a "millwheel" murmur, and it is distinctly different from baseline heart sounds.

18. *Construct a systematic treatment for VAE.*

    Upon detection of VAE, notify the surgeon to flood the surgical area with saline, saline-soaked sponges, or gel foam to prevent further venous entrainment of air. If possible, lower the patient's head to increase venous pressure and slow air entrainment. Turning off anesthetic agents, administration of 100% oxygen, fluids, and push-dose vasopressors are warranted. Immediately aspirate blood and air with a 60-mL syringe from the central line that has been placed preoperatively. The distal end of the central line catheter is optimally positioned at the entrance to the right atria. Avoiding the use of nitrous oxide is indicated, as it will diffuse into the venous air bubble, increase the size, and worsen the condition.

19. *Describe the main goals associated with the anesthetic management of patients for tumor debulking.*

    The main anesthetic goals for tumor debulking are cerebral protection and facilitation of surgical exposure. The reduction of ICP and $CMRO_2$ to reestablish adequate cerebral oxygenation is the main goal. Elevation of ICP >20 mm Hg is associated with increased morbidity and mortality. Anesthetic management of increased ICP focuses on decreasing the amount of the three main constituents of the cranial vault: blood, brain, and CSF.

20. *List the three main components of the cranial vault and differentiate how interventions focused on each of the three components of the cranial vault may affect ICP.*
    - **Blood component:** Hyperventilate in order to lower $PaCO_2$, which decreases CBV. Attempt to minimize stimuli to avoid elevations in blood pressure by administering narcotics and beta-blockers.
    - **Brain component:** Decrease brain fluid content by administering mannitol and/or furosemide. Limit IV fluids to prevent increases in brain fluid and therefore brain volume. Administer barbiturates to decrease $CMRO_2$ by suppressing neuronal activity. Corticosteroids may also be given preoperatively for extended antiinflammatory effects and reduction of brain tissue water content (vasogenic edema).
    - **CSF component:** A ventriculostomy for supratentorial, or a lumbar CSF drain for infratentorial, skull base lesions may be placed to drain CSF. At any given time, 75 mL of CSF is located in the cranial vault, and drainage aids in lowering ICP. Elevating the head facilitates venous outflow and helps reduce ICP.

21. *Explain appropriate methods for treating intraoperative hypertension.*

    Medications that have a rapid onset of action and a short duration are often best for treating intraoperative episodes of hypertension. Hypertension increases blood volume in the cranial vault, which elevates ICP and can increase bleeding. Hypertension may also make surgical exposure and visualization more difficult. IV beta-blockers, such as esmolol and labetalol, are beneficial.

TABLE 28.2	Cranial Nerve Functions	
Cranial Nerve	**Innervation/Function**
IX: Glossopharyngeal nerve	Tongue, larynx; swallowing, larynx elevation
X: Vagus nerve	Most larynx and pharyngeal muscles, thoracic and abdominal organs; airway patency, parasympathetic effects, hemodynamics
XI: Accessory nerve	Neck and upper shoulders; some respiratory accessory muscle function, swallowing
XII: Hypoglossal	Tongue/airway patency, swallowing

Direct-acting vasodilators will increase CBF, whereas enalapril, an angiotensin-converting enzyme inhibitor, has been found to have little effect on CBF. The short-acting calcium channel blocker nicardipine is useful for treating hypertensive periods. Calcium channel blockers have been shown to effectively lower hypertension, to decrease the potential for cerebrovascular spasm, and to be neuroprotective. Intermittent boluses of propofol or a narcotic may aid in attenuating increases in blood pressure related to noxious stimuli. Acute perioperative hypertension is associated with specific periods of noxious stimuli, including intubation, skin incision, outer periosteal scraping of the skull bone, skin closure, and emergence. Increasing the anesthetic depth before surgical stimulation attenuates sympathetic discharge. Hypotension should also be avoided, as a decrease in CBF dilates cerebral vessels, which increases CBV. Maintenance of an appropriate MAP is important to preserve an adequate CPP. Often recommended is a CPP of at least 60 mm Hg (preferably 70 mm Hg).

22. *Differentiate the Cushing response and the Cushing triad.*

The Cushing response is the periodic increase in blood pressure and reflex bradycardia that occurs when the ICP exceeds 30 mm Hg. The associated decrease in CBF causes cerebral ischemia, leading to further edema and elevating the ICP. This is a vicious cycle that leads to the Cushing triad. The Cushing triad is hypertension, bradycardia, and respiratory variability that occur with sustained elevations in ICP. The Cushing triad is a hallmark feature of severe elevated ICP, which can lead to herniation through the foramen magna.

23. *Discuss the different IV anesthetic agent choices for use in tumor debulking procedures in reference to CBF and CMRO$_2$.*

Propofol and etomidate both lower CBF and CMRO$_2$ in a dose-dependent fashion. Cerebral autoregulation, as well as CO$_2$ responsiveness, are maintained with these agents at anesthetic doses. Total intravenous anesthesia (TIVA) using propofol has been used for intracranial procedures. The advantages of TIVA include:

- Decreases CBF and CMRO$_2$
- Lowers CBV
- Lowers ICP
- Possible neuroprotection from antioxidant activity, activation of GABA type A receptors, and alterations in glutamate uptake and release
- Easily titratable
- Attenuates EP monitoring waveforms less than VAAs
- Metabolizes rapidly, allowing for quick emergence and assessment

Propofol lowers MAP and therefore will lower CPP. Care must be taken to maintain adequate CPP. Benzodiazepines decrease CBF and CMRO$_2$ and also possess anticonvulsant properties. Dexmedetomidine is used during intracranial tumor debulking procedures because of its sedative effects and its ability to cause cerebral vasoconstriction and decreases in CBF. Dexmedetomidine decreases CBF but not CMRO$_2$ and is associated with improved hemodynamic stability during craniotomy.

Narcotics have little to no direct effect on ICP, CBF, and CMRO$_2$ but will attenuate sympathetic response to noxious stimuli. Narcotics are a useful adjunct to volatile and IV anesthetic agents. Shorter-acting narcotics, such as remifentanil and alfentanil, facilitate quick emergence.

24. *Evaluate the effect of emergence on ICP.*

Emergence from anesthesia is associated with increases in heart rate and blood pressure. Increased cardiac output increases CBF, which in turn increases ICP. Increased cerebral activity also increases CMRO$_2$, which further increases CBF. Bucking or coughing causes increased intrathoracic pressures, which impede cerebral venous drainage and cause acute increases in ICP. Smooth emergence with normal blood pressure and heart rate is desirable. Elevated ICP is usually no longer a significant concern after tumor debulking, but hemorrhage remains a potential risk. Extubation of the patient "deep" while still anesthetized but with adequate respiratory function is beneficial unless other contraindications exist.

25. *Formulate a plan to accomplish a smooth emergence in patients after a craniotomy for tumor debulking.*

VAAs that have low blood–gas solubility are beneficial for quick emergence after general anesthesia. Titration of narcotics and IV lidocaine has been helpful at attenuating the stimulatory effects of an endotracheal tube but may slow awakening and delay the time before the patient is fully alert. Laryngeal tracheal anesthesia (LTA) provided by administering lidocaine spray is helpful at the time of intubation, but its duration of effect is approximately 90 minutes. The lidocaine can be instilled into the endotracheal cuff at the time of intubation to help anesthetize the trachea and improve tolerance of the endotracheal tube during periods of light anesthesia such as emergence. This technique's duration of effect is quite long, as lidocaine has been shown to diffuse through the polyvinylchloride membrane over time. Switching from one agent, such as a VAA, to a propofol drip, or vice versa, has not been proven to speed emergence.

Postoperative Period

26. *Discuss goals associated with the recovery phase of anesthesia.*

Pain control and maintenance of adequate blood pressure is important postoperatively. If the patient is extubated, the anesthetist should observe for changes in mental status or any signs and symptoms that may suggest an intracranial event such as increased ICP, vasospasm, or hemorrhage. If the patient is to remain intubated, sedation using central nervous system depressant medications is imperative.

Review Questions

1. Which is not considered a component of the cranial vault?
   a. Blood
   b. Brain
   c. Bone
   d. CSF
2. Which factor can decrease ICP?
   a. Hypoxia
   b. Hyperventilation
   c. Delivery of VAAs
   d. Hypercarbia
3. Which is not a potential consequence of elevated ICP?
   a. Confusion or lethargy
   b. Cushing reflex
   c. Cushing syndrome
   d. Cushing triad
4. Which is the mechanism of action by which mannitol protects brain tissue?
   a. Venous engorgement and increased permeability
   b. Osmotic diuresis and free radical scavenging
   c. Hypotension and decreased tissue perfusion
   d. Osmotic diuresis and decreased $CMRO_2$
5. Which events cause physiologic stimulation during a tumor debulking procedure?
   a. Induction, intubation, skin incision, bone sawing, brain tissue resection
   b. Intubation, skin incision, skull periosteal scraping, brain tissue resection
   c. Intubation, skin incision, skull periosteal scraping, emergence
   d. All events during tumor debulking are equally stimulating

Suggested Readings

Abcejo AS, Pasternak JJ, Perkins WJ. Urgent repositioning after venous air embolism during intracranial surgery in the seated position: a case series. *J Neurosurg Anesthesiol* 2019;31(4):413-421.

Batra A, Verma R, Bhatia VK, et al. Dexmedetomidine as an anesthetic adjuvant in intracranial surgery. *Anesth Essays Res* 2017;11(2):309-313.

Bonow RH, Young CC, Bass DI, et al. Transcranial Doppler ultrasonography in neurological surgery and neurocritical care. *Neurosurg Focus* 2019;47(6):E2.

Cardim D, Robba C, Czosnyka M, et al. Noninvasive intracranial pressure estimation with transcranial Doppler: a prospective observational study. *J Neurosurg Anesthesiol* 2020;32(4):349-353.

Grau SJ, Löhr M, Taurisano V, Trautner H, et al. The choice of anaesthesia for glioblastoma surgery does not impact the time to recurrence. *Sci Rep* 2020;10(1):5556.

He H, Peng W, Luan H, et al. The effect of dexmedetomidine on haemodynamics during intracranial procedures: a meta-analysis. *Brain Inj* 2018;32(13-14):1843-1848.

Menon D, Wheeler D. Neuronal injury and neuroprotection. *Anaesth Int Care Med* 2005;6:184-188.

Mishra LD. Cerebral blood flow and anaesthesia: a review. *Indian J Anaesth* 2002;46:87-95.

Prathapadas U, Hrishi AP, Appavoo A, et al. Effect of low-dose dexmedetomidine on the anesthetic and recovery profile of sevoflurane-based anesthesia in patients presenting for supratentorial neurosurgeries: a randomized double-blind placebo-controlled trial. *J Neurosci Rural Pract* 2020;11(2):267-273.

Ranalli LJ, Taylor GA. Neuroanatomy, neurophysiology, and neuroanesthesia. In: Nagelhout JJ, Elisha S, eds. *Nurse Anesthesia*, 6th ed. St Louis, MO: Elsevier, 2018: 645-681.

Stocchetti N, Maas AIR, Chieregato A, et al. Hyperventilation in head injury: a review. *Chest* 2005;127:1812–1827.

Zhang HB, Tu XK, Chen Q, Shi SS. Propofol reduces inflammatory brain injury after subarachnoid hemorrhage: involvement of PI3K/Akt pathway. *J Stroke Cerebrovasc Dis* 2019;28(12):104375.

29

Transsphenoidal Hypophysectomy

KEY POINTS

- A thorough preoperative evaluation is necessary to identify abnormalities resulting from abnormal pituitary hormone secretion or mass effect of the pituitary tumor.
- Vigilant postoperative observation is needed to identify life-threatening complications.
- Perioperative complications of a transsphenoidal hypophysectomy include hemorrhage, increased intracranial pressure (ICP), cranial nerve palsy, diabetes insipidus (DI), and

syndrome of inappropriate antidiuretic hormone secretion (SIADH).
- Intubation by direct laryngoscopy will be difficult in 12% to 30% of acromegalic patients as a result of physiologic changes that occur to the airway.

Case Synopsis

A 36-year-old man who recently moved to the United States has been diagnosed with acromegaly. Presently, he has received no treatment. He is scheduled for transsphenoidal hypophysectomy.

Preoperative Evaluation and Demographic Data

Past Medical/Surgical History

- Acromegaly diagnosed outside the United States several years prior

List of Medications

- None

Diagnostic Data

- Imaging studies
  - Pituitary mass identified on magnetic resonance imaging (MRI)
- Physical assessment
  - Hypertrophy of facial and cranial bones
  - Macroglossia, prognathism, and enlarged hands and feet
  - Deep voice without hoarseness
  - Mallampati Class 2, thyromental distance <6 cm, and no limitations in range of motion of neck and temporomandibular joint
- Laboratory testing
  - Plasma growth hormone (GH), 12.1 ng/mL (normal 0.7 to 6.0 ng/mL; level may be within normal limits, as secretion is pulsatile)

- Insulin-like growth factor 1 (IGF-1), 1282 ng/mL (normal 100 to 402 ng/mL)
- Hemoglobin, 15.9 g/dL; hematocrit, 48.4%
- Platelet count, 299,000/mm^3
- Electrolytes: sodium, 139 mEq/L; potassium, 4.2 mEq/L; chloride, 101 mEq/L; serum bicarbonate, 22 mEq/L

Height/Weight/Vital Signs

- 185 cm, 128 kg, body mass index (BMI) 37 kg/m^2
- Blood pressure, 147/87; heart rate, 72 beats per minute; respiratory rate, 18 breaths per minute; temperature, 36.3°C; room air oxygen saturation, 99%
- Electrocardiogram (ECG): Normal sinus rhythm

Pathophysiology

The pituitary gland, consisting of a large anterior lobe, the adenohypophysis, and a smaller posterior lobe, the neurohypophysis, is located at the base of the brain and is confined to a bony depression in the base of the skull called the *sella turcica*. The floor and anterior wall of the sella turcica adjoin the sphenoid air sinus. The lateral walls surrounding the pituitary gland are adjacent to the cavernous sinuses, which house the internal carotid arteries and cranial nerves III, IV, V, and VI, as seen in Fig. 29.1.

The anterior portion of the pituitary gland secretes six hormones, each by a specific cell type: prolactin, secreted by lactotrophs; adrenocorticotropin, secreted by corticotrophs; GH, secreted by somatotrophs; follicle-stimulating hormone and luteinizing hormone, both secreted by gonadotrophs; and thyroid-stimulating hormone, secreted by thyrotrophs. The secretion of these hormones is regulated by the hypothalamus. The posterior portion of the pituitary

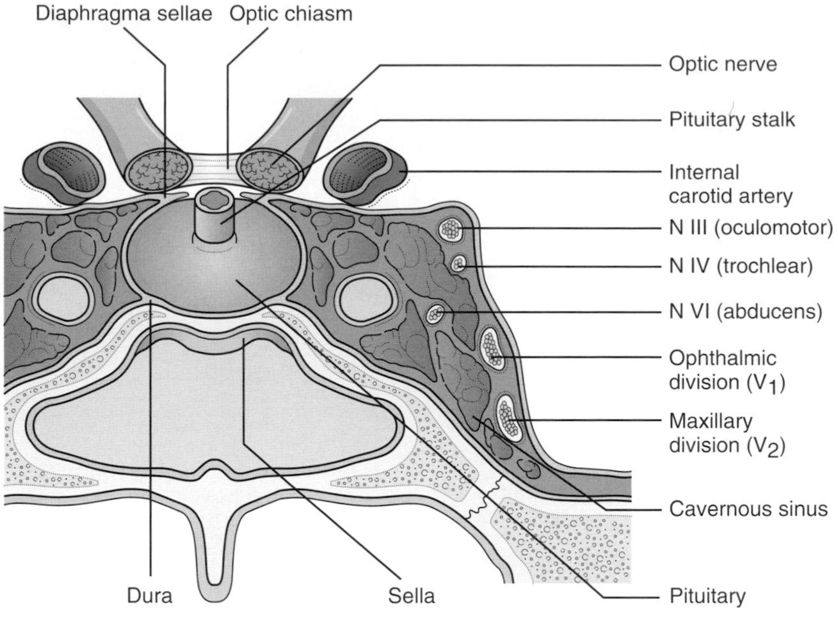

• **Fig. 29.1** Anatomic relationships of the pituitary gland. A coronal section through the sella turcica shows the pituitary gland in relation to surrounding structures: the cavernous sinuses; carotid arteries; and cranial nerves II, III, IV, V1, V2, and VI. (From Ellenbogen RG, Sekhar LN, Kitchen ND: *Principles of neurological surgery*, ed 4, St. Louis, 2018, Elsevier.)

gland, which is also regulated by the hypothalamus, secretes vasopressin and oxytocin. The hormones of the pituitary influence target organs, which are therefore affected by pathology of the pituitary gland.

Almost all pituitary tumors originate in the anterior lobe, and most are benign adenomas. Seventy-five percent of these adenomas cause an inappropriate amount of hormone secretion. Pituitary adenomas are most commonly found in adults in their fourth to sixth decade of life, and they are classified as to their size and functionality. Functioning tumors usually consist of a single cell type and therefore secrete a single hormone, defining the disease process, such as acromegaly and Cushing disease. Nonfunctioning tumors do not secrete excess hormones and are therefore usually not discovered until they are larger. When these tumors reach a critical mass, they impinge on adjacent structures, which leads to specific symptomatology directly related to the structures affected. Pressure on the optic chiasm can lead to vision changes. Numerous other effects can occur as a result of pituitary tumor, including headache, increased ICP due to obstruction of the third ventricle, cranial nerve palsy, and neurologic changes due to vascular occlusion. Tumors may also impinge on the normal pituitary tissue and cause a decrease in hormone secretion.

Acromegaly and Cushing disease are conditions that have many significant implications for the management of anesthesia. Acromegaly results from an excess production of GH when the individual develops the condition in adulthood, and gigantism if the condition develops before epiphyseal closure. The most common cause of acromegaly is a pituitary somatotroph adenoma that releases GH. An excessive amount of GH stimulates the production of IGF-1 by the liver. Supraphysiologic concentrations of these two

hormones contribute to the signs and symptoms of the disorder, characterized by increased growth and increased carbohydrate, fat, and protein metabolism. The onset of the defining characteristics can evolve over 10 years before fully developing. As a result, the signs and symptoms of acromegaly may be very subtle, which makes this endocrine disorder difficult to correctly diagnose.

Excessive amounts of growth hormone cause an overgrowth of the bony and soft tissues, which can be seen in the mouth, tongue, and laryngeal cartilages. The resulting prognathism, macroglossia, and enlargement of the uvula can hinder ventilation and intubation. Other anatomic changes associated with acromegaly include thickening of the vocal cords, reduced size of the laryngeal aperture, and hypertrophy of the periepiglottic folds. Obstructive sleep apnea (OSA) is seen in 60% to 75% of individuals who have acromegaly. Recurrent laryngeal nerve palsy has been observed and attributed to tissue overgrowth and the subsequent tension exerted on the nerve. Compression of the trachea as a result of an enlarged thyroid has also been described. Hypertension is seen in 30% of acromegalic patients and is commonly associated with myocardial hypertrophy. Diabetes mellitus is observed in 25% of these patients and can drastically affect perioperative care.

The pituitary gland secretes adrenocorticotrophic hormone (ACTH or corticotropin), which causes cortisol secretion by the adrenal gland. Cushing syndrome results from excessive secretion of cortisol. The etiology of Cushing syndrome includes medications that stimulate the production of glucocorticoids, adrenal tumors, ectopic ACTH production, and Cushing disease, resulting from ACTH-secreting pituitary tumors. Hypersecretion of cortisol has dramatic and systemic effects on the body, which include truncal obesity, redistribution of fat ("moon face"), proximal myopathy, osteoporosis, hypertension, left ventricular hypertrophy, hypernatremia, hypervolemia, hypokalemia, OSA, gastrointestinal reflux, glucose intolerance, insomnia, and depression.

The diagnosis of Cushing syndrome is based on assessing free cortisol levels, which are measured in urine (>250 mcg/24 hr). Other assays that are used to measure plasma corticotropin are utilized to differentiate between corticotropin-dependent and corticotropin-independent hypercortisolism. Nearly 70% of the cases of corticotropin-dependent hypercortisolism are the result of Cushing disease. The diagnosis of an ectopic cortisol source can be excluded by using a high-dose dexamethasone suppression test.

Surgical Procedure

The treatment of choice for a well-circumscribed pituitary tumor is a transsphenoidal hypophysectomy, which accounts for approximately 20% of the intracranial surgeries done in academic institutions. This procedure debulks the pituitary mass and, as a result, endocrine function improves. Access to the pituitary gland is best achieved via the transsphenoidal approach, although this technique may not be possible if very large tumors exist. This technique is achieved either from a sublabial or endonasal approach. It minimizes surgical trauma to the brain and has the least incidence of complications. Once the sphenoid sinus is traversed, access to the sella turcica is achieved by removing the inferior portion. The surgeon is able to remove the tumor using a microscope. The imaging techniques that are employed include fluoroscopy, ultrasound, frameless stereotaxis, three-dimensional computer-assisted neuronavigation, or MRI. The free space created by excision of the tumor can be packed with synthetic reabsorbing material, fat, fascia, or muscle that is harvested from the abdomen or thigh. This graft also seals the dura. The bone fragment from the floor of the sella turcica and the sphenoid sinus is packed.

Anesthetic Management and Considerations

Preoperative Period

1. *Discuss the preoperative evaluation of a patient with a pituitary tumor.*

   Evaluation of the prolactin concentration, thyroid function test, and an MRI should be performed preoperatively. Although thyroid gland dysfunction is rarely caused by a pituitary adenoma, it is important to determine if the patient is euthyroid. An MRI yields superior results compared with a computed tomography (CT) scan because of its capability for differentiating soft tissues. This difference allows the surgeon to identify the presence of microadenomas. Depending on the disease process, a more in-depth evaluation should be performed based on the target organs affected, such as the musculoskeletal, cardiovascular, and respiratory systems.

2. *Discuss the neurologic abnormalities possible in a patient with a pituitary tumor.*

   Functional tumors rarely extend beyond the sella turcica and therefore they seldom produce symptoms by mass effect. Nonfunctional tumors are usually not diagnosed until the tumor is outside the sella, causing impingement on adjacent structures. A pituitary tumor is the most common cause of bitemporal hemianopsia due to its close proximity to the optic chiasm. The cavernous sinuses exist lateral to the sella and contain cranial nerves III, IV, V, and VI, as shown in Fig. 29.1. Cranial nerve palsy can result from compression of these nerves. Increased ICP due to the tumor mass may cause symptoms such as headache, papilledema, and altered level of consciousness.

3. *Discuss the anatomic airway abnormalities and associated anesthetic implications that are observed in a patient with acromegaly.*

   Distinct abnormalities in the airway anatomy of patients with acromegaly were first described in 1896, when a dying patient was described to have respiratory failure. The autopsy of this patient described a narrow glottic opening, thickened laryngeal cartilages, and soft tissue hypertrophy. Further investigation showed the presence of laryngeal stenosis, subglottic narrowing, and vocal cord paralysis, resulting from recurrent laryngeal nerve stretching. These changes, in conjunction with prognathism, macroglossia, and hypertrophy of the lips and epiglottis, can make airway management challenging. It has been estimated that 12% to 30% of acromegalic patients will be difficult to intubate by direct laryngoscopy. It has been suggested that glottic or subglottic involvement can be suspected if hoarseness, stridor, or OSA is observed. These findings strongly suggest the need for alternative airway management strategies such as an awake intubation. The use of a smaller endotracheal tube than what would be expected is prudent to avoid soft tissue trauma, bleeding, and subsequent edema.

Intraoperative Period

4. *Describe the positioning considerations for transsphenoidal hypophysectomy.*

   Because the approach of a transsphenoidal hypophysectomy involves either a sublabial or endonasal approach, the surgeon must have access to the upper lip and nose. The operating table and patient are rotated 180 degrees. The patient's head is slightly elevated and secured in a headrest. This head position increases the potential for a venous air embolus to occur. The surgeon typically stands to the left of the patient, and the patient's head is therefore turned to the left. The endotracheal tube should be secured to the left side of the mouth and taped to the patient's cheek or lower lip.

5. *Discuss the potential cardiovascular abnormalities for a patient with acromegaly and Cushing disease.*

   Half of all untreated acromegalic patients die before the age of 50, and the increased mortality is attributed to cardiac disease. Approximately half of normotensive patients with acromegaly have left ventricular hypertrophy. Increases in cardiac output and stroke volume may also be observed in conjunction with the increased ventricular mass. Diastolic dysfunction evidenced by decreased left ventricular compliance and resulting in increased left ventricular filling pressure is characteristic of acromegalic cardiomyopathy. Large proximal coronary arteries are rarely affected in acromegalic patients, but distal branches may become stenotic. An increased incidence of supraventricular and ventricular ectopy with exertion has been described in this patient population. ECG abnormalities associated with acromegaly include bundle branch block, ST-segment depression, and T-wave abnormalities.

It is estimated that nearly 80% of all patients with Cushing disease have hypertension, and 50% of those untreated have a diastolic blood pressure >100 mm Hg. Considering these findings, ECG abnormalities are common, such as high-voltage quick release system (QRS) complexes, inverted T waves, and left ventricular hypertrophy, as evidenced by strain patterns. Diastolic dysfunction is prevalent in over 40% of patients with Cushing disease.

6. *Discuss the intraoperative anesthetic considerations when caring for the patient with Cushing disease.*

Obstructive sleep apnea is present in over one half of all patients with Cushing disease. Hyperglycemia frequently occurs, and intraoperative blood glucose assessment is imperative. One-third of patients with Cushing disease exhibit exophthalmos, which predisposes these patients to developing corneal abrasions. Thinning skin, resulting from hypercortisolism, leads to the presence of superficial veins, which can make vascular cannulation difficult. Pathologic fractures occur in approximately 20% of these patients due to the development of osteoporosis. Therefore careful positioning and padding all pressure points are vital. Due to protein catabolism, muscle hypermetabolism resulting in weakness occurs. The dose of muscle relaxant medication should be decreased and subsequently dosed based on the response to peripheral nerve stimulation. The presence of hypokalemia should be corrected preoperatively to avoid the untoward cardiac effects and inhibit further skeletal muscle weakness.

7. *Describe the anesthetic complications that can be encountered during a transsphenoidal hypophysectomy.*

Because vital neurologic structures exist within close proximity of the pituitary gland, adequate muscle relaxation should be maintained throughout surgery to avoid inadvertent patient movement and subsequent trauma. Such trauma may produce cranial nerve damage, injury to the optic chiasm, or vascular injury. The internal carotid arteries exist lateral to the pituitary gland, and massive hemorrhage can occur as a result of accidental dissection. In the event of internal carotid hemorrhage, deliberate hypotension may be necessary during surgical repair. The expected blood loss is usually minimal but

may be significant if the tumor is large or involves the suprasellar region. The surgeon may request a Valsalva maneuver to assess for a cerebrospinal fluid (CSF) leak. If a CSF leak is discovered, the sella turcica is often packed with autologous fat.

Postoperative Period

8. *Explain the anesthetic considerations related to emergence and extubation for a patient undergoing transsphenoidal hypophysectomy.*

A significant amount of blood can passively enter the patient's stomach during surgery. Because blood has known emetogenic effects, it should be removed at the conclusion of the case by orogastric suctioning. An oral airway should be placed before emergence to encourage the patient to breathe through his or her mouth because the nasal cavity is packed. Although deep extubation can be performed in neurosurgical patients, awake extubation is most often appropriate, especially if ventilation and intubation were difficult. If airway management was difficult, extubation can occur using an endotracheal tube changer. Pharyngeal suctioning should occur before emergence to avoid excessive stimulation and coughing. During emergence, intravenous lidocaine can be administered to blunt hyperreactive airway reflexes.

A postoperative assessment of the patient's neurologic status needs is performed expeditiously. This can be facilitated by administering drugs that produce short clinical effects, such as propofol and remifentanil, and inhalation agents with low blood solubility, such as sevoflurane.

9. *Explain the importance of a comprehensive neurologic examination postoperatively.*

An in-depth neurologic assessment needs to be done postoperatively to evaluate the involvement of structures in close proximity to the surgical site such as the internal carotid arteries; cranial nerves III, IV, V, and IV; and the optic chiasm. Complications involving these structures include carotid artery spasm and hemorrhage, cranial nerve damage, and visual changes, respectively. Postoperative bleeding may impinge on the brainstem causing visual changes and altered level of consciousness. If deficits or abnormalities are discovered, an immediate direct assessment utilizing CT, MRI, or reexploration is indicated.

10. *Discuss the postoperative complications that may have a delayed onset after transsphenoidal hypophysectomy.*

Complications involving neuroendocrine abnormalities may not be detectable in the immediate postoperative period. Disruption of the posterior pituitary can lead to diabetes insipidus (DI) or syndrome of inappropriate antidiuretic hormone (SIADH) secretion. These conditions usually become evident in the first 24 to 48 hours after surgery and are rarely seen in the immediate postoperative period. DI occurs in approximately 25% of these patients; however, DI is usually transient.

A urinary catheter may be placed intraoperatively and maintained postoperatively for assessment of urinary output. Treatment of DI includes fluid and electrolyte replacement and administration of vasopressin.

Assessing the patient for the presence of fluid draining into their throat, frequent swallowing, or continuous drainage can be indicative of a CSF leak. Nausea and vomiting occur in nearly 40% of neurosurgical patients and can have detrimental consequences on increased ICP. The use of prophylactic antiemetic medication should be incorporated into the plan of care. Hypopituitarism can also occur in the postoperative period. Plasma cortisol levels may decrease significantly after micro-adenomectomy, and this situation will require corticosteroid administration to avoid the development of acute adrenal crises.

Review Questions

1. Which statement regarding an acromegaly is false?
   a. The etiology is excess secretion of growth hormone.
   b. The signs and symptom develop rapidly.
   c. A narrow glottic opening and subglottic stenosis should be anticipated.
   d. A gradual change in voice occurs.
2. Which comorbid factor is uncommon in a patient with acromegaly?
   a. Biventricular hypertrophy
   b. Obesity
   c. Insulin resistance
   d. Sleep apnea
3. Which complication is least frequently observed in the immediate postoperative period after transsphenoidal hypophysectomy?
   a. Diabetes insipidus
   b. Altered level of consciousness
   c. Cranial nerve palsy
   d. Visual changes
4. Which anesthetic consideration is most appropriate for a patient having transsphenoidal hypophysectomy?
   a. Muscle relaxation should be used to avoid patient movement
   b. Placement of a laryngeal mask airway is suggested to avoid coughing on emergence
   c. Long-acting analgesics are beneficial to ensure a smooth emergence and analgesia in the postoperative period
   d. Either an oral or nasal endotracheal tube is acceptable
5. Which cardiovascular abnormality is least likely associated with Cushing disease?
   a. Aortic stenosis
   b. Diastolic dysfunction
   c. Inverted T waves
   d. Hypertension

Suggested Readings

Bernabeu I, Aller J, Álvarez-Escolá C, et al. Criteria for diagnosis and postoperative control of acromegaly, and screening and management of its comorbidities: expert consensus. *Endocrinol Diabetes Nutr* 2018;65(5):297-305.

Ezzat S, Caspar-Bell GM, Chik CL, et al. Predictive markers for postsurgical medical management of acromegaly: a systematic review and consensus treatment guideline. *Endocr Pract* 2019;25(4):379-393.

Holdaway IM, Rajasoorya CR, Gamble GD. Factors influencing mortality in acromegaly. *J Clin Endocrinol Metab* 2004;89:667-674.

Hong GK, Payne SC, Jane JA Jr. Anatomy, physiology, and laboratory evaluation of the pituitary gland. *Otolaryngol Clin North Am* 2016;49(1):21-32.

Kim JH, Hur KY, Lee JH, et al. Outcome of endoscopic transsphenoidal surgery for acromegaly. *World Neurosurg* 2017;104:272-278.

Melmed S, Bronstein MD, Chanson P, et al. A Consensus Statement on acromegaly therapeutic outcomes. *Nat Rev Endocrinol* 2018;14(9):552-561.

Parolin M, Dassie F, Alessio L, et al. Obstructive sleep apnea in acromegaly and the effect of treatment: a systematic review and meta-analysis. *J Clin Endocrinol Metab* 2020;105(3). pii: dgz116.

Pazarlı AC, Köseoğlu Hİ, Kutlutürk F, et al. Association of acromegaly and central sleep apnea syndrome. *Turk Thorac J* 2017;20(2):157-159.

Ranalli LJ, Taylor GA. Neuroanatomy, neurophysiology, and neuroanesthesia. In: Nagelhout JJ, Elisha S, eds. *Nurse Anesthesia*, 6th ed. St Louis, MO: Elsevier, 2018:645-681.

Seidman PA, Kofke WA, Policare R, et al. Anaesthetic complications of acromegaly. *Br J Anaesth* 2000;84:179-182.

Smith M, Hirsch NP. Pituitary disease and anaesthesia. *Br J Anaesth* 2000;85(1):3-14.

Wall RT. Endocrine disease. In Hines RL, Marschall KE, eds. *Anesthesia and Co-Existing Disease*, 7th ed. St. Louis, MO: Elsevier, 2018:345-475.

30

Asleep-Awake Craniotomy

KEY POINTS

- Asleep-awake craniotomies are necessary in only a small percentage of patients—those in whom seizure focus may be suppressed during general anesthesia or may be adjacent to the "eloquent" cortex.
- The eloquent cortex is defined as areas of the cortex that, if removed, will result in loss of sensory processing or linguistic ability, minor paralysis, or paralysis.
- The most common areas of the eloquent cortex are in the left temporal and frontal lobes for speech and language, bilateral occipital lobes for vision, bilateral parietal lobes for sensation, and bilateral motor cortex for movement.

- When these conditions exist, an awake craniotomy may be the best/only option to identify the seizure focus and minimize brain injury.
- One of the most important elements for a successful asleep-awake craniotomy is a highly motivated and well-informed patient.
- Factors that mitigate the successful conduct of an asleep-awake craniotomy include intraoperative confusion, nausea, and seizures.

Case Synopsis

A 59-year-old white female presents with a left frontal oligodendroglioma tumor that has recurred in various areas of the eloquent cortex. She has also experienced several recent seizures. Due to the recurrence in the eloquent cortex and seizure history, the neurosurgeon elects to proceed with an asleep-awake craniotomy with intraoperative mapping of the eloquent cortex and electrocorticographic identification of the seizure nidus.

Preoperative Evaluation and Demographic Data

Past Medical/Surgical History

- Hypertension
- Seizures
- Smoking history of 25 years
- Left frontal craniotomy with partial tumor resection in 1986 under general anesthesia; no anesthetic complications
- Gamma knife treatment of tumor recurrence

List of Medications

- Phenytoin
- Depakote
- Metoprolol
- Dexamethasone
- Famotidine

Diagnostic Data

- Hemoglobin, 12.8 g/dL; hematocrit, 38%
- Glucose, 176 mg/dL (week before surgery)

- Electrolytes: sodium, 132 mEq/L; potassium, 3.6 mEq/L (week before surgery)
- Phenytoin level, 12 mcg/dL; Depakote level, 86 mcg/mL (week before surgery)

Height/Weight/Vital Signs

- 160 cm, 81 kg
- Blood pressure, 164/88; heart rate, 58 beats per minute; respiratory rate, 21 breaths per minute; room air oxygen saturation, 96%; temperature, 37.1°C

Pathophysiology

Representing approximately 10% of all primary brain and central nervous system tumors, oligodendroglioma is a well-differentiated, diffusely infiltrating tumor that occurs in adults and is typically located in the cerebral hemispheres. These tumors are predominantly composed of cells that morphologically resemble oligodendroglia. In 50% to 80% of the cases, patients with oligodendrogliomas present with seizures reflective of increased intracranial pressure. Because of the typically slow growth of oligodendrogliomas, the elapsed time between the initial symptoms and clinical diagnosis may vary from 1 week to 12 years. Oligodendrogliomas, like all other infiltrating gliomas, have a very high rate of recurrence. Historically, surgery has been the mainstay of treatment for oligodendrogliomas. The extent of resection depends in large part on the location of the tumor and its proximity to the eloquent cortex. If possible, the goal is total resection of the tumor. In patients who undergo total gross resection, no further treatment may be necessary, but the patient must be followed up for clinical or radiologic recurrence.

Surgical Procedure

The removal of an oligodendroglioma recurrence is accomplished by a left frontotemporal craniotomy. After adequate exposure of the cortical surface is achieved, mapping of areas which, when stimulated via Ojemann stimulator, produce aphasia is accomplished. Ojemann stimulation results in an inability to speak, and this apparatus is marked with numbered plastic indicators and recorded (areas of aphasia). After the mapping of the areas of aphasia, Ojemann stimulation is used to identify areas where stimulation results in an inability to name the playing card shown to the patient while stimulation is occurring (areas of aphasia and anomia), as depicted in Fig. 30.1. Placement of cortical electrodes are used to electrocortigraphically identify areas of seizure activity, as is also shown in Fig. 30.1. Surgical removal of the tumor is guided by the boundaries identified by cortical mapping and includes areas identified by electrocorticography.

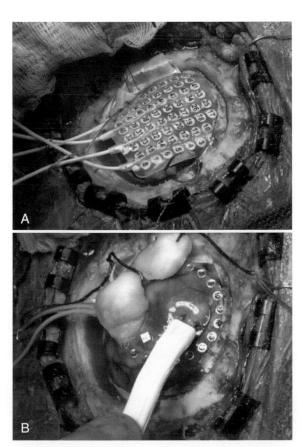

• **Fig. 30.1** Brain electrocorticography and mapping. Images of a left-sided frontal craniotomy showing intraoperative brain mapping during an awake craniotomy. (A) Electrocorticography with a high-density grid to identify cortical epileptogenic discharges. Patients are monitored during 6 to 8 minutes of (B) electrocorticography for continuous monitoring along with cortical stimulation with the Ojemann stimulator for brain mapping to identify eloquent areas of the brain. (From Chaichana K, Quinones-Hinojosa A: *Comprehensive overview of modern surgical approaches to intrinsic brain tumors*, St. Louis, 2019, Elsevier.)

Anesthetic Management and Considerations

Preoperative Period

1. *Discuss the role, contents, and timing of preoperative education surrounding asleep-awake craniotomy.*

It is essential that preoperative education for a patient undergoing an asleep-awake craniotomy be thorough, frank, and conducted in such a manner that both the patient and the anesthetist believe that the anticipated procedure should and can be accomplished in an awake state. The anesthetist, who is directly responsible for the conduct of the asleep-awake craniotomy and will be present throughout the procedure, should meet with the patient at a date before the surgery.

The preoperative education should allow first for the anesthetist to assess the suitability of the patient for an asleep-awake craniotomy. Only those patients with the ability to clearly understand risks and benefits and who, in the opinion of the neurosurgeon and the anesthetist, will cooperate during surgery should be considered as candidates for an asleep-awake craniotomy. The preoperative education of the patient should focus on what the patient is to expect from a sensory standpoint. Visually, they are to be instructed in what to expect in the operating room, what they will be seeing when they emerge under the drapes, who they will see, and how they will be dressed. The odors can be especially offensive to some patients and should be explained, especially regarding use of the electrocautery. Tastes regarding use of airway devices and medications should also be explained. The sensation of feeling and touch should focus on how the patient will be positioned and the use of the Mayfield head holder, the awkward body positioning with the need for minimal movement, and the potential for significant discomfort. Special emphasis should be placed on the sounds that may be heard. Usually patients are emerging from anesthesia during removal of the bone flap. The drilling sound is conducted directly to the ear and can be quite loud and disturbing to the patient. The preoperative education should focus next on the required activities of the patient during the surgery.

The mapping of aphasia and anomia should be clearly explained to the patient with attention for the potential of Ojemann stimulation to result in temporary aphasia and anomia. The preoperative education should focus on how intraoperative issues will be addressed. The patient's seizure history should be thoroughly addressed to assess the presence of "aura," time of day when most seizures occur, and medications. The anesthetist must have a clear understanding of the type of seizure the patient has historically and its presentation.

The patient should be fully informed of all plans for dealing with seizures encountered during the procedure. The potential for emergent intubation and general anesthesia should the patient become uncooperative or have persistent seizure activity, airway compromise, or hemo-dynamic instability should also be discussed. All additional questions should be addressed, and a written outline of all these details should be provided to the patient for further review. Arguably, the single most important element in the successful awake craniotomy is the well-informed patient.

Intraoperative Period

2. *Describe the induction of and maintenance of the "asleep" portion of the awake craniotomy.*

The purpose of the "asleep" portion of the awake craniotomy is to minimize patient discomfort and facilitate placement of invasive monitoring, patient positioning, local anesthetic injection, removal of the cranium, and placement of Mayfield pins. This patient is given appropriate prophylactic antibiotics before arrival in the operating room. Ondansetron is administered before the induction of anesthesia to decrease the potential for nausea and vomiting.

After monitors are placed, induction is accomplished using propofol followed by a remifentanil-and-propofol infusion. A laryngeal mask airway (LMA) is placed and secured. The patient is manually ventilated to achieve a rate and tidal volume that is sufficient to produce an end tidal carbon dioxide ($ETCO_2$) representative of low normocarbia ($ETCO_2$ 28 to 32 mm Hg). Increases in CO_2 levels above normal concentrations, regardless of whether the patient is awake or asleep, will cause an increase in cerebral blood flow that will increase intracranial pressure (ICP). Anesthesia is maintained with the propofol-and-remifentanil infusion while all invasive monitoring is accomplished.

The patient is placed in a Mayfield headrest after local infiltration and secured to the operating table with straps across the chest, hips, and legs. The surgical field is infiltrated with local anesthesia, surgical prepping and draping are accomplished, and surgery is initiated. Careful attention is placed to the head positioning to assure:

- Access to the airway is always maintained
- The LMA is secured and positioned such that it can be rapidly reinserted should the need arise
- The patient can see the anesthetist and is able to see the pictures/playing cards necessary for anomia mapping
- Patient comfort is maximized
- The patient's joints are flexed and the body is secured to avoid movement when turning the table from side to side

A light is placed under the drapes and positioned to provide light to the patient at all times. At this time an arterial blood gas, electrolyte levels, and antiseizure medication levels are collected and administered as indicated.

3. *Cite various methods that can be used to reduce intracranial pressure during an awake craniotomy.*

Controlling ICP is vitally important during an awake craniotomy. The primary method that is used to reduce ICP in awake craniotomies is accomplished by using osmotic diuretics and hypertonic saline. Immediately after the central line is secured and the urinary catheter has been placed, 1 to 1.25 gm/kg of mannitol is administered. Additionally, 150 mL of 7.5% normal saline are administered over a 2-hour period. Both of these medications facilitate the movement of fluid from the extravascular space into the intravascular space, which decreases the total brain fluid volume and ICP.

These patients often develop cerebral edema associated with the lesion, and dexamethasone 10 mg. It is prudent to avoid medications/techniques that increase ICP, and these are listed in Box 30.1.

4. *Describe the interventions that can be used to treat intraoperative nausea, confusion, and seizures during an awake craniotomy.*

Any anesthetic plan for an asleep-awake craniotomy must account for management of nausea, confusion, and seizures.

- **Nausea:** Treatment of intraoperative nausea focuses on avoiding factors that contribute to nausea such as hypotension, pain, and medications that are especially emetogenic. Rapid movement of the patient subsequent to the administration of anesthetic agents can result in nausea. Moving the patient during the procedure should be done slowly after requesting that the patient close their eyes before movement. Additional prophylaxis for nausea includes the administration of ondansetron before induction, the use of propofol for anesthesia induction and maintenance, and administration of dexamethasone and the use of ephedrine to treat nausea related to hypotension. Acute episodes of nausea that are unrelated to hypotension may be treated with additional doses of ondansetron. If hypotension occurs, additional doses of ephedrine or vasopressor agents can be administered.
- **Anesthetic management:** Local anesthesia is the primary anesthetic during the awake phases of the operation. The local anesthesia that is injected subcutaneously contains epinephrine, which causes vasoconstriction of local vessels, and, after absorption, the systemic effects including tachycardia and increased blood pressure can occur. The maintenance

---

• BOX 30.1   Factors That May Increase Intracranial Pressure

- Hypercarbia
- Hypoxia
- Coughing/straining
- Venous outlet obstruction from improper positioning
- Trendelenburg position
- Hypertension
- Fluid overload

of anesthesia during the period when the skull cap is removed is accomplished by using short-acting anesthetic agents so that hemodynamic instability can be rapidly treated and emergence can occur quickly. Pain can be alleviated by administering short-acting narcotics and augmentation of the field block by the surgeon.

- **Level of consciousness:** Treatment of confusion focuses on avoiding anesthetic agents that contribute to amnesia and can often cause confusion. Medications such as benzodiazepines (midazolam), hypnotics such as diphenhydramine, antidopaminergics such as droperidol or haloperidol, and phenothiazines such as Phenergan or Thorazine should be avoided if possible. Appropriate preoperative preparation is crucial for preventing confusion. Because most patients having an awake craniotomy are emerging from general anesthesia during the removal of the bone flap, explaining to the patient that there will be noise from surgical interventions such as drilling is imperative. Additionally, it is well recognized that any preoperative focal neurologic deficits will be enhanced immediately upon emerging from general anesthesia.

This patient exhibited difficulty with verbal expression soon after emergence; however, she was prepared that expressive aphasia, receptive aphasia, or both might occur. Immediately upon emergence, she was unable to speak although she would hold up fingers appropriately. This possibility had been discussed with the patient preoperatively and resulted in minimal discomfort.

- **Seizures:** The treatment of all intraoperative seizures is predicated on the assumption that the potential for seizures has been adequately treated preoperatively, as evidenced by therapeutic blood concentrations of antiseizure medications. Blood should be drawn immediately after the induction of anesthesia to determine the phenytoin and Depakote concentrations. Also, cold irrigating fluid placed on the brain by the surgeon has been used to inhibit seizure activity.

This patient's phenytoin level is low, 5 mcg/dL (normal range 10 to 20 mcg/dL) and after induction she was treated with phenytoin 500 mg before emergence. The diagnosis and treatment for intraoperative active seizures must address the following:

- Is the activity being exhibited a seizure?
- Is it a focal seizure or consistent with the seizures reported in the preoperative visit?
- Is the seizure progressing to a grand mal seizure?

During Ojemann stimulation, it may be difficult to determine the onset of aphasia compared with "absence" seizure activity. The treatment for seizures is to stop the stimulation, and frequently no further treatment is routinely necessary. A thorough preoperative seizure history will also determine the presence of any "aura," which the patient is instructed to report to the anesthetist if they occur. The treatment of the aura is

the same as for a seizure: stopping brain stimulation. Should the twitching continue, 10 to 20 mg of propofol may be given. If the seizure activity is inconsistent with that reported preoperatively and/or appears to be progressing to uncontrollable movements of the head and neck after withdrawal of stimulation, application of cold saline to the cortical surface by the neurosurgeon is indicated. If seizure activity continues, administration of propofol 100 to 200 mg and reinsertion of the LMA are indicated.

The major concerns if a grand mal seizure occurs and is sustained during awake craniotomy are that the violent movement may result in cervical trauma or the head springing free from the Mayfield apparatus and lacerating the scalp on the sharp pins. Also, the increased cerebral neuronal activity will increase the cerebral metabolic rate of oxygen consumption and can also result in swelling of the brain and increased ICP.

5. *Describe one technique for awakening the patient while their head is in a Mayfield headrest.*

When the patient emerges from general anesthesia, they are in a confined, draped, and dark environment. Their movements are restrained by multiple straps, and their head is fixed in the three pins of the Mayfield headrest. Because it takes longer to emerge from propofol than remifentanil, after completing the skin flap, during the creation of burr holes, the propofol infusion is discontinued and the remifentanil drip is decreased and then stopped. The patient emerges from general anesthesia, and the LMA is removed just before the bone flap removal. Continuation of the propofol and remifentanil infusions until the bone flap is removed can result in hypoventilation, causing hypercarbia, and the brain can become swollen at the dural incision.

6. *Discuss appropriate sedation techniques after the awake data have been gathered.*

When the neurosurgeon determines that patient participation is no longer essential, sedation may be established. The use of medications and dosages that can contribute to confusion and dysphoria should be avoided. If sedation is to be established before dural closure, respiratory depression will result in cerebral edema and closure of the dural will be difficult. Nausea can be triggered by use of narcotics such as morphine, and these are avoided. Tailoring the depth of sedation should be determined by the individual's current level of anxiety and discomfort. Administering dexmedetomidine may be useful to produce sedation without causing significant respiratory depression.

7. *Develop an anesthetic plan for airway management during an asleep-awake craniotomy.*

Any plan for managing the airway during an asleep-awake craniotomy must take into account the three distinct times of the surgery: the asleep phase, the awake phase, and the sedation phase.

The asleep phase of the surgery must account for the physiologic stimulation that occurs during fixation of the head in the Mayfield headrest. Coughing and bucking during extubation while the patient's head is fixed to this apparatus is contraindicated. Because the LMA is situated above the vocal cords, subglottic nociceptive reflexes are minimally stimulated, and bucking may be minimized compared with an endotracheal tube.

The awake and sedation phases of the procedure do not frequently require airway manipulation. The placement of a nasal cannula with $ETCO_2$ monitoring is sufficient during these phases. Airway obstruction is usually associated with a medication overdose, and this situation is easily relieved by pulling the chin forward. Talking to the patient and simply requesting that they take a breath may be sufficient. If the patient will require sustained hyperventilation and muscle relaxation, usually an unforeseen surgical event has occurred. In this instance, additional anesthesia personnel will be needed. Reinsertion of the LMA should be accomplished as soon as possible. When the surgical events permit, an endotracheal tube should be placed using a fiber-optic approach, or if removal of the head from the Mayfield headrest is permitted, under direct vision. If the LMA is not able to be reinserted, the patient must be removed from the Mayfield headrest immediately and bag–mask ventilation established. An induction agent and muscle relaxant are indicated during intubation in order to rapidly facilitate airway management and avoid increases in ICP.

Postoperative Period

8. *Discuss the potential causes of nausea, confusion, and seizures during the immediate postoperative period.*

Upon the completion of surgery, the patient's head is removed from the Mayfield headrest and the drapes are removed. The patient should be cautioned against exaggerated head movement. Due to the removal of the tumor and associated tissue, intracranial volume is decreased. Shearing of cerebral venous complexes can lead to the development of a subdural hematoma. Nausea, confusion, and lethargy can be symptoms associated with a subdural hematoma. The presence of iatrogenic intracranial pathology should be excluded during the evaluation.

Presentation of seizures immediately postoperatively should be evaluated and managed as in the intraoperative portion of the procedure. Auras and small focal seizures consistent with preoperative history and intraoperative experience should be observed, noted, and reported to the surgeon. The decision to administer supplemental antiseizure medication during the postoperative period is at the discretion of the surgeon. If focal seizures occur and progress to grand mal seizures, administration of an induction dose of propofol should be administered and airway management initiated. Valsalva maneuvers and jerking movements can lead to intracerebral bleeding and cerebral edema, which both increase ICP.

Review Questions

1. The single most important factor in a successful awake craniotomy is:
   a. A low-grade tumor in the Broca area.
   b. Maintaining normocarbia.
   c. Decreasing ICP.
   d. A highly motivated, well-informed patient.
2. All of the information should be discussed during preoperative education except:
   a. The patient's seizure history.
   b. The limitations regarding the head being placed in a fixed position.
   c. The options communicated by the surgeon should the asleep-awake option fail.
   d. The activities that the patient will be required to perform while they are awake.
3. A patient undergoing an awake craniotomy experiences a focal seizure that is resistant to two small doses of propofol and then progresses to generalized tonic/clonic seizures. The most appropriate initial intervention includes:
   a. Instilling cold irrigation solution to the brain.
   b. Increasing the dose of ketamine.
   c. Administering diazepam.
   d. Administering succinylcholine.
4. The patient emerging from the "asleep" part of the "asleep-awake" craniotomy, if properly prepared, will encounter all of the following except:
   a. Their head fixed to a rigid frame.
   b. A loud drilling noise.
   c. A dark and confined space.
   d. A sharp pain on the left side of the chest.
5. The indications for awake craniotomy include:
   a. Patients with receptive aphasia.
   b. Patients with tumors in areas of the eloquent cortex.
   c. Patients without an opinion as to whether they have general or local anesthesia.
   d. Patients who have very high pain tolerance.

Suggested Readings

Abaziou T, Tincres F, Mrozek S, et al. Incidence and predicting factors of perioperative complications during monitored anesthesia care for awake craniotomy. *J Clin Anesth* 2020;64:109811.

Erickson KM, Cole DJ. Anesthetic considerations for awake craniotomy for epilepsy. *Anesthesiol Clin* 2007;25(3):535-555.

Eseonu CI, Rincon-Torroella J, Lee YM, et al. Intraoperative seizures in awake craniotomy for perirolandic glioma resections that undergo cortical mapping. *J Neurol Surg A Cent Eur Neurosurg* 2018;79(3):239-246.

Frost EA, Booij LH. Anesthesia in the patient for awake craniotomy. *Curr Opin Anaesthesiol* 2007;20(4):331-335.

Manninem PH, Mrinalini B, Lukitto K, et al. Patient satisfaction with awake craniotomy for tumor surgery: a comparison of remifentanil and fentanyl in conjunction with propofol. *Anesth Analg* 2006;102(1):237-242.

Natalini D, Ganau M, Rosenkranz R, et al. Comparison of the asleep-awake-asleep technique and monitored anesthesia care during awake craniotomy: a systematic review and metaanalysis. *J Neurosurg Anesthesiol* 2020 Jan 16. doi:10.1097/ANA.0000000000000675

Palese A, Skrap M, Fachin M, et al. The experience of patients undergoing awake craniotomy: in the patients' own words. A qualitative study. *Cancer Nurs* 2008;31(2):166-172.

Petrovich Brennan NM, Whalen S, deMorales Branco D, et al. Object naming is a more sensitive measure of speech localization than number counting: converging evidence from direct cortical stimulation and fMRI. *Neuroimage* 2007;37 Suppl 1:S100–S108.

Piccioni F, Fanzio M. Management of anesthesia in awake craniotomy. *Minerva Anestesiol* 2008;74(7–8):393-408.

Raimann FJ, Adam E, Strouhal U. et al. Dexmedetomidine as adjunct in awake craniotomy - improvement or not? *Anaesthesiol Intensive Ther* 2020;52(1):15-22.

Ranalli LJ, Taylor GA. Neuroanatomy, neurophysiology, and neuroanesthesia. In: Nagelhout JJ, Elisha S, eds. *Nurse Anesthesia*, 6th ed. St Louis, MO: Elsevier, 2018:645-681.

Sewell D, Smith M. Awake craniotomy: anesthetic considerations based on outcome evidence. *Curr Opin Anaesthesiol* 2019;32(5): 546-552.

Sitnikov AR, Grigoryan YA, Mishnyakova LP. Awake craniotomy without sedation in treatment of patients with lesional epilepsy. *Surg Neurol Int* 2018;9:177.

Tachibana S, Tanaka S, Yamakage M. Successful anesthetic management using dexmedetomidine sequentially with propofol in the asleep-awake-asleep technique for elderly patients undergoing awake craniotomy. *Case Rep Anesthesiol* 2020;2020:6795363.

31

Retinal Surgery

KEY POINTS

- Retinal detachments (RDs) are the result of three main causes that include but are not limited to:
  - A hole, break, rip, or tear in the neuronal layer.
  - Exudation of fluid into the subretinal space from retinal vessels.
  - Traction of adhesions between the vitreous gel and the retina.
- Patients presenting for RD surgeries frequently have a constellation of coexisting diseases.

- Many factors influence the type of anesthesia given to the RD patient, and a team approach between the patient, surgeon, and anesthetist is imperative for a successful intraoperative course.
- Nitrous oxide (N_2O) use during general anesthesia will increase the size and pressure of intravitreal tamponading agents.

Case Synopsis

A 73-year-old woman who experienced a spontaneous loss of vision in her right eye is scheduled for a vitrectomy.

Preoperative Evaluation and Demographic Data

Past Medical/Surgical History

- Obesity, body mass index (BMI) of 38 kg/m^2
- Tobacco use history: 1 pack a day for 40 years
- Poor exercise tolerance
- Hypertension
- Non–insulin-dependent diabetes
- Gastroesophageal reflux disease (GERD)
- Previous surgeries: bilateral cataracts
- She has no anesthetic problems, blood transfusions, or familial anesthetic problems.

List of Medications

- Amlodipine (Norvasc)
- Metformin (Glucophage)
- Pantoprazole (Protonix)

Diagnostic Data

- Hematocrit, 39.1%; platelets 240,000/microliter; prothrombin time, 11.1 seconds; partial thromboplastin time, 28 seconds; international normalized ratio, 1.0
- Electrolytes: sodium, 135 mEq/L; potassium, 4.2 mEq/L; chloride, 108 mEq/L; bicarbonate, 31 mEq/L; blood urea nitrogen, 20 mg/dL; creatinine, 1.3 mg/dL; glucose, 190 mg/dL
- Finger stick blood glucose was 187 mg/dL on the morning of surgery
- Electrocardiogram (ECG): normal sinus rhythm with nonspecific T-wave abnormalities
- Stress echocardiogram: left ventricular ejection fraction of 50% with no wall motion abnormalities
- Chest x-ray: small right pleural effusion

Height/Weight/Vital Signs

- 165 cm, 104 kg, BMI 38.2 kg/m^2
- Blood pressure, 149/87; heart rate, 89 beats per minute; respiratory rate, 18; temperature, 36.8°C; room air oxygen saturation, 97%

Pathophysiology

Approximately 1 in 10,000 patients will develop an RD in any given year, with odds of 1 in 300 over a lifetime, and a broad spectrum of symptoms can occur. Most patients will report sensations of flashing lights (related to retinal traction), vision loss, shadows, clouds, or a curtain-like blackness that comes into the field of vision. It can occur spontaneously, when the patient reportedly was straining (working out, running, etc.) or as a result of a trauma such as a motor vehicle accident. Fig. 31.1 represents the anatomic structures that comprise the retina. Approximately 40% to 50% of patients presenting with RDs are myopic, 30% to 40% have had cataract

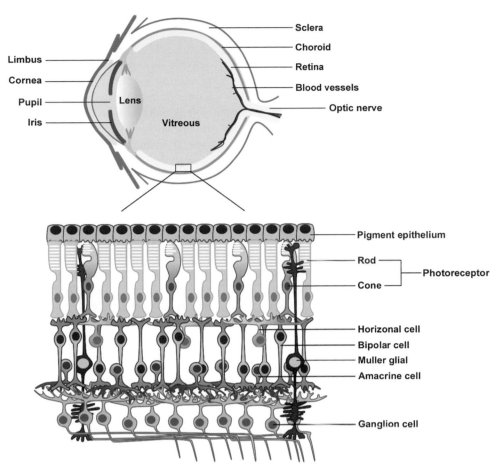

• **Fig. 31.1** Schematic diagram of the anatomy of the eye and layers of the retina. (From Narayan R: *Encyclopedia of biomedical engineering*, Philadelphia, 2019, Elsevier.)

extractions, and 10% to 20% have incurred a direct ocular trauma.

Predisposing factors for the development of an RD include:
- Advanced age (66% of people over 70 years of age will develop an RD)
- Prior eye surgery (especially cataract extraction with or without lens implantation)
- Vitreal diseases such as glaucoma
- RD in the opposite eye
- Metabolic disorders such as diabetic retinopathy
- Vascular disorders such as sickle cell disease
- Tumors
- Myopia

There are three different types of RDs that are based on the etiology of retinal damage: *rhegmatogenous, exudative,* or *tractional.* Rhegmatogenous RDs are the most common form of RD, in which a hole, break, rip, or tear in the neuronal layer allows fluid that is present in the vitreous cavity to separate the sensory and retinal pigment epithelium (RPE) layers. Exudative (serous) detachments occur when subretinal fluid accumulates and causes a detachment without a break or tear in the retina. Tractional RDs occur as a result of adhesions between the vitreous gel and the retina and mechanical forces that cause the separation of the retina

from the RPE without a retinal break. If a greater concentration of adhesions exists, there is a higher incidence that a tear or break may occur in the retina. Fig. 31.1 shows the cross-sectional anatomy of the eye with an associated enlarged retina.

Surgical Procedure

The primary surgical goal of an RD is to restore and/or preserve vision in the affected eye. Two types of surgical procedures, a vitrectomy or scleral buckle, are used to repair RDs and can be utilized separately or in combination, depending on the type and severity of detachment, etiology, or disease process.

A vitrectomy is an intraocular procedure in which three 19- to 25-gauge openings are made into the vitreous cavity. The opening in the inferotemporal quadrant is used to infuse a balanced salt solution throughout the case, while the openings at 10 and 2 o'clock are used to insert a fiber-optic light source and other instruments such as scissors, picks, forceps, and suction. This operation is performed using a microscope with a lens that is either sutured into or held in place over the eye. Once the retina is repaired, a tamponade is needed to rehabilitate sight by securing the retina in the

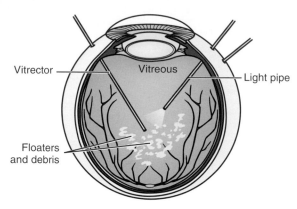

• **Fig. 31.2** Surgical instrumentation orientation for a vitrectomy. (From Phillips N: *Berry & Kohn's operating room technique*, ed 13, St. Louis, 2017, Elsevier.)

Labels on figure: Vitrector, Vitreous, Light pipe, Floaters and debris

proper orientation. An internal tamponading gas bubble is introduced during a vitrectomy to seal a retinal detachment when a scleral buckle alone is not adequate for the repair. These patients must sometimes remain in the prone position postoperatively for several days to facilitate improved retinal reattachment. Silicone oil is utilized as a long-term tamponading agent, and it is injected only in those patients that are at increased risk of developing another retinal detachment. The oil will be removed several months later during a second operation. Silicone oil does not usually necessitate a prone position to elicit its tamponading effect and therefore is particularly useful in patients who cannot cooperate with a prone postoperative position (i.e., children). Surgical instrumentation used for a vitrectomy is shown in Fig. 31.2.

A scleral buckle involves localizing and repairing retinal breaks with a cryoprobe or laser and supporting the damaged retina with an extraocular scleral buckle that consists of a solid or sponge silicone piece. For surgical optimization, a rectus muscle is severed to gain access to the sclera. The retinal tear is then repaired, the silicone buckle is sewn onto the sclera to create an indentation or buckle effect inside the eye, and the muscle is then repaired over the buckle. The buckle is positioned so that it pushes in on the diseased retina (an external tamponading effect), causing the tear to close. Once the break is closed, the subretinal fluid will usually spontaneously resolve over a few days. Sometimes the surgeon elects to drain the subretinal fluid at the time of surgery. Fig. 31.3 illustrates a scleral buckle procedure.

Anesthetic Management and Considerations

Preoperative Period

1. *Define the types of retinal detachments, the coexisting diseases, and anesthetic concerns associated with retinal surgery.*

Rhegmatogenous, exudative, and tractional are the three different types of RDs commonly seen in patients that require treatment. Rhegmatogenous RDs can occur

from stressful activities, straining, or advanced age. Exudative RDs occur as a result of inflammatory processes or tumors. Tractional RDs are usually associated with diabetic retinopathy and sickle cell disease. All patients presenting for repair of RDs, emergently or not, should have a thorough preoperative examination.

It is important to evaluate the patient's cardiovascular status due to the physiologic stress associated with general endotracheal anesthesia (GETA), medications utilized during ophthalmic surgery, and the side effects that can occur with regional blocks. An in-depth preoperative evaluation may be indicated, if time permits, to establish a thorough understanding of any cardiac disease state or altered functional capacity. Many patients with tractional RDs present with diabetes; blood glucose levels should be considered when monitoring throughout the perioperative period. Depending on the patient's normal glucose levels, preoperative optimization in glucose readings may be indicated. Because no absolute consensus has been determined as an ideal glucose value, a range of 90 to 180 mg/dL is an appropriate goal. The risks and benefits associated with the administration of high-dose steroids for preventing postoperative nausea and vomiting (PONV) or edema should also be considered when dealing with diabetic patients, as these medications can dramatically increase blood glucose levels. The anesthetist should also keep in mind that diabetic patients are at increased risk for silent myocardial ischemia (MI). A continuous ECG should be monitored for ischemic changes throughout the perioperative period. Measures such as preoperative aspiration prophylaxis and rapid sequence induction (RSI) should be considered to prevent aspiration caused by diabetic gastroparesis.

Renal and hepatic function must be considered when dealing with patients who have RD. An electrolyte panel is prudent for any patient, especially those that may have renal disease. Several of the medications used in ophthalmic procedures can drastically alter electrolytes and lead to cardiac dysrhythmias, including severe sinus bradycardia, atrial flutter and fibrillation, supraventricular tachycardia, junctional rhythms, and sinus arrest. Altered metabolism and potentially prolonged effects of anesthetics and analgesics should be considered in patients with increased cytochrome P450 enzyme induction or decreased liver function.

Hematologic factors should be considered when coagulopathies are present or specifically with patients who have sickle cell disease. Coagulopathies, either pharmacologically induced or because of a disease state, need to be discussed with the surgical team to determine if a regional technique would be contraindicated due to the risk of hematoma with needle placement.

The patient's level of anxiety needs to be assessed, considered, and treated appropriately. When faced with the possibility of vision loss, many patients develop high levels of anxiety and apprehension. Additionally, they are

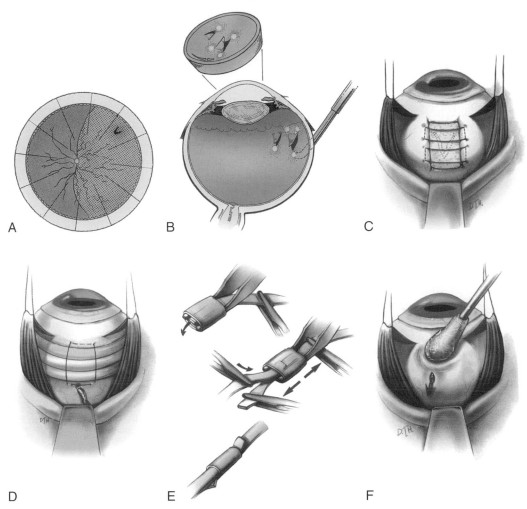

• **Fig. 31.3** Scleral buckling operation for treatment of retinal detachment. (A) Diagram of retina showing detachment of retina of temporal half of left eye, with retinal tear at equator of the globe at 1:30 o'clock position. (B) Examination of the fundus by means of ophthalmoscope and handheld lens and depression of sclera with diathermy electrode. Surgeon visualizes the field and places an electrode beneath the retinal tear; a burn mark is made on the sclera at the site of the retinal tear with a diathermy electrode. (C) A sponge is sutured in place over the treated site of the retinal tear. (D) Band and tire are used to encircle the eye. (E) Placement of Watzke silicone sleeve is one method to secure the edges of the encircling band. (F) Small incision is made through the sclera, and the choroid is finely incised to allow subretinal fluid to drain. (From Ryan SJ, et al: *Retina*, ed 4, St. Louis, 2006, Mosby.)

anxious about the possibility of being conscious or aware during a procedure, can become claustrophobic under the operating room drapes, or are afraid of the pain they might feel during the operation. It is estimated that up to 90% of patients having a vitrectomy experience visual sensation without pain during their procedure that they found frightening if they were not properly informed that these experiences could occur. Appropriate education and preparation, with proper reassurance from both the anesthesia and surgical teams, is indicated before any regional technique.

2. *Identify drugs commonly used during retinal detachment surgery that may affect coexisting diseases in this patient population.*

   The effects of several drugs that are important for the ophthalmologist must be used with caution for patients who present for retinal surgery. Topical phenylephrine, when used in the concentrated 10% solution, may cause severe hypertension and should be used with caution or avoided in patients with severe coronary artery disease, history of MI, dysrhythmias, or those with cerebral aneurysms. Patients with borderline renal and cardiovascular function should be evaluated before an infusion of mannitol, an osmotic diuretic, is administered. Large doses of mannitol can be used to decrease intraocular pressure (IOP), but this intervention can also result in serious side effects such as renal failure, congestive heart failure, pulmonary congestion, electrolyte imbalances, extremes in blood pressures, MI, and allergic reactions. Acetazolamide (Diamox) is a carbonic anhydrase inhibitor used to decrease aqueous humor production and lower IOP. Its use is relatively contraindicated in patients with renal and hepatic dysfunction due to its propensity to cause electrolyte imbalances and metabolic acidosis. These patients may develop cardiac dysrhythmias from electrolyte abnormalities. Patients with chronic lung diseases and CO_2 retention may develop severe acidosis from administration of Diamox. The pharmacologic agents commonly used in retinal surgery and their physiologic effects and anesthetic concerns are listed in Table 31.1.

Intraoperative Period

3. *Discuss the differences between anesthetic techniques for retinal detachments and the challenges each poses for the anesthetist.*

Regional techniques are increasingly popular because they offer increased safety for high-risk patients. They decrease operating room time, provide patients with prolonged analgesia, and are associated with rapid recovery time. Regional techniques, such as retrobulbar, peribulbar, and sub-Tenon nerve blocks, are reserved for vitrectomies lasting less than 2 hours. The use of regional anesthesia varies according to the patient's willingness to participate, communicate, and cooperate; the patient's coagulation status; and the surgeon's preference. Squinting of the eyes can raise

IOP over 25 mm Hg. A facial nerve block can be placed in addition to the regional technique to block these effects by anesthetizing the orbicularis oculi muscle. Topical anesthetic drops, used as the only anesthetic in other anterior segment ophthalmic procedures, unfortunately do not provide the akinesis necessary for a vitrectomy and are frequently used as an additional adjunct for perioperative pain control. Once a retrobulbar block is in place, control of anxiolysis and any necessary supplementation of analgesia should be continued with caution. Because the patient's airway is not readily accessible to the anesthetist, caution should be used to avoid oversedation and airway obstruction. Conversely, a semi-awake, disoriented patient who is moving poses a risk of serious damage to the surgical site and can make it impossible to utilize a microscope to repair the detached retina. Intraoperative expectations of the surgical and anesthesia teams, as well as the patient, need to be discussed preoperatively in order to devise a safe and smooth plan of intraoperative care.

GETA is usually reserved for vitrectomies requiring muscle paralysis (as is the case with some scleral buckles) and when the length of the surgery will exceed the estimated duration of local anesthetic action. Other indications for general anesthesia include the inability of patients to remain motionless, patients who refuse a

TABLE 31.1 Pharmacologic Agents Commonly Used During Retinal Surgery

Name and Route	Class of Drug	Mechanism of Action	Side Effects	Intended Use
Diamox (IV)	Carbonic anhydrase inhibitor	Acts on sodium pump that is part of the mechanism of aqueous humor secretion	Potassium depletion, transient choroidal congestion, diuresis	Decreases IOP
Mannitol (IV)	Osmotic diuretic	Increases plasma oncotic pressure relative to aqueous humor	Transient choroidal congestion, renal failure, congestive heart failure, pulmonary congestion	Decreases IOP
Atropine (Topical)	Anticholinergic	Blocks acetylcholine at ciliary and circular muscles of the iris	Tachycardia, agitation, flushing	Causes mydriasis and cycloplegia
Phenylephrine (Topical)	Alpha-adrenergic agonist	Capillary decongestion	Tachycardia, palpitations, hypertension	Causes mydriasis
Epinephrine (Topical)	Sympathetic agonist	Decreases aqueous secretion, improves aqueous humor outflow	Tachycardia, hypertension, palpitations	Decreases IOP
Cyclogyl (Topical)	Anticholinergic	Blocks acetylcholine at ciliary and circular muscles of the iris	Central nervous system toxicity, incoherence, slurred speech, hallucinations, convulsions in children	Short-acting mydriatic and cycloplegia

regional technique, and the surgeon's preference. The overall goal of the anesthetist during GETA for repair of an RD should be to minimize hemodynamic variability, maintain normocarbia, and avoid abrupt increases in IOP by providing a smooth anesthetic induction, maintenance, and emergence. The anesthetist should administer medications that inhibit PONV and minimize the use of emetogenic agents, if possible, because vomiting dramatically raises IOP. Patients should be adequately premedicated with an anxiolytic and should take chronically prescribed calcium-channel blocker or beta-blocker medications to control heart rate and blood pressure. If gastroparesis is a possibility, administering metoclopramide and an H_2 antagonist during the preoperative period is prudent.

The "time-out" procedure should be followed before induction to identify and mark the correct surgical eye. Caution should be used when applying the mask for preoxygenation and during ventilation via the mask so as not to apply pressure on the affected globe. A smooth anesthetic induction with an appropriate intravenous (IV) agent, administration of a nondepolarizing muscle relaxant for paralysis, and the use of 4% lidocaine administered using a laryngeal tracheal anesthesia (LTA) kit before placement of a preformed right-angle oral Ring–Adair–Elwyn (RAE) endotracheal tube (ETT) is recommended. If N_2O is administered during the case, its use should be discontinued a minimum of 15 minutes before a tamponading gas agent is injected, because continued N_2O use may increase the size of the gas bubble and result in an increase in IOP. Intraoperative antiemetics such as dexamethasone, droperidol, and ondansetron can help in the prevention of postoperative retching and vomiting that can raise IOP to greater than 40 mm Hg. Intraoperative insertion of a nasogastric tube to empty the stomach may possibly reduce the incidence of PONV. The use of IV lidocaine upon emergence should also be considered to decrease the incidence of coughing during the return of airway reflexes, providing a smooth emergence and thus avoid a subsequent rise in IOP. Box 31.1 lists specific challenges associated with anesthesia management for retinal surgery.

• BOX 31.1   Challenges Associated With Anesthesia Management for Retinal Surgery

- Patient safety and preference
- Akinesia of the eye
- Appropriate levels of analgesia, amnesia, and anxiolysis
- Minimal bleeding
- Maintenance of normal IOP and hemodynamics
- Smooth induction and emergence
- Postoperative course void of PONV
- No access to the patient's airway intraoperatively

---

4. *Discuss whether retinal detachment surgery should be considered an emergency.*

Although time-sensitive surgical concerns are associated with this surgery, it is of paramount importance that a cautious approach is undertaken when dealing with these ophthalmologic emergencies. The patient's safety is the primary goal, and life-threatening risks associated with common comorbidities must be minimized before proceeding with anesthesia to preserve eyesight. The urgency of the surgery and the risk to vision should be discussed with the surgical team to devise a plan for safe anesthesia within a time frame that is conducive to preserving the patient's sight.

If it is not possible to perform a regional technique for a patient with a full stomach, then a modified RSI for control and protection of the airway during GETA is indicated. It is not recommended to insert a nasogastric tube in patients with RD who are awake because of the distress and increase in IOP that may occur. Preoperative blood glucose should be corrected if necessary in patients with diabetes mellitus and beta-blockers titrated as indicated in patients with cardiovascular disease. Once standard monitors are applied, preoxygenation should be implemented without the mask compressing the affected globe. Cricoid pressure should be applied during induction using a rapid-acting IV hypnotic and muscle relaxant of choice tailored to the individual patient. Muscle relaxation monitoring is useful to ensure that full paralysis is present before direct laryngoscopy (DL) to prevent coughing, which can dramatically increase IOP. The use of succinylcholine for RSI in urgent cases is still controversial because of the transient rise in IOP caused by fasciculations. In the closed-eye RD patient, succinylcholine has been shown to increase IOP 6 to 8 mm Hg for 1 to 4 minutes after administration. IOP returns to baseline in 5 to 7 minutes. Although the rise in IOP may be mild and abrupt, the use of succinylcholine should only be used after collaboration with the surgeon to avoid patient injury.

5. *What monitors are imperative to patient safety during RD repairs?*

Regardless of whether a regional or GETA technique is utilized to correct an RD, all standard monitors should be implemented.

- An ECG is imperative to monitor for ischemic changes, the oculocardiac reflex (OCR), and any changes indicative of electrolyte imbalances caused by coexisting illnesses or medications commonly used for ophthalmic purposes.
- Blood pressure measured frequently via an automated cuff must be continually monitored to assess for adequate perfusion and effects on IOP. Studies have shown ocular ischemia and retinal artery occlusion can occur if low systolic blood pressures can persist throughout the case. Heart rate and blood pressure deviations from baseline can be used to

monitor for increasing anxiety or lightening levels of anesthesia.

- Pulse oximetry is essential to assure adequate oxygenation, considering the distance and inaccessibility of the patient's airway.
- Continual end tidal carbon dioxide ($ETCO_2$) monitoring will help avoid hyperventilation or hypoventilation, which is important because of the effect hypercarbia has on IOP, as well as serving as a safety monitor for airway/circuit disconnects.
- Neuromuscular blockade monitoring should be utilized to assure adequate muscle relaxation and to prevent acute IOP increases from "bucking" or coughing in GETA cases.
- Bispectral index (BIS) monitoring provides information to help the anesthetist assess the patient's depth of anesthesia by evaluating the electromyelogram to determine central nervous system activity.

6. *Discuss the effect of ocular physiology on IOP.*

The normal range for IOP varies between 10 and 22 mm Hg and increases by several mm Hg in the supine position, varies 1 to 2 mm Hg with each cardiac contraction, and changes 2 to 5 mm Hg during sleep and upon awakening. IOP contributes to the shape and optic properties of the eye and is determined by many anatomic and physiologic factors, including a balance between production and drainage of aqueous humor and by changes in intraocular blood volume.

Aqueous humor is similar to blood plasma and occupies the anterior chamber, or front third of the eye. In addition to helping shape the eye, it serves to nourish structures such as the cornea and lens, but also carries away waste materials with drainage through the trabecular network, the Schlemm canal, the episcleral venous system, and a system of venous pathways that lead to the superior vena cava. Aqueous humor is formed at a rate of 2 microliters/min and drains at a similar rate through the venous system. When venous congestion increases, such as during a Valsalva maneuver or upon coughing, the outflow of aqueous humor is impeded and IOP rises significantly. Changes in venous pressure have been shown physiologically to have the most profound effect on IOP.

Intraocular blood volume is controlled by vessel dilation and contraction of the choroid layer that lies between the retina and the sclera. As choroidal arterioles dilate in response to hypercapnia and constrict in response to hypocapnia, IOP and volume fluctuate.

Minimal changes in IOP occur when normocarbia is maintained. Hypoxemia may minimally increase IOP through choroidal dilation. Changes in arterial blood pressure also have minimal effects on IOP, although abrupt hypertension and/or profound induced hypotension can affect IOP. It is an elevation in venous pressure that most profoundly increases IOP through an increase in intraocular blood volume and distention of the orbital

TABLE 31.2	Physiologic Influences on Intraocular Pressure	
Physiologic Variable	**Effect on Intraocular Pressure**
Central Venous Pressure	
Increase	Marked increase
Decrease	Marked decrease
Arterial Blood Pressure	
Increase	Mild increase
Decrease	Mild decrease
$PaCO_2$	
Increased through hypoventilation	Moderate increase
Decreased through hyperventilation	Moderate decrease
PaO_2	
Increase	No effect
Decrease	Mild increase
Other Physiologic Influences	
Coughing/Bucking	Marked increase
Vomiting	Marked increase
Deep Inspiration	Mild decrease

vessels. Physiologic factors that affect IOP are listed in Table 31.2. Vigilance in maintaining hemodynamic stability with a venous pressure consistent with baseline values is crucial for successful retinal surgery.

7. *Describe the effect of anesthetic agents on IOP.*

Most general anesthetic agents cause a decrease in IOP. Potential explanations include:

- Reduced choroidal blood volume from a decreased blood pressure
- Decreased extraocular muscle tension from muscle relaxation resulting in a lower ocular wall tension
- An increase in papillary muscle constriction that increases aqueous outflow

Succinylcholine raises IOP up to 8 mm Hg for a total of 7 minutes after administration secondary to prolonged extraocular muscle contraction, and its use is controversial during RSI for RD surgery. A summary of the effects of anesthetic medications on IOP is listed in Table 31.3.

8. *Discuss the OCR, possible causes, and treatment.*

The OCR is a response caused by traction on ocular muscles (medial rectus) or by pressure exerted on the globe. The afferent pathway is initiated through the trigeminal nerve (cranial nerve [CN] V) from the ciliary ganglion to the ophthalmic division of the trigeminal nerve through the gasserian ganglion. The main sensory nucleus is located in the fourth ventricle of the brain.

TABLE 31.3	Anesthetic Medications and Their Effects on Intraocular Pressure	
Drug	**Effect on Intraocular Pressure**	
Inhaled Anesthetics		
Volatile	Moderate decrease	
N_2O	Mild decrease	
Intravenous Agents		
Barbiturates	Moderate decrease	
Benzodiazepines	Moderate decrease	
Ketamine	Controversial	
Narcotics	Mild decrease	
Propofol	Decrease	
Etomidate	Controversial because of myoclonus	
Muscle Relaxants		
Depolarizers	Moderate increase	
Nondepolarizers	No to mild decrease	

TABLE 31.4	Retinal Tamponading Agents	
Agent	**Blood: Gas Partition Coefficient**	**Avoid N_2O**
Air	Nitrogen in air 0.015	5 days
Sulfurhexafluoride (SF_6)	0.004	10 days
Perfluoropropane	0.00125	30 days

• BOX 31.2 Treatment for Initiation of the Oculocardiac Reflex

- Immediately notify the surgeon to temporarily stop the surgical stimulus until heart rate increases.
- Confirm adequate ventilation and oxygenation of patient.
- Treat with anticholinergic if conduction disturbances continue.
- Ask for surgical application of local anesthetics to rectus muscles for persistent episodes.

Activation of the efferent pathway via the vagus nerve (CN X) can cause cardiac dysrhythmias that can include sinus arrest, heart block, bradycardia, and asystole. This reflex can be stimulated by any number of surgical maneuvers, most commonly during the administration of a retrobulbar block or during muscle manipulation during a vitrectomy.

Attempts to block the OCR with anticholinergics before retrobulbar blockade are controversial. Pretreatment has not been shown to consistently be effective, safe, or reliable for blocking the OCR. However, it should be noted that the OCR will usually stop after repeated traction on the medial rectus muscles due to reflex fatigue. Treatment for the OCR is presented in Box 31.2.

9. *List the anesthetic implications for gases that are utilized for retinal tamponading.*

Several agents are used as tamponading agents and are included in Table 31.4. When using N_2O during general anesthesia, it is imperative that N_2O be discontinued at least 15 minutes before the gas tamponading agent is injected. If N_2O is not discontinued before the gas injection, the gas bubble will increase in size. This occurs because the N_2O is significantly more soluble than nitrogen or other molecules in the tamponading agent—the N_2O molecules diffuse into the gas bubble and increase its size. If the bubble continues to increase in size after the eye is surgically closed, IOP increases and may decrease the effectiveness of the retinal repair by jeopardizing ocular perfusion. Additionally, once N_2O molecules diffuse from the tamponading bubble postoperatively, the enlarged gas tamponade bubble will shrink, which increases the potential for RD due to the variability of the IOP gradient.

Postoperative Period

The surgery was performed utilizing a retrobulbar block with monitored anesthesia care (MAC), with minimal hemodynamic changes throughout 42 minutes of surgery. Six hours after surgery, the patient was still in the recovery room and was complaining of severe pain. Her vital signs include blood pressure, 168/90; heart rate, 101 beats per minute; and respiratory rate, 28.

10. *Discuss possible explanations for the patient's current status.*

Pain is the most likely cause of the patient's change in hemodynamic status. The most probable causes of pain after RD surgery include:
- Pain from a distended bladder and inability to urinate
- Pain in the lower extremities from a deep vein thrombosis
- Chest pain from MI, angina, shortness of breath from a pulmonary embolism, or other thromboembolic event

Unlikely causes of the pain because of the delay in symptoms are:
- Pain in the eye from the injected antibiotics and steroids placed at the end of the case
- Pain in the orbit from a retrobulbar hemorrhage

It is most important to determine the specific cause of the patient's pain and then to provide interventions that treat the distinct problem.

Review Questions

1. Which is the initial intervention if the oculocardiac reflex is suspected?
   a. Administer an anticholinesterase drug
   b. Wait for the reflex to fade and a normal rhythm to resume
   c. Immediately intubate the patient
   d. Notify the surgeon to stop surgery
2. During general anesthesia for a retinal detachment repair using sevoflurane, 50% air and 50% oxygen, and vecuronium, one could expect:
   a. Increased venous pressure.
   b. Increased incidence of the oculocardiac reflex.
   c. Increased IOP in healthy individuals.
   d. Ocular akinesia.
3. A patient emergently comes to the operating room for an appendectomy after undergoing a vitrectomy with a tamponading agent 1 week ago. Which is the best choice of inhalational maintenance during the case to maintain a safe anesthetic?
   a. 50% air, 50% O_2 with 1 MAC of sevoflurane
   b. 70% air, 30% O_2 with 0.3 MAC of desflurane
   c. 50% N_2O, 50% O_2 with 0.7 MAC isoflurane
   d. 70% N_2O, 30% O_2 with 0.5 MAC sevoflurane

4. Which is true regarding tamponading agent reabsorption?
   a. Air is reabsorbed in 5 days.
   b. Sulfurhexafluoride (SF_6) is reabsorbed in 30 days.
   c. Silicone oil is reabsorbed in 10 days.
   d. Perfluoropropane is absorbed in 10 days.
5. Which factor increases IOP to the greatest degree?
   a. Lying in the supine position
   b. Decrease in central venous pressure
   c. Use of succinylcholine
   d. Deep inspiration

Suggested Readings

Abdeldayem OT, Amer GF, Abdulla MG. Postoperative analgesic efficacy of sub-Tenon's block with levobupivacaine in retinal surgery under general anesthesia. *Anesth Essays Res* 2019;13(3): 437-440.

Charles S, Fanning GL. Anesthesia considerations for vitreoretinal surgery. *Ophthalmol Clin North Am* 2006;19:239-243.

Fang ZT, Keyes MA. A novel mixture of propofol, alfentanil, and lidocaine for regional block monitored anesthesia care in ophthalmic surgery. *J Clin Anesth* 2006;18:114-117.

Harvey RR. Anesthesia for ophthalmic procedures. In: Nagelhout JJ, Elisha S, eds. *Nurse Anesthesia,* 6th ed. St Louis, MO: Elsevier, 2018:925-945.

Kelly DJ, Farrell SM. Physiology and role of intraocular pressure in contemporary anesthesia. *Anesth Analg* 2018;126(5): 1551-1562.

Loriga B, Di Filippo A, Tofani L, et al. Postoperative pain after vitreoretinal surgery is influenced by surgery duration and anesthesia conduction. *Minerva Anestesiol* 2019;85(7):731-737.

McCannel CA, Nordlund JR, Bacon D, et al. Perioperative morbidity and mortality associated with vitreoretinal and ocular oncologic surgery performed under general anesthesia. *Trans Am Ophthalmol Soc* 2003;101:209–213.

Van Wicklin SA. Systematic review and meta-analysis of prone position on intraocular pressure in adults undergoing surgery. *Int J Spine Surg* 2020;14(2):195-208.

Vann MA, Ogunnaike BO, Joshi GP. Sedation and anesthesia care for ophthalmologic surgery during local/regional anesthesia. *Anesthesiology* 2007;107:502-508.

Yannuzzi NA, Swaminathan SS, Hussain R, et al. Repair of rhegmatogenous retinal detachment following globe perforation by retrobulbar anesthesia. *Ophthalmic Surg Lasers Imaging Retina* 2020;51(4):249-251.

32
Ruptured Globe

KEY POINTS

- There is an increased incidence of ruptured globe injuries in young athletic patients and elderly patients with multiple comorbidities.
- A traumatic accident that results in a ruptured globe may be associated with an acute head injury, cervical spine instability, and thoracoabdominal disruption requiring immediate resuscitation and stabilization.
- Increased intraocular pressure (IOP) can occur during the perioperative period as a result of coughing, straining, and pressure. There is an increased risk of leakage of vitreous humor and intraocular contents during the induction of anesthesia and intraoperative repair of the ruptured globe.

Case Synopsis

An 88-year-old woman has fallen at home, resulting in the following injuries: ruptured left globe, fractured left hip, and fractured right mandible. The patient is admitted to the emergency department. She is evaluated by ophthalmology, orthopedics, oral maxillofacial, and medicine services. The patient specifically denies loss of consciousness before or after the injury and describes the cause of the fall as tripping over a rug. The first surgical procedure that the patient will undergo is repair of the left ruptured globe.

Preoperative Evaluation and Demographic Data

Past Medical/Surgical History

- Essential hypertension
- Hypothyroidism
- History of breast cancer with resulting left breast mastectomy

Medications

- Aspirin
- Vicodin
- Synthroid
- Fexofenadine (Allegra)
- Escitalopram (Lexapro)

Laboratory Values and Diagnostic Data

- Hemoglobin, 11.2 g/dL; hematocrit, 34.4%; glucose, 100 mg/dL; blood urea nitrogen, 24 mg/dL; creatinine, 0.9 mg/dL
- Electrolytes: sodium, 140 mEq/L; potassium, 4.5 mEq/L; chloride, 108 mEq/L; carbon dioxide, 23 mEq/L

- Electrocardiogram (ECG): normal sinus rhythm without abnormality
- Chest x-ray (CXR): no acute disease
- Left hip x-ray: fractured femoral head
- Interpretation of the computed tomography (CT) of the head:
  1. Acute fracture at the junction of the right mandibular head and neck with displacement from the mandibular fossa.
  2. Biconvex, well-circumscribed area of hyperdensity in the left lateral globe suggests subretinal hemorrhage; area of irregular density in the left globe likely vitreous hemorrhage; intact intraocular muscles and optic nerve. There is no evidence of cerebral hematoma or other abnormalities.

Pathophysiology

It is estimated that more than 2 million people per year within the United States sustain ocular injuries involving the globe, which results in visual impairment or complete loss of vision in approximately 2% of this patient population. Approximately 33% of childhood blindness occurs as a result of trauma to structures of the eye. There is an increased incidence of ocular injuries associated with young male patients who engage in sports and strenuous physical activities.

A ruptured globe can be defined as loss of the integrity of the outer membranes of the eye. Globe rupture commonly occurs as a result of traumatic injury to a normal eye. Impact from blunt objects can cause anterior posterior compression of the globe, which raises IOP (normally 10 to 20 mm Hg) high enough to cause rupture of the ocular tissues. The rupture typically occurs in regions where the

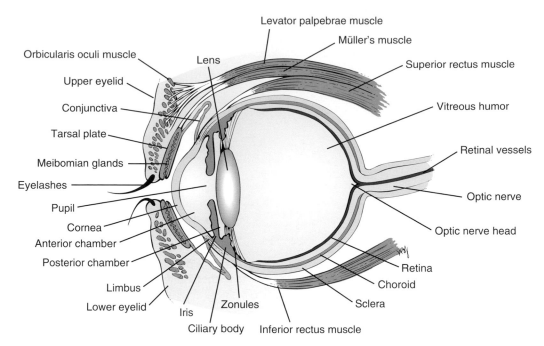

• **Fig. 32.1** Anatomic representation of the structures that comprise the globe. (From Swartz MH: *Textbook of physical diagnosis: history and examination*, ed 8, St. Louis, 2021, Elsevier.)

scleral covering is thinnest, including the insertion points of the extraocular muscles, limbus, and around the optic nerve. An anatomic diagram of the globe and the associated structures is included in Fig. 32.1. Perforation of the globe can occur as a result of impalement by sharp objects, and the severity of the injury is proportional to the velocity of the penetrating object. Foreign bodies may remain within the globe. The anterior or posterior segment of the globe may lose surface integrity after eye surgery if external pressure is exerted on the eye.

Because trauma to the globe is often caused by a forceful blow to the head, there is the potential for concurrent injuries, such as acute head injuries that may be associated with neurologic damage. Contusions and fractures of orbital and facial bones can occur. Dental fractures can cause bleeding in oral structures and can become dislodged, complicating airway management. Patients who sustain head trauma should have a comprehensive evaluation to determine if cervical spine disruption has occurred before nonemergency airway manipulation. If the eye injury is associated with falling down, the patient's body should be surveyed for the presence of injuries to the thorax, abdomen, and bony skeleton.

Surgical Procedure

Ruptured globe injuries require surgical repair. Basic first aid measures include gentle cleansing of the periorbital area with an antiseptic, irrigation of the globe with sterile saline, and then application of a dressing and shield to prevent external ocular pressure. Patients are counseled to avoid coughing, sneezing, or initiating the Valsalva maneuver to limit the potential for increased IOP.

During surgery, the globe will be gently fixated with the lids elevated. Every effort will be made to avoid exerting pressure on the globe to prevent extrusion of intraocular contents. The eye will be thoroughly examined for the location and extent of injuries. Meticulous assessment and methodical repair of the structures of the globe will occur. These structures include the following: conjunctiva, cornea, sclera, anterior and posterior chambers, iris, lens, and retinal structures (see Fig. 32.1).

Anesthetic Management and Considerations

Preoperative Period

1. *Discuss the type and frequency of various coexisting diseases that are associated with patients presenting for repair of a ruptured globe.*

    The presence of coexisting diseases is dependent on the circumstances of injury and the patient population that is affected. In young, athletic patients injured during sports or high-risk physical activities, good medical health is likely, but coexisting neurologic, orthopedic, and organ damage is possible, depending on the nature and extent of the traumatic injury. The comorbidities and injuries associated with a ruptured globe are listed in Box 32.1. In elderly patients with a ruptured globe after intraocular eye surgery or a fall, a more extensive list of coexisting medical disease processes associated with the ocular disorders is common.

2. *Examine the basic anatomy of the intact eye (anterior and posterior segments); the physiology of aqueous fluid generation, pressure, and flow; and the motor, sensory,*

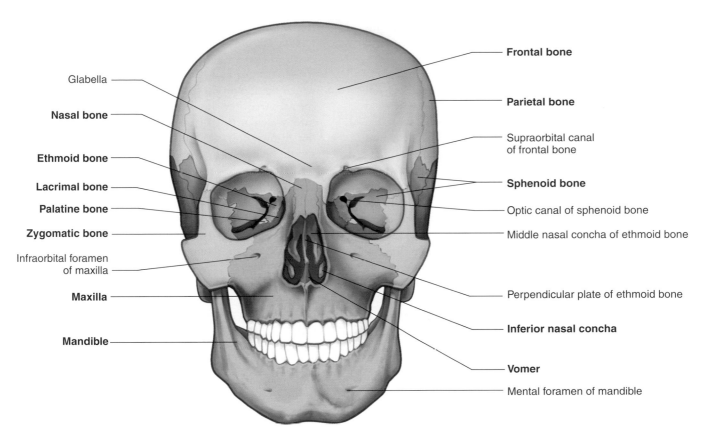

Glabella

Nasal bone

Ethmoid bone

Lacrimal bone

Palatine bone

Zygomatic bone

Infraorbital foramen
of maxilla

Maxilla

Mandible

Frontal bone

Parietal bone

Supraorbital canal
of frontal bone

Sphenoid bone

Optic canal of sphenoid bone

Middle nasal concha of ethmoid bone

Perpendicular plate of ethmoid bone

Inferior nasal concha

Vomer

Mental foramen of mandible

• **Fig. 32.2** The cranium with emphasis on the bony orbital structures. (From Patton KT: *Anatomy & physiology*, ed 10, St. Louis, 2019, Elsevier.)

• **BOX 32.1** **Comorbidities and Injuries Associated With Ruptured Globe**

- Orbital bone fractures
- Head injuries: intracerebral hemorrhage, neurologic trauma
- Neck and cervical spine injuries
- Skeletal fractures
- Cardiac arrhythmias
- Recent eye surgery

and autonomic innervation of the eyeball and its associated muscles.

Understanding the underlying ophthalmologic motor, sensory, and autonomic structure and function will assist the anesthetist to understand the anesthetic implications of the planned surgical repair. The eye is a globular structure, consisting of fluids, intricate internal membranes, and a proteinaceous crystalline lens, surrounded by a tough, fibrous outer coat of tissue and muscle, nestled within the protective cavity of the bony orbit (Figs. 32.1 and 32.2).

Multiple extraocular structures surround the globe. The eyelids protect and lubricate the eye and consist of thin skin supported by a fibrous layer called the *tarsal plate,* which helps maintain the lids' shape and strength.

Various muscles contribute to eyelid movement, including the orbicularis oculi and levator palpebrae. The outermost covering of the eye is a mucous membrane called the *conjunctiva* that extends from the edge of the cornea to the posterior aspect of the eye, looping back to form the inside of the eyelids. Accessory glands in the eyelids produce most of the liquid tears, which keep the eye moist and drain through the puncta into the nose.

The globe itself is divided into two segments. The anterior segment includes structures that lie anterior to the vitreous humor, a sphere of clear, gel-like material in the posterior globe. Comprising approximately 33% of the eye, the anterior segment includes the cornea (clear front surface of the eye), iris (the colored part of the eye that controls the pupil opening size), ciliary body (membranes derived from the pupil that control lens shape by tension on the lens zonules and secrete nutrient-containing aqueous humor bathing anterior segment structures), and lens. There are two fluid-filled spaces: the anterior chamber lying between the cornea and iris and the posterior chamber between the iris and vitreous, containing the lens. The lens is a proteinaceous structure that consists of three layers: a tough outer capsule, a middle cortex, and a hard nucleus, all of which are suspended by zonule ligaments.

The posterior segment of the globe, which comprises 66% of the eye, consists of the anterior hyaloid membrane, the gel-like vitreous body, the retina, the choroid layers, and the optic nerve. The vitreous body is surrounded by a clear hyaloid membrane. Vitreous is a microfibrillar netlike structure; the gel consistency derives from mucopolysaccharides and hyaluronate acid components. This consistency serves to keep the retina firmly engaged against the lower layers of the eye and maintains the shape of the globe. The retina, the innermost surface, is an extension of the optic nerve, which corresponds to the pia mater meningeal membrane. This region converts light into electrical impulses that are relayed to the brain for interpretation. The choroid layer, immediately inferior to the retina, corresponds to the arachnoid mater meningeal membrane and supplies the retina with oxygen and nutrients. The outermost covering of the eye, called the *sclera*, corresponds to the dura mater in other areas of the central nervous system (CNS). Thus the optic nerve sheathe is an extension of the CNS bathed in cerebrospinal fluid. Medications that are injected into this sheath are rapidly transported to the brain.

Aqueous humor is the major determinant of the IOP, which normally ranges from 10 to 20 mm Hg. This fluid is formed by the ciliary body in the posterior chamber by passive filtration from blood vessels and by an active process requiring the enzyme carbonic anhydrase. The fluid moves through the pupil into the anterior chamber, and there it is drained via numerous interconnected venous channels associated with the canal of Schlemm. Thus any factor that obstructs this drainage—elevated venous pressure from coughing or straining, or the mechanical obstruction associated with glaucoma—will cause acute elevations in the IOP. If increases in IOP are extreme, nutrient supply to the avascular structures of the globe such as the lens and retina can become compromised.

The innervation to the eye is composed of motor, sensory, and autonomic functions. There are six extraocular muscles controlling movement of the eyeball: the superior, medial, and inferior rectus muscles, all controlled by the oculomotor nerve (cranial nerve [CN] III); the lateral rectus, controlled by the abducens nerve (CN VI); the superior oblique nerve, controlled by the trochlear nerve (CN IV); and the inferior oblique innervated by oculomotor nerve (CN III). Eyelid motor function is controlled by branches of the facial nerve (CN VII). Sensory innervation to the periorbital area and eye structures is derived from the ophthalmic division of the trigeminal nerve (CN V). The oculomotor nerve sends parasympathetic fibers to the ciliary ganglion that constricts the pupil (miosis), and sympathetic fibers arising from the superior cervical sympathetic ganglion and carotid plexus cause pupillary dilation (mydriasis). The *light reflex* refers to pupillary constriction in response to increased light exposure via oculomotor nerve activation of the preganglionic parasympathetic fibers, which originate in the Edinger–Westphal nucleus of the rostral midbrain.

3. *Discuss the preoperative evaluation of the patient with a ruptured globe.*

The patient should undergo an in-depth interview in which the significant past medical history is elicited, and special attention should be directed toward the CNS, cardiovascular (CV), and respiratory systems. The existing disease processes and their severity and treatment should be investigated, along with any previous difficulties with anesthesia and surgery. The cause of the ruptured globe should be thoroughly investigated. Patient falls that are accompanied by loss of consciousness may be associated with CNS or CV abnormalities that can affect the anesthetic management. The patient should be subjected to a thorough physical examination. An airway assessment should be accompanied by a search for occult neck or head injury. A general survey of the body should be undertaken to rule out previously unsuspected injuries, especially when the ruptured globe was caused by trauma. Information gathered from the medical history and physical assessment, appropriate laboratory tests, ECG, CXR, and other diagnostic tests should be obtained and interpreted before the induction of anesthesia in order to ensure a safe and individualized plan of care.

Intraoperative Period

4. *Describe the controversial issues associated with anesthetic management for patients with a ruptured globe.*

Patients who have sustained a ruptured globe because of a traumatic accident are not ideal candidates to receive retrobulbar or peribulbar nerve blocks. Regional anesthesia is relatively contraindicated for several reasons. Insertion of the needle into the infraorbital foramen may cause further damage to traumatized tissue and increase the size and density of a hematoma. This event could result in increased IOP and extrusion of the intraocular contents. Additionally, a regional block may provide inadequate anesthesia, as periorbital blood ameliorates the effectiveness of the local anesthetic by preventing the diffusion of anesthetic molecules to cause blockade of sensory nerves. These patients may sustain associated injuries, including orbital fractures, soft tissue contusions or lacerations, and periorbital hematomas. Therefore this patient will receive general anesthesia.

Patients with open globe injury requiring general anesthesia have two primary airway considerations: potential for pulmonary aspiration with lack of fasting and potential for increased IOP during laryngoscopy. In considering appropriate measures to secure the airway in nonfasted patients for emergent repair, prevention of aspiration is a priority; if airway examination reveals significant abnormality with potential inability to intubate or ventilate after induction, then awake fiber-optic intubation can be considered with excellent topicalization

TABLE 32.1	Effects of Anesthetic Agents on Intraocular Pressure	
Drug	**Effect on Intraocular Pressure**	
Induction agents, benzodiazepines, opioids	Decreases IOP	
Ketamine	No effect on IOP with lower doses (3 mg/kg); increases IOP in high doses (6 mg/kg)	
Succinylcholine	Increases IOP (5–8 mm Hg) due to prolonged contraction of extraocular muscles	
Inhaled anesthetics	Decreases IOP	
Nondepolarizing muscle relaxants	Decreases IOP	
Dexmedetomidine	Decreases IOP	

TABLE 32.2	Effects of Various Anesthetic Interventions on Intraocular Pressure	
Intervention/Physiologic Alteration	**Effect on Intraocular Pressure**	
Airway instrumentation	Increases IOP with light levels of anesthesia	
Hypoventilation, hypoxemia	Increases IOP	
Coughing, vomiting, Valsalva maneuver	Increases IOP	
Trendelenburg position	Increases IOP	
Deep plane of anesthesia	Decreases IOP	
Decreased sympathetic nervous system activation	Decreases IOP	

and appropriate sedation to reduce coughing and increased IOP.

If asleep orotracheal intubation is deemed appropriate in the nonfasted patient, there is some controversy surrounding the use of succinylcholine as a component of a rapid sequence induction. This depolarizing muscle relaxant is associated with an elevation in IOP of approximately 8 mm Hg lasting 5 to 7 minutes. Several mechanisms are hypothesized to explain this effect: specific tonic response of unique morphologic structures in the extraocular muscles, drug effects on cerebral blood flow, and alterations in the formation of aqueous humor. Nondepolarizing muscle relaxants lower IOP and thus are the paralytic drugs of choice for these cases, if deemed safe to use for intubation. A summary of the effects of anesthetic agents on IOP is included in Table 32.1.

5. *Describe factors that influence IOP during anesthetic management.*

Various anesthetic interventions and the alterations in physiology associated with general anesthesia can have pronounced effects on IOP, as listed in Table 32.2. The most profound effect is a rise that can be associated with direct laryngoscopy and intubation due to sympathetic nervous system stimulation. To minimize severe increases in IOP, patients should receive adequate anesthesia before airway instrumentation. It is imperative that intraoperative ventilation is adequate in order to avoid hypercarbia and hypoxemia because both factors will increase IOP.

6. *Discuss the rationale for using intraoperative neuromuscular blockade.*

Patients with "open-eye" conditions—a physical opening between the atmosphere and inner eye—are at risk for loss of intraocular contents with coughing, straining, or Valsalva maneuver when IOP increases due to increased sympathetic tone and increased venous pressure in periorbital veins. Thus during general anesthesia, such patients should receive nondepolarizing neuromuscular blockade to prevent sudden increases in IOP.

7. *Develop an anesthetic care plan to include management of fluid therapy, changes in vital signs, oculocardiac reflex, and appropriate monitoring.*

Fluid therapy for patients with ruptured globe should meet patient needs identified on preoperative assessment; the ophthalmologic injury and surgery for repair are not associated with fluid shifts or blood loss. Patients may be hypovolemic or hypervolemic due to coexisting injury or medical comorbidities, and crystalloid or colloid administration should be titrated to euvolemia.

Basic intraoperative monitors as recommended by the American Association of Nurse Anesthetists (AANA)—ECG, blood pressure, pulse oximetry, end tidal CO_2—are usually sufficient. Regional anesthesia via retrobulbar or peribulbar block may be associated with unintended intravascular or subarachnoid administration of local anesthetic drug, requiring resuscitation from unconsciousness, seizure, or hypotension. Intraoperative administration of local anesthetic block to patients receiving general anesthesia may be associated with hypotension due to decreased surgical stimulus. Vasodilation associated with potent inhaled anesthetics may produce hypotension requiring vasopressor treatment. Nitrous oxide (N_2O) should be avoided if the surgeon plans intravitreal gas injection; N_2O molecules will diffuse into the bubble, producing increased IOP.

Tension on the extraocular muscles during injury repair may serve as an afferent stimulus arc, via the ciliary ganglion to the ophthalmic branch of the trigeminal nerve, for the oculocardiac reflex. Efferent vagal discharge produces bradycardia, which can be profound. Treatment consists of stopping the stimulus, administering anticholinergic drugs, and infiltrating periorbital local anesthetics if appropriate.

8. *Examine the indications for antiemetic therapy in the patient with a ruptured globe.*

The Society for Ambulatory Surgery has issued consensus guidelines on the prevention and management of postoperative nausea and vomiting (PONV), and several risk factors were identified that potentially apply to this specific patient population. Increased risk of PONV is associated with the use of volatile anesthetics, strabismus (extraocular muscle) repair, maxillofacial surgery, and the use of intraoperative and postoperative opioids. Furthermore, the guidelines state that preventive measures were appropriate in patient populations in which PONV might pose a risk to surgical outcome, and increases in IOP associated with retching and vomiting may well pose a risk to the surgical repair of intraocular structures. Thus prophylactic treatment for the prevention of PONV should be considered in all patients with ruptured globe. Though numerous medications are available, a combination of dexamethasone within 1 hour before induction of anesthesia combined with a 5-hydroxytryptamine (5-HT) receptor-blocking medication at conclusion of surgery would appear to be reasonable choices with minimal side effects.

9. *Discuss issues related to extubation of the patient with a ruptured globe with or without a full stomach.*

Extubation is ideally accomplished without straining or coughing to avoid increases in IOP. In fasting patients, "deep" extubation before reflex return is ideal in the absence of airway abnormality or aspiration risk. At the conclusion of surgery, inhaled anesthetics are maintained at surgical levels while administering 100% oxygen and muscle relaxants are reversed; after return of spontaneous respiration intravenous (IV) lidocaine, dexmedetomidine, or propofol can be administered to inhibit the cough reflex. After oropharyngeal suctioning, the endotracheal tube cuff is slowly emptied, and the endotracheal tube is removed gently. The patient may be transferred to the postanesthesia recovery area with insufflated oxygen, positioned on the side to allow for secretion drainage.

In a nonfasting patient, a variation of this technique may avoid excessive coughing and straining yet assure adequate reflex return before extubation. All steps outlined in the previous paragraph are followed. At the conclusion of oropharyngeal suctioning, a soft catheter is left in the oropharynx. The patient's head is elevated to 45 degrees, the inhalation agent is discontinued, and the patient is not disturbed again until he or she is responsive, at which time the pharynx is suctioned and the tube is removed.

10. *Case management: induction, maintenance of anesthesia, emergence, and extubation.*

The patient was induced with etomidate using a modified rapid sequence induction with cricoid pressure. She was paralyzed with rocuronium and intubated using video laryngoscopy. Anesthesia was maintained with sevoflurane, oxygen, and air. A brief period of hypotension was treated with ephedrine and a fluid bolus, and rocuronium was titrated to a single twitch on nerve stimulator. Fentanyl was administered incrementally for analgesia. Ondansetron was administered for emetic prophylaxis. After surgery completion, residual relaxation was reversed with neostigmine and glycopyrrolate, spontaneous respiration resumed, lidocaine was administered with 100% oxygen, and the oropharynx was suctioned. When the patient opened her eyes to command, the endotracheal tube was removed without coughing, and she was transported to the postanesthesia recovery area.

Postoperative Period

11. *List the potential complications after repair of a ruptured globe.*

Acute increases in IOP can occur due to edema, intraocular, or periorbital hemorrhage, which may manifest as pain and nausea or sudden decrease in vision in the affected eye. Periorbital hemorrhage may occur from unsuspected orbital trauma or fracture, resulting in exophthalmos, swelling, and epistaxis. Emesis associated with pain and PONV may result in damage to the surgical repair through acute increases in IOP associated with retching.

12. *Discuss the management of postoperative pain in this patient population.*

Postoperative pain may be effectively prevented and treated by perioperative peribulbar or retrobulbar block. When local anesthetic block is contraindicated, pain may be persistent, severe, and associated with PONV. Patients should receive opioid analgesic drugs intraoperatively and in the postoperative anesthesia care unit to decrease postoperative pain. Antiemetic prophylactic therapy should be administered intraoperatively to help prevent PONV. The head of the bed should remain elevated to facilitate venous drainage and prevent excessive swelling, and an ice pack may be applied to the operative eye. Severe and persistent postoperative pain that is resistant to high-dose opioid therapy is indicative of increased IOP or periorbital hemorrhage. These findings warrant immediate surgical evaluation and possible reexploration of the globe to prevent damage to the eye.

13. *Explain the pathophysiology related to increased intraocular pressure that occurs in the postoperative period after ruptured globe repair.*

One of the most serious postoperative complications associated with repair of a ruptured globe is increased IOP. Increased pressure in the globe can rapidly compress vessels supplying oxygen and nutrients to intraocular structures. The pain is likely caused by a release of acidic metabolites and other mediator molecules. Neurons in the trigeminal ganglia project onto emetogenic nuclei in the vagal nucleus tractus solitarius in the brainstem. Facial and eye pain can cause nausea and vomiting via this pathway.

Review Questions

1. Why is the use of succinylcholine controversial in the anesthetic management of the patient with ruptured globe injury?
   a. The possibility of abnormal pseudocholinesterase may lead to prolonged neuromuscular blockade.
   b. Global rupture may lead to hyperkalemia in susceptible patients.
   c. Prolonged contraction of extraocular muscles may cause elevated IOP.
   d. Fasciculations may lead to decreases in IOP.

2. Which is a contraindication to the use of regional anesthesia for repair of a global rupture?
   a. Periorbital hemorrhage
   b. Decreased IOP
   c. Fractured mandible
   d. Decreased vision in affected eye

3. Neuromuscular blockade during anesthetic management of patients with ruptured globe injury ensures:
   a. Adequate retinal perfusion.
   b. Successful surgical repair.
   c. Control of retinal hypoperfusion due to hemorrhage.
   d. Preventing increased IOP due to the Valsalva maneuver.

4. Which intervention may interrupt the oculocardiac reflex?
   a. Relaxing tension on the extraocular muscles
   b. Pressure on the globe
   c. Tetracaine topical anesthesia on the globe
   d. Irrigation of the periorbital space

5. Deep extubation is often not possible after repair of a ruptured globe because:
   a. Regional anesthesia is usually employed.
   b. Hypotension may ensue.
   c. Of the risk of aspiration.
   d. IOP may increase.

Suggested Readings

Beshay N, Keay L, Dunn H, Kamalden, et al. The epidemiology of Open Globe Injuries presenting to a tertiary referral eye hospital in Australia. *Injury* 2017;48(7):1348-1354.

Colyer MH. Open-globe injuries: a global issue of protection. *Clin Exp Ophthalmol* 2019;47(4):437-438.

Fahling JM, McKenzie LK. Oculocardiac reflex as a result of intraorbital trauma. *J Emerg Med* 2017 Apr;52(4):557-558

Harvey RR. Anesthesia for ophthalmic procedures. In: Nagelhout JJ, Elisha S, eds. *Nurse Anesthesia,* 6th ed. St Louis, MO: Elsevier, 2018:925-945.

Joo J, Koh H, Lee K, Lee J. Effects of systemic administration of dexmedetomidine on intraocular pressure and ocular perfusion pressure during laparoscopic surgery in a steep Trendelenburg position: prospective, randomized, double-blinded study. *J Korean Med Sci* 2016;31(6):989-996.

Rozentsveig V, Yagev R, Wecksler N, et al. Respiratory arrest and convulsions after peribulbar anesthesia. *J Cataract Refract Surg* 2001;27(6):960-962.

Scott IU, Mccabe CM, Flynn HW, et al. Local anesthesia with intravenous sedation for surgical repair of selected open globe injuries. *Am J Ophthalmol* 2002;134(5):707-711.

Singh RB, Choubey S, Mishra S. To evaluate the efficacy of intravenous infusion of dexmedetomidine as premedication in attenuating the rise of intraocular pressure caused by succinylcholine in patients undergoing rapid sequence induction for general anesthesia: a randomized study. *Anesth Essays Res* 2017;11(4):834-841.

33

Open and Laparoscopic Approaches for Hysterectomy

KEY POINTS

- For many patients, gynecologic procedures may bring about feelings such as fear, shame, anxiety, guilt, and embarrassment regarding the surgical procedure.
- Patients undergoing hysterectomy are at high risk for postoperative nausea and vomiting (PONV).
- Nerve injuries associated with positioning can occur during open and laparoscopic hysterectomy.
- Creation of a pneumoperitoneum using carbon dioxide (CO_2) may cause pronounced physiologic changes such as

decreased respiratory compliance, increased airway pressure, and impaired cardiac function.
- Complications such as venous gas embolism (VGE), endobronchial intubation, extraperitoneal insufflation, and pneumothorax may occur during a laparoscopic hysterectomy.

Case Synopsis

A 49-year-old African American woman has developed painful uterine fibroid tumors. She has been scheduled by her gynecologist for a laparoscopic vaginal hysterectomy.

Preoperative Evaluation and Demographic Data

Past Medical/Surgical History

- Past medical history unremarkable; no previous surgical history

Medication List

- No routine medications
- No history of smoking; denies alcohol and recreational drug use

Diagnostic Data

- Human chorionic gonadotropin (hCG) urine pregnancy test, negative
- Hemoglobin, 13 g/dL; hematocrit, 39%; platelets, 240,000/mm³
- Electrolytes: sodium, 139 mEq/L; potassium, 4.1 mEq/L; chloride, 104 mEq/L; CO_2, 23 mEq/L
- Type and screened for two units blood of packed red blood cells

Height/Weight/Vital Signs

- 163 cm, 102 kg
- Blood pressure, 128/64; heart rate, 72 beats per minute; respiratory rate, 20 breaths per minute; room air oxygen saturation, 99%; temperature, 36.8°C
- Electrocardiogram (ECG): normal sinus rate, no abnormalities

Pathophysiology

Uterine leiomyomas (fibroids) are the most common benign tumor that occurs in women; indications for a hysterectomy are listed in Box 33.1. These tumors may grow rapidly, particularly in the perimenopausal-age woman. Fibroids may cause excessive uterine size, ureteral obstruction, and occasionally, first-trimester miscarriage. The most common symptoms associated with fibroids are menorrhagia, pelvic pain, or abdominal pressure. Fibroids may develop in any one of three uterine locations: (1) submucosal (within the innermost layer of the uterus), (2) intramural (within the myometrial layer), and (3) subserosal (within the outermost uterine layer).

Although the exact cause is unknown, genetic alterations and hormones such as estrogen and progesterone may be factors in the growth of fibroids. For patients older than 45 years of age, bilateral salpingo-oophorectomy (BSO) is often performed simultaneously during a hysterectomy to

- Leiomyoma 38%
- Malignancy 15%
- Ovarian tumors 10%
- Abnormal bleeding 13%
- Adenomyosis 9%
- Pelvic pain or adhesions 5%
- Endometriosis 3%
- Uterine prolapse 1%

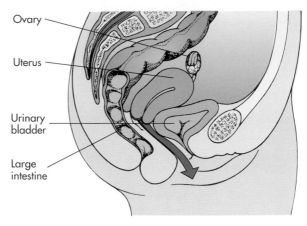

• Fig. 33.2 Anatomic structures associated with vaginal hysterectomy. Uterus is removed through vagina and there is no abdominal incision. (From Monahan FC, Sands JK, Neighbors M, et al: *Phipps' medical-surgical nursing: Health and illness perspectives*, ed 8, St. Louis, 2007, Elsevier.)

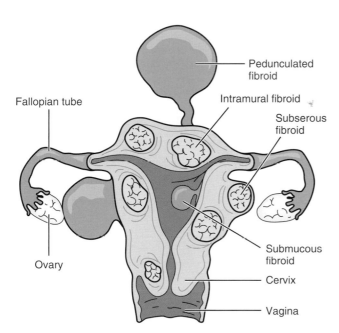

• Fig. 33.1 Fibroids within the uterus. (From Phillips N: *Berry & Kohn's operating room technique*, ed 13, St. Louis, 2017, Elsevier.)

decrease the potential for ovarian cancer. Fig. 33.1 provides an illustration of fibroids within the uterus.

Surgical Procedure

Two surgical approaches are possible when performing a hysterectomy: vaginal and abdominal. The specific technique may be further divided into variations according to the specific disease process, the patient's individual anatomic characteristics, and the surgeon's preference. The vaginal approach is performed with the patient in a dorsal lithotomy position with steep head-down tilt (Trendelenburg). This procedure is advantageous due to surgical visibility, and it is associated with decreased morbidity and mortality. Recovery time is more rapid, is associated with less pain, and has a lower rate of complications involving the surgical site compared with the abdominal approach. Its use is limited by anatomic and pathophysiologic factors such as uterine size, pelvic adhesions, or the presence of gynecologic cancer, all of which may require an abdominal approach. A laparoscopic-assisted vaginal hysterectomy

(LAVH) is a variation in which the hysterectomy is initially accomplished via a laparoscopic technique but the remainder of the surgery is performed vaginally. Fig. 33.2 illustrates the anatomic structures and removal of the uterus during vaginal hysterectomy.

The abdominal approach is performed with the patient in the supine position. Factors such as uterine size and possible need for lymph node dissection will determine whether a Pfannenstiel or low midline is used. The abdominal hysterectomy approach may be further delineated into (1) subtotal or supracervical, (2) total, or (3) radical. A subtotal hysterectomy is the removal of part or all of the uterine fundus with the preservation of the lower uterine segment or uterine cervix. A total hysterectomy includes removal of the uterus and the uterine cervix but not the removal of fallopian tubes or ovaries. A total hysterectomy compared with a subtotal hysterectomy is performed whenever possible because it decreases the possibility of cervical cancer that may occur in the future. A radical hysterectomy is accomplished if cancer is present, and it involves the removal of the uterus, upper vagina, and all the parametrial tissues to the pelvic side wall. Fig. 33.3 provides an illustration of the functional anatomy and surgical intervention during an abdominal hysterectomy.

Anesthetic Management and Considerations

Preoperative Period

1. *Discuss the potential psychological components for patients having a hysterectomy.*

   Fear, anxiety, embarrassment, shame, and guilt may be associated with gynecologic surgery. Patients who have chronic pain may have concerns regarding postoperative pain management. Women who have urinary incontinence may be embarrassed about their condition, and those who have a pelvic mass may have anxiety or

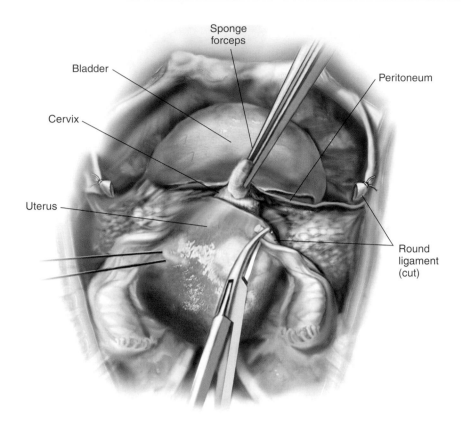

• **Fig. 33.3** Functional anatomy and surgical intervention during an abdominal hysterectomy. (From Baggish M, Karram M, eds: *Atlas of pelvic anatomy and gynecologic surgery*, Philadelphia, 2016, Elsevier.)

fear of disfigurement and concern over the loss of sexual function and desirability. In addition, religion, ethnicity, family dynamics, educational level, gender identity, and the value placed on a woman's reproductive ability all may influence the patient's thought process. The potential psychological ramifications of the surgery should be acknowledged, respected, and managed with sensitivity.

2. *Identify the available anesthetic techniques for abdominal or vaginal hysterectomy.*

General anesthesia is the most commonly used technique for patients having a hysterectomy. Regional anesthesia offers advantages such as rapid recovery, a decreased incidence of PONV, postoperative pain management, shorter postoperative stay, cost-effectiveness, and decreased hemodynamic variability. However, the use of regional technique may be limited by factors such as surgical requirements and surgeon and/or patient preference. Spinal, epidural, or combined spinal-epidural (CSE) anesthesia is appropriate for patients undergoing simple hysterectomy through a Pfannenstiel incision or vaginal hysterectomy. Spinal anesthesia may be less desirable in the younger population due to the increased propensity for postdural puncture headache (PDPH). If spinal anesthesia is used, a pencil-point needle should be used to decrease the incidence of PDPH. A blockade of the T4–T6 sensory dermatome level is sufficient to provide anesthesia for uterine procedures.

3. *Determine the anesthetic technique most commonly used for a laparoscopic hysterectomy.*

General anesthesia with neuromuscular blockade is most commonly utilized. The airway is maintained and protected by an endotracheal tube. Neuromuscular blockade allows for maximal insufflation of the abdomen during pneumoperitoneum and results in lower intraabdominal pressures (IAPs) and improved surgical visualization and access.

4. *Summarize the disadvantages of nitrous oxide during a laparoscopic hysterectomy.*

The use of nitrous oxide (N_2O) during laparoscopic surgery is controversial. Because N_2O is highly diffusible, concerns about bowel distension that will limit surgical vision and access, as well as potentially increasing the incidence of PONV, are limitations. There are limited scientific data that definitively help link the use of N_2O to these disadvantages. The decision to include or omit N_2O from a general anesthetic is best determined by the individual anesthesia provider.

Intraoperative Period

5. *Describe the pertinent physiologic changes that are associated with the lithotomy position.*

The lithotomy position is often associated with Trendelenburg (head of the surgical table tilted downward) during a hysterectomy to increase visualization of the perineum and to improve the surgical access. Elevation of the legs above the thorax acutely increases venous return. Mean arterial blood pressure (MAP) and cardiac filling pressures such as central venous pressure (CVP) and pulmonary artery pressure (PAP) increase.

In patients with normal cardiovascular functioning, vascular physiologic reflexes compensate for these transient increases in filling pressures. However, those patients who have cardiovascular disease states may not tolerate the lithotomy or Trendelenburg positions. Patients who have peripheral vascular insufficiency can develop venous stasis and peripheral ischemia. Those patients with a hiatal hernia, gastroesophageal reflux disease, or who are obese may have decreased lower esophageal sphincter tone and gastric barrier pressure, increasing the risk for regurgitation and aspiration of gastric contents. Acute and significant hypovolemia may not be observed during the lithotomy position due to increased venous return. Lowering of the legs into the supine position is accompanied by a redistribution of blood volume, which can result in severe hypotension.

Pulmonary side effects that are associated with the lithotomy position are minimal, but with the addition of Trendelenburg, functional residual capacity (FRC) is decreased. Obese patients and those who are having general anesthesia experience ventilation–perfusion (V/Q) mismatching and atelectasis, thus decreasing lung aeration.

6. *Discuss risk factors associated with positioning and nerve injury during laparoscopic hysterectomy.*

The most common reason for nerve injuries during laparoscopy are caused by pressure that is applied directly to peripheral nerves. Risk factors that may lead to injury from pressure or stretching of the nerves include the length of surgery, the type of leg support used to place patients in the lithotomy position, and preexisting systemic diseases that decrease peripheral blood flow such as diabetes. The "candy cane" stirrup offers minimal control over the positioning of the hips and the lower legs. This device has been implicated in an increased incidence of lower extremity nerve injuries, especially the common peroneal nerve. The use of leg supports ("boot-type" stirrups) that hold the entire posterior aspect of the leg are currently used more frequently. Slender patients or those with a body mass index (BMI) of less than 20 kg/m^2 are thought to be at increased risk due to lack of subcutaneous tissue padding from external pressure.

7. *Assess the various types of nerve injuries that are associated with laparoscopic and open abdominal hysterectomy.*

- **Brachial plexus injuries** are the most commonly reported peripheral nerve injury related to positioning. During laparoscopy, the risk of brachial plexus injury is increased for patients with outstretched arms or when they are placed in steep Trendelenburg position.

These injuries result in sensory deficits extending to the medial aspect of the hand, forearm, and arm.

- **Femoral nerve injury** is the most commonly reported nerve injury after gynecologic surgery. The damage is presumed to be caused by pressure-related surgical instrument retraction on the femoral nerve during an open hysterectomy. However, during laparoscopy the femoral nerve can be injured as a result of protracted nerve stretching during the lithotomy position as a result of prolonged hip flexion, abduction, and external rotation. This injury may be decreased by positioning the patient in low lithotomy and using "boot-type" stirrups. Because the femoral nerve contains both sensory and motor components, nerve injury often results in a loss of sensation over the anterior thigh and medial aspect of the lower leg, motor weakness of the quadriceps muscle, and decreased patellar reflexes.
- **Lateral femoral cutaneous nerve injury** is similar to femoral nerve injury because of its near-identical anatomic path. In contrast to the femoral nerve, which has mixed sensory and motor function, it is solely a sensory nerve. Injury to this nerve causes numbness or pain in the proximal-lateral aspect of the thigh.
- **Obturator nerve injury** results from prolonged hip flexion in the lithotomy position. This nerve has both sensory and motor function. Damage may lead to loss of sensation in the medial aspect of the thigh. Obturator nerve injury that causes weakness of the adductor muscle group and results in an impaired ability to walk is a rare event.
- **Sciatic nerve injury** may result from excessive abduction and external rotation of the hip in combination with flexion of the knee. The sciatic nerve both supplies the motor innervation to the hamstring muscle and provides motor and sensory transmission to the lower leg through the common peroneal nerve. Sciatic nerve injury may manifest as a loss of sensation over the calf and on the sole, dorsum, and lateral side of the foot. Foot drop is also possible due to anterior and lateral compartment muscle weakness.
- **Common peroneal nerve injury** may result from direct pressure such as from the use of candy cane stirrups and excessive stretch due to prolonged flexion of the knee. Excessive external rotation of the hip may also increase the risk of injury. The common peroneal nerve contains both sensory and motor functions. Injury may be manifested as a loss of cutaneous sensation in the lateral and anterior aspect of the lower leg. More serious injuries may result in foot drop.

8. *Describe the pertinent cardiovascular effects associated with a pneumoperitoneum.*

Abdominal insufflation alters MAP and heart rate (HR). The extent of these and other cardiovascular changes are multifactorial and are dependent on the IAP that is achieved, the volume of CO_2 that is absorbed systemically, the intravascular volume, and the mode and pressure during artificial ventilation. However, one of the most important determinants of cardiovascular function during laparoscopy is IAP. At an IAP below 15 mm Hg, cardiac output is increased due to increased venous return and increased cardiac filling pressures. At IAP values greater than 15 mm Hg, venous return decreases, leading to a decrease in cardiac output, which may result in hypotension. An increase in systemic vascular resistance (SVR), MAP, CVP, and mean PAP is associated with a pneumoperitoneum for laparoscopic hysterectomy.

Bradyarrhythmias such as bradycardia, atrioventricular dissociation, and asystole can occur during the creation of a pneumoperitoneum and traction on the abdominal viscera or intraperitoneal structures during an open hysterectomy. These phenomena have been attributed to vagal stimulation, which initiates the celiac reflex caused by insertion of the Veress needle or trocar, pneumoperitoneum-induced peritoneal stretch, or CO_2 embolization. Conversely, tachyarrhythmias may occur due to increased concentrations of CO_2 and catecholamines.

9. *Describe the pertinent respiratory effects of a pneumoperitoneum.*

Changes in respiratory function during laparoscopic surgery include a reduction in lung volume, increased peak airway pressures, and decreased pulmonary compliance due to increased IAP and patient positioning. Elevated IAP reduces diaphragmatic excursion and shifts the diaphragm cephalad, leading to early closure of smaller airways (increased closing capacity), causing atelectasis and decreased FRC. This upward shift of the diaphragm may lead to preferential ventilation of the nondependent portions of the lung, which results in V/Q mismatch and increased intrapulmonary shunting.

10. *Discuss the use of CO_2 to the creation of a pneumoperitoneum.*

Carbon dioxide gas is most commonly used during laparoscopic surgery because it is nonflammable, rapidly absorbed from the vascular space, and easily excreted from the respiratory system. CO_2 is readily available and inexpensive. The disadvantages that are associated with the use of CO_2 gas for the pneumoperitoneum include increased risk of hypercarbia resulting in respiratory acidosis. It is theorized that CO_2 causes peritoneal and diaphragmatic irritation, which has been linked to postoperative shoulder pain. Air and oxygen both support combustion when bipolar diathermy or lasers are used. Nitrogen, argon, and helium have been studied but are considered more hazardous due their low blood gas solubility and potential to create a VGE.

11. *List four respiratory complications associated with a pneumoperitoneum.*
    - **Endobronchial intubation** may occur due to cephalad displacement of the diaphragm and the carina during pneumoperitoneum and migration of the endotracheal tube (ETT) during Trendelenburg positioning. The result may include decreased oxygen saturation, increased peak airway pressure, and the potential for bronchospasm from stimulation of the carina from the distal end of the ETT. The treatment for this situation involves manual ventilation with 100% oxygen; assessing the adequacy of bilateral, equal, and clear breath sounds; and finally, manipulating the ETT into the proper position.
    - **Extraperitoneal insufflation** may be diagnosed by identifying a dramatic increase in end tidal carbon dioxide ($ETCO_2$) and the presence of subcutaneous emphysema. Treatment includes immediately notifying the surgeon and exsufflation until the CO_2 is eliminated. This complication frequently resolves rapidly after surgery. The anesthetist should be cautious and determine if subcutaneous emphysema is present in the neck region. If so, ventilation and reintubation may be difficult or impossible to accomplish.
    - **CO_2 gas embolism** is a rare complication, but it can result in death. Carbon dioxide gas enters the venous system by placement of a trocar into a vein or an abdominal organ. An "air lock" is created at the junction between the inferior vena cava and the right atrium, which disrupts blood flow into the heart. It may manifest as a sudden loss of $ETCO_2$, tachycardia, arrhythmias, hypotension, hypoxia, increased CVP, altered heart tones (mill-wheel murmur), and cardiovascular collapse. The treatment for VAE includes exsufflation, ventilation with 100% oxygen, discontinuing anesthetic agents, administration of fluids and vasopressors to augment the patient's blood pressure, aspiration from a CVP line, and placing the patient in a head-down left lateral position to increase blood flow into the heart by preventing a right ventricular outflow obstruction.
    - A **pneumothorax** may occur due to diaphragmatic or pleural trauma, or through a defect in the aortic or esophageal hiatus. Increased airway pressures, absence of breath sounds over the affected lung, precipitous oxygen desaturation, hypoxemia, hypercarbia, and hemodynamic instability may be seen. The definitive treatment used for a pneumothorax that causes physiologic compromise is immediate thoracentesis.

Postoperative Period

12. *Compare various pharmacologic and nonpharmacologic methods used to attenuate PONV.*

Various nonpharmacologic methods are used to minimize the potential for developing PONV, and these strategies are listed in Box 33.2.

Traditional antiemetic drugs used to prevent PONV include anticholinergics (atropine, scopolamine), antihistamines (cyclizine, diphenhydramine), steroids (dexamethasone), and phenothiazines (promethazine, prochlorperazine). Other antiemetics include:
- Benzamide (metoclopramide), which blocks dopamine receptors centrally within the vomiting center and chemoreceptor trigger zone (CTZ), as well as

- Use of regional anesthesia technique if possible
- Administration of medications used for PONV prophylaxis
- Gastric decompression with oral or nasogastric tube
- Adequate perioperative IV hydration
- Avoid/minimize use of N_2O
- Minimize use of neostigmine if muscle relaxation is necessary
- Pain control using nonsteroidal antiinflammatory drugs and local anesthesia infiltration

peripherally in the gastrointestinal tract. The drug also increases gastric emptying, increases lower esophageal sphincter tone, and lowers gastric fluid volume. Rapid intravenous (IV) administration may cause abdominal cramping, dystonia, and extrapyramidal reactions. Metoclopramide is contraindicated in patients with intestinal obstruction and should be avoided in patients with Parkinson disease.

- Butyrophenones (droperidol and haloperidol) act as a dopamine receptor antagonist within the CTZ. Droperidol has an onset of action from 30 to 60 minutes after administration and an extended duration of action from 4 to 24 hours. However, the use of droperidol has been limited due to the US Food and Drug Administration (FDA) black box warning because of reports of QTc prolongation and torsades de pointes. This warning contained administration guidelines, which include:
  - Droperidol should not be given to those patients with known or suspected QTc prolongation.
  - It is also held in those patients at risk for QTc prolongation, such as those with congestive heart failure, bradycardia, cardiac hypertrophy, hypokalemia, hypomagnesemia, or those taking medications that may increase QTc.
  - If droperidol is to be given, a 12-lead ECG is to be done before treatment to determine the QTc interval.
  - Post-droperidol administration, continuous ECG monitoring for 2 to 3 hours is necessary to observe for arrhythmias.
  - The lowest dose of droperidol is to be given, with small increases to effect.

- Haloperidol has an onset of 30 minutes after administration with a duration of about 4 hours. Adverse effects to butyrophenones include extrapyramidal side effects, orthostatic hypotension, neuroleptic malignant syndrome, and adverse ECG changes.
- Dexamethasone is a synthetic steroid that is frequently used as a prophylactic measure against PONV. The exact mechanism by which dexamethasone exerts an antiemetic effect has not been determined; however, it may have an inhibitory effect on prostaglandin synthesis or antagonize neurokinin type 1 receptors present in the CTZ. It is most efficacious when given concomitantly with other antiemetic medications. Due to its slow onset of action (2 hours) and long half-life (46 to 72 hours), dexamethasone is most efficacious if it is administered early in the perioperative phase, within 1 hour before induction, and the antiemetic effects prolonged.
- Hydroxytryptamine type 3 receptor antagonists ($5HT_3$) such as ondansetron, dolasetron, and granisetron are medications that are commonly used for PONV prophylaxis. Ondansetron has a half-life of 3 to 4 hours and is thus best given toward the completion of surgery for PONV prophylaxis. The time of administration of dolasetron has not been shown to decrease PONV. All $5HT_3$ antagonists have similar efficacy at equipotent doses, and the side effects include headache, abdominal pain, increased liver enzymes, and possible QT prolongation.

13. *Discuss the mechanism of shoulder pain commonly seen after laparoscopic surgery.*

    Shoulder pain is a common type of discomfort that is experienced on the first postoperative day after laparoscopic surgery. The visceral-type pain that is reported by patients is thought to be caused by the pneumoperitoneum rather than the use of trocars in the peritoneal space. The pneumoperitoneum is thought to induce pain by distension of the peritoneum and abdominal wall, leading to traction of the nerves and injury to blood vessels. Carbon dioxide contributes to pain by decreasing the intraperitoneal pH, leading to acidosis. The resulting inflammation is believed to irritate the phrenic nerve, which is perceived as shoulder pain. Ketorolac (Toradol) is an effective treatment for shoulder pain after laparoscopic surgery.

Review Questions

1. Which nerve injury results in a loss of sensation over the anterior thigh and medial aspect of the lower leg and motor weakness of the quadriceps muscle?
   a. Common peroneal
   b. Lateral femoral cutaneous
   c. Obturator
   d. Femoral

2. Sensory blockade at the ____ dermatome should be achieved if a spinal or epidural anesthetic technique is administered for hysterectomy?
   a. T4–T6
   b. T6–T8
   c. T1–T2
   d. T8–T10

3. Which hemodynamic parameter is decreased with creation of a pneumoperitoneum?
   a. Mean arterial pressure
   b. Stroke volume
   c. Systemic vascular resistance
   d. Pulmonary artery pressure

4. Which of the following respiratory parameters is increased with pneumoperitoneum?
   a. Peak inspiratory pressure
   b. Functional reserve capacity
   c. Vital capacity
   d. Pulmonary compliance

5. Which best describes the mechanism of action associated with metoclopramide?
   a. Enhances release of acetylcholine
   b. Inhibits prostaglandin synthesis
   c. Antagonizes hydroxytryptamine type 3 receptors
   d. Blocks dopaminergic receptors in the vomiting center, CTZ, and gastrointestinal tract

Suggested Readings

Abdalmageed OS, Bedaiwy MA, Falcone T. Nerve injuries in gynecologic laparoscopy. *J Minim Invasive Gynecol* 2017;24(1):16-27.

Dabush-Elisha I, Goren O, Herscovici A, Matot I. Bradycardia during laparoscopic surgeries: a retrospective cohort study. *World J Surg* 2019;43(6):1490-1496.

Dedden SJ, Geomini PMAJ, Huirne JAF, Bongers M. Vaginal and laparoscopic hysterectomy as an outpatient procedure: a systematic review. *Eur J Obstet Gynecol Reprod Biol* 2017;216:212-223.

Moriber N. Anesthesia for laparoscopic surgery. In: Nagelhout JJ, Elisha S, eds. *Nurse Anesthesia,* 6th ed. St Louis, MO: Elsevier, 2018:743-751.

Nguyen, NT, Wolfe BM. The physiologic effects of pneumoperitoneum in the morbidly obese. *Ann Surg* 2005;241(2):219-226.

Sandberg EM, Twijnstra ARH, Driessen SRC, Jansen FW. Total laparoscopic hysterectomy versus vaginal hysterectomy: a systematic review and meta-analysis. *J Minim Invasive Gynecol* 2017;24(2):206-217.

Thompson J. Positioning for anesthesia and surgery. In: Nagelhout JJ, Elisha S, eds. *Nurse Anesthesia,* 6th ed. St Louis, MO: Elsevier, 2018:380-396.

Wallis CJD, Peltz S, Byrne J, Kroft J, et al. Peripheral nerve injury during abdominal-pelvic surgery: analysis of the National Surgical Quality Improvement Program database. *Am Surg* 2017;83(11):1214-1219.

Yong J, Hibbert P, Runciman WB, Coventry B. Bradycardia as an early warning sign for cardiac arrest during routine laparoscopic surgery. *Int J Qual Health Care* 2015;27(6):473-478.

34

Dilation and Curettage

KEY POINTS

- Dilation of the cervix and curettage of the uterine lining is a common gynecologic procedure performed for diagnostic or therapeutic indications.
- Most patients who have a dilation and curettage (D&C) are discharged on the same day as the procedure.

- Risks associated with a D&C include a perforated uterus, cervical laceration, infection, and hemorrhage.

Case Synopsis

A 43-year-old woman with infertility and intervention with in vitro fertilization (IVF) 7 weeks ago has been experiencing vaginal bleeding for the past 2 weeks. She is scheduled by her gynecologist to have a D&C procedure.

Preoperative Evaluation and Demographic Data

Past Medical/Surgical History

- No significant past medical history
- D&C for spontaneous abortion 2 years ago

List of Medications

- Prometrium (fertility drug)
- Serophene (fertility drug)

Diagnostic Data

- Hemoglobin, 9.1 g/dL; hematocrit, 27.3%
- Beta-hCG level, 150 mIU/mL, indicating pregnancy at approximately 1 month gestation
- Ultrasound: negative for fetal activity

Height/Weight/Vital Signs

- 160 cm, 77 kg; body mass index (BMI), 30.1
- Blood pressure, 140/90; heart rate, 92 beats per minute; respiratory rate, 18 breaths per minute; room air oxygen saturation, 97%; temperature, 37.1°C

Pathophysiology

Abnormal uterine bleeding is often a result of benign fibroid tumors (myomas), polyps, hormonal imbalances of progesterone and estrogen, retention of the placenta post-childbirth, or early pregnancy failure. The uterus is a muscular, pear-shaped, hollow organ lined by the endometrium, which thickens in response to estrogen, and once ovulation occurs, progesterone prepares the lining for implantation of an embryo, as shown in Fig. 34.1. The IVF process includes administering hormonal medications to the patient, harvesting several eggs after ovulation, egg retrieval and fertilization in a petri dish, incubation, and transfer of the embryo 2 to 5 days later into the uterus. Approximately one-third of all women have mild to moderate cramping or light bleeding during the first trimester of pregnancy; however, if the bleeding is followed by severe cramping, miscarriage is likely. Miscarriages occur most often during the first 3 months of pregnancy and result in 15% to 20% of all clinically recognized pregnancies. Ultrasound examinations and beta-hCG tests are done when vaginal bleeding is present and early termination of the pregnancy is suspected. The term *missed abortion* is used to define a nonviable pregnancy retained for a minimum of 8 weeks. An *incomplete abortion* is the term used to define the passage of some fetal or placental tissue; however, some of the tissue is retained within the uterus. Anatomic representation of the uterus and cervix is shown in Fig. 34.1.

Surgical Procedure

The patient is positioned in the lithotomy position with her legs in stirrups. A tenaculum is inserted into the vagina to provide stability and expose the cervix. A uterine sound is inserted into the cervix to determine the safe depth that the cervical dilators and curettes can be inserted. When an incomplete abortion occurs, the cervix is frequently open.

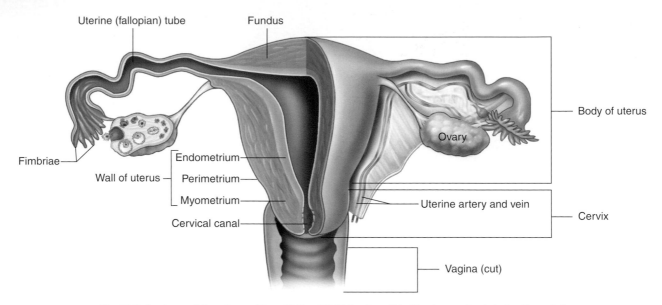

• **Fig. 34.1** Anatomy of the uterus. (From Patton KT, Thibodeau GA: *The human body in health and disease*, ed 7, St. Louis, 2018, Elsevier.)

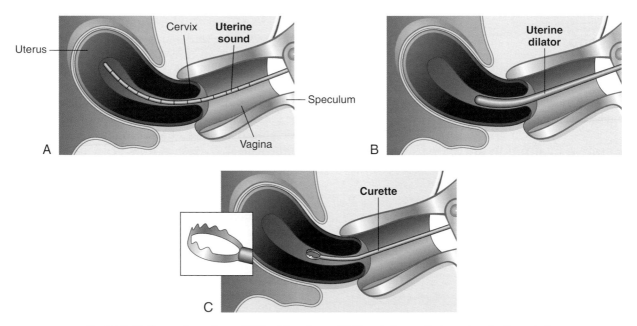

• **Fig. 34.2** Dilation and curettage (D&C) of the uterus. (A) The uterine cavity is explored with a uterine sound (a slender instrument used to measure the depth of the uterus) to prevent perforation during dilation. (B) Uterine dilators (Hanks or Hagar) in graduated sizes are used to gradually dilate the cervix. (C) The uterus is gently curetted and specimens are collected. (From Chabner DE: *The language of medicine*, ed 12, St. Louis, 2021, Elsevier.)

When the cervix is closed, it must be dilated. Metal dilators of increasing diameter are inserted into the cervix to dilate it approximately 1.5 cm. Once this opening is achieved, either a sharp curette is used to scrape the lining of the uterus or vacuum aspiration is used to evacuate the contents of the uterus. Suction aspiration can be done via electric vacuum or manual aspiration with a 60-mL syringe and a cannula. This process is illustrated in Fig. 34.2.

Anesthetic Management and Considerations

Preoperative Period

1. *Discuss the common coexisting diseases of women who present for D&C.*

   Women of all ages and with varying medical conditions present for D&C. Women under the age of 40 may have unexplained bleeding due to hormonal imbalance, and oftentimes coexisting endocrine pathology is present. Menstrual abnormalities have been linked to obesity in young women. Women over the age of 40 may have abnormal bleeding due to endometrial cancer. Cardiac disease is associated with the postmenopausal period and is often present. Anemia is often present in women who have experienced hemorrhage. Because this patient has experienced vaginal bleeding for the past 2 weeks, she is anemic. Physiologic compensation in response to mild to moderate degrees of anemia that develops gradually in a healthy female frequently does not pose additional surgical and anesthetic risk.

2. *Discuss the impact of anemia on tissue oxygenation.*

Each gram of hemoglobin binds with 1.39 mL of oxygen. A normal hemoglobin for women ranges from 12.1 to 15.1 g/dL. Excessive vaginal bleeding from any cause can result in decreases in hemoglobin and, because of that decrease, a lowering of arterial content of oxygen (CaO_2). The decrease in CaO_2 will affect delivery of oxygen to the tissues. Compensation occurs due to the production of 2,3-diphosphoglycerate as a result of anaerobic metabolism and results in a rightward shift of the oxygen–hemoglobin dissociation curve, which facilitates release of oxygen from hemoglobin. Increased sympathetic nervous system tone stimulates the myocardium to increase cardiac output to provide more oxygen at a tissue level. The patient has a 9.1 g/dL hemoglobin and a hematocrit of 27.3% and an elevated heart rate in response to anemia. It is critical that the anesthetist maximize the oxygenation to assure adequate tissue delivery. A higher fraction inspired oxygen delivery should be considered.

3. *Describe the potential link between obesity and infertility.*

The incidence of obesity has dramatically increased over the last decade and has reached epidemic proportions within the United States. The presence of obesity is associated with all age groups, and its incidence is increasing rapidly in women in their childbearing years. Researchers have found that obese women of reproductive age have up to a 67% higher incidence of miscarriage compared with women of normal weight. The risk of miscarriage further increases in obese women who receive infertility treatment. Obese women also have a higher incidence of polycystic ovaries, abnormal ovulation, and hormonal imbalances. These factors affect the ability of a woman to become pregnant and to sustain the pregnancy to full term.

4. *Explain the implications of BMI and anesthetic risk.*

BMI is a calculation of body fat based on height and weight. The formula to calculate BMI = (weight in pounds/[height in inches] × [height in inches]) × 703, or in the metric system BMI = (weight in kilograms/[height in meters] × [height in meters]). A normal BMI is between 18.5 and 24.9. Overweight individuals have a BMI between 25 and 29.9, 30 to 34.9 represents obesity, 35 to 39.9 is defined as severe obesity, 40 to 44.9 is

morbid obesity, and super obesity is a BMI >45. Obesity increases the morbidity and mortality associated with anesthesia due to its impact on the various physiologic systems. Obese individuals have an increased metabolic demand, oxygen consumption, incidence of sleep apnea, abdominal pressure, the volume of distribution for lipid-soluble drugs, cardiac output, and risk of developing arrhythmias due to myocardial hypertrophy. These patients have a decreased functional residual capacity and gastroesophageal sphincter tone. There is an increased risk of gastric aspiration, and preoperative prophylaxis accompanied with a rapid sequence induction is indicated. Preoperative data that should be assessed before surgical intervention include an electrocardiogram to identify any ischemia, arrhythmias, and hypertrophy and a chest x-ray to evaluate heart size and evidence of pulmonary hypertension. Consultation with a cardiologist to evaluate the patient's cardiovascular status is warranted if the patient has a history of cardiac-related symptoms.

5. *Discuss the physiologic and hormonal changes associated with pregnancy that may increase the risk of gastric aspiration.*

During pregnancy, there is an increase in progesterone. Progesterone antagonizes the effects of motilin, which is an amino acid peptide that is secreted into the mucosa of the proximal portion of the small intestine and results in the onset of uterine contractions. This substance facilitates gastric emptying. Thus increased progesterone secretion delays gastric emptying. Furthermore, placental gastrin secretion results in increased gastric acidity, decreased lower esophageal tone, and increased intragastric pressure. Patients who present for anesthesia who are between 12 and 14 weeks pregnant should be considered a "full stomach" and are believed to be at increased risk of gastric aspiration.

Intraoperative Period

6. *Discuss the airway management concerns for a patient who is obese.*

The anesthetic technique that can be utilized for this procedure includes general anesthesia, spinal anesthesia, or sedation with paracervical block. If general anesthesia is indicated due to the specific patient situation, a mask technique or insertion of a laryngeal mask airway (LMA) is unsuitable for airway management for obese patients. Because the obese patient is at risk for aspiration, the potential for a difficult airway, and obstructive sleep apnea, placement of an endotracheal tube should be accomplished. The head-elevated laryngoscopy position (HELP), in which the head and neck are elevated above the chest and abdomen, improves the view of laryngeal structures by aligning the airway axes during direct laryngoscopy. The reverse Trendelenburg position allows for increased diaphragmatic excursion and functional residual capacity. This maneuver allows for more effective preoxygenation before the induction of anesthesia.

7. *Describe the anesthetic considerations associated with the lithotomy position.*

Improper positioning may lead to nerve injuries in the lower extremities. The nerves that are predisposed to compression and damage include the femoral, sciatic, obturator, lateral femoral cutaneous, and common peroneal. Nerve injury in the lithotomy position has been reported to be 1:3608 patients. Of these injuries, 78% involve the common peroneal nerve, 15% the sciatic nerve, and 7% the femoral nerve. These nerve injuries are most common among patients who are thin, endure a prolonged surgical procedure, and smoke cigarettes. The common peroneal nerve is a branch of the sciatic nerve, which is responsible for sensory and motor innervation to the lower leg, feet, and toes. It is anatomically positioned lateral to the neck of the fibula below the knee. Injury can occur with compression of the lateral aspect of the knee against the stirrup, which can result in foot drop and paresthesia to the lower extremity. To avoid common peroneal nerve damage, it is essential to pad the stirrup and properly place the lower leg to avoid compression.

Injury to the hip joints can also occur when patients are placed in the lithotomy position. Proper care while initiating the lithotomy position includes raising or lowering both legs simultaneously and avoiding external rotation and hip flexion beyond 110 degrees. Injury to the common peroneal nerve will result in foot drop, the inability to evert the foot, and the loss of dorsal extension of the toes. Sciatic nerve injury can result from excessive external rotation and pressure in the region of the sciatic notch. Sciatic nerve injury results in weakness or paralysis of muscles below the knee and numbness of the foot and lateral half of the calf. The anesthetist must be vigilant when raising the foot of the operating table to avoid injuries to the fingers and hands when the arms are tucked on the either side of the body.

8. *Discuss the ventilatory and cardiovascular changes that are associated with the lithotomy position.*

In a ventilated patient, peak inspiratory pressure and end tidal carbon dioxide ($ETCO_2$) values will increase, and vital capacity and functional residual capacity decrease. Depending on the degree of hip flexion, abdominal contents are displaced upward on the diaphragm and impede lung excursion, especially when patients are placed in the Trendelenburg position. These physiologic changes are amplified for patients who are obese, and significant ventilation–perfusion mismatch resulting in hypoxemia and hypercarbia can occur. The risk of gastric aspiration increases during general anesthesia when patients are placed in the lithotomy position.

The estimated blood volume contained in both legs is between 250 and 500 mL. When placed in the lithotomy position, gravity increases the flow of blood from the legs, increasing the central blood volume. Perfusion to the lower extremities is reduced, and central venous pressure and pulmonary capillary wedge pressure are increased. This position also promotes venous stasis, increasing the potential for deep vein thrombus formation. When the lithotomy position is combined with Trendelenburg, cardiac output decreases as afterload is increased.

9. *Discuss the advantages and disadvantages of providing regional anesthesia for a D&C.*

A major advantage of a spinal or epidural regional technique is that airway maintenance and artificial ventilation are frequently unnecessary. Other advantages include decreased anesthetic requirements for providing sedation, postoperative analgesia, decreased cardiopulmonary depression, and a lower incidence of postoperative nausea and vomiting (PONV).

A disadvantage for using neuraxial anesthesia during a D&C procedure is the duration of the anesthetic relative to the short length of the procedure. In obese patients, a regional technique may be technically challenging to perform due to difficulties identifying the iliac crests or the spinous processes, problems with depth of needle insertion, and epidural catheter migration associated with changes in position. Another issue may be an unexpected high block due to different dosing requirements in the obese patient population. Researchers have found a direct positive correlation with an increase in weight and the height of the block with any given dose. It is theorized that increased abdominal tissue mass exerts pressure on the abdominal vasculature, which directly increases the blood volume within the epidural venous plexus. The engorged veins push inward on the dura mater, decreasing the volume of cerebrospinal fluid within the subarachnoid space. Because the patient is awake when a regional technique is performed, premedication and continuous sedation with a benzodiazepine and/or an opioid should be considered, as the patient is often anxious and may be emotionally distraught.

10. *Discuss the advantages and disadvantages of providing general anesthesia for a D&C.*

An advantage associated with general anesthesia is that the patient is unconscious and not aware of the sounds of the suction, which can be bothersome for a woman who has endured a miscarriage. Furthermore, the pelvis is completely relaxed and the pelvic examination by the gynecologist can be accomplished most effectively.

Disadvantages associated with general anesthesia include an increased risk of aspiration and nerve injury, the potential for difficult airway management, and an increased incidence of PONV. If inhalation agents are administered, there is a dose-related increased risk for uterine atony or relaxation that may increase the incidence of bleeding. Anesthetic-related complications are considered greatest with general anesthesia for D&C.

11. *Discuss the effects of inhalation agents on uterine smooth muscle.*

All inhalation agents relax uterine smooth muscle by decreasing the availability of intracellular free calcium and inhibiting contraction. The degree of uterine relaxation is dependent on the dose that is administered. Uterine atony is associated with increased blood loss. Desflurane and sevoflurane cause a greater uterine relaxation compared with isoflurane at 1.5 MAC.

12. *Explain the pharmacologic properties of oxytocin (Pitocin).*

Oxytocin is a hormone that is produced in the paraventricular nuclei of the hypothalamus and is secreted from the posterior pituitary. The physiologic action associated with oxytocin includes stimulation of uterine contractions. A synthetic form is administered to increase the frequency and force of uterine contractions. When a spontaneous abortion is associated with uncontrolled bleeding, the surgeon will ask the anesthetist to administer 10 units of oxytocin to enhance uterine contraction. Side effects associated with pitocin administration include headache, bradycardia, tachycardia, and nausea and vomiting.

13. *Describe the technique that is used to correctly administer a paracervical block.*

A paracervical block is considered a nerve block and is usually performed by the gynecologist. The technique for the block involves the use of a local anesthetic, usually 1% lidocaine, 1% lidocaine with 0.005 mg/mL epinephrine, or 3% chloroprocaine. To enhance the comfort of the patient and to decrease anxiety, sedation using a benzodiazepine and small doses of propofol should be considered. Under sterile technique, in the lithotomy position, the cervicovaginal joint is identified with the index finger. A 10-mL syringe and 23-gauge needle with a needle extender are used to inject 1- to 3-mL volumes of local anesthetic at 0.5 cm depth, 1 cm depth, and 1.5 cm depth slowly in the cervicovaginal joint at the 4 or 5 o'clock and 7 or 8 o'clock positions (5 to mL total at each location) to reach the sacrouterine ligaments. This intervention, as shown in Fig. 34.3, anesthetizes the Frankenhauser ganglion, which is the location for the visceral sensory nerve fibers to the upper vagina, cervix, and uterus. The anesthetist should be aware of volumes of local anesthetic injected and vigilant for possible signs of local anesthetic toxicity when large volumes of local anesthetic are used.

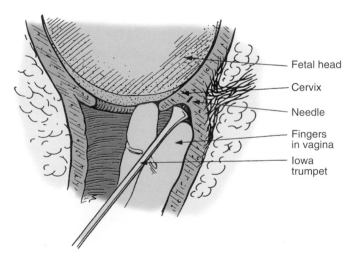

• **Fig. 34.3** Technique of administering a paracervical block. (From Pfenninger JL, Fowler GC: *Pfenninger & Fowler's procedures for primary care,* ed 3, St. Louis, 2011, Elsevier.)

14. *Discuss the possible complications associated with the D&C procedure.*

As with any procedure, the anesthetic risks are determined by the patient's preoperative comorbid diseases and overall health status. The risks related to anesthesia for a D&C are usually related to airway management difficulties, light anesthesia, or nerve injury. The risk of surgical complications associated with the D&C procedure is relatively low. The surgical complications include uterine perforation, cervical tear, infection, and bleeding. The anesthetist must be prepared for periods of peak surgical stimulation. For example, when uterine dilators are inserted into the cervix, the anesthetic depth should be appropriate so that there is no patient movement, which could increase the possibility of uterine perforation. The concentration of inhalation agent that is used should be decreased when possible to lessen the potential for uterine relaxation and bleeding.

Postoperative Period

15. *Discuss PONV management for patients having a D&C procedure.*

The occurrence of PONV is associated with general anesthesia, and gynecologic surgical procedures increase the risk. Certain factors have been associated with a higher incidence of PONV, and unfortunately these factors apply to the patient scheduled for a D&C. They include female gender, outpatient, young adult, and gynecologic surgery. The patient presented here also has an additional risk factor, which is obesity. Adequate intravenous volume replacement is also essential to help reduce the possibility of PONV.

Most patients scheduled for a D&C are at high risk for PONV. In the past low-dose droperidol was considered a low cost-efficient agent to combat PONV. However, due to the black box warning issued in 2001 by the US Food and Drug Administration (FDA) related to cardiac QT prolongation and abnormal rhythms, it is no longer considered the drug of choice used for PONV prophylaxis. Dexamethasone has been found to be as effective as droperidol in preventing PONV. The exact mechanism of the antiemetic properties of steroids is unknown; however, it is postulated that decreasing prostaglandin synthesis or inhibiting neurokinin-1 receptors in the vomiting center has an antiemetic effect. The serotonin antagonist ondansetron is effective in prevention and treatment of PONV.

Combination therapy using dexamethasone and a serotonin antagonist has been found to be of benefit for PONV prophylaxis, as the emetogenic effects induced by anesthetic agents involve a variety of receptors and neurologic pathways. By antagonizing these various receptors and pathways, decreased PONV is frequently achieved.

16. *Discuss the postoperative pain management for a patient who has had a D&C.*

The character of the pain that is most frequently experienced after a D&C procedure is uterine cramps, and the duration extends for 24 hours. Oral acetaminophen with codeine is usually prescribed. Continuous administration of aspirin and ketorolac should be avoided to decrease the potential for uterine bleeding. Patients who experience persistent and severe pain should be evaluated for the possibility of a uterine perforation.

Review Questions

1. The patient presenting for a D&C has a low hemoglobin value, which shifts the oxyhemoglobin dissociation curve to right and:
   a. Decreases the affinity between oxygen and hemoglobin.
   b. Increases epinephrine release from the adrenal medulla.
   c. Decreases the CO_2 production in peripheral tissues.
   d. Increases baroreceptor stimulation in the carotid body and aortic arch.

2. The nerve that is most likely to be damaged from compression of the lateral aspect of the fibula immediately below the knee is the:
   a. Sciatic nerve.
   b. Obturator nerve.
   c. Common peroneal nerve.
   d. Femoral nerve.

3. The hormone that increases the risk of maternal gastric aspiration is:
   a. Estrogen.
   b. Motilin.
   c. Gastrin.
   d. Progesterone.

4. A paracervical block anesthetizes the:
   a. Uterus and cervix.
   b. Cervix and vagina.
   c. Uterus, cervix, and upper portion of the vagina.
   d. Cervix, upper portion of vagina, and urethral orifice.

5. Which is true regarding the effect of inhalation agents on uterine tone?
   a. The degree of atony is dose dependent.
   b. It increases uterine contraction.
   c. It induces minimal effects.
   d. It increases intracellular calcium, causing contractions.

Suggested Readings

Aksoy H, Aksoy U, Ozyurt S, Ozoglu N, et al. Comparison of lidocaine spray and paracervical block application for pain relief during first-trimester surgical abortion: a randomised, double-blind, placebo-controlled trial. *J Obstet Gynaecol* 2016;36(5):649-653.

Allen RH, Kumar D, Fitzmaurice G, et al. Pain management of first-trimester surgical abortion: effects of selection of local anesthesia with and without lorazepam or intravenous sedation. *Contraception* 2006;74:407-413.

Biel FM, Marshall NE, Snowden JM. Maternal body mass index and regional anaesthesia use at term: prevalence and complications. *Paediatr Perinat Epidemiol* 2017;31(6):495-505.

Kason BJ. Obstetric anesthesia. In: Nagelhout JJ, Elisha S, eds. *Nurse Anesthesia,* 6th ed. St Louis, MO: Elsevier, 2018:1064-1091.

Krough, MA. Obesity and anesthesia practice. In: Nagelhout JJ, Elisha S, eds. *Nurse Anesthesia,* 6th ed. St Louis, MO: Elsevier, 2018:998-1014.

Renner RM, Edelman AB, Nichols MD, et al. Refining paracervical block techniques for pain control in first trimester surgical abortion: a randomized controlled noninferiority trial. *Contraception* 2016;94(5):461-466.

Thomas JS, Maple IK, Norcross W, Muckler VC. Preoperative risk assessment to guide prophylaxis and reduce the incidence of postoperative nausea and vomiting. *J Perianesth Nurs* 2019;34(1):74-85.

Wilson SF, Gurney EP, Sammel MD, Schreiber CA. Doulas for surgical management of miscarriage and abortion: a randomized controlled trial. *Am J Obstet Gynecol* 2017;216(1):44.e1-44.e6.

Yoo KY, Lee JC, Shin MH, et al. The effects of volatile anesthetics on spontaneous contractility of isolated human pregnant uterine muscle: a comparison among sevoflurane, desflurane, isoflurane, and halothane. *Anesth Analg* 2006;103:443-449.

35

Cesarean Section

KEY POINTS

- Spinal anesthesia is considered an ideal choice for parturients undergoing cesarean section.
- Preeclampsia is a systemic disease process with multiple anesthetic considerations.
- A complete physical examination and history are critical when assessing the parturient with preeclampsia.
- The anesthetist must explain to the parturient in detail what to expect during a cesarean section.

- A plan of treatment for inadequate spinal analgesia must be outlined before the cesarean section.
- Postoperative treatment of a parturient with preeclampsia includes maintenance of adequate analgesia, hemodynamic control, maintenance of appropriate fluid and electrolyte balance, and seizure prophylaxis.

Case Synopsis

A 28-year-old parturient with an estimated fetal gestational age of 39 weeks presents to the labor and delivery unit, where she is diagnosed with preeclampsia. During an attempt at induction of labor, the fetus demonstrates a decline in fetal heart rate. It is decided that a cesarean section will be performed.

Preoperative Evaluation and Demographic Data

Past Medical/Surgical History

- Previous cesarean section 22 months ago
- Tonsillectomy as a child—no anesthetic complications
- Gestational gastroesophageal reflux disease (GERD)
- Allergy to penicillin; develops rash

List of Medications

- Prenatal vitamins
- Magnesium sulfate
- Tums

Diagnostic Data

- Hemoglobin, 10 g/dL; hematocrit, 30%; platelets, 125 mm^3
- Glucose, 139 mg/dL
- Blood urea nitrogen, 13 mg/dL; creatinine, 0.8 mg/dL
- Electrolytes: sodium, 140 mEq/L; potassium, 3.9 mEq/L; chloride, 104 mEq/L; carbon dioxide, 24 mEq/L
- 24-hour urine protein, 320 mg/L

Height/Weight/Vital Signs

- 163 cm, 100 kg
- Blood pressure, 150/98; heart rate, 90 beats per minute; respiratory rate, 18 breaths per minute; room air oxygen saturation, 98%; temperature, 36.8°C
- Fetal heart rate, 130 to 140 beats per minute

Pathophysiology

Preeclampsia is a systemic disease process that does not have a clearly defined pathogenesis. The exact etiology of preeclampsia is unknown, but the condition affects 5% to 9% of all pregnancies, with 85% of cases of preeclampsia affecting women in their first pregnancy. This condition is one of the most common comorbidities found in parturients. Risk factors that are associated with preeclampsia are included in Box 35.1. Multiple etiologic explanations exist for the development of preeclampsia, including immunologic factors, genetic factors, a molecular variant of angiotensinogen, factor V Leiden mutation, excessive maternal inflammatory response to pregnancy, endothelial factors, abnormal increases of intracellular free calcium concentration, promotion of endothelial expression of procoagulants, and altered handling of fatty acids by the liver.

Regardless of the exact etiology of preeclampsia, endothelial damage causes increased platelet aggregation, decreased production of vasodilatory substances, increased glomerular capillary permeability, and increased sensitivity to norepinephrine and angiotensin. The manifestations of these pathologic changes include thrombocytopenia, increased

- History of preeclampsia
- Family history of preeclampsia
- Nulliparity
- Age <20 years and >35 years
- Chronic hypertension and vascular and/or renal disease
- Obesity
- Insulin resistance
- Gestational diabetes
- Sickle cell disease
- Multiple pregnancies

liver enzymes, increased systemic vascular resistance, proteinuria, and edema.

Surgical Procedure

Delivery by cesarean section accounts for approximately one-third of all births in the United States, at about 1 million cases per year; it is one of the most common surgical procedures in the United States. Cesarean section is indicated for maternal factors such as arrested labor, prior cesarean section, abnormalities of placentation, or deteriorating maternal health (as in severe preeclampsia). Fetal factors—for example, macrosomia, malpresentation, and questionable fetal status—may lead to delivery by cesarean section. Cesarean section involves entry of the peritoneal cavity using a Pfannenstiel incision followed by incision of the lower uterine segment. After delivery of the fetus and placenta, the uterus and abdomen are closed. Complications can include hemorrhage, infection, and laceration of the uterus or bladder.

Anesthetic Management and Considerations

Preoperative Period

1. *Define the diagnostic criteria of mild and severe preeclampsia.*
   Mild preeclampsia is diagnosed during pregnancy if the following criteria are met:
   - **Blood pressure:** Sustained systolic pressure of 140 mm Hg or sustained diastolic blood pressure at least 90 mm Hg after the twentieth week of pregnancy in a parturient who had previously normal blood pressure
   - **Proteinuria:** Greater than 300 mg in a 24-hour period
   - **Edema:** Not a reliable sign of preeclampsia, as it is present in approximately 30% of all parturients
   Severe preeclampsia is diagnosed during pregnancy if at least one of the following criteria is met:
   - **Blood pressure:** Systolic pressure greater than 160 to 180 mm Hg or a diastolic pressure greater than 110 mm Hg

- **Proteinuria:** >5 g over a 24-hour period or a "dipstick" urine of +3 or +4
- **Oliguria:** Urine output of less than 500 mL in a 24-hour period
- **Neurologic symptoms:** Headache, visual disturbances, or other cerebral symptoms; the presence of grand mal seizures that are not related to other neurologic or metabolic conditions is diagnostic of eclampsia
- **Other associated symptoms:** Epigastric pain, pulmonary edema, liver dysfunction of unknown etiology, and thrombocytopenia

2. *Identify appropriate assessment interventions commonly used to evaluate the parturient with preeclampsia.*
   - Vital signs: blood pressure, heart rate, oxygen saturation, temperature, respiratory rate
   - Physical examination/history: headache, epigastric pain, visual disturbances, seizures
   - Laboratory assessment:
     - Hematocrit and hemoglobin should be assessed for hemoconcentration—a common finding in the hypertensive patient and one that supports the diagnosis of preeclampsia.
     - Platelet counts are obtained to assess for thrombocytopenia.
     - Renal function can be assessed with measures of serum uric acid and creatinine levels. Uric acid levels during pregnancy are typically lower than normal range, and levels of 5 mg/dL are considered abnormal. Likewise, creatinine levels during pregnancy are approximately 0.5 mg/dL, and levels of 0.9 mg/dL are considered abnormal during pregnancy. Urine protein is collected over a 24-hour period and serves as a marker for renal dysfunction.
     - Increasing serum transaminase levels can suggest progression of the disease. Decreased serum albumin levels occur due to capillary leakage and can be used to help quantify the extent of the disease. Increasing levels of lactic acid dehydrogenase (LDH) are suggestive of hemolysis. Any patient with signs or symptoms of severe preeclampsia, clinical signs of coagulopathy, or right upper quadrant pain should have coagulation studies completed (prothrombin time [PT]/activated partial thromboplastin time [aPTT], fibrinogen, and D-dimer).

3. *List the major teaching points the anesthetist should address with both the parturient and their significant other before cesarean section.*
   A thorough explanation of the sequence of events during the spinal anesthetic placement and the surgical procedure has a tremendous benefit to both the patient and the patient's significant other. When patients and their families know what to expect, they frequently experience less anxiety before the surgery. Additionally, a thorough explanation builds patient confidence between the patient and the anesthetist.

The parturient should inform the anesthetist of any symptoms of low blood pressure such as feelings of anxiety, diaphoresis, or nausea. The patient should be informed that they will feel pressure and pulling during the cesarean section, especially during the period immediately before delivery. The patient should be made aware of the possibility of nausea and vomiting associated with the exteriorization of the uterus.

4. *Discuss the preoperative medications that are commonly administered before a cesarean section.*

The American Society of Anesthesiologists Practice Guidelines recommend the timely administration of nonparticulate antacids, H2 receptor antagonists (60 to 90 minutes before surgical intervention), and/or metoclopramide for aspiration prophylaxis. In addition to the gastrokinetic effects associated with metoclopramide, it has been shown to decrease the incidence of postoperative nausea and vomiting (PONV) in obstetric patients having a cesarean section.

Intraoperative Period

5. *Explain the clinical effects of spinal anesthesia in a patient with preeclampsia.*

Spinal anesthesia can usually be safely administered in a patient with mild preeclampsia. A common side effect of the administration of spinal anesthesia is hypotension. In patients who have intravascular volume depletion, such as those with preeclampsia, hypotension can rapidly ensue because of the abrupt onset of the sympathectomy from preganglionic beta-fiber blockade. To reduce the chance of rapidly developing and severe hypotension after the placement of a subarachnoid block (SAB), IV fluid administration is indicated before SAB. Due to the short intravascular half-life of balanced salt solutions, if administration is accomplished more than 15 minutes before the SAB, intravascular volume expansion may be inadequate.

Patients will typically have at least a T10 sensory nerve block 4 minutes after spinal placement and a T4 sensory nerve block 8 minutes after placement. As the spinal anesthesia becomes established, the patient will feel warmth, tingling, numbness, and heaviness in their lower extremities, and these sensations will move up their torso. Inactivation of proprioceptive nerves at the level of the T6 dermatome, which innervates the intercostal muscles, will cause some patients to feel as though they cannot breathe. This can provoke feelings of claustrophobia; however, informing the patient preoperatively that this sensation may occur can reduce the likelihood of anxiety.

In the event of a significant drop in blood pressure, typically 20% below the baseline values, the patient will often report feelings of restlessness and nausea before the blood pressure monitor will display a reading. This symptom is associated with central medullary hypoxia. In addition to the sympathectomy that results from the

SAB, the gravid uterus can cause aortocaval compression, especially if the mother is in the supine position. Sustained left uterine displacement (SLUD) decreases the degree of compression and can restore adequate preload and reduce afterload. Fig. 35.1 depicts the aorta and inferior vena cava in relation to the uterus. It is reasonable to administer vasopressors to avoid severe hypotension. Intravenous (IV) fluids should be infused rapidly if hypotension occurs.

6. *Identify the dermatome level of sensory blockade needed if neuraxial anesthesia is used during cesarean section.*

Typically, a T4–T5 dermatome sensory blockade is desirable. Patients who have a sensory block as low as T6 (located at the tip of the xiphoid process) can usually tolerate the manipulation involved in cesarean section.

7. *Construct a plan of treatment for a patient who experiences inadequate sensory blockade during cesarean section.*

Multiple steps should be taken when assessing an inadequate spinal and deciding on an appropriate course of action. Some patients experience fear and anxiety, and any sensation (e.g., pressure, pulling) may be interpreted as pain. If the patient confirms that she feels pressure or pulling and not sharp pain, reassure her that these sensations are normal. Also, encourage the patient's significant other to talk with the patient, thereby providing a distraction from the sensations. If it is determined that the patient is having pain, determine the location. If it is near the incision site, the surgeon has the option of injecting low concentrations of local anesthetic medication at the incision site. If this intervention is ineffective, or if the pain is not located at the incision site, the anesthetist has a few options.

If the surgery has not started, an epidural may be placed and dosed slowly to achieve an appropriate sensory block. Another option is to postpone the case until the SAB completely recedes and administer a second

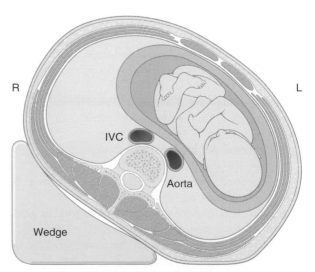

• **Fig. 35.1** Sustained left uterine displacement. *IVC,* Inferior vena cava; *R,* right; *L,* left. (From Pardo MC Jr, Miller RD: *Basics of anesthesia,* ed 7, St. Louis, 2018, Elsevier.)

SAB. The optimum time to wait for a second attempt has not been definitively determined, and a second SAB can result in a high or complete spinal.

If the surgery has already commenced and the patient feels pain, the anesthetist can administer small doses of ketamine (10 to 40 mg IV). Ketamine is a potent analgesic; however, it should be used with caution because it can provoke a significant increase in blood pressure due to the drug's sympathomimetic activity. Administration of midazolam is prudent after the baby has been delivered to decrease the potential for emergence delirium. Rapid-acting narcotics such as IV fentanyl in 25- to 50-mcg boluses and/or administering nitrous oxide in a 50% mixture with oxygen can also be used, but only after delivery and clamping of the umbilical cord have occurred.

General anesthesia is the final and definitive option but is associated with a greater probability of airway difficulties, especially in the edematous, preeclamptic patient. General anesthesia can also provoke significant hemodynamic variability, as well as neonatal respiratory depression.

8. *Compare the advantages and disadvantages of spinal and epidural anesthesia in the parturient with preeclampsia.*

The advantages associated with SAB include:
- Rapid onset
- Relative ease of placement
- Reliability

The disadvantages associated with SAB include:
- Rapid onset of a sympathetic blockade
- Hypotension
- Potential for a postdural puncture headache
- High SAB resulting in severe hypotension, loss of consciousness, and severe bradycardia
- Inadequacy of sensory blockade

The advantages associated with epidural anesthesia include:
- Gradual, controlled onset of sympathetic blockade
- Ability to titrate the volume of local anesthetic to the desired dermatome level
- Improved intervillous blood flow

The disadvantages associated with epidural anesthesia include:
- Possibility of sudden-onset hypotension
- Potential for inadequate, patchy, or unilateral blockade
- Potential for local anesthetic toxicity
- Potential for intravascular injection
- Increased level of technical difficulty during placement compared with spinal anesthesia
- Increased risk of epidural hematoma in patients who develop coagulopathies

9. *Compare the use of phenylephrine and ephedrine when treating hypotension after SAB.*

Ephedrine has long been considered the drug of choice for treatment of neuraxial anesthesia–induced hypotension. Administering phenylephrine may be preferable compared with ephedrine for hypotension that ensues during routine pregnancies. Phenylephrine and ephedrine result in similar fetal acid–base balance after administration. The use of phenylephrine in patients with bradycardia, especially during the period in which the level of the SAB is still variable, can worsen bradycardia. Blockade of sympathetic outflow at the level of the cardio-accelerator fibers (T1–T5) combined with arterial constriction, which initiates the baroreceptor response, is the physiologic rationale for this response.

It is estimated that nearly 70% of obstetric patients develop clinically significant hypotension (systolic blood pressure [SBP] <90 mm Hg). Ondansetron 4 to 8 mg IV may help decrease the incidence of hypotension by inhibiting vasodilation. It is postulated that the antiserotonin effects of ondansetron inhibit the Bezold–Jarisch reflex.

10. *Describe the pharmacologic treatment for uterine atony.*

After delivery of the fetus, an IV infusion of oxytocin, 20 units, is typically administered. In the setting of uterine atony, an additional 20 units of oxytocin can be added to the existing oxytocin infusion. If this intervention fails to increase uterine tone, methylergonovine (methergine) (0.2 mg intramuscularly [IM]) can be administered. It must be used with caution in patients with hypertension, particularly when used concomitantly with ephedrine or phenylephrine. An additional pharmacologic agent, prostaglandin F2-alpha (250 mcg IM), can also be used to treat uterine atony. Like methylergonovine, prostaglandin F2-alpha can cause exaggerated hypertension. This medication can provoke bronchospasm in asthmatic patients. After the use of either methylergonovine or prostaglandin F2-alpha, the anesthetist should consider ordering antidiarrheal medications, as these agents cause diarrhea.

11. *Describe the therapeutic range and the side effects of increasing plasma levels of magnesium sulfate.*

It is vitally important to maintain magnesium sulfate plasma levels within the therapeutic range. Subtherapeutic levels can result in seizures caused by inadequate treatment of preeclampsia, and high levels can result in complete paralysis. Magnesium levels and the associated physiologic response are included in Box 35.2.

• BOX 35.2 Side Effects Associated With Increasing Plasma Levels of Magnesium Sulfate

- 1.5–2.0 mg/dL: Normal plasma concentration
- 4.0–8.0 mg/dL: Therapeutic range
- 5–10 mg/dL: ECG changes (widened QRS complex, PQ interval prolongation)
- 10–15 mg/dL: Loss of deep tendon reflexes
- 15–20 mg/dL: SA and AV block, respiratory paralysis
- 20–25 mg/dL: Cardiac arrest

AV, Atrioventricular; *ECG*, electrocardiogram; *SA*, sinoatrial.

12. *Examine the anesthetic implications associated with magnesium sulfate therapy.*

Magnesium sulfate therapy can exacerbate hypotension associated with neuraxial anesthesia. In the majority of preeclamptic patients, a decrease in blood pressure can be treated by fluid and vasopressors. Magnesium sulfate also prolongs the effects of nondepolarizing muscle relaxants (NDMRs). If paralysis is necessary during general anesthesia, NDMRs should be carefully titrated to effect, and assessment via nerve stimulation is prudent. Although magnesium sulfate may prolong the duration of action of succinylcholine, the standard intubating dose of succinylcholine should not be reduced to facilitate rapid paralysis.

13. *Explain the mechanism of action and the effects of magnesium sulfate in the patient with preeclampsia.*

Magnesium sulfate is considered a first-line treatment for preeclampsia. It exerts anticonvulsant, vasodilator, and tocolytic effects. Magnesium sulfate likely exerts its anticonvulsant actions by reducing cerebral vasoconstriction and by centrally mediating cerebral N-methyl-D-aspartate receptors. Its peripheral vasodilatory effects are attributed to directly or indirectly competing with calcium, by increasing cyclic guanosine monophosphate, by decreasing angiotensin-converting enzyme levels, and by increasing endothelial cell production of PGI2.

Calcium gluconate 10% can be administered over 3 to 5 minutes IV if signs and symptoms associated with magnesium toxicity occur. Signs and symptoms associated with magnesium toxicity include:
- Absent deep tendon reflexes
- Decreased respiratory rate or respiratory arrest
- Unexplained hypotension
- Fetal distress
- Loss of consciousness

14. *Describe the unique communication aspects of the operating room environment during a cesarean section.*

During cesarean section, the patient is not sedated, and their significant other is present. The expectant parents likely have little to no experience in an operating room environment and are not accustomed to the sights, sounds, and smells that accompany surgery. The anesthetist must keep in mind these facts, as they contribute to a situational disorientation on the part of the patient and their significant other. Additionally, the anesthetist will be communicating with the surgeon throughout the procedure.

Postoperative Period

15. *Explain the importance of maintaining magnesium sulfate therapy in the postoperative period.*

Magnesium sulfate therapy is typically continued for 24 to 48 hours after cesarean delivery. Postpartum convulsions are uncommon; however, continuation of magnesium sulfate reduces the risk of seizures.

16. *Describe the goals of the postoperative management of preeclamptic patients who have had a cesarean section.*
- **Adequate analgesia:** Patients receiving spinal anesthesia for cesarean section may receive 0.1 to 0.2 mg of intrathecal preservative-free morphine as well as nonsteroidal antiinflammatory drugs such as ketorolac intravenously. The disadvantages associated with intrathecal narcotics include delayed respiratory depression, pruritus, and nausea and vomiting.
- **Maintenance of hemodynamic control**
- **Maintenance of intravascular volume:** Magnesium sulfate therapy is continued until the patient begins to recover from the signs and symptoms of preeclampsia such as hypertension, coagulopathy, or oliguria.
- **Assessment of electrolyte values**

Review Questions

1. At which serum magnesium value(s) does the loss of deep tendon reflexes occur in parturients?
   a. 10 mEq/L
   b. 20 to 25 mEq/L
   c. 15 mEq/L
   d. 4 to 6 mEq/L
2. Which is not a reliable sign of preeclampsia?
   a. Proteinuria greater than 300 mg in a 24-hour period
   b. Systolic blood pressure greater than 140 mm Hg
   c. Edema
   d. Diastolic blood pressure of 90 mm Hg or higher
3. One possible site of action of the anticonvulsant effect of magnesium sulfate is:
   a. Gamma-aminobutyric acid receptors.
   b. Muscarinic receptors.
   c. Cerebral N-methyl-D-aspartate receptors.
   d. Oxytocin receptors.
4. Which agents are used to treat maternal hypotension and may provide improved fetal acid–base balance compared with ephedrine?
   a. Epinephrine
   b. Ondansetron
   c. Oxytocin
   d. Phenylephrine
5. Which medication is associated with bronchospasm in patients with asthma?
   a. Magnesium sulfate
   b. Prostaglandin F2-alpha
   c. Methylergonovine
   d. Pitocin

Suggested Readings

Aya AG, Vialles N, Tanoubi I, et al. Spinal anesthesia induced hypotension: a risk comparison between patients with severe preeclampsia and healthy women undergoing preterm Cesarean delivery. *Anesth Analg* 2005;101(3):869-875.

Heesen M, Klimek M, Hoeks SE, Rossaint R. Prevention of spinal anesthesia-induced hypotension during cesarean delivery by 5-hydroxytryptamine-3 receptor antagonists: a systematic review and meta-analysis and meta-regression. *Anesth Analg* 2016;123(4): 977-988.

Kason BJ. Obstetric anesthesia. In: Nagelhout JJ, Elisha S, eds. *Nurse Anesthesia*, 6th ed. St Louis, MO: Elsevier, 2018:1064-1091.

Mohta M, Duggal S, Chilkoti GT. Randomised double-blind comparison of bolus phenylephrine or ephedrine for treatment of hypotension in women with pre-eclampsia undergoing caesarean section. *Anaesthesia* 2018;73(7):839-846.

Ni HF, Liu HY, Zhang J, Peng K, Ji FH. Crystalloid coload reduced the incidence of hypotension in spinal anesthesia for cesarean delivery, when compared to crystalloid preload: a meta-analysis. *Biomed Res Int* 2017;2017:3462529.

Practice guidelines for obstetric anesthesia: an updated report by the American Society of Anesthesiologists Task Force on Obstetric Anesthesia and the Society for Obstetric Anesthesia and Perinatology. *Anesthesiology* 2016;124(2):270-300.

Reed A, Lombard C, Leann K, et al. Hemodynamic changes associated with spinal anesthesia for cesarean delivery in severe preeclampsia. *Anesthesiology* 2008;108(5):802-811.

Sivevski A, Ivanov E, Karadjova D, et al. Spinal-induced hypotension in preeclamptic and healthy parturients undergoing cesarean section. *Open Access Maced J Med Sci* 2019;7(6):996-1000.

Šklebar I, Bujas T, Habek D. Spinal anesthesia induced hypotension in obstetrics: prevention and therapy. *Acta Clin Croat* 2019; 58(Suppl 1):90-95.

Visalyaputra S, Rodanant O, Somboonviboon W. Spinal versus epidural anesthesia for cesarean delivery in preeclampsia: a prospective randomized, multicenter study. *Obstet Gynecol Surv* 2006; 61(2):84-85.

Wilson RD, Caughey AB, Wood SL, et al. Guidelines for antenatal and preoperative care in cesarean delivery: Enhanced Recovery After Surgery Society recommendations. *Am J Obstet Gynecol* 2018; 219(6):523.e1-523.e15.

36
Cervical Cerclage

KEY POINTS

- Anesthetists need to minimize fetal drug exposure.
- Maintenance of placental perfusion by avoidance of maternal hypotension is critical.
- Specific interventions can help avoid maternal complications: aspiration and aortocaval compression.
- Addressing maternal anxiety is imperative.

Case Synopsis

A 32-year-old woman, gravida 3 para 0, presents from the OB/GYN's office. She is now at 18 weeks' gestation and has evidence of cervical shortening and dilation to 1 cm and is scheduled to undergo an emergent cervical cerclage.

Preoperative Evaluation and Demographic Data

Past Medical/Surgical History

- Two prior second-trimester pregnancy losses at 19 and 21 weeks' gestation
- No previous medical or surgical history

List of Medications

- Prenatal vitamins

Diagnostic Data

- Hemoglobin, 12.2 g/dL; hematocrit, 33.4%
- Electrolytes: sodium, 139 mEq/L; potassium, 4.1 mEq/L; chloride, 104 mEq/L; carbon dioxide, 21 mEq/L

Height/Weight/Vital Signs

- 165 cm, 78 kg
- Blood pressure, 112/64; heart rate, 71 beats per minute; respiratory rate, 16 breaths per minute; room air oxygen saturation, 98%, temperature, 37°C

Pathophysiology

Incompetent cervix can be the result of trauma or an inherent deficiency in the structure or function of the cervix that leads to repeated second-trimester spontaneous abortions. These second-trimester losses often have three specific characteristics: painless cervical dilation, herniation followed by rupture of membranes, and short labor ending in delivery of a living but extremely immature fetus.

The incidence of cervical incompetence ranges from 0.001% to 1.84%. Diagnosis of cervical incompetence is accomplished by observation of cervical shortening or dilation or protrusion of membranes through the cervical os. Diagnosis can also be determined by past history, such as in this patient, who had recurrent pregnancy loss. Serial examinations utilizing a variety of methods that include manual examination, ultrasound, or magnetic resonance imaging (MRI) may be used to evaluate cervical dilation and length and subsequent changes to determine whether cervical cerclage is warranted.

Surgical Procedure

The majority of pregnant women with an incompetent cervix will undergo a transvaginal placement of a cervical cerclage. Two common types of transvaginal techniques for cerclage are McDonald and Shirodkar. The Shirodkar sutures are placed within the cervical mucosa after dissection of the bladder to the level of the internal cervical os, resulting in slightly greater blood loss. The McDonald suture, which leaves the mucosa intact, is illustrated in Fig. 36.1.

In rare instances—patients with a failed transvaginal cervical cerclage or those with little cervical structure—a transabdominal cerclage may be used. Transabdominal cervical cerclage (TAC) was first described in 1965 with an open laparotomy approach to insert a suture above the cardinal and uterosacral ligaments. There have been some reports of laparoscopic placement, and the most recent case studies include the use of da Vinci robot and other robotic-assisted laparoscopic surgeries for placement of the suture. Pre-pregnancy TAC can be accomplished to avoid the complications of manipulation of the pregnant uterus and increased bleeding. The overall use of TAC is low, being limited by the need for a clear diagnosis of cervical pathology and the technical challenges and learning curves associated with the surgery. A cervical cerclage needs to be removed before or at the onset of labor if a vaginal delivery is to occur; however, the usual

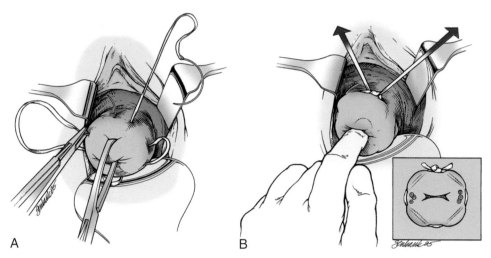

• **Fig. 36.1** Placement of sutures used for the McDonald cervical cerclage. (From Landon MB, Galan HL, Jauniaux ERM, et al: *Gabbe's obstetrics: normal and problem pregnancies*, ed 8, Philadelphia, 2021, Elsevier.)

mode of delivery after the transabdominal approach is via a cesarean section. There is a low incidence of cervical dystocia or failure of dilation secondary to cerclage.

Anesthetic Management and Considerations

Preoperative Period

1. *Describe the physiologic changes of pregnancy that affect anesthesia management of the parturient during the second trimester.*
   - **Cardiovascular:** Increases in heart rate (↑25%), stroke volume (↑25%), and cardiac output (↑50%), begin as early as 2 to 3 weeks' gestation and continue to rise into the second trimester. No further increases in cardiac performance occur until the labor and delivery process. Despite the increase in cardiac output, maternal blood pressure declines due to decreases in systemic vascular resistance, with the greatest decline occurring around the twentieth week. Increased perfusion to the uterus, kidneys, skin, and skeletal muscle occurs throughout gestation. Aortocaval compression syndrome results in a 50% increase in femoral venous pressure, indicating decreased blood return to the heart (preload). This can be observed as early as 13 to 16 weeks' gestation and can result in severe hypotension and uteroplacental insufficiency.
   - **Respiratory:** The increases in oxygen consumption as a result of the increased metabolic demands of the fetus and placenta result in changes within the respiratory system that occur when a woman is likely to undergo cervical cerclage. Approximately half of the 45% increase in tidal volume occurs in

the first trimester, with a corresponding rise in minute ventilation, which results in a decrease in $PaCO_2$ and an increase in pH. Reduction in functional residual capacity begins in the fifth month of pregnancy, and this change is not a primary determinant of decreased lung volume at the time of gestation when a cerclage would be performed.
   - **Gastrointestinal:** The barrier pressure or difference between the lower esophageal high-pressure zone and the intragastric pressure decreases during pregnancy, placing the parturient at increased risk for pyrosis (heartburn) and pulmonary aspiration if undergoing general anesthesia. The rotation and displacement of the gastroesophageal junction as pregnancy progresses are believed to contribute to the increasing incidence of gastroesophageal reflux. Therefore the parturient should be treated as a full stomach with the appropriate precautions regardless of the method of anesthesia selected.

2. *Differentiate between early and late pregnancy with respect to the need for:*
   - **Gastric aspiration precautions:** Early in pregnancy, the gastroesophageal junction has not been displaced, so the risk of aspiration and pyrosis is lower compared with late pregnancy. However, oral administration of a nonparticulate antacid is recommended for each parturient. In late pregnancy, additional treatment for gastric volume and acidity may be needed. Rapid sequence induction is standard practice for pregnant women.
   - **Left uterine displacement (LUD):** Aortocaval compression can be detected as early as 13 to 16 weeks of gestation, and therefore LUD should be initiated for all pregnant women. The anesthesia provider must be aware that in late pregnancy, the vascular effects

associated with aortocaval compression remain present even with LUD due to the increased weight of the fetus, placenta, and amniotic fluid.

- **Fetal monitoring:** In early pregnancy confirmation of fetal heart rate (FHR) before a cerclage is sufficient. There is evidence to suggest that continuous FHR monitoring should be performed if the cerclage is performed after 16 to 20 weeks of gestation.
- **Avoidance of teratogenicity:** Although no current anesthesia drugs have been conclusively proven to be teratogenic in humans when administered in therapeutic doses, there have been studies that suggest the existence of an association. It is prudent to minimize fetal exposure when possible.

3. *Evaluate the advantages and disadvantages of regional/neuraxial and general anesthesia for surgical procedures in pregnancy.*

When the surgical procedure permits, regional techniques offer the advantage of minimal exposure of anesthetic medications to the fetus and the ability of the patient to spontaneously breathe without the need for endotracheal intubation. Peripheral tissues, including those in the airway, become edematous due to the increase in blood volume that occurs during pregnancy, which can make intubation more difficult to accomplish. Spinal anesthesia is most advantageous due to the low amount of drug required that will be administered to provide adequate sensory blockade and optimal surgical conditions. The primary disadvantage of regional anesthesia is caused by the sympathectomy that results from beta-preganglionic sympathetic fiber blockade. As a result, maternal hypotension can occur, decreasing placental perfusion.

General anesthesia, when needed, provides superior uterine relaxation to facilitate replacement of bulging membranes before cervical cerclage when early cervical dilation has occurred. The uterine relaxation may decrease uterine irritability and premature uterine contraction. Disadvantages associated with general anesthesia include increased fetal drug exposure, the potential for difficult intubation, and increased risk of maternal aspiration. Postoperative vomiting may put undue strain on the suture.

4. *Recognize the psychologic impact of prior pregnancy losses and anxiety over outcome of this pregnancy in the patient undergoing cervical cerclage.*

Many women undergoing cervical cerclage have already suffered one or more miscarriages due to extreme prematurity at birth. Understandably, they may be very anxious at the time of this procedure due to the uncertainty of being able to successfully carry the pregnancy to term. Anxiety may be heightened in cases where cervical dilation or bulging of membranes is already present. Establishing a rapport is important, as little to no premedication for anxiolysis or intraoperative sedation is utilized to minimize fetal exposure.

5. *Describe the selection of preoperative medications for the pregnant woman undergoing cervical cerclage.*

Use of preoperative medications is usually minimal and frequently limited to a nonparticulate antacid (Bicitra) or other aspiration precautions (H_2 blocker, cimetidine; gastrokinetic, metoclopramide). Although no particular anesthetic agents or techniques have been proven teratogenic in humans, it is best to avoid unnecessary exposure during the period of organogenesis (15 to 56 days' gestation). A cerclage is not frequently performed beyond this period, but emergency surgery may be required during pregnancy.

Intraoperative Period

6. *Describe the physiologic changes that are associated with the lithotomy position.*

Circulatory changes that occur as a result of lithotomy include an increase in the central blood volume and a decrease in perfusion pressure in the extremities. The higher the legs are placed above the heart, the greater the effect. The Trendelenburg position further amplifies the shifts in blood volume and perfusion.

Sympathectomy resulting from spinal or epidural anesthesia can contribute to the shift in blood volume. Hypotension may occur when the patient is returned to the supine position. Because placental perfusion is dependent on maternal blood pressure, avoiding hypotension is vitally important. Inappropriate positioning or pressure from leg holders can result in a nerve injury, which necessitates proper padding and positioning. Care should be taken to return both legs to midline before replacing them in the supine position to avoid injuring the patient's hips.

7. *Identify the level of sensory blockade needed if neuraxial anesthesia is used during transvaginal placement of a cervical cerclage.*

Cervical cerclage does not require neuraxial blockade above T10, so a low spinal or "saddle block" is sufficient. A transabdominal approach to cerclage will require a higher dermatome level of blockade; however, it is less than a T4 block used for cesarean delivery.

8. *Formulate a plan to maintain placental perfusion.*

Uterine blood flow (UBF) is dependent on uterine arterial and venous pressure and uterine vascular resistance. The formula that is used to calculate UBF is:

Uterine blood flow = Uterine arterial pressure − Uterine venous pressure / Uterine vascular resistance

UBF is decreased if a decrease in uterine arterial pressure or an increase in uterine vascular resistance occurs. To avoid fetal hypoperfusion and maintain UBF, the anesthetist can support the maternal blood pressure by administering intravenous fluid. If vasopressors (ephedrine or phenylephrine) need to be administered for prolonged and severe hypotension, these medications should be used judiciously because the sympathomimetic effects will increase uterine vascular resistance.

Postoperative Period

9. Discuss the potential adverse maternal and fetal outcomes after cervical cerclage.

The risks of aspiration, hypotension, and positioning injuries are all potential complications. Additional maternal risks include those related to anesthesia (nausea, vomiting) and those related to the procedure (infection, premature uterine contractions, bleeding, tearing, or scarring with subsequent failure of the cervix to dilate in labor). There is the potential for amniotic membrane rupture, chorioamnionitis, and premature delivery. Cervical cerclage is not as effective in the prevention of preterm delivery as once believed, particularly in cases of shortened cervix. Although cervical cerclage does reduce the incidence of delivery before 34 weeks, neonatal mortality is unchanged and the risk of maternal postpartum fever is increased.

10. Describe a method for performing cerclage if advanced cervical dilation and/or ballooning of membranes has occurred.

Emergency cerclage can be performed if advanced dilation or bulging of fetal membranes has occurred. This is accomplished by using a sterile inflatable balloon to gently push the fetal membranes into the cavity, allowing placement of a cerclage over the balloon introducer. The balloon is deflated and the cerclage is tightened as the introducer is withdrawn. Use of balloons that can be inflated up to 10 cm and the protection provided by the introducer may result in greater use of the technique in the future. Risks that are associated with this procedure include maternal infection, chorioamnionitis, rupture of membranes, and premature delivery.

Review Questions

1. An advantage of neuraxial blockade for the patient having cervical cerclage placement is:
   a. Minimizing the amount of drug that is administered.
   b. Decreasing the blood loss during the procedure.
   c. Distinguishing the signs and symptoms of bladder perforation.
   d. Reducing postoperative pain.

2. Maternal blood pressure normally decreases during the first and second trimester of pregnancy due to:
   a. Decreased blood viscosity.
   b. Increased placental perfusion.
   c. Decreased vascular resistance.
   d. Increased heart rate.

3. Which intervention is recommended for all parturients to decrease the risk of gastric aspiration?
   a. Use of a high-pressure-cuff endotracheal tube
   b. Nasogastric suctioning before extubation
   c. Metoclopramide
   d. Nonparticulate antacid

4. Changes in gastroesophageal junction barrier pressure during pregnancy result from:
   a. Increased acidity of gastric secretions.
   b. Decreased gastric pressure.
   c. Displacement of the junction.
   d. Decreased progestin.

5. Which formula is most representative of UBF?
   a. Uterine arterial pressure $\times$ uterine venous pressure $-$ O_2 placental consumption
   b. Uterine (arterial pressure $-$ venous pressure) / uterine vascular resistance
   c. CO $\times$ 0.04
   d. SV $\times$ HR/CO

Suggested Readings

Barmat L, Glaser G, Davis G, et al. Da Vinci-assisted abdominal cerclage. *Fertil Steril* 2007;88(5):1437e1-e3.

Iavazzo C, Minis EE, Gkegkes ID. Robotic assisted laparoscopic cerclage: a systematic review. *Int J Med Robot* 2019;15(1):e1966.

Ioscovich A, Popov A, Gimelfarb Y, et al. Anesthetic management of prophylactic cervical cerclage: a retrospective multicenter cohort study. *Arch Gynecol Obstet* 2015;291(3):509-12.

Kason BJ. Obstetric Anesthesia. In: Nagelhout JJ, Elisha S, eds. *Nurse Anesthesia*, 6th ed. St Louis, MO: Elsevier, 2018:1064-1091.

Krispin E, Danieli-Gruber S, Hadar E, et al. Primary, secondary, and tertiary preventions of preterm birth with cervical cerclage. *Arch Gynecol Obstet* 2019;300(2):305-312.

Simcox R, Shennan A. Cervical cerclage: a review. *Int J Surg* 2007; 5:205-209.

Tsatsaris V, Senat MV, Gervaise A, et al. Balloon replacement of fetal membranes to facilitate emergency cervical cerclage. *Obstet Gynecol* 2004;98(2):243-246.

Tyan P, Mourad J, Wright B, et al. Robot-assisted transabdominal cerclage for the prevention of preterm birth: a multicenter experience. *Eur J Obstet Gynecol Reprod Biol* 2019;232:70-74.

Wolfe L, DePasquale S, Adair CD, et al. Robotic-assisted laparoscopic placement of transabdominal cerclage during pregnancy. *Am J Perinatol* 2008;25:653-655.

37

Intraoperative Maternal Hemorrhage Caused by Uterine Rupture

KEY POINTS

- Uterine rupture is a potentially catastrophic complication of pregnancy.
- Uterine rupture may result from abnormalities of uterine anatomy, forceps delivery, external version procedure, connective tissue disease, or other causes; the most widely recognized cause is a uterine scar from previous surgery.
- Cesarean delivery represents the most common nondiagnostic surgery in the United States, accounting for over 1 million births annually.
- To reduce the complications associated with cesarean delivery and to enjoy the benefits of a vaginal birth, approximately 10% of women who have had a cesarean

delivery will deliver a subsequent child vaginally. This practice of "vaginal birth after cesarean" is abbreviated as VBAC.
- VBAC may increase the risk of uterine rupture or failed labor.
- Uterine rupture, although infrequent, calls for an immediate response by the anesthetist to assist with maternal and fetal rescue.
- Uterine rupture may likely be associated with severe hemorrhage, and the anesthetist will be responsible for a challenging fluid resuscitation in this situation.

Case Synopsis

A 30-year-old woman presents to the obstetric unit. The obstetrician reports that she is in early labor but that the labor will be augmented with oxytocin. An order is written for the patient to be administered an epidural, upon her request.

Preoperative Evaluation and Demographic Data

Past Medical/Surgical History

- History of endometriosis with pelvic adhesions
- Five-pack/year smoking history, but quit since becoming pregnant
- Heartburn with gastroesophageal reflux 1 time per week
- Noninsulin-dependent diabetes mellitus, well controlled by diet
  - Obstetric history: gravida 3 para 2
  - Cesarean delivery; epidural anesthesia
- Laparoscopy for endometriosis; general anesthesia without complications
- Table 37.1 provides the patient's obstetric history.

List of Medications

- Prenatal vitamins daily
- Calcium carbonate as needed for heartburn/reflux

Diagnostic Data

- Hemoglobin, 12 g/dL; hematocrit, 36%; white blood count, 12,000/mm^3; platelet count, 120,000/mm^3
- Airway is assessed as Mallampati class III

Height/Weight/Vital Signs

- 163 cm, 84 kg
- Blood pressure, 110/64; heart rate, 82 beats per minute; respiratory rate, 16 breaths per minute; temperature, 36.9°C

Pathophysiology

Cesarean delivery is accomplished by making an incision in the uterus to allow delivery of the fetus. The most common approach is through the Pfannenstiel (bikini line) incision in the abdominal wall, followed by a transverse cut across the lower segment of the uterus, not far above the cervix. Previously common was the vertical, or classical, abdominal incision. Despite the larger access provided for delivery of the baby by the vertical incision, this approach has become less popular due to the resulting increased potential for uterine rupture with subsequent pregnancies. The classical incision is associated with increased rupture risk because the myometrial fibers are separated longitudinally, and the incision extends upward toward the fundus of the uterus, where the strongest contractions occur during labor.

TABLE 37.1	Obstetric History		
Pregnancy	Date	Mode of Delivery	Notes
1	3.5 years ago	Vaginal	
2	22 months ago	Cesarean	Prolapsed cord
3	Current; 41 weeks' gestational age		Macrosomia

Several physiologic changes occur during pregnancy to foster favorable maternal and fetal hemodynamics. Maternal blood volume rises, with a disproportionate rise in plasma volume, in relation to red blood cell mass. This change produces the "physiologic anemia of pregnancy," which serves to promote blood flow to the placenta and to also limit red cell loss during the inevitable bleeding that occurs with delivery. Another physiologic change that occurs in anticipation of this bleeding is an increase in blood coagulation factors.

Surgical Procedure

During the prenatal period, uterine rupture is treated by emergency cesarean delivery to separate the fetus from the dysfunctional uterus and to control maternal bleeding. A rupture that is diagnosed postnatally is treated by a laparotomy to repair or remove the damaged uterus. A wide retractor called a *bladder blade* is commonly used to prevent trauma to the bladder, which overrides the lower uterus. There is an increased incidence of bladder damage during cesarean surgery after uterine rupture, so the anesthetist must be vigilant for lack of urine output or for blood in the urine during this procedure.

Anesthetic Management and Considerations

Preoperative Period

1. *Discuss the pertinent points in the preanesthetic evaluation and planning for a patient undergoing VBAC.*

   In addition to the typical assessment of the labor patient, some special factors should be considered when the patient planning vaginal delivery has had a previous cesarean (this process is referred to as a *trial of labor after cesarean* [TOLAC]). The risk factors for failure of TOLAC or for uterine rupture should be assessed to determine the appropriate level of vigilance and monitoring due the patient. Uterine rupture can result in significant blood loss, and it is imperative that blood products are available for infusion. Established policy

and logistics of blood acquisition in the institution must be considered in determining whether the patient should be tested for blood type and antibody screen or whether blood should be cross-matched. Staff availability is another crucial factor in the safe treatment of patients undergoing TOLAC.

2. *Identify risk factors that may predict complications or failure of VBAC.*

   Certain factors increase the success of VBAC, including history of previous vaginal delivery (particularly if it was a VBAC), spontaneous onset of labor, cervical effacement >75%, no more than one previous uterine incision, and clinically adequate pelvis. Although models to predict uterine rupture in each patient lack reliability, the following factors are associated with increased rates of uterine rupture or failure of vaginal delivery in patients undergoing TOLAC:
   - Vertical (or *classical*) uterine incision
   - Potentially recurring indication for previous cesarean section
   - Increasing number of uterine incisions
   - Interval is less than 24 months since prior cesarean section
   - No history of a previous vaginal delivery
   - Dystocia, or need for induction or augmentation of labor
   - Macrosomia (>4000 g)
   - Post term or multiple gestations
   - Obesity

   The current patient has three favorable historical factors: she is in spontaneous labor, she has had a vaginal delivery previously, and her first cesarean delivery was for prolapsed umbilical cord. The previous vaginal delivery indicates a proven uterus, as opposed to the scenario where unsuitable pelvic dimensions were the cause of the prior cesarean section. Likewise, prolapsed cord is a nonrecurring indication. Unlike cephalopelvic disproportion, it would not be expected that the underlying condition for the first cesarean section would also complicate this pregnancy. However, this patient has several factors that detract from her chance of success, including:
   - Obesity, her body mass index is 31.8 kg/m^2.
   - Large fetus (not uncommon among diabetic patients).
   - It has been just less than 24 months since her previous cesarean surgery, which suggests less-than-optimal time for uterine scar strengthening.
   - Although she is in spontaneous labor, her labor will be augmented by oxytocin. The need for augmentation, as well as the increased muscle tension it produces, confer negative risk factors.

3. *Compare and contrast the advantages of different anesthetic techniques in managing VBAC.*

   As with several obstetric complications that forebode emergency cesarean delivery, it is valuable to have a functioning epidural in place in a VBAC situation. Catastrophic uterine rupture may not allow time, nor may it be appropriate for epidural anesthesia for the cesarean surgery. However, in the case of a lesser uterine rupture, it is beneficial to have the option of using a functioning epidural. A combined spinal-epidural technique typically does not employ the epidural catheter during the initial period after subarachnoid injection. It may be favorable to utilize a traditional epidural technique, so that any deficiencies in epidural function may be identified and remedied immediately. In the present case, the patient has diabetes, which is associated with abnormal vascular development of the uteroplacental unit. This may make uteroplacental insufficiency more likely when her contractions increase in intensity. Her obesity also places her at higher risk for epidural catheter malfunction.

There is a theoretical concern that because abdominal pain is a sign of uterine rupture, epidural analgesia may mask this important sign and delay diagnosis of the complication. Experience shows that the visceral pain of uterine rupture, like that of bladder distention, is difficult to obliterate with moderate epidural analgesia. Therefore concerns that providing epidural analgesia will prevent diagnosis of uterine rupture are unfounded.

4. *Formulate a plan for management of a VBAC patient during labor.*

Anesthetic management for VBAC need not be significantly different from that of routine patients, other than assuring availability of a rapid response in case of emergency. The anesthetist should be assured of prompt availability of blood products because uterine rupture is frequently associated with significant blood loss. Depending on institutional logistics, this may warrant cross-matching type and screen only, or if emergency blood is rapidly available, no additional preparation. As with all obstetric patients, the preanesthetic evaluation includes an assessment of the airway in anticipation of the possibility of emergency surgery. As noted previously, epidural analgesia is acceptable. Although the literature lends little objective information regarding the possibility of an epidural to mask signs of uterine rupture, prudence would suggest that the level of sensory blockade should allow for some awareness of abdominal sensation. The anesthetist should maintain lines of communication with the obstetric provider and labor nurse and also maintain availability for a rapid response when caring for a VBAC patient.

5. *Recognize the unique factors that should heighten the anesthetist's awareness and surveillance of a VBAC patient.*

Any sign that natural labor is not progressing well may indicate a heightened level of awareness for complications of uterine rupture. Such signs include fetal heart rate abnormalities, dystocia or prolonged labor, and the need for high-dose oxytocin. Dystocia occurs in approximately one-half of uterine ruptures, and variable or late decelerations occur as prodromal signs in most cases of uterine rupture.

An epidural catheter is inserted and a T10 level of sensory block is achieved, with pain score of 0/10. The epidural infusion of 0.1% bupivacaine with fentanyl

2 mcg/mL is infusing at 10 mL/hr. The first stage of labor lasted 5 hours, and the patient is now pushing in the second stage. She begins to complain of breakthrough pain, and she is given a rest from pushing while you are called in to redose her epidural. As you arrive, she complains of increasingly severe pain.

6. *Differentiate between various causes of pain that may exist in this patient.*
   • **Inadequate analgesia**: Epidural coverage of sacral dermatomes needed for second-stage analgesia may be lacking. Preservation of sacral motor function (plantar flexion via S1/superficial peroneal nerve) bolsters this supposition.
   • **Placental abruption**: Vascular compromise from smoking history or diabetes in this patient increases her risk of placental abruption. Abnormally copious vaginal bleeding may be an accompanying sign.
   • **Uterine rupture**: Pain is a less reliable sign of uterine rupture than is a change in the fetal heart rate. Uterine rupture typically manifests as diffuse, nonlocalized pain, which may break through moderate epidural analgesia. A uterine hyperstimulation pattern or an abrupt cessation of contractions may be noted on the tocodynamometer. The fetal heart rate will likely show abnormalities such as repetitive late or variable decelerations progressing to a prolonged (terminal) deceleration and fetal bradycardia. Loss of fetal station may also occur.
   • **Fetal malposition**: Dystocia and continuous back pain can result from fetal malposition, such as being in the occiput posterior (OP) position. Similar to pathologic conditions, this pain may not subside between contractions. However, its recognition is suggested by pain in the dermatomes of the lumbar plexus or sacrum and a fetal head that is identified on vaginal examination to be in the OP position.
   • **Other causes**: These include acute appendicitis, rupture of the abdominal rectus muscles, bladder rupture, hepatic rupture (right upper quadrant pain associated with severe HELLP syndrome), and vascular thrombosis (mesenteric, iliac, etc., due to the hypercoagulable state of pregnancy).

You evaluate the fetal heart rate and uterine monitor and observe the pattern is consistent with variable decelerations, as shown in Fig. 37.1. The patient is complaining of severe abdominal pain. Uterine rupture is diagnosed.

Intraoperative Period

7. *Describe the expected obstetric management of a patient with uterine rupture.*

A patient with symptomatic uterine rupture, particularly if accompanied by fetal distress, will require an emergent cesarean delivery to provide the best opportunity for survival of the fetus. Many cases of uterine rupture are of a mild degree, often asymptomatic, and termed uterine dehiscence. These may not be recognized unless failure of vaginal delivery leads to a cesarean

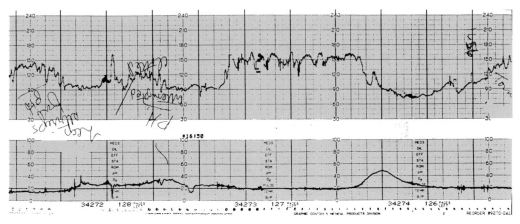

• **Fig. 37.1** Fetal heart rate tracing showing variable decelerations after uterine rupture. (From Gabbe SG, Niebyl JR, Simpson JL, et al: *Obstetrics: Normal and problem pregnancies*, ed 6, St. Louis, 2012, Elsevier.)

delivery and the dehiscence is diagnosed upon visualizing the uterus. A uterine rupture that is severe may lead to cessation of placental perfusion, thus necessitating immediate cesarean delivery. If the uterus is severely damaged or if uncontrollable bleeding occurs, a hysterectomy may also be carried out after delivery of the infant.

Although potentially catastrophic, the overall incidence of uterine rupture is close to only 1%, and better still, the incidence of fetal injury is only around 10% after uterine rupture. Nonetheless, a significant uterine rupture presents a true emergency, and maternal and neonatal well-being will be best served by a very expeditious delivery and resuscitation. In the routine cesarean delivery, uterine incision may disrupt the life-sustaining milieu of the fetus, so it is desirable for the surgeon to expeditiously deliver the infant within 2 minutes after uterine incision. This time frame is supported by animal models that demonstrate physiologic compromise in this interval, after umbilical cord occlusion. Also carrying the potential to disrupt placental perfusion (particularly if the placenta has implanted anteriorly on the site of the eventual rupture), a uterine rupture should likewise demand extreme haste in delivering the infant.

The American College of Obstetricians and Gynecologists recommends that in the case of urgent or emergent cesarean delivery, the delivery should be accomplished within 30 minutes of the decision to do so ("decision-to-incision" time). However, in the case of uterine rupture, 30 minutes may be too long to ensure survival for a fetus with severely compromised perfusion. Therefore effective management of a uterine rupture requires availability of the obstetric, anesthesia, and surgical nursing team to achieve delivery within a time frame closer to 15 minutes. Overall, there is a low incidence of significant neonatal injury or death if delivery is effected within this time frame. Institutional practice and logistics will influence the feasible response time, but when possible, the anesthetist managing a patient undergoing VBAC should not be required to become involved in

other anesthetics, lest they lose the ability to respond rapidly in the case of a uterine rupture. Staff availability for rapid response is the most important asset to ensure effective management of a catastrophic uterine rupture.

8. *Describe the sequence of intervention for anesthetic management of uterine rupture.*

As indicated previously, rapid delivery of the fetus is paramount in the case of uterine rupture. Anesthesia intervention should begin as soon as rupture is identified and may include intensifying the epidural anesthesia before transport to the operating room, preparation for possible or planned general anesthesia, and procurement of blood products. Uterine rupture is associated with significant bleeding and may lead to rapidly developing disseminated intravascular coagulation (DIC). For these reasons, anesthesia care should prepare for an emergent hysterectomy after the delivery and assess the need for red blood cell and clotting factor administration. The anesthetist must estimate the anticipated blood loss to decide whether epidural anesthesia will be sufficient or if general anesthesia will facilitate better control of physiologic parameters. Having a history of gastroesophageal reflux and obesity, the present patient has additional risk factors for aspiration pneumonitis. It would be worthwhile to utilize a regional technique, if appropriate. Box 37.1 summarizes the anesthetic management for a patient who has experienced a uterine rupture.

9. *Formulate a plan to manage blood replacement.*

Whereas vaginal delivery is typically associated with approximately 500 mL of blood loss and cesarean delivery is associated with 1000 mL, a uterine rupture can be expected to typically lead to 1500 to 2000 mL blood loss. Approximately 25% to 50% of women who experience uterine rupture will require blood products. Shock occurs in a similar incidence. In this case, her history of endometriosis and previous laparoscopy suggests that the cesarean delivery may be associated with even more surgical challenges and resultant bleeding.

• BOX 37.1 Anesthetic Management of Uterine Rupture

1. Assess severity of maternal and fetal compromise to determine the type of anesthesia indicated.
2. Assist with transport to the operating room as quickly as possible.
3. If epidural anesthesia is appropriate and a catheter is in place, begin dosing immediately with 3% chloroprocaine or 2% carbonated lidocaine.
4. Obtain 2–4 units of packed red blood cells and plasma.
5. Ensure, through general or regional anesthesia, that surgery can proceed in the shortest amount of time after entering the operating room.
6. Anticipate the need for aggressive fluid and blood replacement due to uterine bleeding and the likelihood of disseminated intravascular coagulation.

Although obstetric patients are generally of good health, the physiologic anemia of pregnancy may prompt practitioners to treat with blood products earlier. Packed red cells will provide oxygen-carrying capacity. In an ideal situation, blood would be type- and cross-matched; however, in the absence thereof, uncrossed type-specific or O negative blood may need to be administered if the patient's condition does not allow time for preparation of other products.

There is a large margin of safety in the amount of clotting factor that can be lost without clinical significance. At the same time, uterine rupture may lead to massive transfusion, and red cells may also need to be supplemented with plasma. Ligation of the uterine arteries may be used by the surgeon to control massive hemorrhage, but at times hemorrhage becomes uncontrollable. The possibility of requiring unconventional approaches, such as administration of recombinant factor VIIA, should be considered. A fluid and blood warmer should be used to maintain body temperature and avoid further compromise of clotting factor function.

10. *Distinguish the anesthetist's responsibility to the mother and to the neonate.*

Being involved in a case where neonatal outcomes are poor is psychologically difficult for everyone involved. In a smaller hospital, staff resources for neonatal resuscitation may not be as ample as in larger institutions. The scenario of a significant uterine rupture may present a quandary for the anesthetist when a hemorrhaging mother and an asphyxiated neonate can both benefit from the anesthetist's intervention. The anesthetist's primary duty is to their original patient, the mother. If the mother is stable and lack of personnel or expertise calls for the anesthetist to become involved with care of the neonate, the decision to divert attention from the primary patient must be made by the anesthetist after weighing the risks and benefits. The guiding principle should be, however, that the primary responsibility is to the mother, even when the health of the neonate is compromised.

11. *Debate the advantages and disadvantages of using salvaged blood in obstetric emergencies.*

Uterine rupture may result in significant amounts of blood loss. Massive transfusions alone, and particularly when involving commingling of maternal and fetal blood, frequently lead to development of DIC. Historically, there has been reluctance to use salvaged blood in obstetrics due to concerns about causing amniotic fluid embolism and alloimmunization of the mother from exposure to fetal antigens, which would be included in the salvaged blood. A mounting body of case report evidence indicates that these fears are largely unfounded, provided that the cell salvage system utilizes a leukocyte filter and a washing process. With these factors in place, the amount of fetal tissue, hemoglobin, and amniotic fluid to be infused into the mother has not demonstrated appreciable increases in hematologic complications. However, many practitioners will limit the amount of blood that is collected for salvage during the period of amniotomy until the placenta is delivered. The American College of Obstetricians and Gynecologists has even recommended blood salvage as a means of managing hemorrhage for placenta accreta. In cases of religious preferences against the receipt of banked blood, cell salvage is an alternative option for managing hemorrhage.

Postoperative Period

The baby was delivered with Apgar scores of 5 (1 minute) and 7 (5 minutes). The neonatal intensive care unit team handled infant resuscitation. The anesthetist administered 6 L of lactated Ringer's solution and 3 units of packed red blood cells. The epidural was left in place for postoperative analgesia.

12. *Describe the potential for uterine rupture postpartum after VBAC.*

The risk of uterine rupture does not exist exclusively during active labor. There have been case reports of uterine rupture antepartum in patients who are not in labor. Likewise, a patient may successfully deliver a VBAC and then experience a uterine rupture postpartum. The anesthetist may be called upon to provide anesthesia for emergency hysterectomy, even after successful VBAC. Hemorrhage is the second most common cause of obstetric complications, and hemorrhage may result from a variety of factors, both anatomic and hematologic. Postpartum bleeding should alert the anesthetist of the possibility of an emergent procedure such as curettage for removal of retained placenta, hysterotomy, placenta accreta, or possibly hysterectomy for uterine rupture.

Review Questions

1. Which is the greatest risk factor for uterine rupture in a patient undergoing VBAC?
   a. Classical uterine incision
   b. History of three previous vaginal deliveries
   c. Oxytocin augmentation of labor
   d. Transmural myomectomy 15 months before VBAC
2. Uterine rupture would most likely be characterized by which signs and symptoms?
   a. Painless vaginal bleeding
   b. Early decelerations of the fetal heart rate
   c. Fetal tachycardia with loss of variability
   d. Variable decelerations and abdominal pain
3. Which is the optimal decision to incision response time for initiating a cesarean delivery for uterine rupture?
   a. 15 minutes
   b. 30 minutes
   c. 45 minutes
   d. 60 minutes
4. What is the most important asset to ensure safe management of a patient for VBAC?
   a. Intrauterine pressure monitoring
   b. Epidural in place immediately upon onset of labor
   c. Staff availability to initiate a cesarean delivery rapidly
   d. Type and cross-matched blood available on the labor ward
5. In the case of maternal hemorrhage and neonatal compromise, the professional *duty* of the anesthetist is to the:
   a. Neonate primarily if intubation of the neonate is indicated.
   b. Mother primarily but may incorporate the neonate if required and if the mother is stable.
   c. Mother only, even if stable and the infant is in cardiac arrest.
   d. Whichever patient has a greater chance of survival.

Suggested Readings

Al-Zirqi I, Daltveit AK, Vangen S. Infant outcome after complete uterine rupture. *Am J Obstet Gynecol* 2018;219(1):109.e1-109.e8.

Baird EJ. Identification and management of obstetric hemorrhage. *Anesthesiol Clin* 2017;35(1):15-34.

Goucher H, Wong CA, Patel SK, Toledo P. Cell salvage in obstetrics. *Anesth Analg* 2015;121(2):465-468.

Grisaru-Granovsky S, Bas-Lando M, et al. Epidural analgesia at trial of labor after cesarean (TOLAC): a significant adjunct to successful vaginal birth after cesarean (VBAC). *J Perinat Med* 2018; 46(3):261-269.

Kaneko M, White S, Homan J, et al. Cerebral blood flow and metabolism in relation to electrocortical activity with severe umbilical cord occlusion in the near-term ovine fetus. *Am J Obstet Gynecol* 2003;188:961-972.

Kason BJ. Obstetric anesthesia. In: Nagelhout JJ, Elisha S, eds. *Nurse Anesthesia*, 6th ed. St Louis, MO: Elsevier, 2018:1064-1091.

Main EK, Goffman D, Scavone BM, et al. National Partnership for Maternal Safety: consensus bundle on obstetric hemorrhage. National Partnership for Maternal Safety; Council on Patient Safety in Women's Health Care. *Obstet Gynecol* 2015;126(1): 155-162.

Sebghati M, Chandraharan E. An update on the risk factors for and management of obstetric haemorrhage. *Women's Health (Lond)* 2017;13(2):34-40.

Truax-Waits SD. Considerations of epidural analgesia in a patient with suspected uterine rupture. *AANA J* 2017;85(2):136-139.

Wu Y, Kataria Y, Wang Z, Ming WK, Ellervik C. Factors associated with successful vaginal birth after a cesarean section: a systematic review and meta-analysis. *BMC Pregnancy Childbirth* 2019; 19(1):360.

38

Labor Epidural

KEY POINTS

- Approximately two-thirds of labor patients in the United States receive epidural analgesia.
- Despite the potential for systemic effects, epidural analgesia can provide more complete pain relief with less maternal somnolence or neonatal respiratory depression than that resulting from parenteral analgesics.
- In the absence of a patient history suggesting otherwise, laboratory evaluation is not required before initiating epidural analgesia.
- The most common risks associated with epidural analgesia include backache, epidural failure, postdural puncture headache (PDPH), and transient neurologic symptoms.
- Testing for improper placement is paramount to safe epidural administration; however, the traditional test dose for intravascular placement may be difficult to interpret and may cause side effects in the laboring patient.
- Inadequate pain relief or total failure of epidural analgesia may occur in 6% to 10% of patients.
- Epidural analgesia for labor should ideally eliminate pain while allowing the maximal amount of motor strength possible and preserving maternal awareness of uterine contractions.

Case Synopsis

A 27-year-old woman presents in early labor. She requests epidural analgesia for labor.

Preoperative Evaluation and Demographic Data

Past Medical/Surgical History

- Protein C deficiency
- History of tobacco use
- Table 38.1 provides the patient's obstetric history

List of Medications

- Prenatal vitamins daily
- Heparin 5000 units subcutaneously, twice daily

Diagnostic Data

- Hemoglobin, 11 gm/dL; hematocrit, 34%; white blood count, 11,500/mm^3; platelet count, 125,000/mm^3
- Airway is assessed as Mallampati class III, short thyromental distance, full range of motion of cervical spine and temporomandibular joint

Height/Weight/Vital Signs

- 157 cm, 110 kg
- Blood pressure, 130/84; heart rate, 85 beats per minute; respiratory rate, 14 breaths per minute; temperature, 36.8°C

Pathophysiology

During gestation, multiple physiologic changes occur to create a favorable environment for embryologic and fetal growth to prepare for the birthing event. These changes include an increase in blood volume, wherein the plasma volume increase is greater than the red blood cell increase, creating an apparent anemia. The minute ventilation is increased almost 50% above normal, but this is in response to an increase in oxygen consumption, so the pH is only slightly elevated within the normal range. Increases in heart rate and stroke volume coupled with a reduction in peripheral vascular resistance lead to an increase in cardiac output of 40% to 50%. This increase can be detrimental to patients with cardiac valvular dysfunction, especially considering that cardiac output may rise to nearly 80% above normal immediately after delivery. Hypercoagulability in pregnancy results from increased levels of most coagulation factors, except for factors XI and XIII, which are slightly decreased. Hormonal changes contribute to sensitivity to general and local anesthetic agents. Gastric function is not significantly altered during pregnancy; however, gastric emptying is delayed during labor. Considering also the presence of reduced lower esophageal sphincter tone and gastric compression from the gravid uterus, the laboring patient should be considered at risk for regurgitation and aspiration.

A term pregnancy is one in which the gestational age of the fetus is 37 to 42 weeks. Although occasional uterine

TABLE 38.1	Obstetric History			
Pregnancy	**Date**	**Mode of Delivery**	**Notes**	
1	4 years ago	N/A	Spontaneous abortion	
2	3 years ago	Vaginal	Blood clot in leg, postpartum	
3	15 months ago	N/A	Spontaneous abortion	
4	Current		39 weeks' gestational age	

TABLE 38.2	Stages of Labor		
Stage	**Characteristic**	**Clinical Endpoints**	**Pain Pattern**
I		Onset of regular contractions until full cervical dilation (10 cm)	T10–L1
(I latent)	Cervix effaces; slow change in dilation	4 cm cervical dilation, rate of dilation increases rapidly to signify transition to active stage I	T10–L1
(I active)	Rapid dilation of cervix	Full dilation of cervix	T10–L1
II		From full cervical dilation until delivery of the fetus	S2–S4
III		From delivery of the fetus until expulsion of the placenta	

contractions may be experienced during the latter stage of pregnancy, onset of labor (including both contractions and cervical effacement) before 37 weeks' gestational age is considered preterm labor. The triggering factor for normal labor onset is not clearly understood, but it may be related to oxytocin released from the posterior pituitary gland or to changes in prostaglandin activity. Labor progresses through distinctive stages, as delineated in Table 38.2. Cervical effacement and dilation, as well as uterine contractions, are responsible for pain in the first stage of labor. Synthetic oxytocin is commonly administered to either induce labor or to augment natural labor contractions. Oxytocin may also be combined with prostaglandin administration for the purpose of encouraging cervical effacement and/or uterine contractions.

Anesthetic Management and Considerations

Preoperative Period

1. *List the indications for epidural analgesia for labor.*

Historically, there existed concern that epidural analgesia impeded the progress of labor, even to the extent of increasing the incidence of forceps or cesarean delivery. Over time, and perhaps due to changing patterns of obstetric anesthesia care, research to describe the relationship between epidural analgesia and instrumented delivery has been equivocal. Although epidural anesthesia may prolong the second stage of labor in some patients, it does so to a degree that is overcome by the benefit of analgesia. By contrast, in some cases (particularly primiparous patients) epidural analgesia with a combined subarachnoid dose may speed the progress of labor. Contemporary practice, supported by the American College of Obstetricians and Gynecologists, utilizes a more liberal indication for epidural analgesia. Epidural analgesia is indicated if the patient is:
- In active labor
- Committed to delivery (i.e., there is not a chance that the patient will be discharged to return to the hospital later)
- In pain
- Desiring epidural analgesia

2. *Consider contraindications to epidural analgesia for labor.*

You evaluate the fetal heart rate and uterine monitor and observe the patterns as shown in Fig. 38.1.

Patient refusal is the absolute contraindication to epidural analgesia. Unlike anesthesia service for surgery, labor epidurals are purely optional. Therefore the anesthetist must take meticulous care to obtain a thorough informed consent from the patient. General contraindications to regional techniques apply to the labor patient as well. Thus, serious coagulopathies, active infection at the site of insertion, increased intracranial pressure, and physiologic factors such as severe aortic stenosis would likely preclude epidural placement. Patients on anticoagulants such as in the present case should be evaluated for the risk of epidural hematoma before deciding on a neuraxial technique. "Mini-dose" heparin, such as 5000 units subcutaneously twice daily, or use of nonsteroidal antiinflammatory medications should not contraindicate a regional technique, unless other confounding factors exist. For patients on

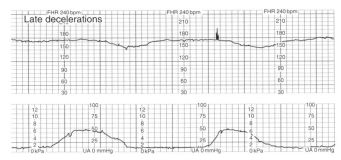

• **Fig. 38.1** Electronic fetal monitor tracing showing late decelerations. *FHR*, Fetal heart rate; *UA*, uterine activity. (From Miller LA, Miller DA, Cypher RL: *Mosby's pocket guide to fetal monitoring*, ed 8, St. Louis, 2017, Elsevier.)

larger doses of heparin or fractionated heparin, accepted guidelines should be followed regarding timing of a neuraxial block in relation to medication administration as set forth by the most current recommendation made by the American Society of Regional Anesthesia.

Regarding obstetric factors, neuraxial blockade carries the side effect of sympathetic block and the resulting potential for hypotension. Placental perfusion is directly related to maternal blood pressure, and initiation of regional anesthesia should be weighed carefully in the presence of an abnormal fetal heart rate. Late decelerations, as pictured in Fig. 38.1, are indicative of uteroplacental insufficiency, and hypotension from a regional block may be detrimental to the fetus in that scenario.

3. *Discuss the necessary laboratory evaluation before initiating a labor epidural.*

The physiologic anemia of pregnancy and benign leukocytosis can be anticipated in every parturient patient, and unless specific factors in the patient history dictate, there are no laboratory studies that must be carried out on a routine basis. In the case of preeclampsia, thrombocytopenic disease, and even possibly pregnancy-induced hypertension, a platelet count would be indicated. Frequently, as in the case presented, pregnant patients present with idiopathic thrombocytopenia. Up to 10% of patients may be found with a platelet count below normal, and in a small number, the count may be less than $100,000/mm^3$. There is much discussion and controversy regarding the lowest platelet count that allows for safe spinal or epidural block placement. A threshold of $100,000/mm^3$ is a conservative cutoff point. In the case of preeclampsia, the rate of drop of the platelet count should be considered as important as the absolute level in determining the best course of action regarding epidural placement. A decreasing platelet count may indicate epidural placement before the level reaches an anticipated point that would preclude placement. Likewise, a rapidly dropping level may give cause for concern that even though the absolute level is adequate, an anticipated significantly low nadir may predispose to bleeding complications after placement or upon removal of the catheter.

4. *Describe the implications of a patient history that includes multiple miscarriages.*

Multiple miscarriages, such as noted in this case, may stem from a variety of causes, commonly including hematologic and anatomic derangements. Abnormal uterine anatomy may prevent normal embryonic implantation or fetal growth. Coagulation abnormalities, specifically, thrombophilias, often lead to miscarriage. Examples of these thrombophilias include deficiencies of protein C or protein S, antiphospholipid (anticardiolipin antibody) syndrome, and factor V Leiden. The main anesthetic concerns of these conditions result from the associated anticoagulation used to suppress the process and the resulting implications for regional anesthesia.

5. *Outline the material risks and the potential benefits of epidural analgesia.*

Risks:
- Failure or incomplete analgesia (6% to 10% of epidurals)
- PDPH (approximately 1% incidence)
- Persistent backache or sensory-motor impairment for up to a few months following discharge
- Infection at the insertion site or in the central nervous system (CNS) (rare)
- Epidural hematoma
- Permanent nerve damage, total spinal/high spinal, and other complications; however, these are sufficiently rare that they may not be considered material risks.

Benefits:
- Potential for complete pain relief
- More complete analgesia than that provided by parenteral agents
- Less CNS depression than experienced with equipotent parenteral agents
- Ability to convert to surgical anesthesia and avoid the dangers of general anesthesia in the case of cesarean delivery

6. *Discuss implications of initiating epidural analgesia either early or later in labor.*

As stated previously, a patient in active labor who is committed to delivery during the present admission may be given epidural analgesia upon request, provided that this plan fits with the obstetric management. The potential for an epidural placed early in labor to cause significant prolongation of labor or dystocia is not a material consideration in timing of delivery of the technique. Instead, practical considerations prevail; in most hospitals, initiation of epidural analgesia automatically relegates the patient to bed rest, unless a "walking epidural" program is in place. The patient considering an epidural early in labor should weigh her desire for pain relief against her desire to walk or even to ambulate only to the lavatory.

On the other end of the spectrum, health care workers frequently inform patients that they may not request an epidural after a point of cervical dilation. Similar to the concern surrounding early epidural placement, there is no absolute rule that precludes epidural placement based upon the stage of labor. However, practical considerations again prevail. In a patient in advanced labor, it may be very difficult to have her remain adequately motionless and cooperative for placement. The sitting position may cause discomfort to the mother and may cause fetal heart rate decelerations due to head compression at the perineum. Finally, there may not be adequate time for establishment of the block before delivery occurs. In this case, a subarachnoid technique seems particularly indicated to provide almost instantaneous pain relief.

The patient is positioned sitting for epidural insertion. A loss of resistance technique is used with saline, which is then injected into the epidural space before catheter insertion. The catheter is inserted 6 cm, but blood backflow on passive drainage occurs. The catheter is withdrawn 1 cm and flushed with saline. No further blood is aspirated. A test dose is administered, consisting of 3 mL of 1.5% lidocaine with epinephrine 1:200,000. No change in motor function or heart rate is observed. After the test dose, the epidural is loaded with 10 mL of 1% lidocaine in divided doses. The patient initially demonstrates a T10 sensory level. An infusion 0.1% bupivacaine with fentanyl 2 mcg/mL is initiated at 10 mL/hr. The patient remains comfortable for 3 hours, but then begins to complain of pain.

7. *Compare the use of air vs. saline in the loss-of-resistance (LOR) syringe.*

The choice between using air or saline for the LOR is often based on the clinician's preference and may be based on their tactile familiarity with one or the other substances as resistance is tested during the procedure. Provided that the volume of air injected is minimized, there are data supporting equivalence of efficacy and side effects between the two materials. However, air in the epidural space can ascend to produce the headache pain of pneumocephalus, and the severity of a PDPH can be increased by ascended epidural air, although the presence of air does not contribute to development of the PDPH initially. There is reasonable conjecture that an air bubble in the epidural space may dwell in space better occupied by local anesthetic solution, and some trials have found greater incidence of inadequate or patchy analgesia when air was used instead of saline for the LOR. Considering numerous factors disfavoring air and that injection of saline reduces paresthesias and vein cannulations from the subsequent catheter insertion, it would be preferable for clinicians to use saline for the LOR technique.

8. *Discuss the process of inserting an epidural catheter.*

The anesthetist should rely on more information than just the loss of pressure resistance to determine needle tip location in identifying the epidural space. A change in resistance accompanied by a gritty feel or

sound during needle advancement can serve to indicate passage through the ligamentum flavum and should indicate more conservative advancements of the needle. Blood return into the needle or catheter obviously indicates penetration of an epidural vein, but more subtly suggests a needle tip position lateral to the midline, as the epidural veins tend not to be situated directly in the midline. In response to initial bloody return via the needle, the needle should be withdrawn and redirected with another LOR technique, with attention to assuring midline placement. In response to blood return via the catheter, the catheter may be withdrawn slightly and flushed with saline. If this maneuver withdraws the catheter from the vein, as evidenced by a lack of blood return and a negative intravenous (IV) test dose, the catheter may be dosed with anesthetic. The incidence of venous cannulation may be decreased by performing the epidural insertion with the patient in a lateral position, as opposed to the sitting position, wherein the epidural veins are more engorged. It is notable that the epidural veins are easily collapsible, and the inability to aspirate blood has little sensitivity for indicating vein cannulation. Passive gravity-assisted flow is a more sensitive indicator of a catheter situated in a blood vessel. Like bloody cannulations, paresthesias may indicate needle tip placement in a lateral epidural space. Paresthesias may indicate direct needle contact with or inside a nerve, and injection should not take place. The needle should be withdrawn. Finally, because the epidural space is occupied by adipose tissue and a venous network, the epidural catheter should be expected to slide easily into the space through the epidural needle. Resistance to catheter advancement, particularly in the first 5 cm of insertion depth, may indicate placement outside of the epidural space. In this case, withdrawal of the entire needle–catheter unit and reinsertion of the needle may be preferable to continuing to secure and attempting to dose the catheter.

9. *Debate the benefits of a shallow or deep catheter insertion depth.*

There is a compromise between inserting the catheter adequately deep to buffer against movement, causing withdrawal from the epidural space, and not inserting the catheter to a depth that promotes coiling or moving to a very lateral situation. The dividing line between these competing intentions is very thin, around the insertion depth of 5 cm. With a multiple-orifice catheter, the most proximate hole is usually situated 2 cm from the catheter tip. This would suggest that 2 to 3 cm is the absolute least depth a catheter may be inserted into the epidural space to have all orifices delivering medication into that space. On the other hand, the cause of many epidural failures is internal withdrawal of the catheter from the epidural space. A deeper insertion depth can provide some buffer against internal mobility of the catheter (in the space between the skin, where secured, and the epidural space). However, insertion depth beyond 4 cm increases the incidence of catheter coiling. This can lead to the catheter moving to one side or out of the lateral vertebral foramen, causing a unilateral block, or it may even lead to catheter knotting. Insertion to a depth of 5 to 6 cm is a good compromise between the competing needs for adequate, but not excessive, depth.

Intraoperative Period

10. *Describe the level of anesthesia required for stage I and stage II of labor.*

During stage I, pain is carried primarily via afferent nerves entering the spinal cord at T10–L1. Therefore adequate sensory block should be reflected in these dermatomes. During stage II, or the pelvic stage, pain is transmitted via the pudendal nerve to S2–S4 roots. As labor progresses, the extent of epidural blockade may need to be widened to assure coverage of the sacral dermatomes. In the absence of perineal pain to assess epidural coverage of sacral dermatomes, absence of plantar flexion of the foot indicates blockade of the S2 dermatome and provides a useful indication of caudal coverage of the epidural block.

11. *Contrast the benefits of different anesthetic medications for a labor epidural infusion.*

A wide variety of anesthetic mixtures may be used to provide epidural analgesia. Optimal epidural analgesia for labor manages the differential block that results from varying sensitivities of different nerves to local anesthetic effects. Differential block refers to blockade, but not all levels of nerve function in affected dermatomes. Ideally,

the epidural will block all pain transmission, while leaving as much motor function preserved as possible, to not interfere with patient positioning and "pushing" during stage II of labor. Lower concentrations of anesthetic help preserve motor function but may be more prone to developing breakthrough pain. Table 38.3 provides some representative epidural solutions, along with potential advantages and disadvantages associated with each of the various mixtures.

12. *Discuss controversies and options related to performing the epidural test dose.*

The epidural test dose is not used to verify optimal positioning of the catheter, but rather to rule out a catheter position that could lead to patient injury: in the intrathecal space or in a blood vessel. The traditional test dose consists of a local anesthetic in a dose that would produce a definitive motor block if administered intrathecally and epinephrine in a dose that would produce a heart rate rise if administered intravascularly. In the laboring patient, the heart rate can be very dynamic, and a rise in heart rate is not specific for epinephrine administration. Furthermore, if the epinephrine is injected intravascularly, it would be expected to cause a brief reduction in placental perfusion, and it could worsen any existing hypertension or preeclampsia. For these reasons, some variants on the test dose are sometimes preferred in the obstetric population.

After an intrathecal dose of anesthetic (when high-volume loading of the epidural is not needed), the IV test dose can be foregone, and a subarachnoid test can be used alone to assure that the infusion will not be

TABLE 38.3 Examples of Medication Solutions Used to Administer Epidural Analgesia

Solution	Advantages	Disadvantages	Representative Use
0.06% bupivacaine + epinephrine 1:800,000	Little to no motor block	Lighter sensory block; may be prone to breakthrough pain	Walking epidural
2 mcg/mL fentanyl	No motor block	Incomplete analgesia; increased opioid side effects apparent	Walking epidural; patient with allergy to all local anesthetics
0.125% bupivacaine + fentanyl 2 mcg/mL	Reliable analgesia; conservative compromise between analgesia and motor block		Typical continuous epidural solution
0.2% ropivacaine + fentanyl 2 mcg/mL	Possibly better analgesia with comparable motor block to 0.125% bupivacaine		Typical continuous epidural solution
0.08% ropivacaine + fentanyl 2 mcg/mL	Reliable analgesia; less toxicity potential than equipotent bupivacaine		Typical continuous epidural solution
0.25% bupivacaine ± opioids or epinephrine	Profound sensory block; resistant to breakthrough pain	Unnecessary motor block; increase in minor transient neurobehavioral deficits of neonate	Malpositioned fetus; "back labor"; opioid allergy

administered into the intrathecal space. Other variants on the test dose include low- then high-volume local anesthetic administration to determine intrathecal and then IV placement. In this case, 2 mL of 2% lidocaine can be given first, with signs of lower extremity weakness after 5 minutes indicating intrathecal administration. Once the intrathecal position is ruled out, 5 mL of 2% lidocaine can be given, with signs of dizziness or other CNS symptoms indicating IV placement. Other drugs suitable for neuraxial administration but with characteristic IV responses may be substituted for epinephrine in the IV test dose under particular circumstances. Fentanyl and isoproterenol are examples of agents that have been used in this way.

13. *Discuss the procedural variants of the traditional labor epidural.*

When the patient needs rapid analgesia without long-term effects or with minimal chance of late complications, a "single-shot spinal" may be used. This approach is useful when the patient is in very advanced labor and will deliver during the 60- to 90-minute duration of effects of the initial injection. With very small needles (27 or 29 gauge), the risk of PDPH may not be appreciably increased if the injection needs to be repeated. The single-shot injection is faster and easier to implement than an indwelling epidural, but it eliminates the benefit of an adaptable technique that can be extended for instrumented or surgical delivery should either of those become necessary.

The combined spinal-epidural (CSE) technique is beneficial in the case of advanced or rapidly progressing labor, intense pain, a history of epidural failure, or the desire to avoid a heavy epidural loading dose (such as in the "walking" epidural). Medications useful for the intrathecal dose include fentanyl 10 to 20 mcg, sufentanil 5 to 10 mcg, bupivacaine 1.5 to 2.5 mg, ropivacaine 2 to 4 mg, or a combination of local anesthetic and opioid, including morphine. After the intrathecal dose, the patient may be started on an epidural infusion, or epidural dosing may be deferred until the effects of the intrathecal dose subside. An intrathecal dose that does not contain morphine will typically provide a significant degree of analgesia for 60 to 90 minutes. If it is anticipated that an epidural infusion will be started eventually, it may be initiated immediately after CSE administration. In this way, the epidural space will be "loaded" by way of the slow infusion over the period during which the intrathecal dose is in effect. The epidural test dose may be used after a CSE, with the understanding that a high-volume test dose procedure may extend the height of spinal blockade and theoretically promote more local anesthetic diffusion through the dural puncture. Some providers omit the IV test dose after a CSE in lieu of initiating the low-concentration infusion. This approach assumes that the low concentration of infusion (e.g., ≤0.125% bupivacaine) does not threaten systemic toxicity even if

it is administered into a vein, while complete recession of the analgesia in the meantime would inform the practitioner that the medication is being delivered somewhere other than the epidural space.

The CSE technique derives analgesia from the intrathecal dose for the first 60 to 90 minutes; therefore a nonfunctional epidural catheter is not discovered until after that period. As a result, although the CSE technique may aid in correct identification of the epidural space, it may also be disadvantageous in patients at risk for surgical delivery, as the anesthetist's ability to recognize catheter malfunctions is delayed. These competing considerations may create a conundrum when caring for an obese patient, such as the one that was presented. In this case, the selection of the CSE approach may be based largely on provider preference.

14. *Discuss the side effects and treatment options for complications of epidural insertion.*

A number of complications may occur during placement, as outlined in Table 38.4.

Epidural catheter dislodgement may occur internally if the catheter is secured to the relatively mobile soft tissue of the patient's back when seated before moving the patient to a recumbent position in bed. This effect is minimal with a thin patient but can be very pronounced with an obese patient. If inserting the catheter with the patient seated, it is advisable to instruct the patient to move to a lateral lying position before securing the catheter to the skin. A similar effect may result from edema formation, which increases the distance from the epidural space to the skin, where the catheter is secured.

TABLE 38.4 Epidural Complications and Management

Complication	Management
Blood in epidural needle	Withdraw needle and redirect.
Blood in epidural catheter	Withdraw catheter (not while still in needle) to extent possible, flush, and use if clear. If continued blood, remove catheter and replace.
Cerebrospinal fluid via epidural needle or catheter	a. Remove needle and/or catheter and reinsert at different level b. Use catheter intrathecally, adjusting dosage accordingly
Paresthesia	Withdraw needle or catheter (not while still in needle) for all but the most transient paresthesias
Resistance on insertion of catheter	Remove catheter and needle as a unit (do not withdraw catheter through needle) and reinsert

15. *Differentiate potential causes of breakthrough pain and their treatment.*
    - **Epidural misplacement:** Block receding bilaterally, perhaps (but not always) visible disconnection of dislodgement at the site of insertion.
    - **Malpositioned fetus:** Fetus is positioned occiput posterior, causing pressure on parturient's sciatic nerve or others. The obstetric team can evaluate fetal position through palpation of the fontanelles.
    - **Labor progression:** Pain from T10 to L1 dermatomes in first stage that transitions to S2–S4 during second stage. Analgesia that does not reach sacral dermatomes may become unmasked as labor progresses to stage II.
    - **Visceral pain:** Bladder distention from sacral anesthesia may not be recognized by the patient and may present as diffuse abdominal pain.
    - **Pathology,** such as placental abruption: Smoking history or vascular compromise from diabetes or thrombophilia in this patient increases her risk of placental abruption. Vaginal bleeding may be an accompanying sign.

    The patient pushed in stage II labor for 3 hours. The obstetrician plans to employ a vacuum extraction and calls for additional epidural dosing.

16. *Formulate a plan for providing anesthesia for an instrumented vaginal delivery (ISV).*

    The use of vacuum extraction, and less commonly forceps delivery, may call for anesthetist intervention to intensify the level of a preexisting epidural block and to stand by for possible complications or conversion to cesarean delivery. With an existing epidural, elevating the patient's head to at least 30 degrees will reduce the incidence of "sacral sparing," or inadequate sacral blockade, as an additional bolus is given. The perineal dose typically consists of 5 to 10 mL of a rapidly acting anesthetic such as 2% to 3% chloroprocaine or 2% lidocaine. If requested to provide anesthesia for ISV without an epidural in situ, an intrathecal dose of 2 to 3 mg bupivacaine followed by elevating the patient's upper body will provide rapid effects, with less sacral sparing than an epidural. However, considering the risk of operative intervention, providing this intrathecal dose as part of a CSE technique provides a useful backup, providing that there is time to perform this procedure.

Postoperative Period

17. *Describe potential removal complications of the epidural catheter.*

    Complications associated with the removal of an epidural catheter are rare. In a patient with coagulopathy, bleeding may be incited by catheter removal. For this reason, catheter removal should be delayed during an interval of significant coagulopathy or therapeutic levels of low-molecular-weight heparin and similar medications. The other class of removal complications involves mechanical problems related to the catheter becoming fixed in place. This can result from a variety of causes and has been reported as occurring even immediately after initial insertion. A soft polyurethane catheter shows a greater propensity for becoming stuck in place, although these catheters perform more favorably in terms of ease of insertion and incidence of vein cannulations. The soft catheter also has a lower breaking strength than the polyamide nylon type. In the case of the inability to remove a catheter, methods to facilitate removal include changing the patient's position, applying steady gentle traction to the catheter, allowing hours to days of rest time before reattempting removal, and general anesthesia with muscle relaxation.

Review Questions

1. Which is absolutely required before insertion of a labor epidural?
   a. Platelet count of 140,000/mm^3
   b. Cervical dilation of 4 cm
   c. Maternal desire for an epidural
   d. Ruptured amniotic sac
2. Which epidural medication would provide the greatest degree of motor block?
   a. Lidocaine 1%
   b. Bupivacaine 0.25%
   c. Fentanyl 2 mcg/mL
   d. Ropivacaine 0.1%
3. Pain from stage I of labor is transmitted through which spinal nerve distribution?
   a. C5–C8
   b. T4–T8
   c. T10–L1
   d. S2–S4
4. Which condition is least associated with pain?
   a. Malpositioned fetus
   b. Placenta previa
   c. Bladder distention
   d. Placental abruption
5. Which complication associated with epidural analgesia occurs with an incidence of approximately 1%?
   a. Inadequate analgesia
   b. Postdural puncture headache
   c. Backache
   d. Nerve damage

Suggested Readings

Bos EME, Schut ME, de Quelerij M, et al. Trends in practice and safety measures of epidural analgesia: report of a national survey. *Acta Anaesthesiol Scand* 2018;62(10):1466-1472.

Chau A, Bibbo C, Huang CC, et al. Dural puncture epidural technique improves labor analgesia quality with fewer side effects compared with epidural and combined spinal epidural techniques: a randomized clinical trial. *Anesth Analg* 2017;124(2):560-569.

Desai N, Gardner A, Carvalho B. Labor epidural analgesia to cesarean section anesthetic conversion failure: a national survey. *Anesthesiol Res Pract* 2019;2019:6381792.

Goodman SR, Smiley RM, Negron MA, et al. A randomized trial of breakthrough pain during combined spinal-epidural versus epidural labor analgesia in parous women. *Anesth Analg* 2009;108(1):246-251.

Halpern SH, Carvalho B. Patient-controlled epidural analgesia for labor. *Anesth Analg* 2009;108(3):921-928.

Hattler J, Klimek M, Rossaint R, Heesen M. The effect of combined spinal-epidural versus epidural analgesia in laboring women on nonreassuring fetal heart rate tracings: systematic review and meta-analysis. *Anesth Analg* 2016;123(4):955-964.

Heesen M, Rijs K, Rossaint R, Klimek M. Dural puncture epidural versus conventional epidural block for labor analgesia: a systematic review of randomized controlled trials. *Int J Obstet Anesth* 2019;40:24-31.

Kason BJ. Obstetric anesthesia. In: Nagelhout JJ, Elisha S, eds. *Nurse Anesthesia,* 6th ed. St Louis, MO: Elsevier, 2018:1064-1091.

Mankowitz SK, Gonzalez Fiol A, Smiley R. Failure to extend epidural labor analgesia for cesarean delivery anesthesia: a focused review. *Anesth Analg* 2016;123(5):1174-1180.

Poma S, Scudeller L, Verga C, et al. Effects of combined spinal-epidural analgesia on first stage of labor: a cohort study. *J Matern Fetal Neonatal Med* 2019;32(21):3559-3565.

Sng BL, Sia ATH. Maintenance of epidural labour analgesia: the old, the new and the future. *Best Pract Res Clin Anaesthesiol* 2017;31(1):15-22.

Thuillier C, Roy S, Peyronnet V, et al. Impact of recommended changes in labor management for prevention of the primary cesarean delivery. *Am J Obstet Gynecol* 2018;218(3):341.e1-341.e9.

Van de Velde M, Dreelinck R, Dubois J, et. al. Determination of the full dose-response relation of intrathecal bupivacaine, levobupivacaine, and ropivacaine, combined with sufentanil, for labor analgesia. *Anesthesiology* 2007;106:149-156.

39

Laparoscopy for Adnexal Mass During Pregnancy

KEY POINTS

- Approximately 2% of pregnant women will require nonobstetric surgery during pregnancy; these are often abdominal surgeries involving laparoscopy.
- If conditions permit, surgery during pregnancy should be accomplished during the second trimester.
- Numerous anesthetic agents can be used safely during pregnancy.

- Maintenance of maternal oxygen saturation and blood pressure during the intraoperative period is critical to avoiding fetal hypoxia from inadequate uteroplacental perfusion.
- Perioperative monitoring of fetal heart rate and uterine tone is prudent.

Case Synopsis

A 26-year-old woman who is at 29 weeks of gestation is evaluated in the anesthesia clinic for a diagnostic laparoscopy for an adnexal mass detected on routine ultrasound.

Preoperative Evaluation and Demographic Data

Past Medical/Surgical History

- Tonsillectomy, without anesthetic complications at 9 years of age

List of Medications

- Prenatal vitamins (folic acid, calcium, iron)

Diagnostic Data

- Hemoglobin, 12.5 g/dL; hematocrit, 37.5%
- Sodium, 139 mEq/L; potassium, 4.1 mEq/L; chloride, 105 mEq/L; carbon dioxide (CO_2), 24 mEq/L
- Blood urea nitrogen, 8 g/dL; creatinine, 0.4 g/dL

Height/Weight/Vital Signs

- 175 cm, 73 kg
- Blood pressure, 110/60; heart rate, 78 beats per minute; respiratory rate, 22 breaths per minute; oxygen saturation on room air, 99%; temperature, 36.9°C

Pathophysiology

An adnexal mass is diagnosed in 2% of pregnancies and can include ovarian cysts and benign or malignant tumors.

Ovarian cysts are often incidental findings noted during routine ultrasonography for pregnant patients. Diagnostic workup for ovarian cysts includes ultrasound and computed tomography (CT) or magnetic resonance imaging (MRI). Ovarian cysts can cause pelvic pain, infertility, nausea, and vomiting. If large enough, cystic masses can obstruct normal labor. If the cyst is small, management involves observation because most cysts will resolve spontaneously. If the cyst is large (>5 to 10 cm), is suspicious for malignancy, or persists for a prolonged time, surgery is indicated.

Surgical Procedure

The need for nonobstetric surgery in the pregnant patient is not a rare occurrence. Approximately 1 in 50 pregnant women will require surgery at some point during their pregnancy. Conditions that predispose to emergent surgery include trauma, appendicitis, cholecystitis, adnexal masses, breast masses, trauma, and cervical incompetence. Although surgery during pregnancy is usually performed to treat maternal pathology, the well-being of the maternal–fetal unit must be considered when planning anesthetic care. Important goals in the care of the pregnant patient for nonobstetric surgery include:

- Mitigating increased maternal risk arising from the physiologic changes of pregnancy
- Minimizing fetal exposure to potentially teratogenic agents
- Prevention of preterm labor
- Avoidance of fetal asphyxia secondary to uterine hypoperfusion or maternal hypoxia

Anesthetic Management and Considerations

Preoperative Period

1. *Discuss how the physiologic changes of pregnancy affect surgical risk.*

   The dramatic anatomic and physiologic adaptations that occur during pregnancy preserve the pregnancy and facilitate labor and delivery. Changes in many maternal organ systems are seen during pregnancy; most important to anesthetic management are changes in the central nervous, pulmonary, cardiovascular, and gastrointestinal systems. The physiologic changes associated with pregnancy are summarized in Table 39.1.

   Due largely to the effect of progesterone on the central nervous system (CNS), the pregnant patient experiences increased sensitivity to inhaled, intravenous, and local anesthetics. Furthermore, the subarachnoid and epidural spaces are reduced in volume due to the anatomic changes of pregnancy, resulting in increased rostral spread of anesthetic agents injected into these spaces.

TABLE 39.1	Physiologic Changes Associated With Pregnancy	
Respiratory System		
• Minute ventilation	• Increased 50%	
• Tidal volume	• Increased 40%	
• Respiratory rate	• Increased 15%	
• Functional residual capacity	• Decreased 20%	
• $PaCO_2$ 32–35 mm Hg	• Decreased	
• Oxygen consumption	• Increased 20%	
• $PaCO_2$–$ETCO_2$ −1 to + 1 mm Hg	• Decreased	
Cardiovascular System		
• Cardiac output	• Increased 40%	
• Stroke volume	• Increased 25%	
• Heart rate	• Increased 25%	
• Systemic vascular resistance	• Decreased	
• Systolic blood pressure	• Unchanged	
• Diastolic blood pressure	• Decreased	
Hematologic System		
• Plasma volume	• Increased 40%–50%	
• Hematocrit	• Decreased	
Central Nervous System		
• Minimum alveolar concentration	• Decreased	
Gastrointestinal System		
• Lower esophageal sphincter tone	• Decreased	
• Barrier pressure	• Decreased	
Metabolic		
• Free drug availability	• Increased	
• Plasma cholinesterase activity	• Decreased	

Oxygen consumption during pregnancy is dramatically increased, whereas functional residual capacity is diminished; this leads to a potential for significant hypoxia in poorly ventilated patients. An increased minute ventilation is normally seen in the pregnant woman as a result of an increase in both tidal volume and respiratory rate. The alveolar hyperventilation that occurs during pregnancy leads to a state of chronic compensated respiratory alkalosis. Difficult endotracheal (ET) intubation and epistaxis (in the case of nasal intubation) can result due to capillary engorgement of the mucosa of the upper airways as early as the first trimester of pregnancy.

The maternal cardiovascular system is dramatically changed by pregnancy. An increase in cardiac output is the product of an increase in heart rate, intravascular volume, and stroke volume. The increased cardiac output, like the increased minute volume, helps the pregnant woman meet the metabolic needs of the fetoplacental unit. The generalized vasodilatation typical during healthy pregnancies leads to decreased systemic vascular resistance during pregnancy and increases sensitivity to the vasodilating effects of anesthetic agents.

The effect of pregnancy on gastric motility and acid secretion remains a subject of debate among experts related to gastrointestinal physiology. What is not in question is that lower esophageal sphincter tone and gastric barrier pressure are decreased in pregnancy, placing pregnant women at increased risk of pulmonary aspiration.

2. *Select the optimal time for surgery in the pregnant patient.*

   In the pregnant patient, elective surgery should be delayed until after delivery. If the need for surgery is pressing, it is preferably performed during the second trimester. If possible, surgery is best avoided during the first trimester because fetal organogenesis occurs during this period. Third-trimester surgery is associated with increased risk of preterm labor and the possibility that the surgeon will experience increased technical difficulty due to the presence of the gravid uterus.

3. *Explain the evaluation and preparation of a pregnant patient for anesthesia and surgery.*

   The preanesthetic assessment of a pregnant patient includes an evaluation of organ systems considering the changes expected in pregnancy. Obstetric consultation should be obtained regarding perioperative monitoring of fetal heart rate and uterine tone. The patient's obstetrician may also be consulted regarding the possible need for tocolysis. In addition, preparation of a pregnant patient for anesthesia and surgery should include aspiration prophylaxis and pneumatic compression devices.

   Pneumatic compression devices are indicated in pregnant patients due to the increased risk of deep vein thrombosis (DVT) resulting from the hypercoagulable state normal in pregnancy, which is exacerbated by surgical trauma. Anxiolytics may be warranted because increased catecholamine levels can cause vasoconstriction, leading to decreased uteroplacental perfusion.

Intraoperative Period

4. Analyze which anesthetic technique is optimal for this surgery.

Research fails to demonstrate improved fetal outcomes associated with any anesthetic technique. A common practice is to employ regional techniques whenever possible because fetal exposure to anesthetic agents is minimized and maternal risk for pulmonary aspiration is reduced. Most surgery during pregnancy is performed for intraabdominal pathology that commonly requires general anesthesia. Increased maternal sensitivity to anesthetic agents necessitates reducing the amount of medication that is administered by approximately 30% to prevent accidental overdosage. Regardless of the technique employed, maintenance of adequate uteroplacental perfusion and maternal oxygenation is essential. Box 39.1 summarizes the most important anesthetic considerations for the pregnant patient undergoing nonobstetric surgery.

• BOX 39.1 Anesthetic Considerations in Pregnant Patients Undergoing Laparoscopic Surgery

Preoperative
- Defer elective surgery until after delivery.
- Urgent surgery should be scheduled during the second trimester, if possible.
- If possible, use of a regional anesthetic technique may be prudent.
- Obstetric consultation should be obtained for recommendations regarding fetal heart rate monitoring and the use of tocolytics in the perioperative period.

Intraoperative
- Patient should be placed in the left uterine displacement to minimize hypotension.
- Recognize and address the increased risk for difficult airway and pulmonary aspiration.
- Reduce dose of anesthetic agents due to increased maternal sensitivity.
- If mechanical ventilation is used, minute volume should be adjusted to maintain $ETCO_2$ at preoperative level.
- Maintain adequate maternal blood pressure and oxygenation to ensure adequate uteroplacental perfusion.
- Intraabdominal pressure should not exceed 15 mm Hg.
- Continuous fetal heart rate monitoring in the intraoperative period should be considered.
- Intraoperative pneumatic compression devices should be employed to minimize venous thrombus.

Postoperative
- Intraoperative pneumatic compression devices should be continued in the postoperative period to minimize risk of venous thrombus.
- Early ambulation should be encouraged to minimize risk of venous thrombus.
- Uterine tone should be monitored and tocolysis instituted if signs of preterm labor are noted.
- Continuous fetal heart rate monitoring should be continued in the postoperative period.

---

5. Examine the advantages and disadvantages of laparoscopic surgery during pregnancy.

A pregnant woman who presents with abdominal discomfort poses a diagnostic challenge for the clinician, who must distinguish between common pregnancy-related symptoms and symptoms resulting from a potential pathology. This process is further complicated by the anatomic changes that are associated with pregnancy. Laparoscopy is valuable in this circumstance, providing a useful tool for both diagnosis and definitive treatment. Other beneficial effects of laparoscopic surgery include decreased intraoperative blood loss, reduced postoperative analgesic requirements, and the fact that the technique tends to facilitate early ambulation, which is important for reducing the risk of thromboembolic complications.

Some clinicians have expressed concern regarding the use of laparoscopy in pregnant patients, and this concern focuses principally on two issues: establishment of the pneumoperitoneum (PnP) and the physiologic effects of the PnP. Establishment of a PnP involves insufflation of CO_2 into the peritoneal space via either blind placement of a Verres needle or open placement of a trocar, either of which has the potential to traumatize organs in the abdomen. Both techniques, when proper precautions are followed, are considered acceptable practice.

The physiologic effects of CO_2 on the PnP have the potential to exacerbate preexisting cardiovascular and pulmonary pathophysiology. The physiologic effects associated with PnP are listed in Table 39.2. Anesthetic considerations for management of the pregnant woman undergoing laparoscopic surgery must take these changes into account and will be discussed in more detail.

6. Describe airway and respiratory management of the pregnant woman undergoing nonobstetric laparoscopic surgery.

General anesthesia should be preceded by denitrogenation. Induction and endotracheal tube (ETT) intubation, using an ETT one size smaller than customarily used in nonpregnant women, should be accomplished expeditiously by the rapid sequence induction with

---

TABLE 39.2 Physiologic Effects Associated With Pneumoperitoneum

Respiratory System

Peak inspiratory pressure	Increased
Pulmonary compliance	Decreased
Vital capacity	Decreased
Functional residual capacity	Decreased
CO_2 delivery to lungs	Increased by 30%
Intrathoracic pressure	Increased

Cardiovascular System

Cardiac output	Decreased
Mean arterial pressure	Increased
Systemic vascular resistance	Increased

Gastrointestinal System

Postoperative emesis	40%–60%

cricoid pressure. Due to decreased functional residual capacity (FRC) and increased oxygen (O_2) demand, pregnant women experience rapid desaturation during even short periods of apnea.

Absorption of CO_2 from the PnP increases the delivery of CO_2 to the lungs. End tidal carbon dioxide ($ETCO_2$) monitoring reliably reflects the partial pressure of arterial CO_2 ($PaCO_2$) in the patient and should be monitored closely. In the pregnant patient undergoing general anesthesia, minute ventilation will need to be adjusted to maintain an $ETCO_2$ in the low-normal range typically seen during pregnancy (32 to 36 mm Hg). Providing adequate minute ventilation can be challenging because a gravid uterus and the presence of the PnP can compromise diaphragmatic excursion, leading to decreased lung compliance. Inadequate ventilation increases the potential risk of fetal and maternal acidosis. Hyperventilation can lead to alkalosis, resulting in a left shift of the oxyhemoglobin disassociation curve and impaired exchange of oxygen between the maternal and fetal circulation.

7. *Review some of the cardiovascular issues seen in this population and appropriate anesthetic management.*

Pregnant women can experience aortocaval compression as early as 20 weeks' gestation; therefore, patients undergoing surgery should be positioned in such a manner that the uterus is displaced to the left, optimizing maternal preload and placental perfusion. In addition to the risk of decreased preload caused by aortocaval compression, insufflation of the abdomen to establish a PnP decreases venous return. Intravascular volume should be optimized before induction of anesthesia. Generalized vasodilation occurs during normal pregnancy, putting the patient at risk for sudden decreases in blood pressure. The development of hypotension may be mitigated by the effects of the PnP, which causes increased systemic vascular resistance. The risk of hypotension can be reduced by avoiding high doses of inhaled agents. If the patient experiences a significant drop in blood pressure (systolic blood pressure below 100 mm Hg or a decrease in mean arterial pressure of >20% of baseline), the hypotension should be treated aggressively to ensure adequate uteroplacental perfusion because the uterus lacks the ability to autoregulate. Both phenylephrine and ephedrine have been used successfully to support the maternal blood pressure and preserve uteroplacental perfusion.

8. *Identify the teratogenic risks of surgery and anesthesia in the pregnant patient.*

Teratogenicity refers to significant structural or functional changes in a newborn resulting from prenatal treatment. This complex phenomenon involves the susceptibility of the species, as well as the dose, duration of exposure, and timing of exposure to the agent during gestation. The risk of fetal harm resulting from anesthetics has been the subject of much concern on the part of the general public and clinicians.

Most anesthetic drugs (except for neuromuscular blocking medications) are highly lipid soluble and therefore cross the placenta and enter the fetal circulation. Despite the potential risk of fetal injury, very few drugs are thoroughly studied to determine whether their use is safe in pregnancy. This is largely due to the multiple scientific and ethical challenges that drug testing in pregnancy presents. A list of widely recognized teratogenic drugs is found in Box 39.2.

Despite many years of clinical experience and several studies, no anesthetic agent has been definitively identified as having teratogenic effects. The ability to conclusively affirm the safety of an anesthetic agent in pregnant women (or, for that matter, most drugs) is constrained by the limited number of studies in this population.

Two anesthetic agents have been implicated as having teratogenic effects. An association between maternal benzodiazepine use and increased risk of cleft lip and palate in newborns was suggested after case reports. This association was not supported by later case-controlled and prospective studies. In laboratory studies involving rodents, exposure to very high levels of nitrous oxide (N_2O) led to abortion and congenital malformations. Observational studies examining human exposure to N_2O in normal concentrations have failed to establish an association between N_2O and abortion or congenital malformation.

9. *Explain the role of fetal heart rate monitoring in the management of patients undergoing nonobstetric surgery.*

Whether or not to use fetal heart rate monitoring is a decision which is best made considering the specific circumstances surrounding the patient and surgery in question and after consultation between obstetric, surgical, and anesthetic practitioners. If a decision is made to employ fetal monitoring in the perioperative period, it is essential to have qualified personnel present to operate and interpret the monitor(s).

Fetal heart rate monitoring can be easily accomplished after 22 to 24 weeks' gestation using surface transducers. Intraoperative monitoring may be problematic because

---

• BOX 39.2 Drugs Reported to Have Human Teratogenic Effects

- Angiotensin-converting enzyme inhibitors
- Aminoglycosides
- Androgens
- Antithyroid medications
- Carbamazepine
- Cocaine
- Corticosteroids
- Cytotoxic agents
- Diethylstilbestrol
- Estrogens
- Ethanol
- Lithium
- Penicillamine
- Phenytoin
- Retinoids
- Tetracycline
- Thalidomide
- Valproic acid
- Warfarin

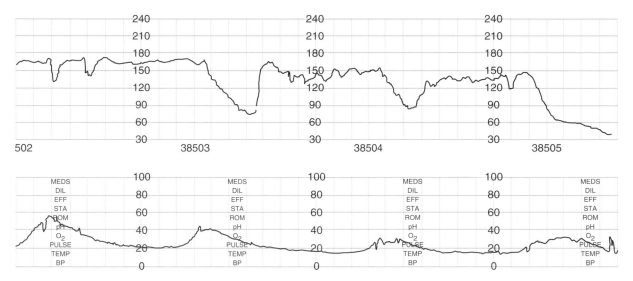

• **Fig. 39.1** Fetal heart rate decelerations with contractions. Bradycardia occurred after the last contraction (only the initial segment is visible). (From Rakel RE, Rakel DP: *Textbook of family medicine*, ed 9, St. Louis, 2015, Elsevier.)

transabdominal monitor placement can interfere with the surgical field. In these cases, options include omitting monitoring during the intraoperative period or the use of a vaginal probe.

Fetal exposure to anesthetic agents has the effect of eliminating beat-to-beat variability and is not of concern. Persistent fetal bradycardia (Fig. 39.1) at any point in the perioperative period indicates fetal compromise and should trigger actions directed toward improving delivery of oxygen to the fetus. Depending on the circumstances, actions to improve fetal oxygenation may include left uterine displacement, tocolysis, release of surgical retraction, and support of maternal blood pressure and oxygenation.

Postoperative Period

10. *Plan the postoperative care of a pregnant patient after nonobstetric surgery.*

Postoperative care of surgical patients should devote considerable attention to managing pain and nausea.

These priorities are of even greater significance in the population under consideration because pregnancy and laparoscopic surgery put the patient at especially high risk for nausea and vomiting and the risk that increased levels of catecholamines accompanying pain can cause decreased uteroplacental blood flow.

Special considerations in the postoperative care of pregnant women undergoing nonobstetric surgery include prophylaxis against venous thrombosis and monitoring of the fetal heart rate and uterine tone. Measures to reduce the risk of venous thromboembolism include sequential compression hose, anticoagulation (avoiding the teratogenic agent warfarin), and early ambulation.

Preterm labor presents a significant risk to the wellbeing of the fetus and accounts for 70% of perinatal morbidity and mortality. Monitoring of the fetal heart rate and uterine activity for 12 to 24 hours after surgery may be warranted, with timely intervention for fetal bradycardia or preterm labor indicated if these conditions are detected.

Review Questions

1. Low maternal blood pressure can lead to poor perfusion of the placenta due to the:
   a. Increased maternal circulating volume.
   b. Lack of uterine vascular autoregulation.
   c. Leftward shift of the oxyhemoglobin curve.
   d. Presence of fetal hemoglobin.
2. Maternal hyperventilation can lead to:
   a. Altered uterine tone.
   b. Decreased cardiac inotropy.
   c. Increased risk of persistent fetal circulation.
   d. Leftward shift of the oxyhemoglobin disassociation curve.

3. Absence of fetal beat-to-beat variability during administration of general anesthesia to the mother is considered:
   a. A normal fetal response.
   b. A sign of damage to the fetal nervous system.
   c. An indication for emergent delivery.
   d. An indication for tocolysis.

4. Which intervention used for thromboembolic prophylaxis is contraindicated during pregnancy?
   a. Early ambulation
   b. Low-molecular-weight heparin
   c. Sequential compression hose
   d. Warfarin

5. In the setting of nonobstetric surgery during pregnancy, the greatest cause of fetal morbidity and mortality is:
   a. Congenital defects.
   b. Maternal death.
   c. Postoperative infection.
   d. Preterm labor.

Suggested Readings

Costa-Martins S, Santos JV, Bernardes J. Laparoscopic surgery during pregnancy. A survey among European Obstetricians and Gynecologists. *Eur J Obstet Gynecol Reprod Biol* 2016;206:247-248.

Heesen M, Klimek M. Nonobstetric anesthesia during pregnancy. *Curr Opin Anaesthesiol* 2016;29(3):297-303.

Hong JY. Adnexal mass surgery and anesthesia during pregnancy: a 10-year retrospective review. *Int J Obstet Anesth* 2006;15(3):212-216.

Kason BJ. Obstetric anesthesia. In: Nagelhout JJ, Elisha S, eds. *Nurse Anesthesia*, 6th ed. St Louis, MO: Elsevier, 2018:1064-1091.

Olutoye OA, Baker BW, Belfort MA, Olutoye OO. Food and Drug Administration warning on anesthesia and brain development: implications for obstetric and fetal surgery. *Am J Obstet Gynecol* 2018;218(1):98-102.

Shigemi D, Aso S, Matsui H, Fushimi K, Yasunaga H. Safety of laparoscopic surgery for benign diseases during pregnancy: a nationwide retrospective cohort study. *J Minim Invasive Gynecol* 2019;26(3):501-506.

Vasco Ramirez M, Valencia G CM. Anesthesia for nonobstetric surgery in pregnancy. *Clin Obstet Gynecol* 2020;63(2):351-363.

Vujic J, Marsoner K, Lipp-Pump AH, et al. Nonobstetric surgery during pregnancy - an eleven-year retrospective analysis. *BMC Pregnancy Childbirth* 2019;19(1):382.

40

Robotic-Assisted Laparoscopic Prostatectomy

KEY POINTS

- Because the average age of men who develop prostate cancer is greater than 50 years, patients presenting for radical prostatectomy frequently have at least one comorbidity.
- The most common intraoperative complications associated with radical prostatectomy are acute hemorrhage and positioning injuries.
- Presently, there are several surgical options and anesthetic choices for patients with prostate cancer.
- Accurate monitoring of blood loss, as well as a plan for fluid and blood replacement, is imperative.

Case Synopsis

A 69-year-old man presents to his urologist with increased urinary frequency and urgency. He undergoes a thorough urologic workup that reveals his prostate-specific antigen (PSA) is elevated. His doctor performs a digital rectal examination and palpates several irregular nodules. The results from a prostate biopsy definitively reveal that the patient has prostate cancer. His urologist recommends a radical prostatectomy and explains the risks and benefits of the various surgical options, which include laparoscopic and robot-assisted laparoscopic technique. The patient chooses the robot-assisted laparoscopic approach.

Preoperative Evaluation and Demographic Data

Past Medical/Surgical History

- Hypertension
- Coronary artery bypass graft (CABG) performed 2 years ago
- Well-controlled asthma
- Osteoarthritis
- 12-pack/year smoker, stopped smoking 2 weeks ago

List of Medications

- Atenolol
- Hydrochlorothiazide
- Singulair inhaler
- Aspirin
- Sildenafil (Viagra)

Diagnostic Data

- Hemoglobin, 14.1 g/dL; hematocrit, 40.9%
- Blood urea nitrogen (BUN), 17 mg/dL; creatinine, 1.0 mg/dL
- Electrolytes: sodium, 141 mEq/L; potassium, 3.4 mEq/L; chloride, 101 mEq/L; carbon dioxide (CO_2), 25 mEq/L
- Glucose, 144 mg/dL
- PSA, 18 ng/mL (reference range 0 to 4.5 ng/mL for age 61 to 70 years)
- Biopsy of the prostate is positive for adenocarcinoma

Height/Weight/Vital Signs

- 185 cm, 86 kg
- Blood pressure, 161/96; heart rate, 78 beats per minute; respiratory rate, 14 breaths per minute; room air oxygen saturation, 99%; temperature, 37.4°C
- 12-lead electrocardiogram (ECG): normal sinus rhythm with a right bundle branch block; heart rate, 72 beats per minute
- Exercise stress test: no evidence of ischemia
- Cardiac Doppler ultrasound: estimated ejection fraction, 55%

Pathophysiology

It is estimated that up to one-third of men develop cellular dysplasia consistent with prostate cancer by 50 years of age. The incidence of prostate cancer increases with age, and at 75 years of age, the possibility rises to approximately 75%. Prostate cancer is the second leading cause of mortality due to cancer-related deaths. Prostate cancer generally occurs in

TABLE 40.1	TNM Staging of Prostate Cancer	
Stage	**Description**	

Primary Tumor

Tx	• Primary tumor cannot be assessed
T0	• No evidence of primary tumor • Clinically unapparent tumor not palpable or visible by imaging
T1	• T1a–Tumor incidental, found in 5% or less of resected tissue • T1b–Tumor incidental, found in more than 5% of resected tissue • T1c–Tumor identified by needle biopsy (because of elevated PSA). Tumor is confined within the prostate gland.
T2	• T2a–Tumor involves one lobe • T2b–Tumor involves both lobes. Tumor extends through the prostatic capsule.
T3	• T3a–Extracapsular extensions (unilateral or bilateral) • T3b–Tumor invades the seminal vesicles
T4	• Tumor is fixed or invades adjacent structures other than seminal vesicles: bladder neck, external sphincter, rectum, levator muscles, and/or pelvic wall

Regional Lymph Nodes

Nx	• Regional lymph nodes have not been assessed
N0	• No regional lymph node metastasis
N1	• Regional lymph node metastasis

Distant Metastasis

Mx	• Distant metastasis has not been assessed
M0	• No distant metastasis
M1	• M1a–Nonregional lymph nodes • M1b–Bone • M1c–Other sites

men over the age of 50. Therefore it is reasonable to expect a high incidence of comorbidities such as hypertension and diabetes in this patient population. Prostate cancer is considered a slowly progressing cancer. Early detection and prompt treatment significantly increase the probability of survival.

The initial routine screening for prostate cancer is achieved by assessing PSA blood test results. It is theorized that if all men lived long enough, they would develop prostate cancer. The information provided by PSA testing has limitations, which include the sensitivity and specificity of the results. Many factors can cause falsely elevated PSA results, such as a urinary tract infection. More recently, the upper limits in the reference range of the PSA are indexed in relation to patient age. A digital rectal examination provided by a urologist and a prostate biopsy are necessary to definitively diagnose the presence of prostate cancer.

Approximately 95% of prostate cancer is caused by adenocarcinoma. Androgens and estrogens affect prostate epithelial proliferation, thereby supporting carcinogenesis. However, not all patients who develop prostate cancer have elevated androgen levels. The incidence of prostate cancer differs according to various ethnic groups. African American men are 60% more likely to develop the disease compared with Caucasian men.

Once a patient is diagnosed with prostate cancer and a prostate sample is obtained, the tumor is staged using the TNM classification system (T5 tumor, N5 nodes, M5 metastasis) and the Gleason grading scale, both of which are included in Tables 40.1 and 40.2. It is believed that several predisposing factors for developing prostate cancer include increased age, race, family history, and a high-fat diet. However, the exact mechanism that triggers prostate cancer remains unknown. Patient symptomatology varies significantly and ranges from no symptoms to those that are associated with benign prostatic hypertrophy (BPH), which include urinary hesitancy, frequency, retention, urgency, and incontinence. If these symptoms are present, it is likely the tumor has grown large enough to partially occlude the urethra, and surgical intervention is necessary.

Surgical Procedure

The procedure involves removing the entire prostate gland, the seminal vesicles, the ejaculatory ducts, and a portion of the bladder neck. Sometimes the surrounding lymph nodes are removed and examined for pathologic staging. There are bilateral neurovascular bundles adjacent to the prostatic capsule. This neural tissue allows a man to achieve a penile

TABLE 40.2	Gleason Grading of Prostate Cancer
Grade	Description
Grade 1	Small, uniform glands with minimal nuclear changes
Grade 2	Medium-sized acini, still separated by stroma but more closely arranged
Grade 3	The most common finding in prostate cancer biopsies, showing marked variation in glandular size and organization with infiltration of stromal and neighboring tissues
Grade 4	Markedly atypical cells with extensive infiltration into the surrounding tissues
Grade 5	Sheets of undifferentiated cancer cells

erection. Surgeons may try to preserve sexual function by preserving the nerve bundles. The procedure is called a *nerve-sparing prostatectomy*. In patients with a history of impotence, these nerve bundles are removed (non–nerve-sparing prostatectomy). Once the prostate gland is removed, the bladder neck and urethra are reanastomosed over an indwelling urinary catheter. The catheter helps surgeons visualize and align the two edges of the urethra as they are rejoined. This reestablishes a path for urine flow.

A subset of the laparoscopic approach is the robotic-assisted laparoscopic prostatectomy, in which the da Vinci surgical robot is employed. The robot offers the surgeon more precise motor movements as well as the ability to obtain a magnified view of the surgical field during dissection. These attributes are particularly beneficial for the intracorporeal anastomoses, which is technically challenging. Three to six trochars are placed in the abdominal wall as a pathway for the camera and instruments. Through these ports, the retroperitoneal space is insufflated with CO_2 gas. Steep Trendelenburg (30% to 45%) is required for the laparoscopic approach, as gravity mobilizes the abdominal contents toward the diaphragm, providing a clear view of the surgical field and ample space to safely dissect the prostate gland. Robotic-assisted prostatectomy is associated with decreased bleeding and decreased incidence of postoperative impotence.

Anesthetic Management and Considerations

Preoperative Period

1. *Describe the comorbidities that are likely found in this patient population.*

   Due to the advancing age of this patient population, these men frequently present with at least one or more coexisting disease process such as hypertension, diabetes mellitus, renal dysfunction, myocardial infarction, arrhythmias, and emphysema. Renal impairment is probable in cases that have had chronic urinary obstruction. It is estimated that patients 65 years and older have at least one comorbid factor. The incidence of commonly occurring pathophysiologic disease states associated with patients who have prostate cancer is listed in Table 40.3.

TABLE 40.3	Incidence of Comorbidities in Patients With Prostate Cancer	
Comorbidity		Incidence of Comorbidity
Chronic obstructive pulmonary disease		10%
Coronary artery disease		10%
Hypertension		10%
Diabetes		5%
Renal failure		1%

2. *Determine a comprehensive plan to ensure this patient's health is optimized preoperatively.*
   - **Cardiovascular System:** Due to the physiologic stress induced by anesthesia and laparoscopic surgery, a comprehensive cardiac evaluation is necessary before the surgical procedure. A degree of cardiac pathology must be suspected because this patient is nearly 70 years of age, has a history of essential hypertension, CABG 2 years prior, and diabetes mellitus. A thorough preoperative workup would include a 12-lead ECG, a treadmill cardiac stress test, and clearance from a cardiologist. Hemodynamic control will be an essential aspect of the anesthetic management for this patient.

     The patient should be instructed to continue taking all of his daily medications, except for the aspirin and Viagra, until the day of surgery. Aspirin should be stopped 2 weeks before surgery to decrease prolonged bleeding. A discussion of the medication Viagra will occur later in this chapter.
   - **Respiratory System:** The patient's bronchial asthma is well controlled, and as a result, pulmonary function tests are not required. This patient also smokes cigarettes, which, along with asthma, further increases the possibility of hyperreactive airway and chronic obstructive pulmonary disease (COPD).
   - **Renal System:** Patients with chronic urinary obstruction may develop renal insufficiency. The BUN and creatinine values for this patient are within limits.
   - **Antibiotic Prophylaxis:** The primary infecting microorganism that results in postoperative infection after

radical prostatectomies are coliforms. A broad-spectrum antibiotic such as cefazolin or an aminoglycoside antibiotic such as gentamicin should be administered immediately before the surgical incision.

- **Preoperative Laboratory Assessment:** Hemoglobin and hematocrit values will be obtained to compare these results to those performed intraoperatively after surgical blood loss and hemodilution have occurred. Depending on the preoperative hemoglobin level, a type and screen are obtained.

     The patient is regularly taking hydrochlorothiazide, a diuretic used to treat hypertension. His electrolytes should be checked to make certain the results are within normal limits. Lastly, his blood sugar should be checked before surgery. His blood glucose value is 144 mg/dL. If this result is elevated when compared with his baseline values, the cause is most probably the result of the stress response and no treatment is warranted at this time. Serial glucose values will be assessed intraoperatively.

3. *Discuss the pharmacology of sildenafil (Viagra) and any physiologic concerns regarding its use within the perioperative period.*

     During sexual arousal, there is an influx of blood into the corpus cavernosum due to the relaxation of smooth muscle causing an erection. This response is mediated by the production of nitric oxide (NO). Cyclic-guanosine monophosphate (cGMP) is responsible for smooth muscle relaxation and is produced from guanosine triphosphate (GTP) when NO activates guanylyl cyclase. Phosphodiesterase controls the length of time the cGMP works. Phosphodiesterase 5 (PDE 5) is the phosphodiesterase isoenzyme that terminates the action of cGMP on the corpus cavernosum. Viagra inhibits PDE 5, thereby allowing the accumulation of cGMP, which sustains penile erection. The use of Viagra is contraindicated with concurrent organic nitrates, such as nitroglycerin, because it potentiates the actions of NO. The synergistic effects of this drug combination could cause a precipitous drop in the patient's blood pressure that is minimally responsive to adrenergic agonists. Considering this patient's history of a CABG, the use of nitroglycerin is a sound pharmacologic choice if hypertension ensues. If the patient has taken Viagra in the 24 hours before surgery, the use of nitroglycerin would be contraindicated, and the safest course of action is to postpone surgery.

Intraoperative Period

4. *State the advantages and disadvantages of administering various antihypertensive medications to this patient.*

     Beta-adrenergic antagonists, commonly referred to as beta-blockers, can be cardioselective, only antagonizing beta-1 receptors, or nonselective, antagonizing both beta-1 and beta-2 receptors. Beta-blocking drugs have negative inotropic (contractility), negative chronotropic (rate), and negative dromotropic (speed of cardiac conduction) effects on the myocardium and result in decreased cardiac output (CO), a component of blood pressure. By increasing

oxygen supply and decreasing myocardial oxygen demand, beta-blocking medications are cardioprotective.

It is important to note that beta-2 receptor blockade in the lungs results in bronchiolar smooth muscle constriction, which can result in bronchospasm. This patient is already predisposed to developing bronchospasm due to his smoking history, COPD, and asthma. Therefore beta-blocking medications must be used with extreme caution in patients with these disease states. Because beta-blockers can cause acute congestive heart failure (CHF), the anesthetist should consider the patient's ejection fraction before administration. This patient's ejection fraction is estimated to be 55%, which is nearly a normal value.

Because anesthesia and surgery are both extremely physiologically stimulating, events such as tachycardia and hypertension can occur. Patients receiving beta-blockers preoperatively should not abruptly discontinue taking medications because hypertension, arrhythmias, angina, and myocardial infarction can occur. Beta-blocking medications that can be administered intravenously during the perioperative period include:

- **Propranolol (Inderal)** is a nonselective beta-1 and beta-2 receptor antagonist. Propranolol has a long duration of action and, for this reason, the oral form is frequently prescribed for chronic therapy.
- **Metoprolol (Lopressor)** is a nonselective beta-1 and beta-2 receptor antagonist. However, due to the intrinsic sympathomimetic effects of metoprolol, patients with decreased ejection fraction may benefit.
- **Labetalol (Trandate)** is a nonselective beta-1, beta-2, and alpha-1 receptor antagonist. Alpha-1 receptor antagonism results in vascular dilation, which results in decreased systemic vascular resistance (SVR). The beta-blocking effects associated with labetalol are significantly more potent than the alpha-1 blocking effects, at a ratio of 7 to 1, respectively.
- **Esmolol (Brevibloc)** is a short-acting selective beta-1 antagonist. It is metabolized in the plasma by nonselective red blood cell esterases, and as a result, this drug's elimination half-life is only 10 minutes. The degree of beta-1 selectivity may be compromised, and beta-2 receptor blockade can occur when the medication is administered as an intravenous bolus.

5. *Compare the anesthetic options for open radical prostatectomy and laparoscopic prostatectomy.*

     The prostate is innervated by sympathetic nerve fibers that originate in the T10–T12 and L1–L2 segments of the spinal cord and by parasympathetic nerve fibers originating from S2–S4. The innervation of the prostate and bladder neck makes neuraxial anesthesia an option for open radical prostatectomy. Spinal and epidural anesthesia have been administered with success, and the benefits of regional anesthesia include decreased blood loss, reduced postoperative pain, and a shorter postanesthesia recovery compared with general anesthesia. Disadvantages associated with neuraxial anesthesia include prolonged surgical length, extremes in positioning (i.e., exaggerated lithotomy for the perineal approach), and the possibility of massive blood loss. A combined epidural and general anesthetic is associated with less blood loss and allows for postoperative pain management.

Neuraxial anesthesia is an anesthetic option for laparoscopic prostatectomy. However, the pressure exerted by the pneumoperitoneum on the diaphragm and the need for steep Trendelenburg positioning make breathing difficult. There is also the potential for bowel injury secondary to patient movement. Therefore general anesthesia is considered the gold standard for open and laparoscopic radical prostatectomy.

6. *Describe the potential nerve injuries that are associated with positioning for radical prostatectomy.*

Most anesthetic-related nerve injuries are the result of overstretching and compression of a nerve or from hypoperfusion. During an open prostatectomy, the patient is positioned supine. The table is flexed at the level of the anterosuperior iliac spine, and the patient's legs are placed in a low lithotomy position.

The two most often reported anesthetic-related nerve injuries are ulnar nerve neuropathy and brachial plexus injury, both of which can result from improper positioning of the upper extremities. The upper extremities are tucked to the patient's side. Care must be taken to avoid damaging the hand and/or fingers when lowering the foot of the operating room table. The entire length of each arm must be padded and secured, including the ulnar groove. Pressure points should be reassessed every 15 minutes during the intraoperative period.

Injuries that occur most often to the nerves of the lower extremities during lithotomy positioning are the common peroneal, sciatic, obturator, and femoral. The length of the legs as well as the popliteal space should be padded and supported. Lateral placement of the knees can stretch the obturator nerves. Lifting and lowering the lower extremities simultaneously can avoid lumbar sacral nerve injuries. In the lithotomy position, damage to the common peroneal nerve results from direct pressure on the posterior and inferior surface of the head of the fibula against the leg support. This is an example of a compression injury. Femoral nerve damage can occur from the lithotomy position when the thigh is hyperextended. This is an example of a stretch injury.

Sensory injuries occur more frequently than motor injuries. If the injury results in numbness or tingling, these symptoms usually resolve within 1 week. Any neurologic injury that is sustained should be evaluated by a neurologist. This patient has osteoarthritis, and proper positioning is imperative to help avoid nerve injury. The prolonged length of the procedure and extreme Trendelenburg position may further predispose him to positioning-related injuries.

7. *Explain the physiologic changes that occur with steep Trendelenburg and lithotomy positioning and laparoscopic surgery.*

The physiologic stress that is experienced during laparoscopic prostatectomy is a dynamic process. The individual's compensatory response for the physiologic changes varies. The most significant changes occur to the cardiovascular system and respiratory system.

- **Cardiovascular System:** The cardiovascular system is affected by laparoscopic surgery and specifically the pneumoperitoneum in the following ways:
  - Increased SVR (increased afterload)
  - Increased pulmonary vascular resistance (PVR)
  - Decreased venous return (decrease preload)
  - Increased mean arterial pressure (MAP)
  - Increased CO due to stress response (most typical) and decreased CO with marginal ejection fraction due to increased afterload

  Increasing the patient's circulating volume by administering intravenous fluid helps offset decreases in CO and venous return. Instrumentation of the airway and surgical trauma increase sympathetic nervous system predominance. Increases in afterload cause increased myocardial oxygen consumption, which is of great concern in patients with preexisting cardiac pathology. Additionally, when the legs are placed in the lithotomy position, there is approximately 300 to 400 mL of blood that passively increases central blood volume. Lastly, the Trendelenburg position further exacerbates this situation. These factors support the need for a comprehensive preoperative cardiac evaluation.

  Inhalation agents, narcotics, and adrenergic antagonists directly or indirectly cause a decrease in SVR, PVR, and sympathetic nervous system tone, resulting in decreased myocardial oxygen consumption. Insufflation during creation of the pneumoperitoneum may initiate the celiac reflex caused by stretching of the abdominal cavity. The response causes increased vagal tone, which can manifest as arrhythmias, hypotension, bradycardia, and possibly asystole. Treatment of the celiac reflex that causes hemodynamic instability includes immediate evacuation of the pneumoperitoneum and then administration of an anticholinergic (atropine or glycopyrrolate) if necessary.

- **Respiratory System:** The pneumoperitoneum increases intraabdominal pressure, and the Trendelenburg position allows the abdominal contents to move cephalad and impinge on the diaphragm. The result is both a decrease in functional residual capacity (FRC) and a decrease in thoracolumbar compliance, which support ventilation–perfusion mismatch. Also, insufflation is accomplished using CO_2 gas. Systemic absorption of CO_2 occurs over time and can result in acidosis. Increasing minute ventilation is imperative to maintain normocapnia and provide oxygenation. Because peak airway pressures (PAP) will be elevated, increasing the tidal volume will further increase PAP. This patient has COPD, and dramatically increasing PAP could result in barotrauma. Ventilation using a set pressure compared with a set volume may help decrease PAP. Therefore increasing the respiratory rate while maintaining PAP to achieve normocapnia and adequate arterial oxygenation is recommended.

8. *Identify potential intraoperative complications that can occur during robot-assisted laparoscopic prostatectomy.*

Robotic-assisted laparoscopic prostatectomy is associated with unique complications. A list of potential complications is listed in Box 40.1.

9. *Review the benefits of this patient's choice of laparoscopy over laparotomy.*

It has been demonstrated that the inflammatory response associated with tissue trauma is decreased with laparoscopic surgical procedures. Measurement of two mediators of inflammation, C-reactive protein and interleukin-6, is decreased during laparoscopic surgery compared with a traditional open approach. Robot-assisted laparoscopic radical prostatectomy results in less intraoperative blood loss, less postoperative pain, greater nerve sparing success, and decreased time until ambulation postoperatively. Together, these factors result in shorter length of hospitalization and a higher rate of patient satisfaction.

10. *Evaluate a fluid management plan for patients having a laparoscopic prostatectomy.*

Hypotension can occur after the induction of anesthesia due to the relative intravascular volume depletion due to "nothing by mouth" (NPO) guidelines and the myocardial depression and vasodilation that occur with anesthetic agents. Fluid replacement must account for the following factors:

- Hourly maintenance rate
- NPO deficit
- Insensible or surgical loss

Administration of isotonic crystalloid solutions such as lactated Ringer's or normal saline should be used. Albumin, a colloid solution, can also be used. The anesthetist must continuously assess the amount of blood loss that occurs. Physiologic signs of intraoperative hemorrhage include tachycardia and hypotension.

• BOX 40.1 Potential Complications Associated With Robot-Assisted Laparoscopic Prostatectomy

- Extraperitoneal insufflation resulting in subcutaneous emphysema
- Potential for hypercarbia resulting in acidosis
- CO_2 gas embolism
- Arterial hypoxemia
- Endotracheal tube migration
- Barotrauma resulting in a pneumothorax
- Stimulation of the celiac reflex resulting in hemodynamic instability
- Increased cardiac workload resulting in myocardial ischemia
- Airway and cerebral edema resulting from prolonged steep Trendelenburg positioning
- Acute and massive hemorrhage
- Unintentional surgical trauma to the bowel, bladder, abdominal organs, and vascular structures
- Retinopathy/postoperative visual loss

In response to blood loss, both SVR and stroke volume increase to compensate for decreased intravascular volume. When physiologic signs associated with hemorrhage begin to occur, the degree of hypovolemia is moderate to severe. The estimated blood loss is frequently between 50 and 100 mL after a laparoscopic prostatectomy. The following equation is used to calculate allowable blood loss for this patient.

$$\frac{EBV \times (Hi - Hf)}{Hi} = ABL$$

ABL, Allowable blood loss; *Hi*, initial hematocrit; *Hf*, final lowest acceptable hematocrit; *EBV*, estimated blood volume = weight in kilograms multiplied by the average blood volume (65–70 mL/kg).

The actual blood loss may be difficult to accurately determine because after the bladder neck is severed, urine flows directly into the surgical field, mixing with blood. Serial assessment of the patient's hematocrit is imperative to most objectively quantify the degree of blood loss. There is no single hematocrit value that necessitates the need for blood transfusion. This decision should be based on the patient's preoperative level of functioning, assessment of hemodynamic factors, and the progress of the surgery. Hemoglobin and hematocrit values should be rechecked in the recovery room and during the patient's hospital stay.

11. *Discuss the importance of maintaining normothermia throughout the procedure.*

Even during laparoscopic surgery, a dramatic and rapid decrease in core temperature can occur. The negative effects associated with hypothermia can adversely affect the patient's surgical and anesthetic outcome. Coagulopathy leading to increased surgical bleeding and altered hemostasis; decreased drug metabolism resulting in prolonged emergence from anesthesia; and postoperative shivering, which greatly increases myocardial oxygen demands, can result from hypothermia.

The primary mode of heat loss that patients experience during surgery is by radiation. Core temperature monitoring should be assessed using an esophageal probe. An esophageal stethoscope also allows for continuous assessment of high-quality breath sounds. Maintaining body temperature can be accomplished by using:

- Heated air warming blanket
- Fluid warming system
- Covering the patient's head
- Avoiding the use of high liter fresh gas flow
- Using warmed irrigation in the surgical field

12. *Describe the reason that indigo carmine or methylene blue is administered during laparoscopic prostatectomy.*

As with other laparoscopic surgical procedures, injury to the ureters is a known complication. A tear or inadvertent damage is difficult to identify during laparoscopic visualization, so it is common for the surgeons to ask the anesthetist to administer indigo carmine or methylene blue to determine ureteral integrity. Hepatic metabolism is minimal, and both dyes are primarily excreted by the kidneys within approximately 10 minutes after intravenous administration. If ureteral damage has occurred or ureteral reanastomosis is necessary, the surgeon can detect the blue-colored urine and then repair the defect.

The choice of which dye to use is dependent on the hospital drug formulary and the surgeon's preference. These medications can produce an increased blood pressure; however, the degree of hypertension is frequently mild and the duration is short. It is proposed that the hypertension occurs due to the inhibition of NO, which is a potent vasodilator. Additionally, the oxygen saturation displayed by the pulse oximeter will artificially decrease due to the blue color of the dyes. The physiologic effects associated with methylene blue and indigo carmine are as follows:

Methylene blue
- Hypertension
- Dysrhythmias
- Hyperthermia
- Anaphylaxis
- Methemoglobinemia if large doses are administered

Indigo carmine
- Bradycardia
- Hypertension
- Methemoglobinemia if large doses are administered

Postoperative Period

13. *Create a postoperative plan for this patient.*

If venous congestion of the airway is suspected, it is appropriate to take the patient to the recovery room intubated. Deflating the endotracheal tube cuff and verifying the presence of an air leak can help confirm the presence of swelling. Administration of sedative and analgesic medications is warranted.

The patient's vital signs should be closely monitored throughout the postoperative period, and as previously mentioned, serum hemoglobin and hematocrit values should be obtained. The urine collection system should be monitored for bleeding.

The CO_2 gas used during laparoscopic surgery is converted to carbonic acid. Carbonic acid has been implicated in causing peritoneal irritation. It has been reported that as many as 80% of patients report neck or shoulder pain in the 24-hour postoperative period. The diaphragmatic peritoneal pain is referred to the shoulder via the phrenic nerve. This pain can be difficult to distinguish from cardiac pain and is effectively treated by administering ketorolac.

Review Questions

1. Which medication decreases heart rate, decreases myocardial contractility, and causes a decrease in SVR?
   a. Esmolol
   b. Labetalol
   c. Metoprolol
   d. Atenolol
2. Elevating the patient's legs into the lithotomy position causes:
   a. A decrease in afterload.
   b. A decrease in SVR.
   c. An increase in myocardial oxygen consumption.
   d. An increase in CO_2 production.
3. Which is an advantage of robotic laparoscopic prostatectomy compared with a traditional open abdominal approach?
   a. Increased blood loss
   b. Decreased risk of infection
   c. Decreased inflammatory mediator response
   d. Decreased ability to maintain normothermia

4. Which physiologic phenomena can occur with both indigo carmine and methylene blue?
   a. Anaphylaxis
   b. Hypotension
   c. Bradycardia
   d. Methemoglobinemia
5. Which condition is associated with perioperative hypothermia?
   a. Decreased drug metabolism
   b. Hypercoagulation
   c. Hypotension
   d. Decreased myocardial oxygen consumption

Suggested Readings

Ackerman RS, Cohen JB, Getting REG, Patel SY. Are you seeing this: the impact of steep Trendelenburg position during robot-assisted laparoscopic radical prostatectomy on intraocular pressure: a brief review of the literature. *J Robot Surg* 2019;13(1): 35-40.

Atallah F, Khedis M, Seguin P, et al. Postoperative analgesia and recovery after open and laparoscopic prostatectomy. *Anesth Analg* 2004;99:1878-1879.

Cao L, Yang Z, Qi L, Chen M. Robot-assisted and laparoscopic vs open radical prostatectomy in clinically localized prostate cancer: perioperative, functional, and oncological outcomes: a systematic review and meta-analysis. *Medicine (Baltimore)* 2019;98(22):e15770.

Chen K, Wang L, Wang Q, et al. Effects of pneumoperitoneum and steep Trendelenburg position on cerebral hemodynamics during robotic-assisted laparoscopic radical prostatectomy: a randomized controlled study. *Medicine (Baltimore)* 2019;98(21):e15794.

Doe A, Kumagai M, Tamura Y, Sakai A, Suzuki K. A comparative analysis of the effects of sevoflurane and propofol on cerebral oxygenation during steep Trendelenburg position and pneumoperitoneum for robotic-assisted laparoscopic prostatectomy. *J Anesth* 2016;30(6):949-955.

Du Y, Long Q, Guan B, et al. Robot-assisted radical prostatectomy is more beneficial for prostate cancer patients: a system review and meta-analysis. *Med Sci Monit* 2018;24:272-287.

Gerges FJ, Kanazi GE, Jabbour-Khoury SI. Anesthesia for laparoscopy: a review. *J Clin Anesth* 2006;18(1):67-78.

Holden M, Parsons JK. Robotic-assisted simple prostatectomy: an overview. *Urol Clin North Am* 2016;43(3):385-391.

Malhorta V. Anesthesia considerations radical prostatectomy. rev esp anestesiol 2006;29(1):S89–S91.

Moncada I, López I, Ascencios J, Krishnappa P, Subirá D. Complications of robot assisted radical prostatectomy. *Arch Esp Urol* 2019; 72(3):266-276.

Morriber NA. Anesthesia for robotic surgery. In: Nagelhout JJ, Elisha S, eds. *Nurse Anesthesia*, 6th ed. St Louis, MO: Elsevier, 2018: 752-759.

41

Transurethral Resection of the Prostate

KEY POINTS

- It is estimated that the majority of patients who present for transurethral resection of the prostate (TURP) have one or more preexisting medical conditions.
- Systemic absorption of irrigation fluid used during TURP can result in fluid volume overload, dilutional hyponatremia, and metabolic acidosis.
- Factors that most significantly influence the volume of irrigating fluid absorbed during TURP include the hydrostatic

pressure of the irrigating solution, the number and size of open venous sinuses during resection, the peripheral venous pressure, and the duration of resection.
- Depending on the severity of dilutional hyponatremia, severe neurologic and cardiac compromise can occur rapidly.
- Perioperative complications that are associated with TURP include TURP syndrome, hemorrhage, hypothermia, sepsis, bladder perforation, and myocardial dysfunction.

Case Synopsis

A 75-year-old man has developed urinary obstruction caused by benign prostatic hypertrophy (BPH). He is scheduled by his urologist to have a TURP procedure.

Preoperative Evaluation and Demographic Data

Past Medical/Surgical History

- Non–insulin-dependent diabetes, hypertension

List of Medications

- Hydrochlorothiazide, terazosin hydrochloride (Hytrin), finasteride (Propecia)

Diagnostic Data

- Hemoglobin, 13.2 g/dL; hematocrit, 39.4%; glucose, 139 mg/dL; blood urea nitrogen, 15 mg/dL; creatinine, 1.1 mg/dL
- Electrolytes: sodium, 139 mEq/L; potassium, 3.9 mEq/L; chloride, 104 mEq/L; carbon dioxide, 24 mEq/L

Height/Weight/Vital Signs

- 180 cm, 78 kg
- Blood pressure, 152/84; heart rate, 61 beats per minute; respiratory rate, 16 breaths per minute; room air oxygen saturation, 98%; temperature, 36.8°C
- Electrocardiogram (ECG): normal sinus rhythm; heart rate, 66; left ventricular hypertrophy; ejection fraction, 50%

Pathophysiology

BPH is a nonmalignant and progressive condition that will occur in approximately 90% of men during their lifetimes. TURP is the second most common surgical procedure performed in men older than 65 years of age.

Urethral obstruction is caused by both a static and a dynamic component. Due to testicular hormones, the median and lateral lobes of the prostate become enlarged and cause a mechanical (static) obstruction that narrows the urethral lumen resulting in urinary retention (Fig. 41.1). The dynamic aspect of urinary obstruction is the result of smooth muscle tension of the prostate and bladder neck that further inhibits urine flow. Depending on the degree of obstruction, the inability to urinate can cause mild to severe discomfort and hydronephrosis.

A complex venous network surrounds the prostatic capsule. This anatomic feature is significant because veins within this complex will be ligated during surgical resection. This will allow irrigating solution to enter systemic circulation. Depending on the amount and rapidity of bleeding and the amount and rapidity of absorption of irrigating fluid, the patient can develop severe anemia, dilutional hyponatremia and hypervolemia, and metabolic acidosis (see Fig. 41.1).

Surgical Procedure

Removal of the hypertrophic prostatic tissue is accomplished via a resectoscope that is placed in the urethra. Irrigating solution is continuously infused during the procedure while the surgeon applies either a cutting current to

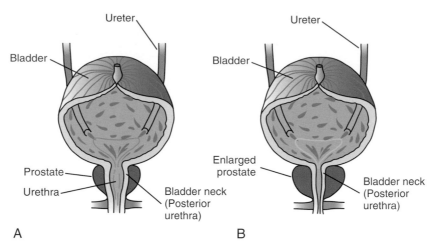

• **Fig. 41.1** (A) Normal prostate gland. (B) Enlarged prostate gland showing the narrowing of the urethra, decreasing urine flow. (From Workman ML, LaCharity L: *Understanding pharmacology*, ed 2, St. Louis, 2016, Elsevier.)

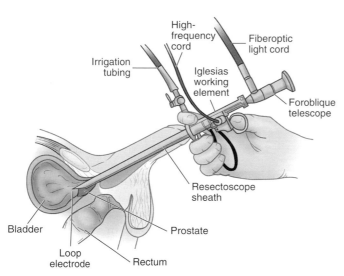

• **Fig. 41.2** Components of a resectoscope that is used to perform TURP. (From Rothrock JC: *Alexander's care of the patient in surgery*, ed 16, St. Louis, 2019, Elsevier.)

resect small pieces of the prostate or a coagulating current to control bleeding. Intraoperative blood loss can be decreased if the surgical technique includes frequent application of a coagulating current. This process is accomplished by using an energized wire loop that is inserted through the resectoscope, as depicted in Fig. 41.2.

Anesthetic Management and Considerations

Preoperative Period

1. *Discuss the type and frequency of various coexisting diseases that are associated with patients presenting for TURP.*

   The speed at which BPH develops is dependent on the individual and is progressive. The average age of male patients with BPH that causes significant urinary obstruction is approximately 70 years. Therefore patients

• **BOX 41.1** Medical History and Frequency of Disease Associated With Patients Having TURP

- Hypertension, 33%
- Ischemic heart disease, 18%
- Myocardial infarction, 12%
- Arrhythmia, 12%
- Chronic obstructive pulmonary disease, 12%
- Diabetes, 11%
- Renal insufficiency, 10%

presenting for TURP often have significant systemic coexisting disease. The type and frequency of pathophysiology associated with patients presenting for TURP are listed in Box 41.1. It is estimated that the majority of these patients have one or more preexisting medical conditions.

2. *Describe the potential link between cardiovascular dysfunction and BPH.*

   In addition to testicular hormones, BPH is thought to be enhanced by metabolic syndrome. The components of metabolic syndrome include hypertension, diabetes, obesity, insulin resistance, and dyslipidemia. These factors are thought to be a predisposition for developing prostate cancer. Men with evidence of increased inflammatory mediator values such as C-reactive protein are also more likely to develop BPH. Another proposed mechanism for BPH is impaired blood flow caused by vascular insufficiency. There is evidence to support an association between hypertension and BPH, which may be caused by sympathetic nervous system hyperactivity. Of those that develop symptoms of urinary obstruction, a higher mean arterial pressure is associated with increased prostate size. Additionally, it is believed that intraprostatic inflammation plays a significant role in the development and progression of BPH.

3. *Examine the autonomic and sensory innervation to the prostate gland.*

Autonomic nervous system responses are initiated via adrenergic, cholinergic, neuromodulator (adenosine), and nonadrenergic noncholinergic (nitric oxide) mechanisms. Sympathetic innervation arises from the superior hypogastric plexus and extends from T10–L2. The autonomic nervous system modulates the growth and secretory function to the prostate gland. These effects are the result of alpha-1 adrenergic stimulation. Beta-2 adrenergic stimulation aids in maintaining normal cellular integrity.

The inferior hypogastric plexus (pelvic nerves) are formed from the division of the splanchnic, hypogastric, pudendal, and sacral nerves. Parasympathetic innervation originates from S2–S4 via muscarinic receptors. It has been postulated that alpha-1 adrenergic overstimulation can lead to prostatic hyperplasia. A combination of other chemical substances such as nitric oxide, adenosine, and vasoactive intestinal polypeptides may influence smooth muscle tone and blood flow.

The exact spinal cord location of the sensory ganglia from the prostate gland is unknown. Sensory information is relayed at two different spinal cord segments. It appears that the majority of sensory innervation originates from the T12–L2 and L5–L6 levels. An illustration that diagrams the autonomic nervous system innervation to the genitourinary system is included in Fig. 41.3.

4. *Explain the mechanism of action and physiologic effects of medications used to treat BPH.*

Terazosin hydrochloride, an alpha-adrenergic antagonist, is predominantly alpha-1 receptor specific and produces minimal alpha-2 blockade. The physiologic effect of this medication on the prostate gland is a decrease in smooth muscle contraction within the prostatic capsule and the bladder neck, thereby decreasing the symptoms associated with urinary obstruction. However, terazosin hydrochloride does not decrease or slow the progression of BPH. Terazosin

hydrochloride is also used as an antihypertensive medication resulting in decreased arterial tone.

A metabolic by-product of testosterone, dihydrotestosterone (DHT) is synthesized by 5-alpha reductase (5AR). DHT binds to androgen receptors on the prostate gland and accelerates cellular proliferation. Finasteride is a 5AR inhibitor (5ARI) that decreases the formation of DHT. Finasteride and other 5ARIs help decrease symptoms of urinary obstruction and decrease prostatic hyperplasia.

5. *Describe the importance of administering antibiotic prophylaxis for TURP.*

The incidence of bacteriuria and urinary tract infections (UTIs) after TURP surgery is approximately 6%. Most of these cases resolve spontaneously after the urethral catheter is removed. For this reason, prescribing antibiotics to all patients having TURP is a controversial practice. However, it is estimated that the incidence of septicemia ranges from 1% to 4%. The mortality rate for patients older than 65 years of age who develop septicemia is 20%.

The cause of UTI after TURP is multifactorial. Sources of infections include inflamed tissue within the prostatic capsule, urethral flora, contamination during surgery, and urethral catheter colonization. The most effective antibiotic regimen has not been determined. Cephalosporins are most commonly administered preoperatively. The use of preoperative antibiotics has been shown to decrease postoperative bacteriuria by nearly twofold. The signs and symptoms of septicemia are discussed later in this chapter.

Intraoperative Period

6. *Describe the anatomic and physiologic changes associated with the lithotomy position.*

Patients are most often placed in low lithotomy for TURP. The lithotomy position is associated with a

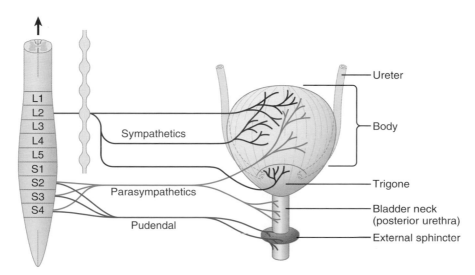

• **Fig. 41.3** Autonomic nervous system innervation to the genitourinary system. (From Hall JE, Hall ME: *Guyton and Hall textbook of medical physiology*, ed 14, St. Louis, 2021, Elsevier.)

decrease in functional residual capacity, and patients who have a history of chronic obstructive pulmonary disease may have difficulty breathing. When the legs are raised, the central venous blood volume is increased by approximately 500 mL. As a result, myocardial workload is increased. Venous stasis and peripheral ischemia occur most often in patients with preexisting vascular insufficiency.

Ligaments in the lower legs and lumbar region are stretched. The lumbar curve is decreased, which can cause the level of spinal anesthesia to spread cephalad potentially resulting in a high spinal. This is most likely to occur within minutes after the spinal anesthetic has been administered. It is imperative to pad areas of the lower leg to avoid injury. The nerves at risk for injury include the common peroneal (lateral knee) and saphenous (inner knee). The obturator, femoral, and lateral femoral cutaneous nerves can be injured if hyperflexion of the thighs occurs.

7. *Examine the differences between various irrigating solutions used during TURP.*

Continuous irrigation through the resectoscope is necessary during TURP in order to dilate the prostatic urethra, provide visibility for the surgeon, and dilute and wash away blood and resected prostatic tissue. The advantages and disadvantages related to various irrigating solutions used for TURP are summarized in Table 41.1.

Normal physiologic osmolarity is approximately 280 mOsm/L. Absorption of irrigating solution that is significantly hyperosmolar or hypo-osmolar can have severe physiologic effects. The definition of osmosis is the movement of water from a higher concentration (low solute concentration) to a lower concentration (high solute concentration) across a semipermeable membrane. Therefore creating extracellular fluid hypotonicity in relation to the intracellular fluid will cause cellular swelling and lysis. If the extracellular fluid is hypertonic in relation to the intracellular fluid, cells crenate (shrink).

- **Glycine 1.5%:** Glycine is the most common irrigating solution used in North America. It is an essential amino acid and inhibitory neurotransmitter that is naturally present in the body. The metabolic by-product of glycine is ammonia, a potent cerebral and myocardial depressant that can cause a decreased level of consciousness and decreased cardiac output.

Glycine is cardiotoxic and has been associated with cardiac hypokinesis and elevated troponin I levels. Ammonia decreases the production and release of norepinephrine from postsynaptic nerve terminals resulting in hypotension. Hyperglycinemia can cause transient visual disturbances ranging from blurred vision to blindness and may last from 24 to 48 hours. It is theorized that the inhibitory effects of glycine interrupt retinal synaptic transmission. Vision improves as glycine is metabolized and excreted.

- **Cytal (2.7% sorbitol/0.54% mannitol):** Mannitol, a sugar alcohol compound, is not metabolized and is rapidly excreted by the kidneys. However, sorbitol is metabolized to fructose, which can result in hyperglycemia. It is theorized that during glycolysis, fructose metabolism occurs preferentially over glucose metabolism. Therefore pyruvate and lactate are liberated, resulting in lactic acidosis.

- **Distilled water:** This solution is rarely used in the United States because of the hypo-osmolarity and the concern over causing cell lysis.

- **Normal saline/lactated Ringer's:** These solutions would seemingly be ideal for TURP due to their relative iso-osmolarity and lack of metabolic by-products. However, due to the electrolytes in these solutions (cations), current dispersion occurs, making it difficult for the urologist to accurately focus on the electrical current.

8. *Cite factors that affect the volume of irrigating fluid absorbed systemically during TURP.*

The four factors that have the most significant influence on the volume of irrigating fluid absorbed during TURP include:

- The hydrostatic pressure of the irrigating solution. The pressure is determined by the height of the irrigating solution container. The ideal height of the irrigation bag to maintain adequate surgical visibility is 60 cm.
- The number and size of open venous sinuses during resection. A larger prostate gland has a greater surface area, and during resection, a greater number of venous sinuses are exposed to irrigant. Also, intermittent coagulation of the bleeding vessels will decrease absorption.
- The peripheral venous pressure. Absorption is greatest when the venous pressure is lowest.

TABLE 41.1	Characteristics of Irrigating Solutions Used for TURP			
Solution	**Osmolarity (mOsm/L)**	**Advantages**		**Disadvantages**
Glycine 1.5%	200	• Decreased TURP syndrome		• Hyperglycinemia • Hyperammonemia
Cytal: 2.7% sorbitol 0.54% mannitol	167	• Decreased TURP syndrome		• Hyperglycemia • Lactic acidosis
Distilled water	0	• Superior visibility		• Hemolysis • Hyponatremia
Normal saline 0.9%	308	• Minimal effects with absorption		• Current dispersion
Lactated Ringer's	274	• Minimal effects with absorption		• Current dispersion

- The duration of resection. Approximately 10 to 50 mL of irrigant can be absorbed into systemic circulation per minute of resection. Ideally, TURP procedures should last no longer than 60 minutes.

9. *Explain the physiologic alterations associated with the absorption of irrigating fluid.*

Absorption of irrigating fluid increases vascular volume and dilutes plasma proteins, which cause a decrease in protein oncotic pressure. This effect results in the movement of fluid from the intravascular to the interstitial compartment. For each 100 mL of fluid diffusing into the interstitial space, 10 to 15 mEq of sodium is lost to the intravascular space, resulting in dilutional hyponatremia. Hypocalcemia can also occur. Serum potassium values can increase by 15% to 25% due to intravascular hemolysis. These cellular changes can result in severe metabolic acidosis known as TURP acidosis. Additionally, hypervolemia can ensue, causing cerebral edema, myocardial ischemia, and congestive heart failure. The cardiac effects are dependent on the amount of fluid absorbed, the rate of fluid absorption, the size of the patient, and the patient's cardiac reserve. Factors that increase the likelihood of TURP syndrome include resection time greater than 60 minutes, prostatic weight greater than 30 g, inexperienced surgeon, and total irrigation volume of greater than 30 L.

10. *Correlate the signs and symptoms associated with TURP syndrome with various serum sodium values.*

It is vital to realize that a specific serum sodium value may result in loss of consciousness and cardiovascular collapse in one patient, whereas another patient that has the identical serum sodium will not exhibit signs and symptoms of TURP syndrome. The best method of avoiding the consequences of TURP syndrome is preventing the situation from occurring. The neurologic and cardiac manifestations associated with acute hyponatremia are listed in Tables 41.2 and 41.3.

11. *Construct a plan of treatment for a patient who develops TURP syndrome.*

The signs and symptoms associated with TURP syndrome vary dramatically and will determine the plan of treatment. Interventions used to treat TURP syndrome are listed in Box 41.2.

12. *Explain the advantages and disadvantages of neural blockade for TURP.*

The individual patient's preoperative profile is most important when determining an anesthetic technique for any surgical procedure. The ideal level of sensory blockade resulting from neural blockade is the T10 dermatome. The advantages and disadvantages of neuraxial blockade are listed in Box 41.3.

13. *Compare and contrast signs and symptoms of an extraperitoneal bladder perforation and an intraperitoneal bladder perforation.*

Bladder perforation can occur as a result of increased pressure from the irrigating solution or from the cutting current of the energized wire loop. Urologists should be aware that the amount of fluid output should be similar to the amount of fluid introduced into the bladder. Bladder perforation can occur in two different regions within the bladder: either intraperitoneal or extraperitoneal. The signs and symptoms associated with bladder perforation are listed in Box 41.4.

The only sign that may be indicative of an intraperitoneal bladder perforation during general anesthesia is bradycardia caused by the leakage of irrigation into the

TABLE 41.3 Neurologic Manifestations Associated With Acute Hyponatremia

Serum Sodium (mEq/L)	
120	Mild signs/symptoms • Dizziness • Headache • Nausea
115	Moderate signs/symptoms • Restlessness • Confusion
110	Severe signs/symptoms • Loss of consciousness • Seizures • Respiratory arrest

TABLE 41.2 Cardiac Manifestations Associated With Acute Hyponatremia

Serum Sodium (mEq/L)	
120	• Hypotension • Decreased myocardial contractility • Initial widening of QRS complex
115	• Bradycardia • Widening QRS complex • Possible ventricular ectopy
110	• Ventricular tachycardia • Ventricular fibrillation • Cardiac arrest

• BOX 41.2 Treatment Plan for TURP Syndrome

- Stop surgery
- ACLS/BLS protocol as needed
- Check electrolytes, specifically serum sodium values, every 20 minutes
- Administer diuretics (furosemide)
- Treat seizure activity (benzodiazepine, propofol, airway management)
- Hypertonic saline (3% or 5%), not to exceed 100 mL/hr infusion rate
- Invasive hemodynamic monitoring

ACLS, Advanced cardiac life support; *BLS,* basic life support.

• BOX 41.3 Advantages and Disadvantages of Neuraxial Blockade for TURP

Advantages

- The major advantage is the ability to assess the patient's level of consciousness as an early monitor to detect TURP syndrome. This is the reason that neural blockade is considered the technique of choice by many practitioners.
- The ability to assess chest pain and/or shortness of breath caused by myocardial ischemia and/or volume overload.
- The ability to assess abdominal pain caused by a bladder perforation.
- Decreased vascular resistance will lessen the possibility of hypervolemia.
- It is controversial if neuraxial blockade decreases blood loss during TURP.

Disadvantages

- Moderate to severe hypotension can occur as a result of peripheral vascular dilation. This effect will be potentiated in patients taking alpha-adrenergic antagonists for BPH.
- Due to arthritic changes associated with aging, placement can be difficult.
- Decreasing venous resistance can increase the amount of irrigation absorption that occurs through open venous sinuses.
- Dysphoria that can result in patient movement when benzodiazepine, narcotics, and other central nervous system depressants are administered.

• BOX 41.4 Comparison of Signs and Symptoms Associated With Extraperitoneal and Intraperitoneal Bladder Perforation

Extraperitoneal Perforation
- Discomfort
  1. Periumbilical
  2. Inguinal
  3. Suprapubic
- Periumbilical/inguinal tissue distention

Intraperitoneal Perforation
- Discomfort
  1. Chest
  2. Upper abdomen
  3. Shoulder tip (diaphragmatic irritation)
- Nausea and vomiting
- Abdominal rigidity
- Shortness of breath
- Diaphoresis
- Hiccups

---

peritoneal cavity, which initiates the celiac reflex. Most small extraperitoneal bladder perforations resolve spontaneously, but urethral catheter placement is used to minimize bladder pressure. The majority of large extraperitoneal perforations or intraperitoneal perforations are treated by direct surgical closure.

14. *Discuss factors that affect the estimated blood loss during TURP.*

    The average estimated blood loss during TURP is 300 to 400 mL. The total blood loss is highly variable but is most closely related to the size of the prostate and duration of resection. Blood loss is increased with prostate size

---

• BOX 41.5 Postoperative Complications Associated With TURP

- TURP syndrome
- Hemorrhage
- Hypothermia
- Sepsis
- Bladder perforation
- Postoperative hemorrhage
- Subclinical disseminated intravascular coagulation
- Myocardial infarction
- Transient myocardial ischemia

---

greater than 45 g and resection time greater than 90 minutes. The average blood loss is estimated to be 10 to 15 mL/g of resected prostate. Having blood available to transfuse is dependent on the size of the prostate and the patient's current hemoglobin value and physiologic condition. Dilution of the blood by the irrigation makes estimating blood loss difficult. The following equation can be used to calculate the estimated blood loss. Tranexamic acid 1 g intravenously (IV) before the start of surgery decreases blood loss during TURP.

$$\text{Blood loss} = (\text{Hct \% of irrigant} \times \text{Total volume of irrigant}) / \text{Preoperative Hct \%}$$

A postoperative subclinical disseminated intravascular coagulation (DIC) syndrome occurs in less than 1% of patients. The exact mechanism is unknown; however, the cause may be related to resected prostate tissue that enters central circulation during resection. Treatment for DIC includes administering fibrinogen, platelets, and cryoprecipitate.

Postoperative Period

The total resection time for this surgery was 105 minutes. In the postanesthesia care unit, the patient exhibits the following acute symptoms: restlessness, confusion, shivering, blood pressure of 80/46, respiratory rate of 32, sinus tachycardia with intermittent unifocal premature ventricular contractions (PVCs) rate of 102, room air oxygen saturation of 93%, and temperature of 35.4°C.

15. *List potential postoperative complications that can occur after TURP.*

    If the bladder irrigation is not warmed, average temperature loss after TURP is 1° to 1.5°C. Hypothermia can inhibit coagulation and increase myocardial oxygen demand. Other postoperative complications associated with TURP are listed in Box 41.5.

16. *Discuss potential causes and diagnostic criteria that could cause this clinical scenario.*

    Potential postoperative complications that can occur after TURP surgery include:

    - Bladder perforation: Discomfort in the abdominal and/or the inguinal region, no urine output from the urethral catheter. A urology consultation is necessary.

- Hyponatremia: Obtain a serum sodium value, treat hyponatremia as discussed previously.
- Hypervolemia: Listen to bilateral lung fields, obtain chest x-ray, consider diuretics.
- Hemorrhage: Obtain hemoglobin/hematocrit value. Administer blood if necessary.
- Hypothermia: Confirm temperature value of 35.4°C, forced-air warming, consider meperidine to decrease shivering when oxygen saturation improves.

- Myocardial ischemia/infarction: Obtain chest x-ray, obtain 12-lead ECG, administer volume if no signs of congestive heart failure, administer phenylephrine, check calcium levels as a potential cause of hypotension, consult a cardiologist.

Treatment for this patient would include providing high-flow oxygen, warming measures, and diagnosing the specific cause(s) of this scenario before definitive treatment.

Review Questions

1. An advantage of neuraxial blockade for monitoring patients having TURP surgery includes:
   a. Assessing neurologic function.
   b. Determining the speed of irrigation absorption.
   c. Distinguishing signs and symptoms of bladder perforation.
   d. Estimating blood loss.
2. Which intervention is indicated for treatment of TURP syndrome?
   a. Administering 3% sodium chloride at a rate of 200 mL/hr
   b. Administering etomidate to decrease the seizure threshold
   c. Administering furosemide
   d. Assessing hemoglobin value every 20 minutes
3. Abdominal rigidity, shoulder tip pain, and shortness of breath are associated with:
   a. Common peroneal nerve compression.
   b. Extraperitoneal bladder perforation.
   c. Intraperitoneal bladder perforation.
   d. Myocardial ischemia.

4. A serum sodium value of _____ mEq/L is associated with confusion, widening QRS complex, and bradycardia.
   a. 110
   b. 115
   c. 120
   d. 125
5. Which irrigation fluid is associated with direct myocardial depression?
   a. Cytal
   b. Glycine
   c. Isotonic crystalloids
   d. Distilled water

Suggested Readings

Berger AP, Bartsch G, Deibl M, et al. Atherosclerosis as a risk factor for benign prostatic hyperplasia. *BJU Int* 2006;98(5):1038-1042.

Hahn RG. Fluid absorption in endoscopic surgery. *Br J Anaesth* 2006;96:8-20.

Kumar V, Vineet K, Deb A. TUR syndrome - a report. *Urol Case Rep* 2019;26:100982.

Marchioni M, Cindolo L, Di Nicola M, et al. Major acute cardiovascular events after transurethral prostate surgery: a population-based analysis. *Urology* 2019;131:196-203.

McGowan-Smyth S, Vasdev N, Gowrie-Mohan S. Spinal anesthesia facilitates the early recognition of TUR syndrome. *Curr Urol* 2016; 9(2):57-61.

Meng QQ, Pan N, Xiong JY, Liu N. Tranexamic acid is beneficial for reducing perioperative blood loss in transurethral resection of the prostate. *Exp Ther Med* 2019;17(1):943-947.

Mishra VC, Allen DJ, Nicolau C, et al. Does intraprostatic inflammation have a role in the pathogenesis and progression of benign prostatic hyperplasia? *BJU Int* 2007;100:327-331.

Morse CY. Renal anatomy, physiology, pathophysiology and anesthesia management. In: Nagelhout JJ, Elisha S, eds. *Nurse Anesthesia*, 6th ed. St Louis, MO: Elsevier, 2018:682-708.

Qiang W, Jianchen WU, MacDonald R, et al. Antibiotic prophylaxis for transurethral prostatic resection in men with preoperative urine containing less than 100,000 bacteria per ml: a systematic review. *J Urol* 2005;173(4):1175-1181.

Riedinger CB, Fantus RJ, Matulewicz RS, et al. The impact of surgical duration on complications after transurethral resection of the prostate: an analysis of NSQIP data. *Prostate Cancer Prostatic Dis* 2019;22(2):303-308.

Sun F, Sun X, Shi Q, Zhai Y. Transurethral procedures in the treatment of benign prostatic hyperplasia: a systematic review and meta-analysis of effectiveness and complications. *Medicine (Baltimore)* 2018;97(51):e13360.

Zhang R, Chen X, Xiao Y. The effects of a forced-air warming system plus electric blanket for elderly patients undergoing transurethral resection of the prostate: a randomized controlled trial. *Medicine (Baltimore)* 2018;97(45):e13119.

Extracorporeal Shock Wave Lithotripsy

KEY POINTS

- Careful monitoring of the electrocardiogram (ECG) for dysrhythmias, such as ventricular tachycardia, is necessary due to the timing of extracorporeal shock waves.
- The shock waves, which are aimed toward the patient's flank region, are painful.
- The location for anesthesia is often outside of the operating room, which may involve poor lighting, small spaces, high noise level, and a safety risk (e.g., radiation exposure).
- Extracorporeal shock wave lithotripsy (ESWL) is noninvasive but may cause bacteremia in susceptible patients.

Case Synopsis

A 57-year-old man complains of right flank pain and hematuria for 4 days. An x-ray shows evidence of a renal calculus located in the right upper calyx. He is scheduled to have ESWL to the right kidney by his urologist.

Preoperative Evaluation and Demographic Data

Past Medical/Surgical History

- Hypercholesterolemia
- Hypertension
- Insulin-dependent diabetes mellitus
- Three-vessel coronary artery bypass graft (CABG) 5 years ago; no anesthetic complications

List of Medications

- Zocor (simvastatin)
- Lopressor (metoprolol)
- Aspirin
- NPH and Lantus insulin

Diagnostic Data

- White blood cell count, 4.7×10^9/L
- Hemoglobin, 13.7 g/dL; hematocrit, 41%
- Platelets, 215 mm^3
- Sodium, 136 mEq/L; potassium, 4.8 mEq/L; chloride, 102 mmol/L
- Blood urea nitrogen (BUN), 21 mg/dL; creatinine, 1.5 mg/dL
- Glucose, 133 mg/dL
- Partial thromboplastin time, 30 s; prothrombin time, 12.3 s; international normalized ratio, 1.1 s
- Kidneys, ureters, bladder (KUB) x-ray: right renal calculi

Height/Weight/Vital Signs

- 183 cm, 104 kg; body mass index, 31 kg/m^2
- Blood pressure, 136/65; heart rate, 71 beats per minute; respiratory rate, 18 breaths per minute; room air oxygen saturation, 97%; temperature, 36.9°C
- 12-lead ECG: Normal sinus rhythm (NSR) with first-degree atrioventricular (AV) block and left axis deviation

Pathophysiology

Renal calculi are hardened crystalline masses often referred to as "kidney stones." They can exist within the kidney, as shown in Fig. 42.1, or the ureter and cause hydronephrosis. Nephrolithiasis, a condition where calculi are present in the kidneys or urinary tract, is more common in men than in women (3:1 ratio) and less common in Asian and African Americans. It is estimated that between 10% and 15% of adults in the United States will develop kidney stones. People who live in the southeastern region of the country have the highest incidence of nephrolithiasis. The potential causes for the development of kidney stones include diet and mineral content and fluoride concentration in drinking water. Frequent episodes of nephrolithiasis may occur in association with a host of metabolic disorders such as renal tubular acidosis, Dent disease, hyperparathyroidism, and medullary sponge kidney. The rate of calcium excretion as well as pH of the urine plays a factor in the composition of the calculus formation. These stones are formed of calcium oxalate (80%), uric acid, calcium phosphate, cystine, and struvite. Compositional analysis of stones can be used as an integral component in the prevention of future stone formation. The signs and symptoms associated with nephrolithiasis are listed in Box 42.1.

Diagnosis of kidney stones is accomplished by assessing signs and symptoms that are commonly associated with

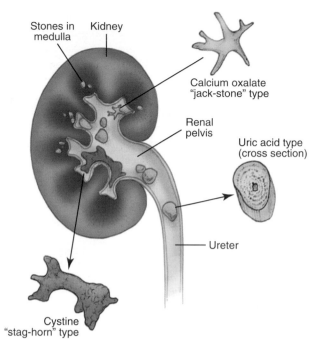

• **Fig. 42.1** Kidney stones present in the renal calyces. (From Nix S: *Williams' basic nutrition and diet therapy*, ed 15, St. Louis, 2017, Elsevier.)

• BOX 42.1 **Signs and Symptoms Associated With Kidney Stones**

- Severe flank/back/groin pain
- Dysuria
- Hematuria
- Pyuria
- Nausea and vomiting
- Hydronephrosis
- Urinary frequency
- Fever and chills

nephrolithiasis; KUB abdominal x-ray; intravenous pyelogram; computed tomography (CT) scan; blood tests (increased white blood cells, hypercalcemia, elevated BUN/creatinine); urinalysis for the presence of red blood cells; bacteria; protein; casts; crystalline formations; and urine culture. Most kidney stones that are less than 4 mm in diameter will spontaneously pass out of the kidney through the ureter and into the bladder. However, if the diameter of the stone is greater than 6 mm in diameter, the need for surgical intervention may be necessary.

Surgical Procedure

Lithotripsy is a therapeutic medical procedure used to disintegrate stones in the urinary tract and renal pelvis. ESWL is a noninvasive technique using a focused, high-intensity acoustic pulse emitted from a water-filled device (shock wave generator), which is in contact with the patient's skin at the level of the kidney (approximately L2 vertebrae), as shown in Fig. 42.2. With older ESWL devices, it was necessary to submerge the patient's entire body in a warm water bath while the procedure occurred. Due to advances in the technologic construction of ESWL units, this process is no longer necessary. If the treatment is to occur outside of the anesthetizing area such as in a mobile trailer, all the necessary anesthesia and emergency equipment must be present. Because the shock waves have the same acoustic density as water, the energy passes through tissue planes and shears the stone instead of damaging tissue. Thousands of pulsatile shock waves of energy are focused on the calculi. The kidney stone is visualized by fluoroscopy or ultrasound. The fragments of stone are then able to pass into the bladder and be eliminated from the body. Care must be used when positioning and securing the patient to the ESWL table. As the table and lithotripter move in response to the stone's position, padding of extremities and frequent visual inspection

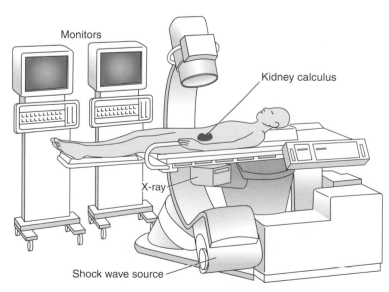

• **Fig. 42.2** Equipment used for ESWL. (From Koesterman JL: *Buck's 2020 step-by-step medical coding*, St. Louis, 2020, Elsevier.)

- Dysrhythmias
- Nausea and vomiting
- Pleural injury
- Renal parenchymal or subcapsular hemorrhage
- Impaired skin integrity
- Hypertension

are warranted to prevent nerve injury. The shock wave generator produces noise, and the patient's ears are covered to avoid acoustic trauma. A temporary ureteral stent is frequently placed at the end of this procedure to maintain urinary flow and ureteral patency. The overall complication rate associated with ESWL is approximately 5% to 15%. The side effects caused by the treatment can be mild or severe, and a list of the potential complications is listed in Box 42.2.

Anesthetic Management and Considerations

Preoperative Period

1. *Discuss the anesthetic options available for ESWL.*

    A number of anesthetic techniques are available for an ESWL procedure. General anesthesia can be utilized as well as intravenous sedation under monitored anesthesia care using a propofol or remifentanil infusion, subcutaneous infiltration of local anesthesia, or application of topical anesthesia such as eutectic mixture of local anesthesia (EMLA) cream and unilateral transversus abdominis plane block.

    If neuraxial anesthesia is chosen (spinal or epidural), a T6 dermatome sensory blockade is desirable because renal innervation by sympathetic fibers is located between T10 and L1. A spinal block can be performed by using local anesthesia and/or sufentanil.

2. *Identify the anesthetic concerns related to this patient's medical history and ESWL.*

    - **Hypertension, hyperlipidemia, and CABG:** Although ESWL is a noninvasive surgical procedure, the patient can experience a significant amount of pain, which has been described by patients as being snapped by a rubber band in the flank region. The number of shock wave pulses that are needed to obliterate the stone varies depending on its composition. However, a typical ESWL treatment results in hundreds of pulses.

    A painful experience activates the sympathetic nervous system, and the cardiovascular response includes tachycardia, increased myocardial contractility, increased rate of cardiac conduction, and vasoconstriction. Because this patient has risk factors that are associated with cardiac dysfunction, increased myocardial oxygen demand without the ability to increase supply can result in ischemia and infarction. His

medication regimen also includes metoprolol (Lopressor), which he should continue taking throughout the perioperative phase.

- **Obesity:** This patient is considered obese as per body mass index. Obesity will increase the difficulty of positioning the patient's kidney area directly over the shock wave generator. Also, due to the association between obesity and the presence of redundant airway tissue, obstruction of the airway during intravenous sedation can occur. Because the patient cannot move during the procedure, dysphoria and agitation are best avoided.

3. *List the contraindications to having an ESWL procedure.* Contraindications to ESWL are included in Box 42.3.

Intraoperative Period

4. *Evaluate the potential for cardiac dysrhythmias in relation to a patient's cardiac morbidity.*

    Because the shock waves can result in cardiac dysrhythmias, the timing of the pulses is linked to the ECG. Referred to as a gated ESWL, the energy is discharged 20 milliseconds after the R wave in the cardiac cycle. The R wave is the electrical event that coincides with ventricular depolarization, and stimulation that occurs before the R wave can result in severe dysrhythmias such as ventricular tachycardia. The event immediately preceding the R wave when the shock wave is emitted correlates with the absolute refractory period. A supramaximal stimulus that is applied to the cardiac myocyte during this period will not result in depolarization, and the potential for dysrhythmia formation is decreased.

    Patients with a cardiac pacemaker or automatic internal cardiac defibrillator (AICD) should be carefully monitored for heart rate and rhythm abnormalities. Although rarely needed, a magnet should be readily available to reprogram the pacemaker if necessary. Before ESWL therapy, placement of a magnet over most types of AICDs will temporarily inhibit the detection of tachyarrhythmias. The focal point of the shock wave generator should be greater than 15 cm away from the cardiac device.

- Obstruction distal to the kidney stone
- Anticoagulation
- Bleeding disorders
- Abdominal aortic aneurysm >5 cm
- Automated internal cardiac defibrillator
- Pacemaker
- Renal artery aneurysm
- Acute urinary tract infection
- Pregnancy
- Morbid obesity

5. Compare the impact of positive pressure ventilation and spontaneous ventilation on the ESWL procedure.

Stone movement is more profound with spontaneous ventilation due to the involvement of structures within the abdomen during diaphragmatic contraction and relaxation to achieve tidal volume respirations. With positive pressure ventilation, stone movement can be decreased and controlled by changing the tidal volume, respiratory rate, and peak inspiratory pressures. Even small changes in location of the calculus as a result of ventilation can prolong the ESWL treatment and increase the number of shocks necessary to effectively eliminate the stone. This predisposes the patient to a greater risk of complications (e.g., bruising, bleeding).

Postoperative Period

6. Summarize the mechanism for hematuria after ESWL.

Although shock waves are focused on the calculus, some tissue damage within the urinary tract and/or renal parenchyma may occur as a result of time and intensity of shock waves. A small amount of hematuria may occur after ESWL, but it is usually limited to approximately 24 to 48 hours after treatment.

Review Questions

1. Which cardiovascular response is most likely to occur during extracorporeal shock wave lithotripsy?
   a. Cardiac dysrhythmias
   b. Hypotension
   c. Hypertension
   d. Congestive heart failure
2. Which is not a contraindication for having an ESWL procedure?
   a. Six-centimeter abdominal aortic aneurysm
   b. Ureteral obstruction distal to the calculus
   c. History of myocardial infarction 2 years prior
   d. von Willebrand disease
3. Anesthetic techniques that can be used for ESWL include all of the following except:
   a. General anesthesia.
   b. Spinal anesthesia.
   c. Regional anesthesia.
   d. Bier block.

4. The shock wave is timed to discharge 20 milliseconds after the _____ wave during gated ESWL to avoid cardiac dysrhythmias.
   a. P wave
   b. R wave
   c. Q wave
   d. T wave
5. Blockade at which dermatome level is necessary to perform an ESWL under spinal anesthesia?
   a. T4
   b. T5
   c. T6
   d. T7

Suggested Readings

Cannata F, Spinoglio A, Di Marco P, et al. Total intravenous anesthesia using remifentanil in extracorporeal shock wave lithotripsy (ESWL). Comparison of two dosages: a randomized clinical trial. *Minerva Anestesiol* 2014;80(1):58-65.

Coe FL, Evan A, Worcester E. Kidney stone disease. *J Clin Invest* 2005;115:2598-2608.

Elnabtity AM, Tawfeek MM, Keera AA, et al. Is unilateral transversus abdominis plane block an analgesic alternative for ureteric shock wave lithotripsy? *Anesth Essays Res* 2015;9(1):51-56.

Lee C, Weiland D, Ryndin I, et al. Impact of type of anesthesia on efficacy of medstone STS lithotripter. *J Endourol* 2007;21:957-960.

Morse CY. Renal anatomy, physiology, pathophysiology and anesthesia management. In: Nagelhout JJ, Elisha S, eds. *Nurse Anesthesia*, 6th ed. St Louis, MO: Elsevier, 2018:682-708.

Semins MJ, Matlaga BR. Strategies to optimize shock wave lithotripsy outcome: Patient selection and treatment parameters. *World J Nephrol* 2015;4(2):230-234.

Silbert BS, Evered LA, Scott DA. Incidence of postoperative cognitive dysfunction after general or spinal anaesthesia for extracorporeal shock wave lithotripsy. *Br J Anaesth* 2014;113(5):784-791.

Sir E, Eksert S, Zor M, et al. The analgesic efficacy of ultrasound guided unilateral transversus abdominis plane block in the pain management of shock wave lithotripsy. *Arch Esp Urol* 2019;72(9): 933-938.

Sorenson C, Chandhoke P, Moore M, et al. Comparison of intravenous sedation versus general anesthesia on the efficacy of the Doli 50 lithotriptor. *J Urol* 2002;168(1):35-37.

Telha KA, Alkohlany K, Alnono I. Extracorporeal shockwave lithotripsy monotherapy for treating patients with bladder stones. *Arab J Urol* 2016;14(3):207-210.

Terlecki RP, Triest JA. A contemporary evaluation of the auditory hazard of extracorporeal shock wave lithotripsy. *Urology* 2007; 70(5):898-899.

Yang YG, Hu LH, Chen H, Li B, et al. Target-controlled infusion of remifentanil with or without flurbiprofen axetil in sedation for extracorporeal shock wave lithotripsy of pancreatic stones: a prospective, open-label, randomized controlled trial. *BMC Anesthesiol* 2015;15:161.

43

Breast Reconstructive Surgery

KEY POINTS

- Preoperative identification of the patient's chemotherapeutic agent regimen is essential. An anesthetic plan must account for the potential physiologic and pharmacologic effects associated with these medications.
- Anesthetic considerations vary related to the type of breast reconstruction performed. The specific surgical technique employed is individualized to the patient's needs and preferences.
- Patients who have comorbidities presenting for breast reconstructive surgery are at increased risk for complications throughout the perioperative period. These comorbidities most typically include hypertension, diabetes mellitus, dyslipidemia, active smoking, and obesity.
- Postoperative complications may require reoperation for debridement and drainage and include hematoma, seroma, infection, skin flap necrosis, and implant exposure.

Case Synopsis

A 59-year-old woman with diagnosed breast cancer is scheduled for modified radical mastectomy with immediate transverse rectus abdominus myocutaneous (TRAM) flap reconstruction.

Preoperative Evaluation and Demographic Data

Past Medical/Surgical History

- Lumpectomy and biopsy for breast mass
- Hypothyroidism
- Chemotherapy as a treatment for breast cancer
- Shortness of breath and fatigue during exertion

List of Medications

- Doxorubicin hydrochloride (Adriamycin)
- Hydrochlorothiazide
- Synthroid
- Phenergan

Diagnostic Data

- Hemoglobin, 12.3 g/dL; hematocrit, 36.6%; platelets, 219/mm³; glucose, 93 mg/dL; blood urea nitrogen, 21 mg/dL; creatinine, 0.9 mg/dL
- Electrolytes: sodium, 137 mEq/L; potassium, 3.9 mEq/L; chloride, 105 mEq/L; carbon dioxide, 24 mEq/L

Vital Statistics

- 170 cm, 79 kg; body mass index, 27.2 kg/m² (overweight)

- Blood pressure, 121/79; heart rate, 78 beats per minute; respiratory rate, 16 breaths per minute; room air oxygen saturation, 99%; temperature, 37°C
- Electrocardiogram (ECG): normal sinus rhythm; heart rate, 72 beats per minute
- Echocardiogram: ejection fraction (EF) = 58% and there are no associated wall motion abnormalities

Pathophysiology

Each year over 211,000 women and 1700 men are diagnosed with breast cancer. Adenocarcinoma is the most common cause of breast cancer, and the process of cellular dysplasia begins in the cells lining the ducts and lobules of the breast. Risk factors for breast cancer include family history, nulliparity, early menarche, advanced age, obesity, and personal history of breast cancer. Women who have the genetic mutation *BRCA1* or *BRCA2* have a 40% to 85% increased risk of developing breast cancer over their lifetimes. Some women with this gene mutation undergo prophylactic mastectomies. Breast cancer is commonly treated with a combination of surgery, radiation therapy, chemotherapy, and hormone therapy. Breast reconstruction may be immediate or scheduled during a subsequent surgery for patients who choose to undergo mastectomies. There are two different types of postmastectomy reconstruction: prosthetic implant–based reconstruction and autologous tissue–based reconstruction. Many factors influence the choice of reconstruction technique, including the type and location of the cancer, the extent of resection necessary, medical and surgical risk factors of the patient, desired size and shape of the reconstructed breast, and patient preference.

Surgical Procedure

Implant-Based Reconstruction

Current prosthetic reconstruction may involve a single-stage implant reconstruction with either a standard or an adjustable implant, a two-stage tissue implant reconstruction, or a combined implant with autologous tissue reconstruction. Immediate single-stage reconstruction is best suited for women with small breasts and women who qualify for skin-sparing techniques. Advantages of skin-sparing techniques include improved symmetry after reconstruction due to preservation of a breast envelope. In some patients, superior results are obtained with a two-stage reconstruction.

With a two-stage reconstruction, a tissue expander is placed in the submuscular pocket during the primary procedure. The deflated expander exerts minimal tension on the mastectomy flap. Complete muscular coverage minimizes the risk of expander exposure in the event of flap necrosis. Postoperatively, the expander can be slowly filled through an internal port until the desired volume is achieved. During the second-stage procedure, the temporary expander is exchanged for a permanent implant. A partial or complete capsulotomy is performed at this time to maximize breast projection and ptosis, as shown in Fig. 43.1.

Combined Implant and Autologous Tissue Reconstruction

A combined implant with autologous or donor tissue reconstruction can allow for complete wound closure. Tissue

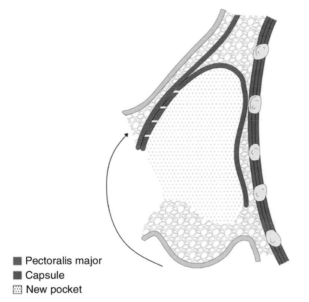

■ Pectoralis major
■ Capsule
▦ New pocket

• **Fig. 43.1** Removal of the breast expander. At this time capsulotomy is performed. The dual plane pocket is created by releasing the muscle, and the implant is covered inferiorly with the advancement of the lower pole skin flap. (From Giudice G, Maruccia M, Nacchiero E, et al: Dual plane breast implant reconstruction in large sized breasts: how to maximise the result following first stage total submuscular expansion, *JPRAS Open* 15:74–80, 2018.)

is most commonly retrieved from the latissimus dorsi myocutaneous flap. The tissue is rotated from the back to the anterior chest to create the breast. This type of flap may not be ample, and the implant is placed between the latissimus and pectoralis muscle to increase the volume of the reconstruction. The duration of implant-based breast reconstructive surgery ranges from 2 to 9 hours (mean 4 hours).

Autologous Tissue Reconstruction

The distinct advantage of autologous tissue breast reconstruction is that the reconstructed breast looks and feels more natural. Results from autologous tissue reconstruction are more consistent over the woman's lifetime. One of the disadvantages of autologous reconstruction is that it is a more complex procedure, requiring a longer surgical procedure and a greater period of convalescence. Three different types of flaps are most commonly used for these procedures: latissimus flaps, TRAM flaps, and deep inferior epigastric perforator (DIEP) flaps.

A TRAM flap procedure is performed to replace the breast tissue with an ellipse of tissue from the rectus abdominus muscle. The pedicle TRAM flap maintains the original blood supply through the superior epigastric artery. The donor tissue is rotated into position, contoured, and then secured in place. A free TRAM flap involves microvascular anastomoses of the inferior epigastric artery to either the thoracodorsal or internal mammary vessels. The blood supply to the flap is temporarily suspended until this reanastomosis occurs. This method allows for transfer of larger amounts of tissue than the pedicle TRAM flap. If TRAM flap hypoperfusion and failure occur, then surgical flap debridement or hematoma evacuation will be instituted. Increased body mass index, smoking, and radiation treatment all increase the potential for TRAM flap failure. The duration for a TRAM flap varies greatly from 5 to 12 hours (mean 7.5 hours).

The DIEP flap has been used recently to minimize donor site morbidities seen with other autologous options such as abdominal wall deformities and muscle weakness. The DIEP flap uses the inferior epigastric artery as the vascular supply that can be dissected without sacrificing any muscle tissue or fascia. Deep inferior epigastric perforator flaps have been shown to improve perfusion to the reconstructed breast and survival. This technique does not require surgical microvascular expertise, longer operative times, and the need for intense postoperative flap monitoring.

Anesthetic Management and Considerations

Preoperative Period

1. *Identify the comorbidities that increase mortality from breast cancer.*

   Mortality from breast cancer significantly increases when it is associated with systemic disease states, including diabetes, renal failure, stroke, liver disease, and previous cancer. Mortality also increases with advanced age.

Women who are older than 65 years of age account for approximately 45% of all new breast cancer cases. Smoking and obesity increase flap failure and decrease wound healing associated with reconstruction.

2. *Describe reasons that obesity complicates the anesthetic and surgical management of patients with breast cancer.*

Obese women are more likely to develop breast cancer due to increased production of estrogen. These patients have a higher incidence of flap complications, flap failure, and impaired wound healing. Obesity causes numerous pathophysiologic processes that affect multiple organ systems, including:

- **Cardiovascular system:** There is an interrelationship between obesity and cardiovascular disease. Hypertension and dyslipidemia can result in the development of concentric hypertrophy and coronary artery disease. As a result, myocardial performance is decreased. There is increased myocardial oxygen demand, and during periods of physiologic stress, myocardial ischemia, myocardial infarction, and congestive heart failure can occur.
- **Respiratory system:** Chest wall compliance is decreased in obese patients, resulting in restrictive lung disease. Total lung capacity and functional residual capacity are also decreased. These effects contribute to the rapid development of arterial hypoxemia from premature airway closure and ventilation–perfusion mismatch.

  Obesity is associated with the presence of redundant airway tissue, which can make ventilation and intubation difficult or impossible. Obstructive sleep apnea and chronic hypercarbia are associated with obesity. Optimal alignment of the laryngeal, pharyngeal, and oral axes by ramping the patient and achieving a sniffing position is warranted. Thorough preoxygenation before the induction of anesthesia is vital to decrease the possibility of hypoxemia.
- **Endocrine system:** People who are obese are at increased risk of developing noninsulin-dependent diabetes. The incidence increases as body mass index increases and results in altered glucose metabolism and impaired insulin receptor sensitivity. Perioperative assessment of blood glucose is warranted.
- **Gastrointestinal system:** Obesity has been associated with decreased gastric emptying time and gastroesophageal reflux disease. Preoperative gastrointestinal prophylaxis with a gastrokinetic agent, histamine receptor type 2 antagonist, and nonparticulate antacid is indicated for obese patients who are at increased risk of gastric aspiration.
- **Hepatic system:** Due to the infiltration of hepatocytes with triglycerides, morbid obesity is associated with nonalcoholic fatty liver disease. The degree of hepatic compromise can be assessed by results from liver function tests. Hepatic dysfunction is associated with coagulopathy and decreased metabolism of anesthetic medications.

3. *Identify commonly used chemotherapeutic agents and discuss the anesthetic implications.*

Chemotherapeutic agents such as bleomycin, Adriamycin, methotrexate, and tamoxifen affect the anesthetic plan and intraoperative care. This patient has taken Adriamycin, which has the potential to cause cardiotoxicity. Even small doses of Adriamycin can cause cardiotoxicity. Myocardial dysfunction can be acute or chronic. Manifestations associated with the acute form that are reversible include arrhythmias, ST-T–wave abnormalities, and decreased EF. The severity of the effects associated with chronic treatment with Adriamycin is dose dependent and can result in congestive heart failure. The frequency of significant cardiomyopathy is estimated to be between 1% and 10% if the total dose of Adriamycin is less than 450 mg/m^2. The proposed mechanism of action by which Adriamycin decreases cardiac performance results from myofibril degeneration and myocardial mitochondrial dysfunction.

Due to the synergy between the cardiotoxic effects produced by Adriamycin, myocardial depression caused by the inhalation anesthetic agents, and physiologic stress produced by surgery and anesthesia, a comprehensive preoperative cardiac evaluation is essential. A list of commonly used chemotherapeutic agents, the physiologic changes, and the associated anesthetic considerations is presented in Table 43.1.

4. *Discuss the anesthetic considerations regarding intravenous (IV) placement.*

It is best to avoid placing IV catheters or taking serial blood pressure measurements on the mastectomy side to avoid the development of lymph edema. If bilateral mastectomies were performed, the anesthetist should place the IV on the side opposite from where the lymph node dissection occurred. If bilateral lymph edema exists, or if bilateral lymph node dissection was performed, external jugular or internal jugular cannulation should be considered. An option for patients without diabetes is to place the IV in a lower extremity.

5. *Discuss the anesthetic considerations for blood pressure assessment, including arterial line placement.*

Patients with heart disease, anemia, bilateral lymph edema, or other comorbid factors may benefit from the placement of an arterial line. An arterial line will allow for easy access for blood sampling and provide real-time and reliable blood pressure measurements. Placing the blood pressure cuff on the leg is also an option in select patients when upper extremity blood pressure monitoring is contraindicated.

6. *Discuss the anesthetic considerations for preoperative sedation.*

Because the surgeon routinely marks the chest wall while the patient is standing during the preoperative phase, caution against providing heavy sedation must be exercised during this time. An example of preoperative chest wall markings is shown in Fig. 43.2. Due to the possibility of redundant airway tissue and the reduction

TABLE 43.1	Common Chemotherapeutic Agents Used to Treat Breast Cancer: Physiologic Effects and Anesthetic Considerations			
	Bleomycin	Doxorubicin Hydrochloride (Adriamycin)	Methotrexate (Trexall, Amethopterin)	Tamoxifen (Nolvadex)
Physiologic effects	• Pulmonary toxicity	• Cardiac toxicity: transient dysrhythmias, ECG changes, irreversible cardiomyopathy, and congestive heart failure • Cardiac risk is increased with increasing dose, prior radiotherapy, and female gender • Myelosuppression resulting in thrombocytopenia, anemia, and leukopenia	• Renal dysfunction • Hepatic dysfunction • Anemia	• Nausea and vomiting • Dehydration
Anesthetic considerations	• Avoid FiO_2 >30% to prevent pulmonary fibrosis and edema • Chest x-ray • Arterial blood gas as indicated by history and physical • Pulmonary function testing as indicated by history and physical	• ECG to evaluate for cardiomyopathy • Complete blood count to evaluate for myelosuppression	• Complete blood count • Blood urea nitrogen • Creatinine • Liver function tests	• Intravenous hydration • Antiemetic medication

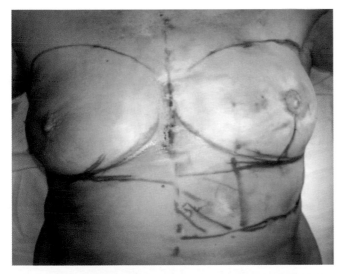

• **Fig. 43.2** Preoperative marking before stage 2 breast reconstructive surgery. (From Bland KI, Copeland EM, Klimberg S, et al: *The breast: Comprehensive management of benign and malignant diseases*, ed 5, St. Louis, 2018, Elsevier.)

of functional residual capacity, oversedation can result in airway obstruction and hypoxemia.

Intraoperative Period

7. *Explain how blood pressure control affects flap perfusion.*

One of the complications of the TRAM flap procedure is postoperative necrosis of the newly constructed breast. Therefore maintenance of mean arterial pressure within 20% of preoperative values allows for adequate perfusion pressure to the flap tissue. Extremes in blood pressure should be avoided. Hypertension frequently causes excessive bleeding, and hypotension can result in hypoperfusion to the graft. It is important to avoid the use of vasopressors to treat hypotension, as vasoconstriction of the arterial vasculature will restrict blood flow to the flap. The blood pressure is most effectively supported by administering fluids.

8. *Identify how volume replacement affects hemostasis.*

In order to avoid infusing a large volume of crystalloid, patients may benefit from the use of albumin. Intraoperative assessment of serial hemoglobin values is necessary to ensure adequate oxygen-carrying capacity. The decision to administer blood, fresh frozen plasma, and platelets should be based on the patient's preoperative physical status, hemodynamic stability, laboratory values, and surgical hemostasis.

9. *Discuss the anesthetic considerations for autologous blood donation and transfusion.*

Autologous blood donation is the collection of the patient's own blood before elective surgery. This blood can be auto-transfused, if necessary, during the intraoperative or postoperative periods. It has not been proven that the risk of transmission of communicable bloodborne diseases is less with autologous blood compared with banked blood. Autologous donation is associated with a higher rate of postoperative transfusion. This phenomenon is most likely due to relative preoperative anemia caused by autologous donation. Transfusions are not routinely required for breast reconstructive surgery, and as a result, autologous blood donation is infrequently performed for reconstructive breast surgery.

10. *Discuss the anesthetic implications of administering nitrous oxide for TRAM flap reconstruction.*

During TRAM flap reconstruction, the abdominal donor site is often closed as though the patient has undergone an abdominoplasty. Because nitrous oxide is highly diffusible, its use should be avoided to prevent abdominal distention. Avoiding the use of nitrous oxide will allow for optimal cosmetic results.

11. *Explain the rationale for maintaining normothermia during breast reconstructive surgery.*

Normothermia should be maintained during breast reconstructive surgery, particularly during flap reconstruction. Hypothermia causes vasoconstriction, thus restricting blood supply to the flap, and therefore maintenance of normothermia is important to optimize flap perfusion. Hypothermia can also result in decreased hemostasis, causing hematoma formation; postoperative shivering, which significantly increases myocardial oxygen demand; and decreased hepatic metabolism and renal excretion of drugs, leading to delayed emergence from anesthesia.

12. *Explain the advantages and disadvantages for using dextran during breast reconstructive surgery.*

Pharmacologic antithrombotic prophylaxis that occurs with the use of dextran can be used during flap reconstructive surgery to minimize the risk of TRAM flap hypoperfusion and necrosis caused by microvascular thrombus formation. However, risks associated with dextran administration include coagulopathy and anaphylaxis. Breast reconstruction is an elective surgery. High-risk patients are frequently offered reconstructive surgery using breast implants rather than flap reconstruction to minimize the risk of microvascular thrombosis. As a result, dextran is not routinely administered intraoperatively.

13. *Identify changes in patient positioning are required during intraoperative breast reconstructive surgery.*

Mastectomies and breast reconstructive surgeries are usually performed in a supine position with mild flexion. In order to gain access for the latissimus dorsi flap harvest, the patient will be placed in the lateral decubitus position. After placement of the implant or flap construction, the patient may be moved to a sitting position to assess the overall appearance and symmetry of the breast reconstruction. Hypotension can occur when the patient is moved abruptly into a sitting position. It is important to secure both arms in order to keep them from falling forward and to avoid brachial plexus and ulnar nerve injury. Lastly, holding the endotracheal tube is important to decrease the potential for accidental extubation or right mainstem intubation.

Postoperative Period

14. *Discuss methods for postoperative pain control.*

Numerous pain management modalities can be used to decrease postoperative pain. These strategies include patient-controlled analgesia, thoracic epidural, intercostal nerve block, thoracic paravertebral nerve block, IV administration of narcotics, and oral pain medication. Decreasing postoperative pain is important because it inhibits sympathetic nervous system hyperactivity and allows patients to breathe deeply in order to prevent atelectasis. A paravertebral block enhances the recovery after anesthesia and provides analgesia throughout the immediate postoperative period.

15. *Discuss the long-term postoperative care necessary after breast reconstructive surgery.*

Many patients will undergo subsequent surgical procedures because breast implants are not considered permanent devices. The implants may need to be replaced over a period of years due to the development of contractures, migration, leakage, or rupture. Reintervention for scar revision and nipple reconstruction is also common. Advancements in surgical techniques for nipple reconstruction can be accomplished using monitored anesthesia care. Breast tissue is reconfigured into a nipple. Tattooing techniques are used, and the new nipple is colored to match the color of the areola.

Review Questions

1. Maintenance of intraoperative blood pressure during breast reconstructive surgery is best controlled by administering:
   a. Ephedrine to maintain preoperative mean arterial pressure.
   b. Lactated Ringer's.
   c. A crystalloid solution and blood.
   d. A phenylephrine bolus.

2. Which preoperative evaluation(s) are indicated for a patient receiving bleomycin?
   a. ECG and echocardiography are obtained to determine potential cardiac toxicity
   b. Liver function tests are obtained to determine potential hepatic impairment
   c. Blood urea nitrogen and creatinine are obtained to determine potential renal impairment
   d. Arterial blood gas and chest x-ray are obtained to determine potential pulmonary impairment

3. A diabetic patient is scheduled for a right mastectomy with lymph node dissection. Which is the best area to place an IV?
   a. Left hand
   b. Right hand
   c. Left leg
   d. Right leg
4. Which patient is at the highest risk for developing breast cancer?
   a. A patient with a negative *BRCA1* and *BRCA2* gene
   b. A positive *BRCA2* gene and history of ovarian cancer
   c. A morbidly obese 30-year-old woman
   d. A woman with a 20-pack/year smoking history

5. Which perioperative intervention(s) will help to ensure TRAM flap perfusion?
   a. Controlled hypothermia and normotension
   b. Normothermia, normotension, normocarbia
   c. Intraoperative dextran infusion
   d. Controlled hypotension to prevent bleeding

Suggested Readings

Andrades P, Fix RJ, Danilla S, et al. Ischemic complications in pedicle, free, and muscle sparing transverse rectus abdominis myocutaneous flaps for breast reconstruction. *Ann Plast Surg* 2008;60(5): 562-567.

Cai A, Suckau J, Arkudas A, et al. Autologous breast reconstruction with Transverse Rectus Abdominis Musculocutaneous (TRAM) or Deep Inferior Epigastric Perforator (DIEP) flaps: an analysis of the 100 most cited articles. *Med Sci Monit* 2019;25:3520-3536.

Carlson GW, Page AL, Peters K, et al. Effects of radiation therapy on pedicled transverse rectus abdominis myocutaneous flap breast reconstruction. *Ann Plast Surg* 2008;60(5):568-572.

Depypere B, Herregods S, Denolf J, et al. 20 years of DIEAP flap breast reconstruction: a big data analysis. *Sci Rep* 2019;9(1):12899.

Erdmann-Sager J, Wilkins EG. Complications and patient-reported outcomes after abdominally based breast reconstruction: results of the Mastectomy Reconstruction Outcomes Consortium Study. *Plast Reconstr Surg* 2018;141(2):271-281.

Fan KL, Luvisa K, Black CK, et al. Gabapentin decreases narcotic usage: enhanced recovery after surgery pathway in free autologous breast reconstruction. *Plast Reconstr Surg Glob Open* 2019; 7(8):e2350.

Kotsopoulos J. BRCA mutations and breast cancer prevention. *Cancers (Basel)* 2018;10(12):524.

Masoomi H, Greives MR, Cantor AD, marques ES. Effect of anemia in postoperative outcomes of autologous breast reconstruction surgery. *World J Plast Surg* 2019;8(3):285-292.

Parikh RP, Myckatyn TM. Paravertebral blocks and enhanced recovery after surgery protocols in breast reconstructive surgery: patient selection and perspectives. *J Pain Res* 2018;11:1567-1581.

Zhu Y, Wu J, Zhang C, et al. BRCA mutations and survival in breast cancer: an updated systematic review and meta-analysis. *Oncotarget* 2016;7(43):70113-70127.

44

Liposuction

Case Synopsis

A 43-year-old woman presents for elective liposuction for body contouring of the flanks, back, inner and outer thighs, and abdomen utilizing the tumescent technique. Intraoperatively, the patient will be placed in the prone position to obtain access to the back and flank area. The planned amount of aspirate is 4000 mL.

Preoperative Evaluation and Demographic Data

Past Medical/Surgical History

- Smoking
- Hypertension
- MWL of 58 kg; status post-bariatric surgery
- Anxiety
- Bilateral tubal ligation and cholecystectomy; no anesthetic complications

List of Medications

- Fexofenadine
- Lexapro
- Hormone replacement therapy
- Multivitamin

Diagnostic Data

- Hemoglobin, 12.7 g/dL; hematocrit, 36.8%
- Electrolytes: sodium, 137 mEq/L; potassium, 3.7 mEq/L; carbon dioxide, 25 mEq/L; glucose, 97 mg/dL

Height/Weight/Vital Signs

- 165 cm, 117 kg

- Blood pressure, 142/87; heart rate, 72 beats per minute; respiratory rate, 18 breaths per minute; room air oxygen saturation, 97%; temperature, 36.2°C
- Electrocardiogram (ECG): normal sinus rhythm with occasional premature atrial contractions; nonspecific T-wave abnormalities
- Chest x-ray (CXR): no acute disease process, heart normal in size

Pathophysiology

Obesity/Lipodystrophy

Body mass index (BMI) is a calculation derived from a patient's height and weight expressed in kilograms per meter squared (kg/m^2). Persons with a BMI greater than 25 kg/m^2 are overweight, and those with a BMI greater than 30 kg/m^2 are classified as obese. Patients with a BMI greater than 40 kg/m^2 are classified as severely obese. A multitude of pathophysiologic changes associated with obesity are summarized in Box 44.1.

Surgical Procedure

Suction-assisted lipoplasty is the most common elective cosmetic procedure performed in the United States. Liposuction involves removing subcutaneous adipose tissue through a cannula with the aid of an external source of suction. Various liposuction techniques are included in Table 44.1. The wetting solution used for liposuction may or may not contain additives such lidocaine with epinephrine, and their significance is discussed further in this chapter. Additionally, the subsequent use of laser-assisted

TABLE 44.1	Commonly Performed Liposuction Techniques			
Technique	Wetting Solution (WS)	WS:Aspirate	Blood Loss	
Dry technique	No wetting solution is utilized	N/A	20%–45% of total aspirate	
Tumescent technique	0.025%–0.1% lidocaine and epinephrine 1:100,000 in normal saline or lactated Ringer's solution	3:1	1% of total aspirate	
Superwet technique	Normal saline or lactated Ringer's solution with epinephrine and sometimes lidocaine	1:1	1% or less of total aspirate	
Ultrasound-assisted technique	Used in conjunction with tumescent or superwet technique	Dependent on technique used in conjunction with ultrasound	1% of total aspirate	

• BOX 44.1 **Pathologic Conditions Associated With Obesity**

Cardiovascular

- Hyperlipidemia
- Hypertension
- Venous insufficiency
- Peripheral vascular disease
- Coronary artery disease
- Ventricular hypertrophy

Respiratory

- Restrictive lung disease
- Obstructive sleep apnea
- Redundant airway tissue
- Hypoventilation syndrome

Other Pathology

- Diabetes
- Gastroesophageal reflux disease
- Cerebrovascular disease
- Cirrhosis
- Cholecystitis
- Impaired wound healing

liposuction may be used in conjunction with the wetting solution to facilitate greater volumes of aspirate. MWL secondary to bariatric surgery has resulted in numerous body contouring procedures being performed in the United States.

Anesthetic Management and Considerations

Preoperative Period

1. *Discuss this patient's preoperative medications and the potential anesthetic concerns.*
   - Potential side effects of beta-blockers are bradycardia, claudication, and sedation.

- Monoamine oxidase inhibitors (MAOIs) result in an increased availability of norepinephrine, which affects the central nervous system as well as the sympathetic nervous system. Potential side effects associated with MAOIs include hypertension and sedation.
- Tricyclic antidepressants may result in seizure-like activity on the electroencephalogram.
- The anticholinergic effects of tricyclic antidepressants increase the likelihood of central anticholinergic syndrome if atropine or scopolamine is administered.
- Oral contraceptives and hormone replacement therapy increase the risk for deep vein thrombosis.
- Venous thrombosis and pulmonary embolism have been associated with the use of third-generation progestins in low estrogen.

2. *Discuss obesity and related coexisting diseases associated with patients having elective liposuction.*

Obesity is present in 50% of the population in America. Patients with a BMI >20% are at increased risk for perioperative complications related to acute and chronic medical conditions such as diabetes, hypertension, and coronary artery disease. Cardiac manifestations related to obesity include an increased myocardial workload, hypertension, and ventricular hypertrophy. Obstructive sleep apnea (OSA) frequently occurs in obese patients, and when coupled with deep sedation, there is an increase in respiratory risk factors. Increases in pulmonary blood flow and pulmonary vasoconstriction due to chronic hypoxia can result in pulmonary hypertension and cor pulmonale in the obese patient with OSA.

Although liposuction is commonly performed with the utilization of local block or tumescent anesthesia, many anesthetists administer sedation to help the patient better tolerate the brief periods of discomfort experienced during the punctures necessary to instill the subdermal infiltration of the local anesthetic. Of concern in the postoperative period is the increased risk of postoperative apnea associated with the use of opioids and sedatives. Gastrointestinal concerns associated with obesity include factors that predispose the patient to aspiration pneumonitis, which includes hiatal hernia, gastroesophageal reflux, decreased gastric emptying, and increased gastric fluid acidity.

Fatty liver infiltrates, which may lead to cirrhosis, can decrease metabolism of medications, increasing the likelihood of local anesthetic toxicity. Strict diets and strenuous exercise resulting in weight loss could cause hypoalbuminemia, electrolyte imbalances, or fluid electrolyte deficiencies.

3. *Discuss the importance of administering prophylactic antibiotics for the patient undergoing liposuction.*
   - Necrotizing fasciitis with overwhelming infection and toxic shock syndrome are known fatal complications associated with liposuction.
   - Causative organisms have been identified as *Streptococcus pyogenes* and *Staphylococcus aureus*.
   - Autopsy reports have shown bacterial invasion from the perineal area.
   - The most common class of antibiotic administered preoperatively for anesthetic procedures is a cephalosporin.
   - Current evidence-based practice recommends that prophylactic antibiotic treatment be instituted within 60 minutes of surgical incision.
   - Subsequent doses of antibiotics are determined based on the antibiotics' half-life and duration of the surgery.

Factors That Contribute to Infection
- **Patient factors:** Extremes of age, malnutrition, obesity, diabetes, hypoxemia, remote infection, corticosteroid therapy, recent operation, chronic inflammation, and prior irradiation
- **Perioperative factors:** Long preoperative hospitalization, no preoperative shower, hair removal, and prior antibiotic therapy
- **Intraoperative factors:** Intraoperative contamination, lengthy operation, excessive electrocautery, foreign material, wound drainage, epinephrine wound injection, intraoperative hypotension, and massive transfusion

Intraoperative Period

4. *Describe the physiologic alterations and potential complications associated with the prone position.*

The prone position is associated with cardiac, respiratory, and cerebral complications. Decreased preload, cardiac output, and blood pressure are associated with venous compression from tension of the abdominal muscles, which causes blood to pool in the lower extremities.

Increased work of breathing results from compression of the abdomen and thorax and decreased lung compliance. In cases of head rotation in the prone position, cerebral venous drainage and cerebral blood flow are also diminished.

5. *Examine the differences for various liposuction techniques.*

Dry Technique
- Performed without infiltrating subcutaneous solutions before suctioning.
- Disadvantages of the dry technique are swelling and discoloration.
- Blood loss is 20% to 45% of the aspirate obtained.
- Transfusion is usually required when large volumes of fat are removed.
- Avoid aspirate volumes greater than 1000 mL because of the risk of large blood loss volumes.
- Never performed in conjunction with ultrasound-assisted liposuction because of the possibility of thermal injuries from the ultrasound.

Wet Technique
- Infiltration of 200 to 300 mL of wetting solution into the operative site before suctioning begins.
- The solution may or may not contain additives such as lidocaine, epinephrine, and/or bicarbonate.
- Epinephrine added to the solution results in a significant decrease in the volume of blood loss to 4% to 30% of the aspirate.

Tumescent Technique
- Tumescent fluid is composed of large volumes of fluid (>4 L) of dilute lidocaine (<1 g/L) and epinephrine (<1 mg/L).
- The segmental injection of tumescent fluid takes place before suctioning.
- Doses of 30 mg/kg of lidocaine have reportedly been safely infiltrated, although the Food and Drug Administration (FDA) recommends the maximum dose of 7 mg/kg of lidocaine with epinephrine in the adult.
- The tumescent technique employs the practice of infiltrating 3 to 4 mL of infiltrate for each 1 mL of aspirate.
- An advantage of this technique is epinephrine-induced hemostasis caused by vasoconstriction, which reduces blood loss to 1% of the volume of aspirate.

Superwet Technique
- The major difference between the superwet technique and the tumescent technique is the amount of aspirate infiltrated.
- Utilizes a 1:1 ratio of aspirate to infiltrate.
- Composition of the infiltrate is either saline or lactated Ringer's with epinephrine and sometimes lidocaine.
- Blood loss with this technique has been found to be comparable to blood loss in the tumescent technique at 1% of the aspirate.

Ultrasound-Assisted Liposuction
- Cannula or probe that delivers fat-liquefying ultrasonic energy to adipose tissue in fibrous areas.
- Adipocytes go through a series of expansion and compression cycles, resulting in implosion of the cell.
- Wetting solution used in conjunction with the ultrasound probe emulsifies fat and aids in cooling the heat generated.

- Blood loss is consistent with the superwet technique at 1% of the aspirate, which is comparable to the tumescent technique.

  Comparisons of the different techniques utilized to perform liposuction are described in Table 44.1.

6. *Explain the physiologic alterations that manifest with intravascular absorption of lidocaine and epinephrine in the tumescent fluid used during liposuction.*

   Local anesthetics have the potential to cause systemic toxicity because these medications cause blockade of cellular sodium channels through the entire body. Untoward effects that occur to the neurologic and cardiovascular systems are dependent on the plasma concentration of the local anesthetic. When a patient begins to develop local anesthetic toxicity, the first signs and symptoms are associated with the neurologic system and include ringing sound in the ears, numbness around the lips, dizziness, and tinnitus. Higher plasma concentrations associated with local anesthetic toxicity manifest as altered level of consciousness, seizures, respiratory arrest, and finally cardiac compromise.

   The greatest determining factor of the lidocaine plasma level during tumescent liposuction is due to hepatic degradation. The liver's maximum clearance capacity is approximately 250 mg of lidocaine per hour. Hepatic enzymes and blood flow are the predominant factors affecting lidocaine metabolism. The plasma half-life of lidocaine is 1.8 hours, but hepatic disease can increase it to 4.9 hours. Decreased hepatic blood flow, as found in congestive heart failure, drastically reduces the rate of elimination of lidocaine. Cardiac and cerebral events occur if the peak metabolic capacity of lidocaine is impaired by drug interactions or hepatic dysfunction. Depression of the intracardiac conduction system and ventricular contractility resulting in asystole can occur. Treatment for cardiac arrest resulting from local anesthetic toxicity includes but is not limited to the infusion of intralipids. The addition of epinephrine to lidocaine-containing solutions reduces the absorption of the local anesthetic by approximately one-third. The anesthetist should be alert to the potential sympathomimetic effects caused by epinephrine. Lidocaine can potentiate the effects of nondepolarizing neuromuscular blocking drugs.

7. *Explain the process of estimating blood loss during liposuction.*
   - Two major determinants of blood loss in liposuction are the amount of blood in each milliliter of aspirate, which can be determined by the technique used, and the total aspirate obtained.
   - Total blood loss can be calculated by multiplying the percentage of blood in the aspirate by the total amount suctioned.
   - Blood loss in the tumescent technique is approximately 1% of the aspirate.

8. *Explain the fluid resuscitation guidelines for the patient undergoing liposuction.*
   - Currently no definitive guidelines exist for fluid management during liposuction.
   - Factors that guide perioperative fluid homeostasis include close monitoring of intravenous (IV) fluid administered, wetting solution infiltrated, amount of aspirate, estimated blood loss, and urinary output.
   - Aspirate is defined as the total volume of fat and fluid obtained during liposuction.
   - Approximately 60% to 70% of wetting solution remains and is absorbed as hypodermoclysis.
   - The volume of fluids to be infused should be guided by the patient's vital signs and urinary output.
   - Patients with greater than 4 L of aspirate removed should receive maintenance fluid only.
   - Patients with greater than 4 L of aspirate removed should receive additional maintenance fluid of 0.25 mL of IV fluid for each mL of aspirate over 4 L.
   - Guidelines for fluid resuscitation are listed in Table 44.1.

Postoperative Period

The total time required to perform the liposuction was 130 minutes. The amount of wetting solution infiltrated was 4300 mL, and the total amount of aspirate obtained was 3800 mL. Fluid resuscitation with crystalloid was 3400 mL, and the urinary output was 625 mL. The dressings and compression garment were applied, and the patient was extubated once she was completely awake after the application. Vital signs in the postanesthesia care unit were blood pressure, 167/92; heart rate, 119 beats per minute; respiratory rate, 26 breaths per minute; and temperature, 35.1°C.

9. *Discuss the following potential complications associated with liposuction.*

Embolism
- Pulmonary embolus is the largest single cause of mortality in patients undergoing liposuction: 4.6 per 100,000 patients.
- Embolism may result from fat or venous thrombosis.
- Pulmonary embolism presents as shortness of breath, pleuritic pain, cough, hemoptysis, palpitations, wheezing, and angina-like pain.
- Deep venous thrombosis (DVT) signs and symptoms include leg pain, Hohmann sign, swelling and erythema, tachycardia, and warmth of the extremity.
- Intermittent pneumatic leg compression devices are recommended for the prophylactic prevention of pulmonary thromboembolism.
- Some of the risk factors for DVT and pulmonary embolism include thrombophlebitis, smoking, obesity, previous DVT, and hormone replacement therapy/oral contraceptives.

- Treatment for pulmonary embolism/DVT includes heparin, thrombolytics, low-molecular-weight heparin, and hemodynamic support.

Pulmonary Edema

- Hyperhydration that results from the infusion of IV fluid for the treatment of hypotension.
- Hypodermoclysis that results from the wetting solution being rapidly absorbed.

Intestinal or Organ Perforation

- Organ perforation has been reported in the presence of an existing abdominal scar on rare occasions.
- Susceptible areas for major damage from perforation include the abdomen, thorax, retroperitoneum, major vessels, and the kidney.
- The signs and symptoms of organ perforation may not manifest for several days; thus the patient presents with an acute abdomen or sepsis requiring an emergency laparotomy to repair the injury.

Hypothermia

- Hypothermia is defined as body temperature <36.5°C.
- The primary mechanism by which patients lose heat within the operating room is by radiation, which occurs

> ### • BOX 44.2 Methods Used to Prevent Intraoperative Hypothermia
>
> - Warming the skin preparation solution, intravenous, and infiltrative fluids
> - Applying forced-air warming blanket
> - Increasing the operating room temperature
> - Warming the infiltration solution to 37°C at the time of injection
> - Covering the patient's head and appendages to help minimize the exposed surface area

rapidly in the operating room. Wetting solutions injected into patients, even if prewarmed, are frequently less than body temperature. Infused IV fluids are also a source of heat loss by way of convection. Perioperative hypothermia can result in increased discomfort, infection, bleeding, decreased metabolism of medications, and shivering, which can prolong discharge. Methods that can reduce the risk of hypothermia are presented in Box 44.2.

Review Questions

1. What is the approximate blood loss for the patient who has undergone tumescent liposuction with 4500 mL of total aspirate obtained?
   a. 450 mL
   b. 1500 mL
   c. 2250 mL
   d. 45 mL
2. Which is an initial sign associated with local anesthetic toxicity?
   a. Seizures
   b. Dizziness
   c. Respiratory arrest
   d. Bradycardia
3. Which physiologic change is associated with the prone position?
   a. Decreased preload
   b. Decreased lung compliance
   c. Increased cardiac output
   d. Increased functional residual capacity

4. Which complication causes the highest mortality for a patient having liposuction?
   a. Hypothermia
   b. Pulmonary embolism
   c. Organ perforation
   d. Necrotizing fasciitis
5. Which class of anesthetic medications can be potentiated by lidocaine?
   a. Inhalation anesthetics
   b. Nitrous oxide
   c. Nondepolarizing muscle relaxants
   d. Benzodiazepines

Suggested Readings

Bellini E, Grieco MP, Raposio E. A journey through liposuction and liposculture: review. *Ann Med Surg (Lond)* 2017;24: 53-60.

Caballini M, Preis F, Casati A. Effects of mild hypothermia on blood coagulation in patients undergoing elective plastic surgery. *Plast Reconstr Surg* 2005;116:316-321.

Cantu CA, Pavlisko EN. Liposuction-induced fat embolism syndrome. *BMJ Case Rep* 2017;2017:bcr2017219835.

Cárdenas-Camarena L, Andrés Gerardo LP, et al. Strategies for reducing fatal complications in liposuction. *Plast Reconstr Surg Glob Open* 2017;5(10):e1539.

Griffin M, Akhavani MA, Muirhead N, et al. Risk of thromboembolism following body-contouring surgery after massive weight loss. *Eplasty* 2015;15:e17.

Klein JA, Jeske DR. Estimated maximal safe dosages of tumescent lidocaine. *Anesth Analg* 2016;122(5):1350-1359.

Kenkel J, Lipschitz A, Luby M, et al. Hemodynamic physiology and thermoregulation in liposuction. *Plast Reconstr Surg* 2004;114:503-513.

Middeldorp S. Oral contraceptives and the risk of venous thrombo-embolism. *Gend Med* 2005;2 Suppl A:S3–S9.

Mohamed AA, Safan TF, Hamed HF, Elgendy MAA. Tumescent local infiltration anesthesia for mini abdominoplasty with liposuction. *Open Access Maced J Med Sci* 2018;6(11): 2073-2078.

Mrad S, El Tawil C, Sukaiti WA, et al. Cardiac arrest following liposuction: a case report of lidocaine toxicity. *Oman Med J* 2019; 34(4):341-344.

Wang G, Cao WG, Zhao TL. Fluid management in extensive liposuction: a retrospective review of 83 consecutive patients. *Medicine (Baltimore)* 2018;97(41):e12655.

45

Mandibular Osteotomy

KEY POINTS

- Maxillofacial surgery is performed for the following pathologic reasons: musculoskeletal and craniofacial abnormalities, dental osseous misalignment, soft tissue deformities, maxillofacial trauma, maxillofacial infection, or tumor growth.
- Airway management for patients having maxillofacial surgery is dependent on the type of surgery that is being performed and the patients' comorbidities. Nasal intubation with a specialized Ring–Adair–Elwyn (RAE) endotracheal tube provides optimal surgical access and visualization.

- Strategies to control postoperative nausea and vomiting (PONV) are extremely important because of the increased potential for aspiration of gastric contents and decreased access to the airway caused by the surgical intervention.
- Blood loss during maxillofacial surgery may be as large as 1500 mL as a result of the complexity and extensive nature of the surgical procedure.

Case Synopsis

A 15-year-old girl with maxillary insufficiency and prognathia is scheduled to have Le Fort I and bilateral sagittal split osteotomies.

Preoperative Evaluation and Demographic Data

Past Medical/Surgical History

- No past surgical history

Medication List

- None

Diagnostic Data

- Hemoglobin, 12.7 g/dL; hematocrit, 37.4%

Height/Weight/Vital Signs

- 173 cm, 86 kg
- Blood pressure, 115/78; heart rate, 82 beats per minute; respiratory rate, 18 breaths per minute; temperature, 37°C; room air oxygen saturation, 99%
- Airway classification Mallampati 1; 7 cm thyromental distance; full range of motion cervical spine without discomfort; both nares appear normal size without any narrowing or obstruction to airflow.

Pathophysiology

Maxillofacial surgery represents a large variety of procedures that range from simple (extraction of teeth) to complex (facial reconstruction after a trauma). There are many indications for

tooth extractions, which include severe caries, pulpal necrosis, odontalgia, aiding orthodontic corrections, removal of impacted molars, and for cosmetic improvement. Orthognathic procedures are carried out on both maxillae and mandibles and are indicated for psychological and/or aesthetic reasons, medical concerns, or functional/developmental abnormalities.

Maxillofacial trauma can be the result of a blunt force, such as a motor vehicle accident, penetrating trauma, or result from a thermal injury. Blunt and/or penetrating trauma may produce extensive injury due to production of secondary projectiles—teeth or bone fragments—that damage surrounding soft tissues. Other indications for maxillofacial surgery include maxillary insufficiency, prognathia, macrognathia, retrognathia, maxillomandibular complex asymmetry, temporomandibular joint/facial pain, and obstructive sleep apnea. This patient presented with maxillary insufficiency and prognathia for surgical correction/resculpting to improve appearance and dentition alignment.

Relevant Anatomy

Twenty-two bones form the head and facial skeleton. The skull is divided into two regions: the *calvaria* and *facial* skeleton. The calvaria is composed of 8 bones: frontal, occipital, temporal (2), parietal (2), sphenoid, and ethmoid—all of which form the rigid structure for the brain. The remaining 14 bones form the face—that part of the skeleton is most closely associated with visual appearance. These bones are nasal (2), lacrimal (2), superior maxillary (2), zygomatic (2), palate (2), inferior turbinate (2), vomer, and mandible. The teeth lend structure and composition and contribute significantly to the facial skeleton. Fig. 45.1 illustrates the complexity of the bones that form the craniofacial skeleton.

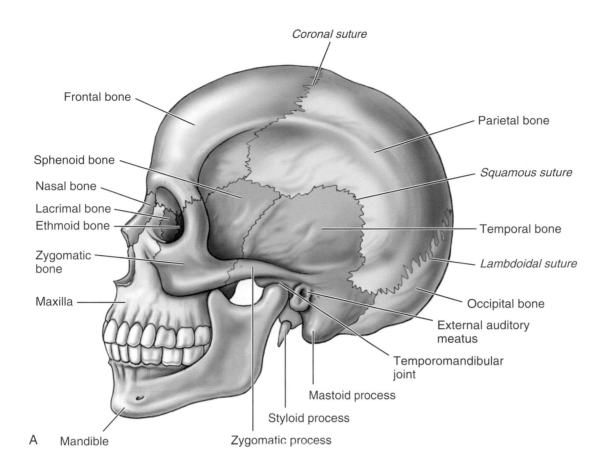

A   Mandible

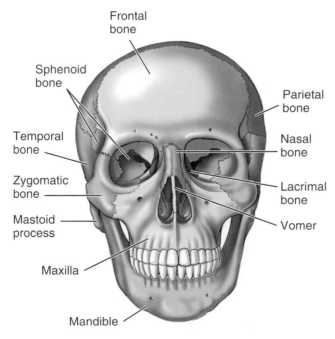

B

• **Fig. 45.1** Bones of the skull. (A) Side view. (B) Front view. (From Herlihy B: *The human body in health and illness*, ed 6, St. Louis, 2018, Elsevier.)

The face is divided into three areas: the upper, middle, and lower face. The upper face is composed of the frontal bone and is bound by the frontozygomatic and frontonasal sutures/articulations. The middle of the face begins with the orbits and extends downward to and includes the upper teeth. The lower face is composed of the lower teeth and mandible.

Surgical Procedure

There are three distinct facial fractures, and the anatomic description is classified into one of three Le Fort categories. Fig. 45.2 depicts the region of the craniofacial skeleton that is characteristic of each type of fracture.

Le Fort I Fracture/Osteotomy

The Le Fort I fracture occurs along the maxillary alveolar rim. This fracture arises from the nasal septum toward the lateral pyriform rims and traverses above the apices of the teeth. The fracture occurs below the zygomaticomaxillary junction and interrupts the pterygoid plates by crossing the pterygomaxillary junction. The Le Fort I osteotomy closely follows the fracture lines and produces separation of the maxilla and the palate.

The surgical incisions are made inside the mouth at the junction of the upper lip and the gum. The bony separation is accomplished with an oscillating saw. The maxilla may be mobilized as a whole or in two or more segments, depending on the anatomic indications, and may be adjusted anteriorly, posteriorly, inferiorly, or any variable combination of these directions, dictated by the presenting anatomic inadequacy. The maxilla is repositioned by several millimeters, then secured with titanium plates and screws. Typically, the duration of surgery is approximately 2.5 to 3.5 hours but may be longer depending on the number of maxillary segments created for the procedure. The patient's age may also contribute to the length of the procedure because of the density of bone that

must be transected. This procedure advances the midface to achieve a more aesthetically pleasing facial construction, as well as more efficient functionality of several facial structures, including dental occlusive alignment and nasal passages/airway. Frequently, this procedure may be completed in an office setting and/or an outpatient/ambulatory care setting.

Le Fort II Fracture/Osteotomy

The Le Fort II fracture forms a pyramidal shape that traverses the nasal bridge via the nasofrontal suture. The bone disruption crosses the maxillae via the frontal process, through the lacrimal bones, inferior orbital floor/rim, frequently through the orbital foramen, and finally through the anterior wall of the maxillary sinus. The base of the pyramid is formed as the fracture lines travel beneath the zygoma, traverse the pterygomaxillary fissure, and extend through the pterygoid plates.

The Le Fort II osteotomy is not commonly performed. Because of the nature of this surgical undertaking, it is reserved for patients in whom growth of the center of the face has been greatly deficient. The target patient is one in whom the facial redesign requires movement of the facial center, maxillae, and nose simultaneously. The Le Fort II osteotomy is a major surgical undertaking requiring surgical incisions in three locations: the junction of the upper lip and gum, a bicoronal incision (from ear to ear across the crown of the head), and either transconjunctival or blepharoplasty incisions. Scalp reflection and surgical manipulation of the nasal and facial bones results in significant blood loss. Blood transfusions may be required intraoperatively and/or postoperatively. Due to the extensive nature of the surgery, extreme bruising and edema are likely to occur. This is compounded by the high level of postoperative pain and potential for nausea and vomiting. Therefore, it is prudent for this patient to remain intubated and sedated and receive assisted or controlled mechanical ventilation for the first 24 hours or more.

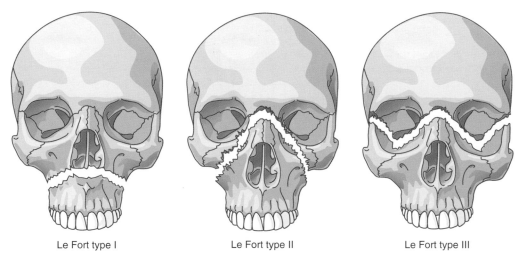

Le Fort type I   Le Fort type II   Le Fort type III

• **Fig. 45.2** Le Fort fractures. Le Fort type I, transverse fracture of the maxillary process from the base of the maxilla and midface. Le Fort type II, triangular fracture involving the entire maxilla and nasal bones. Le Fort type III, craniofacial-midface disassociation. (From Good VS, Kirkwood: *Advanced critical care nursing*, ed 2, St. Louis, 2018, Elsevier.)

Le Fort III Fracture/Osteotomy

The Le Fort III fracture produces separation of the face from the calvaria. As a result of the Le Fort III fracture, the skull has three "mobile" components—the calvaria, face, and mandible—rather than the normal two segments: the mandible and the skull. The Le Fort III fracture is also called *craniofacial dysjunction*. The Le Fort III begins in a fashion similar to the Le Fort II fracture: the nasofrontal and frontomaxillary sutures are separated, and the fracture traverses the medial orbit walls through the nasolacrimal groove and the ethmoid bone. Extension of the fracture line into the optical canals is generally prevented by the thick sphenoid bone. This results in fracture lines that traverse the orbital floor and across the lateral orbital wall via the zygomaticofrontal junction and zygomatic arch. The fracture lines are completed via the base of the ethmoid bone's perpendicular plate, through the vomer, and the sphenoid bone's pterygoid plates.

The Le Fort III procedure is reserved for patients with extremely deficient midfacial growth and development. This procedure is accomplished via incisional approaches described in the Le Fort II procedure. Other procedural aspects that are similar to the Le Fort II procedure include the extensive dissection required, the lengthy duration of the procedure, the high degree of bruising and edema, and the large blood loss that is frequently associated with potential for blood transfusions. As with the Le Fort II, this patient should remain intubated and sedated with assisted or controlled mechanical ventilation for at least the first 24 hours postoperatively. The potential complications that are associated with Le Fort osteotomies are listed in Box 45.1.

Mandibular Sagittal Split Osteotomy

In terms of complexity, the mandibular sagittal split osteotomy (MSSO) may be one of the "simpler" orthognathic procedures. This procedure involves incisions, usually two, at or near the third molars. These molars are frequently extracted about 6 months before this surgical procedure. The mandible is split bilaterally. The splits are the locations where a few millimeters of bone may be removed or added to produce the desired correction in mandible length. The splits are stabilized

in their new position using titanium plates and screws. The MSSO is the least time-consuming orthognathic procedure, usually requiring about 1.5 to 2.5 hours. Frequently, the MSSO is combined with various forms of the Le Fort I procedures to correct various facial growth disparities. Potential complications that are associated with an MSSO procedure and maxillofacial procedures are listed in Boxes 45.2 and 45.3.

Anesthetic Management and Considerations

Preoperative Period

1. *Identify the structural components that comprise the airway.*
   The airway begins within the face/facial skeleton. The airway originates at the external nares and vestibulum oris (mouth), through the nasal and oral cavities, continuing to the nasopharynx and oropharynx, then on to the larynx and glottis to enter the trachea. From the trachea, the airway divides into numerous subdivisions of the bronchial tree to culminate in the alveoli. Three concha or turbinates are present on the lateral walls of the nasal cavity opposite the nasal septum: superior, middle, and inferior. The superior and middle turbinates are formed from the ethmoid bone, while the inferior turbinate is an osseous formation that articulates with the ethmoid, lachrymal, maxillae, and palatine bones. These bony formations disrupt airflow and

---

• **BOX 45.1** **Potential Complications Associated With Le Fort Osteotomies**

- Arteriovenous fistulas
- Fractures to pterygoid plate, sphenoid bone, and middle cranial fossa
- Infraorbital nerve traction injury
- Lacrimal duct injury
- Stensen duct injury
- Velopharyngeal insufficiency
- Vascular necrosis
- Axillary sinusitis
- Nasal–septal buckling
- Nasal–septal deviation
- Ophthalmic duct injury

• **BOX 45.2** **Potential Complications Associated With Mandibular Sagittal Split Osteotomy**

- Avascular necrosis
- Inferior alveolar artery bleeding
- Mental nerve injury
- Proximal segment malposition
- Condylar resorption
- Gingival recession
- Unanticipated fractures
- Inferior mandibular border contour irregularity
- Masseteric artery bleeding
- Unfavorable sagittal split

• **BOX 45.3** **Potential Complications Associated With Maxillofacial Surgery**

- Bleeding
- Devitalization of teeth
- Gingival recession
- Hardware exposure
- Malocclusion
- Malunion/nonunion of bone
- Postoperative infection
- Respiratory decompensation
- Dental injury
- Unanticipated fractures

redirect air into the various sinuses within the facial skeleton. The turbulence that is created prolongs the time the air is in contact with the mucosa of the turbinates. As a result, there is increased moisture and heat as air moves into the lungs.

2. *List the important factors necessary to determine the airway management technique to be used for patients having maxillofacial surgery.*

Airway management for patients having maxillofacial surgery is dependent on the type of surgical procedure that will be performed. A discussion with the surgeon regarding the surgical requirements is imperative. Orthognathic procedures—those producing reshaping/resculpting of the bony structures of the face—require general anesthesia. Due to the nature and complexity of orthognathic procedures, airway management will require a nasal intubation.

3. *Describe the preparation process for nasotracheal intubation.*

Tracheal intubation via the nasal approach differs from the oral approach in that the anesthetist must prepare both nares before intubation. Factors that need to be assessed during the preoperative evaluation include:

- The amount of airflow via the nares/nasal passages
- Is one nare narrower than the other?
- Is the nasal septum deviated significantly in one direction?
- Does the patient perceive a restriction to inspiration or exhalation via the nasal passages?
- Does this patient have unilateral choanal atresia?

Despite the assessment to determine the degree of patency of the nasal passages, both nares should be prepared for endotracheal tube placement. Medications applied directly to the nasal mucosa produce vasoconstriction, which reduces the thickness of the mucosal tissue and decreases the potential for bleeding during intubation. This can be accomplished by using a decongestant nasal spray such as dilute phenylephrine, oxymetazoline nasal, a 4% cocaine solution, azelastine, ipratropium, or cromolyn nasal sprays. Utilizing a 4% cocaine solution offers the added action of anesthetizing the mucosal surfaces and local vasoconstriction.

Before nasotracheal intubation, the right or left nare that the anesthetist determines to be most patent should be further dilated using nasal airways. To help facilitate nasal intubation, it is reasonable to insert a nasal airway that is equal to or slightly larger than the endotracheal tube that will be placed. Nasal passage dilation can be done before entering the operating room, but insertion of the nasal airways may produce significant discomfort despite the use of the lidocaine jelly. Typically, dilation of the nasal passage is undertaken immediately after induction of anesthesia. Any of the three turbinates may be dislodged or injured during dilation or intubation, which will result in significant bleeding. The blood can obscure visualization during the direct laryngoscopy process and increase the risk of aspiration.

4. *Explain the importance of the "golden triangle" in relation to intubation for maxillofacial surgery.*

The "golden triangle" is the facial region outlined by the nose and a portion of the maxilla. The apex of the triangle originates at the frontonasal sutures with the base angles at or near the corners of the mouth. This area is nicknamed the "golden triangle" because it is a highly vascular region. The nose is central to this triangular area. As such, relatively mild trauma in this area can produce a seemingly disproportionate amount of bleeding. The anesthetist must be as gentle as possible during the insertion of nasal airways and the endotracheal tube to minimize the degree of trauma produced during endotracheal tube placement.

Intraoperative Period

5. *Identify the potential complications associated with nasal intubation.*

The most common complications associated with nasal intubation include epistaxis, turbinectomy, and dental trauma. If an unintended turbinectomy occurs during nasal dilation or intubation, blood will pool in the oropharynx and may obstructing the anesthetist's view of the epiglottis and glottis. The endotracheal tube may tamponade the nasal bleeding. However, after extubation, the bleeding can resume. This blood causes aspiration and may initiate a laryngospasm at the end of surgery.

One potential injury that may occur is a pressure injury to the forehead due to constant contact of the endotracheal tube connector. For this reason, during the process of securing the endotracheal tube, padding should be placed between the forehead and the universal connector. If a specialized nasal RAE tube is not used, the placement of a standard endotracheal tube can cause pressure on the nare and surrounding tissues, causing necrosis.

Cerebral injury is another rare but potential complication associated with nasal intubation for patients who have sustained a Le Fort II or Le Fort III fracture as a result of a traumatic injury. The cribriform plate separates the superior portion of the nasal cavity from the cranial vault. If it is damaged, placement of a nasogastric tube or endotracheal tube can result in direct neurotrauma. Nasal intubation is absolutely contraindicated for patients who have sustained these fractures.

6. *Discuss interventions that can be used to decrease blood loss during maxillofacial surgery.*

Due to the intricacy, complexity, and anatomic region associated with maxillofacial surgery, the amount of blood loss can range from 250 to 1500 mL. If the surgery requires bone grafting and the graft(s) are taken from the patient, then the iliac crest or ribs are frequently the preferential sites. The amount of blood loss may be increased as the result of the additional incisions and bone harvesting. Currently, there is no absolute hemoglobin value at which the patient should receive a transfusion. The decision to initiate a transfusion should be based on the patient's comorbid factors and anesthetic course. Blood should be made available for patients having moderate and major craniofacial surgical procedures. Methods that the anesthetist can employ to help decrease blood loss include:

- *Reverse Trendelenburg* positioning to facilitate venous drainage from the head.
- Maintain *normothermia* to preserve adequate platelet function.
- *Deliberate hypotension* can be employed to maintain the patient's mean arterial pressure (MAP) between 60 and 65 mm Hg. In patients who have cardiovascular or neurovascular insufficiency, coronary and cerebral perfusion as determined by autoregulation is increased. Therefore decreasing MAP to this degree may result in myocardial and/or cerebral ischemia/infarction.

Deliberate hypotension can be achieved by administering increased doses of anesthetic agents (narcotics, inhalation agents, propofol infusion), beta-blockers or vasodilators (nitroprusside infusion). A combination of medications is most frequently used.

Postoperative Period

7. *Identify strategies to reduce/prevent PONV for a patient having maxillofacial surgery.*

Retching, with or without vomiting, can disrupt the alignment of the jaw and increase bleeding. The patient's jaws may be secured together using either rubber bands or, less frequently, wires. The limited access increases the potential for aspiration of gastric contents. The anesthetist must balance the need to influence operative blood loss with efforts to reduce or eliminate PONV.

Hypotension, hypovolemia, and narcotic administration are all factors that contribute to the development of PONV. Interventions that can be used to prevent PONV

> **• BOX 45.4 Considerations Before Extubation**
>
> - Respiratory function
> - Return/presence of protective airway reflexes
> - Soft tissue edema
> - Surgical time
> - The presence of pathology
> - Hemodynamic stability
> - Intermaxillary fixation
> - Level of consciousness
> - Pain management requirements
> - Potential for postoperative bleeding

may entail administration of any of several different classes of medications such as gastrokinetic medications (metoclopramide), steroids (dexamethasone), 5-HT3-receptor antagonists (ondansetron or dolasetron), or combination of these medications. Other factors that should be assessed include the degree of hypovolemia that can be treated by administrating intravenous fluids and the presence of pain.

8. *Relate crucial factors to consider for extubation after maxillofacial surgery.*

A significant amount of facial and tracheal edema develops during extensive maxillofacial procedures due to fluids that have entered the interstitial space and from surgical trauma. Careful assessment of the degree of tracheal edema can be achieved by deflating the endotracheal tube cuff immediately before extubation to determine whether a leak occurs during a positive pressure breath. If tracheal edema is present or ventilation and intubation were difficult during the induction, it is prudent to keep the patient intubated. Airway management will almost certainly be more difficult or impossible postsurgically. Box 45.4 lists factors that should be considered before tracheal extubation.

Review Questions

1. Which is not a valid indication to perform an orthognathic procedure?
   a. Improved aesthetics
   b. Alleviation of obstructive sleep apnea
   c. Myofascial pain relief
   d. Temporal arteritis
2. Which description is indicative of a Le Fort II fracture?
   a. Disarticulation of the mandible at the temporomandibular joints
   b. Nasofrontal and frontomaxillary sutures are separated and the fracture traverses the medial orbit walls through the nasolacrimal groove
   c. Fracture forming a pyramidal shape that extends from above the nose and traverses the zygomatic arches
   d. Separation of the midfacial skeleton from the maxilla associated with sphenoid sinus disruption
3. Which intervention may reduce blood loss during maxillofacial surgery?
   a. Elevating the patient's head 15 degrees
   b. Maintaining hypothermia
   c. Maintaining normotension
   d. Decreasing the depth of anesthesia
4. Which complication is not associated with a nasal intubation?
   a. Turbinectomy
   b. Esophageal intubation
   c. Epistaxis
   d. Cranial intubation
5. Which is the most crucial reason to administer PONV prophylaxis for patients having maxillofacial surgery?
   a. Decreased/limited access to the patient's airway
   b. Excess blood loss
   c. Increased postoperative sedation
   d. Facial numbness

Suggested Readings

Chen CM, Lai S, Chen KK, Lee HE. Intraoperative hemorrhage and postoperative sequelae after intraoral vertical ramus osteotomy to treat mandibular prognathism. *Biomed Res Int* 2015;2015:318270.

Choi WS, Samman N. Risks and benefits of deliberate hypotension in anaesthesia: a systematic review. *Int J Oral Maxillofac Surg* 2008;37(8):687-703.

Dobbeleir M, De Coster J, Coucke W, Politis C. Postoperative nausea and vomiting after oral and maxillofacial surgery: a prospective study. *Int J Oral Maxillofac Surg* 2018;47(6):721-725.

Durão N, Amarante J. Osteosynthesis in the surgical treatment of prognathism: state of the art. *Acta Med Port* 2017;30(3):224-232.

Ghabach MB, Abou Rouphael MA, Roumoulian CE, Helou MR. Airway management in a patient with Le Fort III fracture. *Saudi J Anaesth* 2014;8(1):128-130.

Ghosh S, Rai KK, Shivakumar HR, et al. Incidence and risk factors for postoperative nausea and vomiting in orthognathic surgery: a 10-year retrospective study. *J Korean Assoc Oral Maxillofac Surg* 2020;46(2):116-124.

Gil CJ. Anesthesia for ear, nose, throat and maxillofacial surgery. In: Nagelhout JJ, Elisha S, eds. *Nurse Anesthesia,* 6th ed. St Louis, MO: Elsevier, 2018:904-934.

Kim SG, Park SS. Incidence of complications and problems related to orthognathic surgery. *J Oral Maxillofac Surg* 2007;65(12):2438-2444.

Krohner RG. Anesthetic considerations for oral and maxillofacial surgery. *Int Anesthesiol Clin* 2003;41(3):67-89.

Schwartz A. Airway management for the oral surgery patient. *Oral Maxillofac Surg Clin North Am* 2018;30(2):207-226.

46

Anterior Cervical Discectomy/Fusion

KEY POINTS

- Patients who require anesthesia for anterior cervical discectomy/fusion (ACDF) may be difficult or impossible to intubate due to the inability to place them in a "sniffing position" and properly align the oral, laryngeal, and pharyngeal axes.
- A comprehensive preoperative neurologic evaluation of the patient's sensory and motor function is imperative.

- There is the potential for damage to critical structures within the neck resulting from surgical trauma.
- Postoperative respiratory distress can occur due to unilateral recurrent laryngeal nerve injury, airway edema, hematoma, tracheal laceration, and pneumothorax.

Case Synopsis

A 45-year-old woman has paresthesias and numbness in the left shoulder, arm, and fingertips. Her electrocardiogram (ECG) and cardiac stress test are normal. The paresthesias and numbness are caused by cervical nerve compression, as shown on magnetic resonance imaging (MRI). She is scheduled for an ACDF by the neurosurgeon.

Perioperative Evaluation and Demographic Data

Past Medical/Surgical History

- Hypertension
- Hysterectomy

List of Medications

- Atenolol

Diagnostic Data

- Hemoglobin, 13.2 g/dL; hematocrit, 39.4%
- Electrolytes: sodium, 139 mEq/L; potassium, 3.9 Eq/L; chloride, 104 mEq/L; carbon dioxide, 24 mEq/L

Height/Weight/Vital Signs

- 168 cm, 65 kg
- Blood pressure, 135/70; heart rate, 61 beats per minute; respiratory rate, 18 breaths per minute; room air oxygen saturation, 98%; temperature, 36.8°C
- ECG: normal sinus rhythm; heart rate, 64 beats per minute
- Cardiac stress test (treadmill): within normal limits; no evidence of ischemia, infarction, or syncope during exertion

Pathophysiology

Adult men and women between the ages of 40 and 55 are most commonly affected by cervical degeneration as part of the aging process. However, degenerative changes are readily documented in many adults with radiography and MRI beginning about 30 years of age. Instability of the cervical disc can result from traumatic or destructive (neoplastic, degenerative, congenital) disruption of stabilizing elements (anterior and posterior longitudinal ligaments, pedicles, and articulations). It remains unclear why some patients have an increased risk of experiencing cervical spine deterioration and nerve compression.

Pain; weakness; paresthesias; and numbness of the neck, shoulder, arms, and hands are the result of a rupture or herniation of the annulus fibrosus of the disc. The annulus tears on the cervical disc, compressing the nerve root or spinal cord at the cervical level. The bulging of the disc allows the softer inner nucleus to compress the nerve root or spinal cord. Narrowing and compression of the nerves in the cervical region can also result from the formation of osteophytes (spondylosis) or congenital narrowing of the space (stenosis), and symptoms associated with disc degeneration will not occur until later in life, as shown in Fig. 46.1. A rupture or tear can be the result of age, degeneration, or traumatic injury. The cervical vertebrae are more susceptible to injury because of a greater range of motion, the small distance between the vertebrae, and the complexity of the anatomy in this region.

Although it is inexplicable why some patients are affected more than others, degenerative cervical disc disease is

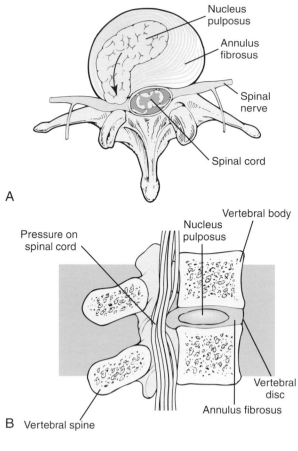

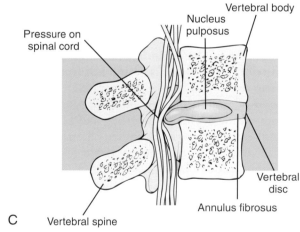

• **Fig. 46.1** Herniated disc. (A) Superior view of herniated disc. (B) Lateral view of bulging disc. (C) Lateral view of herniated disc. (From Frazier M, Drzymkowski J: *Essentials of human diseases and conditions*, ed 6, St Louis, 2016, Elsevier.)

thought to be the result of fibrous changes to the gelatinous disc resulting in less pliability. Degeneration occurs most commonly at the vertebral segments extending from C5–C7. The resulting cervical compression can hinder blood flow and result in narrowing of the cervical canal. The diminished blood flow can produce myelopathy and neural injury, which can be progressive and can result in permanent spinal cord damage if left untreated. Patients who have cervical degeneration can have further numbness, pain, or

irritation by flexion, extension, or rotation of the head and neck. Therefore even minimal manipulation of the head and neck could produce serious and/or permanent injury.

Conservative Treatment Options

Treatment options range from conservative and palliative to emergency surgical intervention. The conservative treatments include rest, use of nonsteroidal medications, cervical traction, physical therapy, pain medication, and instructional exercises used to strengthen the muscles of the neck, upper back, and shoulders. Some patients benefit from conservative treatment; however, patients who continue to experience pain and functional limitations are candidates for ACDF.

Surgical Procedure

The anterior approach is the most common surgical technique used for ACDF. A skin incision is made on the anterior aspect of the neck and then tissue is retracted to expose the anterior cervical spine. The surgical approach occurs between the esophagus and trachea medially and the sternocleidomastoid muscle and carotid sheath laterally. The omohyoid muscle and recurrent laryngeal nerve are retracted inferiorly. Handheld retractors or self-retaining retractors are utilized to provide initial exposure of the anterior vertebral column and the adjacent longus colli muscles. Tissue is removed from the disc to relieve the pressure that is exerted on the nerve root. After the discectomy, the vertebra is fused to the superior or inferior vertebra with bone, mechanical plates, and/or screws in order to prevent dislocation. The anatomy and muscles surrounding the cervical spine are included in Fig. 46.2.

Once removal of the disc occurs, there are several methods surgeons use in order to fill or secure the intervertebral space with instruments called *pituitaries, curettes,* and/or *Kerrison rongeurs.* These techniques use either an autograft (patient's bone) or allograft (cadaver bone) and are placed between the vertebral bodies. One such surgical method for ACDF is the Smith–Robinson technique. The bone graft is inserted into the disc space in order to maintain a neutral position, as shown in Fig. 46.3. Vertebral fusion results over time as the bone graft heals. However, the implantation of plates and screws provides additional vertebral stabilization, as shown in Fig. 46.4.

Surgical Complications

The most common complications resulting from ACDF surgery include:
- Thrombophlebitis
- Infection
- Nerve damage
- Graft inadequacy (migration, erosion, degradation)
- Nonunion of the cervical vertebrae
- Chronic pain

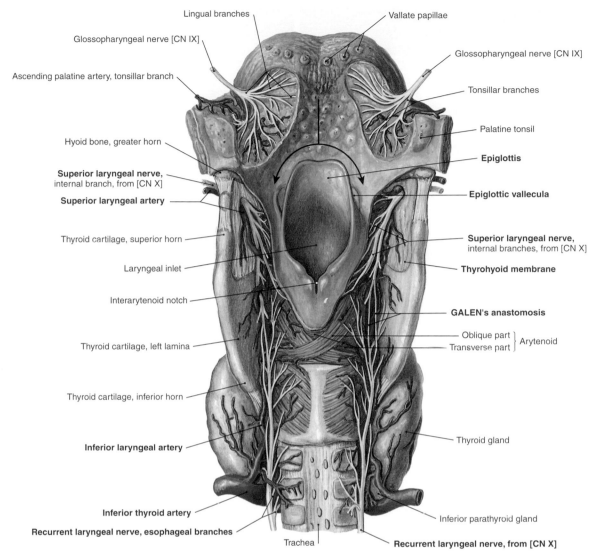

Lingual branches

Glossopharyngeal nerve [CN IX]

Ascending palatine artery, tonsillar branch

Hyoid bone, greater horn

Superior laryngeal nerve, internal branch, from [CN X]

Superior laryngeal artery

Thyroid cartilage, superior horn

Laryngeal inlet

Interarytenoid notch

Thyroid cartilage, left lamina

Thyroid cartilage, inferior horn

Inferior laryngeal artery

Inferior thyroid artery

Recurrent laryngeal nerve, esophageal branches

Trachea

Vallate papillae

Glossopharyngeal nerve [CN IX]

Tonsillar branches

Palatine tonsil

Epiglottis

Epiglottic vallecula

Superior laryngeal nerve, internal branches, from [CN X]

Thyrohyoid membrane

GALEN's anastomosis

Oblique part ⎫
Transverse part ⎭ Arytenoid

Thyroid gland

Inferior parathyroid gland

Recurrent laryngeal nerve, from [CN X]

• **Fig. 46.2** Anterior view of anatomy and muscles of the neck covering the cervical spine. (From Hombach-Klonisch S, Klonisch T, Peeler J: *Sobotta clinical atlas of human anatomy*, Munich, 2019, Urban & Fischer.)

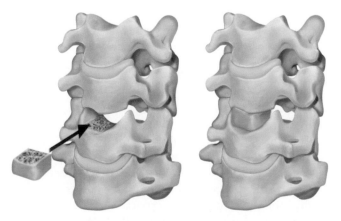

• **Fig. 46.3** Placement of the graft between vertebrae. (From Kim DH, Vaccaro AR, Dickman CA, et al: *Surgical anatomy & techniques to the spine*, ed 2, St. Louis, 2013, Elsevier.)

Anesthetic Management and Considerations

Preoperative Period

1. *Discuss the coexisting diseases that are associated with patients presenting for ACDF.*

   A thorough preoperative evaluation is a standard of care, and it is one of the most important components of providing anesthesia for any patient. Specific information and documentation of symptoms should include the following: sensory and motor function and factors that cause an exacerbation of the symptoms. There is also the potential for gastric immobility caused by parasympathetic and sympathetic dysfunction that occurs at the level of the cervical vertebra.

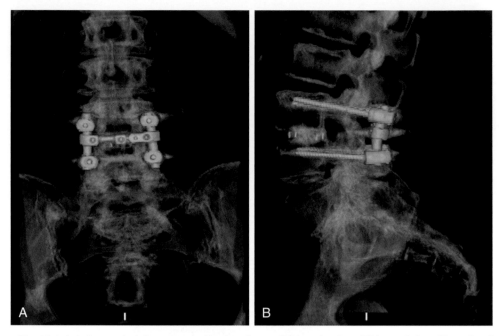

• **Fig. 46.4** Anterior cervical discectomy with plate fixator. **(A)** Anterior view. **(B)** Lateral view. (From Small JE, Noujaim DL, Ginat DT, et al: *Neuroradiology: Spectrum and evolution of disease*, St. Louis, 2019, Elsevier.)

The type and amount of medications that are used to treat pain should be investigated to determine the extent of the patient's perceived discomfort and the potential for increased anesthetic requirements due to the development of functional and/or dispositional tolerance. Patients should remain on their current pain medication regimen until the morning of surgery. Abrupt withdrawal of narcotics for patients with severe pain will increase sympathetic nervous system innervation, leading to tachycardia, hypertension, and seizure activity.

2. *Describe the importance of a thorough assessment of the patient's cardiovascular function before ACDF surgery.*

Anesthesia and surgery can cause significant hemodynamic variability throughout the perioperative period. Optimizing the patient's cardiac status before the day of surgery is necessary to decrease the possibility of cardiovascular dysfunction, which includes labile blood pressure, dysrhythmias, myocardial ischemia, myocardial infarction, and heart failure.

This patient has a history of hypertension, which is being treated with atenolol. She states that she takes her medication every day, and she was instructed to take her atenolol the day of surgery. The ECG that was obtained during exertion showed that by increasing heart rate and myocardial oxygen demand, coronary artery reserve (supply) was sufficient and there was no evidence of ischemia, infarction, or syncope.

3. *Explain the anesthetic concerns related to airway management and ACDF surgery.*

Airway assessment is vitally important for all patients having anesthesia; however, there are added concerns for patients having ACDF surgery. If the patient has sustained a traumatic injury or if it is determined that the cervical spine is unstable, the patient may be placed in an external fixation device. Prophylactic neck immobilization and/or traction using the in-line manual axial stabilization technique may be necessary during airway management. In this circumstance, elevating the patient's head to achieve a "sniffing" position is absolutely contraindicated. In a nonacute situation, certain movements of the neck may cause an exacerbation of the existing symptoms or cervical nerve root and/or spinal cord damage. Positioning the patient's head before the anesthetic induction allows the anesthetist to ensure that the position does not cause pain in the neck or in the arms, which is indicative of pressure on the brachial plexus. Care must be taken not to move the neck or head far from the position that was comfortable. The less extension and manipulation of the neck, the less likely injury to the cervical spine during airway management and surgery will occur. The anesthetist must be cautious with neck mobility and airway management with all patients who have had previous ACDF surgery. Alternative plans for ventilation and intubation must be available for patients who have either acute or nonacute cervical spine injuries.

A meticulous preoperative examination assessing the mobility of the neck, ability to open the mouth, and feasibility of intubation should be considered before the anesthetic induction. The application of cricoid pressure is controversial and should be initiated with caution, as downward pressure of the cricoid ring in order to occlude the esophagus against the cervical vertebrae can cause neurologic damage. Administration of succinylcholine is contraindicated for patients with chronic myopathies that result in muscle wasting. Proliferation of extrajunctional acetylcholine receptors occurs, and due to the depolarizing effects of succinylcholine, this response may result in severe hyperkalemia that is life threatening.

Regional anesthesia can be used to supplement anesthesia for ACDF, but the use of this technique does not provide adequate anesthetic and surgical conditions. Retraction of the trachea and the esophagus is extremely stimulating; therefore general anesthesia is the technique of choice for ACDF. A superficial and deep cervical plexus block provides analgesia during the intraoperative and postoperative period.

Intraoperative Period

4. *Describe the importance of proper positioning for patients having ACDF.*

The patient's arms are most frequently tucked at their sides to allow for adequate surgical access. Proper patient positioning and padding must occur before the surgical incision because it will be more difficult to assess pressure on the bony prominence during the surgical procedure. Ensuring that the arms are abducted less than 90 degrees and that all pressure points are padded decreases the potential for nerve injury.

A gel roll is frequently placed under the shoulders by the surgeon to hyperextend the neck and to maximize the surgical exposure. The patient's head should be properly supported to decrease the pressure exerted on the cervical vertebrae and the patient's occiput. Careful positioning of the endotracheal tube, which should be shifted to the corner of the mouth contralateral to the incision and free from traction, is suggested.

5. *Describe the monitoring considerations and techniques used for the ACDF patient.*

Neurologic monitoring may be used during the ACDF, but these techniques are not commonly employed during an anterior approach in the neck because nerve roots are more readily identifiable compared with the posterior approach. If neurologic monitoring is to be used, the anesthetist should discuss the anesthetic plan with the surgeon and the neurophysiologist so that the anesthetic management and interdisciplinary communication can be optimized.

- **Somatosensory evoked potentials (SSEPs)** are sensitive to the neurologic depressant effects of the inhalation agents at a concentration of >0.5% (volume percent) of the minimal alveolar concentration (MAC). Typically, 0.5 MAC of any volatile agent with the addition of 50% nitrous oxide decreases the amplitude and increases the latency of the SSEP waveforms, which can produce unreliable results. Intravenous anesthetic medications such as narcotics do not affect the evoked potential waveform to the extent associated with the inhalation agents. Thus total intravenous anesthesia (TIVA) can be used as an alternative anesthetic technique. Because SSEP monitoring is used to assess the dorsal or posterior sensory

component of spinal cord transmission, paralytics will not adversely affect the evoked potential.

- **Motor evoked potentials (MEPs)** can be used to assess the integrity of the ventral or anterior portion of the spinal cord during ACDF. MEPs are not affected by the inhalation or intravenous anesthetic agents; however, MEPs are affected by neuromuscular blocking agents. Incomplete paralysis as assessed by the neuromuscular blocking monitor, train of four ratio of 3 out of 4, can allow for adequate monitoring of MEPs. Frequently, SSEP and MEP monitoring are used in conjunction to simultaneously assess the ascending (SSEP) and descending (MEP) neural pathways.

6. *Examine the fluid requirements necessary for patients having ACDF.*

The estimated blood loss that is most often associated with ACDF is less than 50 L. However, due to the proximity of major arterial and venous structures to the surgical site, there is the potential for significant bleeding. If a large amount of blood loss is anticipated, autologous blood infusion, cell saver blood salvage, and normovolemic hemodilution are all methods that can be employed.

Intraoperative and postoperative tissue swelling surrounding the surgical site is always a concern during ACDF procedures. Excessive administration of fluid should be avoided because it will increase edema formation and increase the possibility of developing superior vena cava syndrome. For procedures that exceed 2 hours, a urinary catheter is indicated to assess urine output and to avoid bladder distention. Intravenous fluids that contain glucose should be avoided because if periods of neurologic ischemia occur, increased lactic acid is produced during anaerobic metabolism.

7. *Describe the anesthetic and surgical complications associated with ACDF.*

Acute spinal cord injury can occur during ACDF as a result of inadvertent pressure, edema formation, or partial or complete disruption. The most severe circumstance that can occur is rapidly developing spinal shock. Efferent sympathetic nervous system impulse transmission will not occur to organ systems below the level of the cervical spinal cord trauma. This will result in parasympathetic nervous system predominance and manifest as bradycardia and vasodilation, causing hypotension and heat loss. The treatment for acute neurogenic shock includes administration of intravenous fluids, vasopressors, and forced-air warming. Invasive monitoring such as an arterial line and central venous pressure catheter should be used to guide fluid therapy.

- **Major vascular injury** can occur as a result of surgical trauma to major vasculature in the neck region, including the internal and external jugular veins, superior and inferior thyroid artery, or carotid artery. Blood loss can be rapid and extensive. If the carotid artery is damaged, the potential for acute dissection and emboli formation increases the potential for a

- Acute spinal cord injury
- Spinal nerve injury
- Dural tear
- Anterior spinal artery syndrome
- Hematoma
- Venous air embolism
- Airway edema
- Unilateral recurrent laryngeal nerve injury
- Pneumothorax
- Superior vena cava syndrome
- Hemorrhage
- Vascular injury
- Tracheal laceration

stroke. The anesthetist should be acutely aware of the potential for postoperative hematoma formation and airway compromise if vascular injury has occurred.

- **Airway compromise** can result from unilateral recurrent laryngeal nerve damage and hematoma formation, which impinges on the trachea; airway edema; and tracheal laceration. The degree of airway and tracheal edema can be directly assessed via fiber-optic examination or indirectly by performing a leak test. The endotracheal tube cuff is deflated, and positive pressure breaths are administered to determine if an air leak occurs. This should be accomplished before the endotracheal tube is removed. If an air leak does not exist, then the patient should not be extubated. If intubation is initially difficult, then extubation can be performed over an Eschmann stylet or a tube exchanger so that immediate reintubation is possible. Lastly, if the surgical procedure was prolonged and associated with excessive traction, it may be most prudent for the patient to remain intubated. A complete list of complications that can occur during the perioperative management of patients having ACDF is included in Box 46.1.

Postoperative Period

Two hours after the surgical procedure is complete, the surgeon calls you from the intensive care units and she states that this patient is having difficulty swallowing. She also has a hematoma at the surgical site. The patient is scheduled for an emergent neck exploration.

8. *Discuss the various airway management techniques that can be safely used in this situation.*

The major focus of this scenario revolves around the potential for the patient to rapidly develop respiratory distress and respiratory arrest due to compression of the trachea by the hematoma. A hematoma can occur rapidly after the neck incision is closed or slowly over a period of hours as blood is sequestered into the tissues. Because there is very little room for blood to exist within tissue planes adjacent to the neck, a small amount of blood can cause severe tracheal impingement. Additionally, tracheal deviation can occur without the presence of a large hematoma that is assessed externally. The definitive and initial intervention to resolve this situation is to have the surgeon remove the sutures and evacuate the hematoma.

There is no single airway management technique that is absolutely contraindicated in this scenario. It is possible that even if a complete view of the glottic opening was visualized during induction that the hematoma has dramatically shifted the anatomic airway structures so that visualization is difficult or impossible. A supraglottic device such as a laryngeal mask airway or mask ventilation may not be an effective method to maintain a patent airway. A fiber-optic intubation may prove challenging if edema and blood are present. Additionally, anesthetizing the airway with nebulized lidocaine can cause complete airway collapse, and maintaining spontaneous respirations is important. Lastly, tracheotomy placement as the initial method for establishing the airway is also an option. Having the supplies and ability to perform an emergency tracheotomy is vital.

Review Questions

1. A symptom that is associated with cervical disc herniation includes:
   a. Dilated pupils.
   b. Paresthesias occurring in the shoulder and neck.
   c. Lower back pain.
   d. Frequent headaches.
2. Which of the following interventions is not appropriate for a patient who has sustained an acute cervical spine injury?
   a. Fiber-optic intubation
   b. "Sniffing" position
   c. Awake intubation
   d. In-line manual axial stabilization
3. Which sign is associated with acute neurogenic shock?
   a. Hypertension
   b. Hyperthermia
   c. Bradycardia
   d. Hypocarbia
4. Which regional anesthetic technique can be administered to decrease postoperative pain after ACDF?
   a. Cervical plexus block
   b. Transtracheal block
   c. Intercostal nerve block
   d. Superior laryngeal nerve block
5. There is an increased risk of stroke from emboli entering the brain associated with damage to the:
   a. Internal jugular vein.
   b. Inferior thyroid artery.
   c. External jugular vein.
   d. Carotid artery.

Suggested Readings

Badhiwala JH, Nassiri F, Witiw CD, et al. Investigating the utility of intraoperative neurophysiological monitoring for anterior cervical discectomy and fusion: analysis of over 140,000 cases from the National (Nationwide) Inpatient Sample data set. *J Neurosurg Spine* 2019;31(1):76-86.

Banoub M. Pharmacologic and physiologic influences affecting sensory evoked potentials: implications for perioperative monitoring. *Anesthesiology* 2003;99(3):716-737.

Bovonratwet P, Fu MC, Tyagi V, et al. Incidence, risk factors, and clinical implications of postoperative hematoma requiring reoperation following anterior cervical discectomy and fusion. *Spine* 2019;44(8):543-549.

Hirsch MT. Anesthesia for orthopedics and podiatry. In: Nagelhout JJ, Elisha S, eds. *Nurse Anesthesia*, 6th ed. St Louis, MO: Elsevier, 2018:946-958.

Imani F, Jafarian A, Hassani V, et al. Propofol-alfentanil vs propofol-remifentanil for posterior spinal fusion including wake-up test. *Br J Anaesth* 2006;96(5):583-586.

Kashkoush A, Mehta A, Agarwal N, et al. Perioperative neurological complications following anterior cervical discectomy and fusion: clinical impact on 317,789 patients from the National Inpatient Sample. *World Neurosurg* 2019;128:e107-e115.

Kelly MP, Eliasberg CD, Riley MS, Ajiboye RM, SooHoo NF. Reoperation and complications after anterior cervical discectomy and fusion and cervical disc arthroplasty: a study of 52,395 cases. *Eur Spine J* 2018;27(6):1432-1439.

Kim M, Rhim SC, Roh SW, Jeon SR. Analysis of the risk factors associated with prolonged intubation or reintubation after anterior cervical spine surgery. *J Korean Med Sci* 2018;33(17):e77.

Lin CK, Feng YT, Hwang SL, et al. A comparison of propofol target controlled infusion-based and sevoflurane-based anesthesia in adults undergoing elective anterior cervical discectomy and fusion. *J Med Sci* 2015;31(3):150-5.

Ma Z, Ma X, Yang H, Guan X, Li X. Anterior cervical discectomy and fusion versus cervical arthroplasty for the management of cervical spondylosis: a meta-analysis. *Eur Spine J* 2017;26(4):998-1008.

Pajewski TN, Arlet V, Phillips LH. Current approach on spinal cord monitoring: the point of view of the neurologist, the anesthesiologist and the spine surgeon. *Eur Spine J* 2007;16:S115–S129.

Smith PN, Balzer JR, Khan MH, et al. Intraoperative somatosensory evoked potential monitoring during anterior cervical discectomy and fusion in nonmyelopathic patients—a review of 1,039 cases. *Spine J* 2007;7(1):83-87.

Wang H, Ma L, Yang D, Cervical plexus anesthesia versus general anesthesia for anterior cervical discectomy and fusion surgery: a randomized clinical trial. *Medicine (Baltimore)* 2017;96(7):6119.

Wilson LA, Fiasconaro M, Poeran J, et al. The impact of anesthesia and surgical provider characteristics on outcomes after spine surgery. *Eur Spine J* 2019;28(9):2112-2121.

Wilson LA, Zubizarreta N, Bekeris J, et al. Risk factors for reintubation after anterior cervical discectomy and fusion surgery: evaluation of three observational data sets. *Can J Anaesth* 2020;67(1):42-56.

47
Posterior Spinal Reconstructive Surgery

KEY POINTS

- A comprehensive preoperative examination is vital in order to determine an individualized plan of care before posterior spinal reconstructive surgery.
- Correct prone positioning can decrease the possibility of nerve injury, decrease intraoperative blood loss, and decrease the possibility of postoperative visual impairment.
- Due to the potential for severe hemorrhage, serial hemoglobin and hematocrit values should be obtained, and various techniques for intraoperative blood salvage should be available.
- Cerebral and coronary artery autoregulation must be considered when providing deliberate hypotensive technique.

- A venous air embolism (VAE) can occur during posterior spinal reconstructive surgery as air is entrained into the complex venous network surrounding the spinal cord.
- The integrity of the sensory or dorsal aspect of the spinal cord can be continuously assessed using somatosensory evoked potentials (SSEPs).
- Anesthetic agents used for maintenance of general anesthesia increase latency and decrease amplitude during SSEP monitoring.

Case Synopsis

A 14-year-old girl has adolescent idiopathic scoliosis (AIS), which limits her functional ability and is also physiologically compromising. She is scheduled by her orthopedic surgeon to have posterior spinal reconstructive surgery.

Preoperative Evaluation and Demographic Data

Past Medical/Surgical History

- Scoliosis with decreased functional limitations
- Asthma

List of Medications

- Albuterol as needed
- Prednisone

Diagnostic Data

- Hemoglobin,17.8 g/dL; hematocrit, 53%
- Glucose: 88 mg/dL; blood urea nitrogen (BUN), 15 mg/dL; creatinine, 1.0 mg/dL
- Electrolytes: sodium, 139 mEq/L; potassium, 4.0 mEq/L; chloride, 104 mEq/L; bicarbonate, 20 mEq/L
- Cobb angle of 80 degrees from T9–L3; the curvature is convex toward the patient's right side
- Arterial blood gas (ABG): pH, 7.36; PCO_2, 33 mm Hg; PaO_2, 76 mm Hg; HCO_3, 21 mEq/L; base excess, 1.8; room air oxygen saturation, 94%

- Pulmonary function test (PFT): forced expiratory volume (FEV_1), 60% of predicted; FEV_1/FVC, 90% of predicted
- Chest x-ray: there is significant overcrowding of the left ribs and a mechanical decrease in lung span of the right lung. A gross estimate of the bone density is normal without evidence of obvious cortical thickness to medullary cavity disproportion. There are no cardiac hypertrophy, masses, air, or fluid collections.
- Electrocardiogram (ECG): normal sinus rhythm; heart rate, 92 beats per minute; ejection fraction, 55%

Height/Weight/Vital Signs

- 163 cm, 58 kg
- Blood pressure, 122/78; heart rate, 94 beats per minutes; respiratory rate, 22 breaths per minute; room air oxygen saturation, 96%; temperature, 36.9°C

Pathophysiology

Spinal reconstructive surgery is performed to correct a curvature that occurs to the spinal column. There are gradations of spinal column deformation, which range from minor to severe. Minor deformations may be improved by the use of an external bracing device. Moderate to severe curvatures are frequently treated utilizing surgical interventions and can limit functions of activities of daily living, affect normal lung development, and alter cardiac and respiratory status. Identifying scoliosis before adolescent growth is vital because the primary vertebral curvature can become more

• BOX 47.1 **Pathophysiologic Conditions Associated With Patients Presenting for Spinal Reconstructive Surgery**

- Muscular dystrophy
- Cerebral palsy
- Spina bifida
- Congenital heart disease
- Gastroesophageal reflux
- Dwarfism
- Myasthenia gravis

severe. In most instances, scoliosis is idiopathic, and it occurs approximately six times more frequently in women than in men. However, there may be a familial genetic predisposition for scoliosis. Other causes of scoliosis include neuromuscular pathology, myopathy, congenital, and spinal column instability. Pathologic conditions associated with scoliosis are included in Box 47.1.

Scoliosis, a lateral curvature of the spine, can be present in both the lumbar and thoracic vertebrae. In addition to the lateral curvature, the vertebrae are malrotated, and thus the ribs can cause impingement on the lung pleura, resulting in inadequate lung development, restrictive lung disease, pulmonary hypertension, and respiratory insufficiency. The alterations that occur to respiratory dynamics include ventilation–perfusion mismatch, decreased vital capacity, decreased expiratory reserve volume, decreased total lung capacity, decreased functional residual capacity, and increased residual volume. Fig. 47.1 depicts scoliosis with thoracic cage involvement.

The severity of scoliosis and degree of functional limitation are routinely quantified by assessing the Cobb angle from an x-ray. Because an x-ray only shows an anterior and posterior view, there are limitations when diagnosing the degree of lateral rotation of individual vertebrae. A Cobb angle of 10 to 15 degrees indicates a minor deformity and, frequently, there is no functional limitation. An angle measuring between 20 and 40 degrees is initially treated using an external bracing device. Treatment for a curvature between 40 and 50 degrees is controversial; however, experts agree that a Cobb angle of ≥50 degrees warrants surgical correction. Respiratory function and vital capacity are significantly decreased for patients who have a Cobb angle greater than 90 degrees, which results in hypoxemia and hypercarbia. Patients with a Cobb angle ≥30 degrees are at risk for postoperative respiratory insufficiency.

In patients with congenital scoliosis, the malformation of the thoracic cage can inhibit normal lung development. As a result of hypoxemia, hypoxic pulmonary vasoconstriction increases pulmonary vascular resistance, which causes increased right ventricular workload. Concentric hypertrophy can occur from pressure overload that, if untreated, will result in right ventricular dysfunction and eventual failure. Additionally, hypoxemia and hypercarbia increase sympathetic nervous system activation, thereby increasing systemic vascular resistance, central catecholamine release, and myocardial

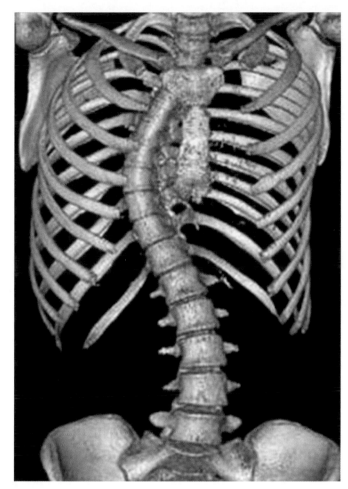

• **Fig. 47.1** Spinal column deformity with associated rib cage abnormality associated with severe scoliosis. (Adapted from Chun EM, Suh SW, Modi HN, et al: The change in ratio of convex and concave lung volume in adolescent idiopathic kyphoscoliosis, *European Spine Journal* 17:224-229, 2008.)

workload. If the vertebral curvature is angled toward the patient's left side, the heart and mediastinal structures can be shifted caudad, which can cause cardiomegaly if pulmonary hypertension or a right ventricular outflow tract obstruction is present.

Numerous physiologic syndromes are associated with patients who have scoliosis, including muscular dystrophy, cerebral palsy, spina bifida, congenital heart disease, gastroesophageal reflux, dwarfing syndrome, and myasthenia gravis. A thorough review of the patient's medical history and comprehensive preoperative examination are necessary to develop an individualized anesthetic plan of care.

Surgical Procedure

The goal of spinal reconstruction surgery is to straighten the spine, achieve improved balance between the torso and pelvis, and maintain surgical correction. However, disadvantages to traditional surgical correction include vertebral fusion resulting in decreased mobility; inhibition of the normal growth process, which can lead to truncal deformity and decreased pulmonary maturation; and chronic pain. For this reason, surgical correction of scoliosis is best attempted before complete skeletal development.

The type of surgical correction performed is dependent on the patient's pathophysiology and the surgeon's experience and preference. The instrumentation that is implanted will cause vertebral fusion within 1-year post-procedure. The hardware can be removed after this time if the patient develops chronic back pain. If a posterior surgical approach is chosen, a midline incision is made from the midthoracic to lower lumbar vertebrae. Once the vertebrae are exposed, pedicle hooks or screws are secured to the lateral aspects of the vertebrae. Pedicle screws are associated with improved surgical correction and improved postoperative pulmonary function. The pedicle hooks or screws anchor the rods that are placed on both sides of the vertebral column. The rods are inserted and then manipulated to cause tension or distract the vertebrae. Distraction causes stimulation and expansion of the growth plate, a phenomenon named the *Hueter–Volkmann principle*. In the past, the gold standard for spinal instrumentation was Harrington rods. Presently, there are numerous other manufacturers of hardware used for posterior spinal instrumentation.

Anterior spinal fusion involves a transthoracic and possibly retroperitoneal approach to the spinal column. Removal of the vertebral discs and implantation of instrumentation occur. Because this approach involves a flank incision, rib resection, and major body cavity intrusion, there is a potential for rapidly occurring massive hemorrhage. There is a need for preferential ventilation of one lung, and therefore a double-lumen endotracheal tube (ETT) is necessary. It has not been definitively determined that anterior spinal fusion yields improved results compared with posterior spinal fusion for adolescents with idiopathic scoliosis.

With the development of minimally invasive surgical procedures, emerging technology and improved techniques result in decreased surgical trauma, decreased blood loss, and equivalent or superior outcomes. Using an anterior vertebral approach using video-assisted thoracoscopic instruments to place large nitinol staples, inserting vertebral bone anchors with flexible ligament tethers, and implanting "growing rods" (which can be elongated and distracted using an external remote control device) are all being investigated as potential future treatment modalities used to treat scoliosis.

Anesthetic Management and Considerations

Preoperative Period

1. *Define the pertinent preoperative assessment data for posterior spinal reconstructive surgery.*
   - **Neurologic:** A thorough neurologic examination of both motor and sensory functioning of the upper and lower extremities is imperative in order to be able to accurately assess limitations that can occur as a result of the surgical procedure and prone positioning. This patient does not have upper or lower body motor or sensory deficits.
   - **Respiratory:** PFT was completed, and her results are indicative of restrictive lung disease. Restrictive lung disease can be divided into two categories: intrinsic, which involves lung parenchyma, or extrinsic, caused by thoracic cage deformation, inadequate respiratory muscle function, or pleural disease. The results of the PFT are estimated by comparing a patient's performance to the performance of healthy subjects who are the same age, weight, and gender. In patients with restrictive lung disease, all measured lung volumes are decreased. FEV_1 is the volume of gas that is forcibly exhaled in 1 second. A normal FEV_1 is 80% of predicted; however, this patient's FEV_1 is only 60%. Forced vital capacity (FVC) is the total volume of gas that is forcibly exhaled in one breath. A normal FEV_1/FVC ratio is 80%, and this patient's ratio is 90%, indicating similar small volumes for both FEV_1 and FVC. A low FEV_1 and a normal or increased FEV_1/FVC ratio is indicative of restrictive lung disease. Decreased FRC and ventilation–perfusion mismatch increase the risk for rapid intraoperative desaturation. Due to the loss of elastic properties of the lungs, vigilant monitoring of peak airway pressures is essential to avoid barotrauma during mechanical ventilation. Furthermore, lung function does not improve dramatically during the postoperative period. The anesthetist and postanesthesia recovery unit staff must be aware of the potential for respiratory distress and failure.

     Her ABG results are indicative of compensated respiratory alkalosis. Her Cobb angle is severe, causing an extrinsic restrictive respiratory defect. Due to the inadequacy of ventilation as evidenced by low PaO_2, there is a compensatory increase in minute ventilation primarily caused by increasing respiratory rate. This results in a low $PaCO_2$. Notice that the low HCO_3 and negative base excess are indicative of compensated respiratory alkalosis.
   - **Cardiovascular:** The patient's ECG shows normal sinus rhythm and near-normal ejection fraction as measured by echocardiography. There is no evidence of cardiac hypertrophy or cardiomegaly on the chest x-ray.
   - **Hematologic:** Her hemoglobin and hematocrit levels indicate polycythemia related to chronic hypoxia.
   - **Endocrine:** The patient is taking prednisone on a regular basis to decrease symptoms associated with bronchial asthma. Knowing that this surgical procedure will cause severe physiologic stress, it is prudent to administer hydrocortisone 100 mg intravenously before surgery to avoid the possibility of acute adrenal crises. The anesthetist should be aware of the possibility of hyperreactive airway during the perioperative period. Her lungs should be auscultated preoperatively, and bronchodilators should be used as needed.

- **Musculoskeletal:** This patient does not have musculoskeletal pathology. Scoliosis is associated with Duchenne muscular dystrophy and spina bifida. Duchenne muscular dystrophy is associated with malignant hyperthermia. In patients with spinal bifida who self-catheterize, there is the potential for the patient to develop a latex allergy.

Intraoperative Period

2. *Summarize the importance of proper prone positioning relative to anatomic and physiologic implications.*

- **Cardiovascular:** During prone positioning, it is important to minimize pressure on the abdomen because pressure on the vena cava and other venous structures will contribute to venous stasis in the lower body and could result in thrombus formation. Also, venous compression will decrease venous return to the heart and cause engorgement of the epidural venous plexus that increases intraoperative blood loss. Due to the long duration of spinal reconstructive surgery, patients frequently develop periorbital, facial, and airway edema.
- **Respiratory:** Chest excursion is decreased, which can result in increased peak inspiratory pressure, decreased FRC, atelectasis, and increased ventilation–perfusion mismatch, which can result in decreased oxygen saturation. For this reason, chest rolls must be positioned properly to minimize pressure on the anterior thoracic cage. Abdominal compression displaces the diaphragm cephalad, further decreasing FRC and thoracic cage expansion. The anesthetist should recheck for equal bilateral and clear breath sounds after the prone position is achieved.

  Before extubation, assessment of the degree of airway edema can be accomplished by direct visualization with a fiber-optic scope, and the patient can be extubated over an ETT exchanger in the event that emergent reintubation is necessary. The decision to extubate the patient upon termination of the surgical procedure must be individualized to the patient. However, if the patient has compromised lung function before surgery; the duration of the procedure is prolonged; an anterior approach is performed; or an extreme volume of crystalloid, colloid, and blood is administered, the patient should remain intubated postoperatively and weaned from artificial ventilation over a 12-hour period.
- **Thoracic outlet syndrome:** Impingement on the nerves that comprise the brachial plexus and the subclavian artery between the first rib and the clavicle can cause permanent nerve damage and decreased perfusion to the arm. Preoperative assessment for the presence of thoracic outlet syndrome is accomplished by having the patient extend their arms above their head. If patients develop paresthesias in their hands or decreased quality of their radial pulses, their arms should be placed at their side throughout the intraoperative period.

- **Intraoperative blindness:** Postoperative visual loss (POVL) can range from partial visual loss to permanent and complete blindness. POVL results from ischemic optic neuropathy (ION). The exact mechanism by which ION occurs has not been conclusively determined. However, possible reasons include extraocular compression, decreased ocular nerve perfusion from microemboli, anemia, and edema formation. Methods to decrease the possibility of POVL include:
  1. Ensuring that there is no pressure on both eyes throughout the procedure, as well as maintenance of the head in a neutral position.
  2. Maintenance of adequate mean arterial pressure (MAP). There is no one specific MAP that will ensure adequate cerebral perfusion pressure. Also, coronary and cerebral autoregulatory pressures are increased in patients with cardiovascular pathology.
  3. An adequate amount of hemoglobin is necessary to facilitate oxygen delivery to peripheral tissues. There is no single minimum hemoglobin value that has been implicated with POVL.
  4. Crystalloids are frequently administered as a component of volume replacement therapy. With judicious use of crystalloids, edema formation can cause ION. It is possible that anemia coupled with edema of the optic nerve can result in a higher incidence of ION.
  5. Peripheral vasoconstriction associated with the use of phenylephrine can further decrease optic nerve perfusion.
- **Miscellaneous concerns:** All joints, including the fingers, hands, elbows, knees, ankles, and toes, as well as genitalia, must be padded and free of continual pressure. Axillary rolls must not impinge on the axillary arteries, and bilateral radial pulses should be palpable. The patient's arms must not be abducted greater than 90 degrees in order to avoid a brachial plexus injury. Specialty positioning devices such as Relton and Wilson frames are used to keep the patient's thorax off of the operating table. Carefully securing the ETT is essential because saliva can decrease the adhesiveness of tape over time. Using a reinforced ETT will decrease the chance of kinking during intraoperative management.

3. *List monitoring equipment that is used during spinal reconstructive surgery.*

  Application of standard monitoring equipment such as pulse oximetry, blood pressure, end tidal carbon dioxide ($ETCO_2$) analysis, and five-lead ECG is used. An esophageal stethoscope will allow for continuous auscultation of breath sounds as well as a core temperature monitor. A urinary catheter is inserted to drain the bladder and to assess volume status. A urine output of 1 to 2 mL/kg/hr is considered ideal. An arterial line is necessary in order to continuously assess blood pressure variability as a result of changes in anesthetic depth, deliberate hypotensive technique, and loss of intravascular volume. Additionally, serial ABG samples can be drawn. The choice to use central venous pressure monitoring should be determined by the patient's physical status. Pulmonary artery catheter placement and monitoring are not indicated for routine use.

4. *Explain various strategies used to maintain adequate hemoglobin levels.*

The estimated blood loss during spinal reconstructive surgery is highly variable, and it is dependent on several factors, including preoperative coagulation status, type of surgical correction, experience of the surgeon, and amount of volume replacement. However, the anesthetist must be prepared to treat rapid and severe hemorrhage. A minimum of two large-bore intravenous lines must be available. Fluid, blood, and blood products are infused through a fluid warming system. Strategies that can be used to preserve hemoglobin include:

- Deliberate hypotension (refer to discussion point #7 in this section).
- Normovolemic hemodilution is accomplished by drawing blood before surgical blood loss.
- The patient's hematocrit has decreased from 28% to 24%. Hypovolemia is treated by administering isotonic crystalloids or colloids at a ratio of 3 mL to each 1 mL of blood lost. The patient is transfused with their own blood after major surgical loss has transpired. Patients must be able to tolerate the physiologic stress associated with acute anemia, and therefore this technique should not be employed in patients with severe cardiovascular or neurovascular pathology.
- Intraoperative blood salvage obtained from the surgical field using a cell saver system allows for transfusion of the patient's own red blood cells. Approximately 60% to 80% of blood loss can be replaced using this technique.
- Autologous or directed donor blood can be collected 2 to 3 weeks before surgery to be transfused as needed during the surgical procedure. For preoperative blood collection to occur, the patient's hemoglobin value should be greater than 11 mg/dL.

Despite the use of preoperative hematologic preparation or intraoperative blood salvage techniques, the patient should be typed and crossed and have a minimum of two units of blood available for infusion.

5. *Discuss the pathophysiologic mechanism of VAE during posterior spinal reconstructive surgery.*

A VAE, although rare, can occur during spinal reconstructive surgery as air is entrained into the complex venous network that surrounds the dura mater and spinal cord. During a posterior surgical approach, surgeons position patients prone with slight flexion in order to improve their vision and access to the operative field. As a result, the venous network is above the level of the heart and therefore air can be entrained into the traumatized veins.

The air that reaches the right atrium creates an air lock, which decreases blood flow into the right heart. As a result, forward blood flow from the right atrium, right ventricle, and then to the pulmonary arteries is impaired.

Left ventricular preload is decreased, resulting in hypotension. This explains the reason that hypotension and decreased ETCO$_2$ are signs that occur during VAE.

6. *List monitoring modalities, signs and symptoms, and treatment for VAE.*

The physiologic effects of VAE are dependent on the speed and amount of air that is entrained into the venous system. Signs and symptoms of VAE will be more severe the more air that is introduced to the venous system over a short period. The monitoring modalities, signs and symptoms, and treatment for VAE are listed in Boxes 47.2, 47.3, and 47.4, respectively.

7. *Describe methods that can be used to induce deliberate hypotension.*

Deliberate hypotension is frequently employed during spinal reconstructive surgery to decrease blood loss. By decreasing the patient's blood pressure, there is less blood loss from the vascular system resulting from surgical trauma. A variety of pharmacologic agents can be used to accomplish continuous hypotension. Anesthetic medications such as inhalation agents and narcotics are used initially to provide an adequate anesthetic depth

---

• BOX 47.2 Monitors Used for Detecting a Venous Air Embolism Listed in Order From Most Sensitive to Least Sensitive

- Transesophageal echocardiography
- Precordial Doppler positioned on the right sternal border between the third and sixth ribs
- Increased pulmonary artery pressures
- Decreased/absent ETCO$_2$
- Increased end tidal nitrogen

• BOX 47.3 Signs and Symptoms of a Venous Air Embolism

- Hypotension
- Millwheel murmur
- Decreased oxygen saturation
- Decreased ETCO$_2$
- Decreased end tidal nitrogen
- Dysrhythmias

• BOX 47.4 Treatment of a Venous Air Embolism

- Notify the surgeon to flood the surgical field with normal saline to decrease air intrusion
- 100% oxygen
- Fluid bolus
- Aspirate from central venous catheter
- Vasopressor administration
- Left lateral decubitus position

and inhibit sympathetic nervous system hyperactivity. A variety of other pharmacologic adjuncts can be used such as vascular dilators, nitroglycerin or nitroprusside, calcium channel blockers, or beta-blockers. It is imperative to use medications that can be titrated and that have a short duration of action for optimum control if hypotension occurs from volume depletion.

Careful consideration must be taken to identify patients who are appropriate candidates for prolonged hypotension. Cerebral autoregulation occurs at MAP between 60 and 160 mm Hg, and coronary artery autoregulation occurs at MAPs between 60 and 140 mm Hg. When the MAP decreases below 60 mm Hg, blood flow to the heart and the brain becomes pressure dependent. For patients with cardiac pathology, the vascular autoregulation curve is shifted to the right, necessitating higher MAP to ensure adequate perfusion. The disadvantages associated with hypotensive technique for spinal reconstructive surgery include cerebral and cardiac ischemia, spinal cord ischemia, optic nerve ischemia, and decreased renal perfusion.

8. *Discuss the advantages and limitations of SSEP monitoring.*

SSEP monitoring is used to detect spinal cord ischemia. If spinal cord ischemia is recognized and treated expeditiously, then spinal cord ischemia and paralysis can potentially be avoided. The risk of iatrogenic paraplegia is approximately 1%.

The major disadvantage associated with SSEP monitoring is the failure to detect ischemia that occurs to the ventral or anterior portion of the spinal cord, which mediates motor function. SSEP monitoring allows assessment of the integrity of the sensory or dorsal or posterior aspect of the cord. Although a rare event, it is possible that adequate SSEP waveforms exist and the patient can still develop postoperative motor paralysis. There is conflicting evidence to support the routine use of SSEP monitoring during spinal reconstructive surgery because it has not been emphatically determined that this monitoring technique decreases morbidity and mortality.

Monitoring SSEP and motor evoked potentials (MEPs) can be accomplished simultaneously. When both modalities are used, the SSEP monitoring electrode must be placed in the epidural space. This technique improves the ability to safely monitor patients.

9. *What are the advantages and disadvantages of performing an intraoperative "wake-up" test?*

The intraoperative "wake-up" test is performed to assess movement to determine that the anterior or ventral portion of the spinal cord is intact. Preoperatively informing the patient that they will wake up momentarily and be instructed to move their feet is essential.

Communication with the surgical team is important so that the patient will regain consciousness at the appropriate time and in a controlled manner. Inhalation agents and neuromuscular blockade will be discontinued. Reassuring the patient as they awake and asking them to move their legs and feet is necessary. After bilateral motor function has been assessed, the patient is reanesthetized. The advantage of the "wake-up" test is confirmation of movement assures that the motor aspect of the spinal cord is undamaged. Disadvantages associated with a "wake-up" test include recall, dislodgement of spinal reconstruction hardware, potential for extubation, and VAE. Additionally, it is possible that permanent and untreatable paraplegia had already occurred before assessing for movement of the lower extremities.

10. *Examine the component parts of an SSEP waveform.*
    - Wave latency is defined as the *time* between the application of a stimulus and the appearance of a neurologic response.
    - Wave amplitude is defined as the *size* or *intensity* of the neurologic response that results from peripheral nerve stimulation.
    - Wave morphology is defined as the general *appearance* of the electrical tracing, as seen in Fig. 47.2.

    Increased waveform latency and decreased waveform amplitude may be indicative of impending spinal cord impairment.

11. *Describe causative factors that can result in increased SSEP waveform latency and decreased SSEP waveform amplitude.*
    - Stretching, torsion, or retraction of the spinal cord
    - Decreased blood flow to the spinal cord
    - Hypoxia

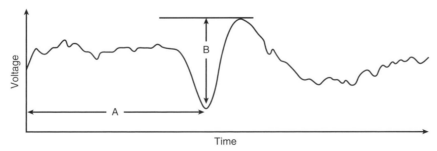

• **Fig. 47.2** The evoked potential waveform is a function of voltage over time. Waveform characteristics that are used to evaluate change in evoked potential signals are *(A)* latency in milliseconds from stimulus onset and *(B)* peak-to-peak amplitude in microvolts. The most commonly accepted SSEP warning criteria are a 10% increase in latency and a 50% decrease in amplitude. (From Errico TH, Lonner BS, Moulton AW: *Surgical management of spinal deformities*, St. Louis, 2009, Elsevier.)

- Hypercarbia
- Anemia
- Anesthetic medications
- Dislodgement of SSEP monitoring probes
- Electrical interference (electrocautery)
- Extreme hypothermia

12. *Cite interventions that should be employed if pathologic SSEP waveforms occur.*
    - Notify the surgeon
    - Increase oxygen concentration
    - Decrease anesthetic depth
    - Ensure adequate blood pressure (as depicted in Fig. 47.3)
    - Assess for anemia

13. *Identify anesthetic medications that have an effect on SSEP waveform monitoring.*

    In order to maintain the integrity of the SSEP waveform during anesthesia, it is desirable to titrate inhalation agents to <0.5 MAC, because neurologic inhibition occurs in a dose-dependent fashion. Nitrous oxide potentiates the cerebral depressant effects of inhalation agents, and this synergy will further increase latency and decrease amplitude during SSEP monitoring, as seen in Fig. 47.4. The effects of anesthetic medications are highly dependent on the dose administered. Higher dose ranges have a greater inhibitory effect on wave latency and amplitude (Table 47.1). In addition, nitrous oxide is highly diffusible and will increase the size of a potential VAE. Lastly, if a transthoracic approach is performed, the use of nitrous oxide is not routinely used during one-lung ventilation. Communication between the anesthetist, neurophysiologist, and surgeon is essential.

Postoperative Period

14. *Describe postoperative pain control strategies for patients having posterior spinal reconstructive surgery.*

    The degree of postoperative pain is intense after postoperative spinal reconstructive surgery. Postoperative pain control is essential in order to facilitate adequate respiratory exchange. Methods that can be used to

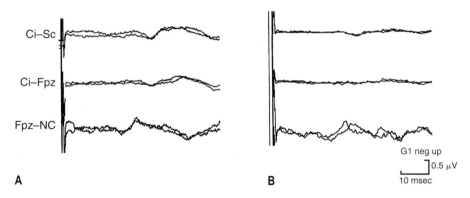

• **Fig. 47.3** Median nerve somatosensory evoked potential. An example of mild hypotension attenuating the cortical response but not substantially affecting the subcortical response. NC represents a noncephalic reference. (A) Blood pressure was 120/70 mm Hg. (B) Blood pressure was 90/50 mm Hg. (From Aminoff MJ: *Aminoff's electrodiagnosis in clinical neurology,* ed 6, St. Louis, 2012, Elsevier.)

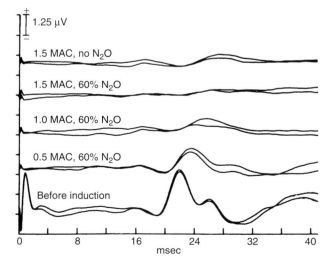

• **Fig. 47.4** The effect of inhalation agent and nitrous oxide on SSEP monitoring. *MAC,* Minimum alveolar concentration; *N₂O,* nitrous oxide. (From Peterson DO, et al: Effects of halothane, enflurane, isoflurane, and nitrous oxide on somatosensory evoked potentials in humans, *Anesthesiology* 65:35-40, 1986.)

TABLE 47.1	Effects of Anesthetic Medications on SSEP Waveforms		
Medication		Latency	Amplitude
Inhaled anesthetic agents		↑	↓
Nitrous oxide		0	↓
Propofol		↑	↓
Etomidate		↑	↑
Ketamine		0	↑
Dexmedetomidine		0	↓
Sufentanil/fentanyl/ remifentanil		↑	↓

decrease postoperative pain include neuraxial opiates or intravenous opioids delivered by a patient-controlled analgesic infusion. If a transthoracic approach is used, intercostal nerve blocks can be performed.

15. *Review the potential postoperative complications that can occur after posterior spinal reconstructive surgery.*

The potential postoperative complications associated with spinal reconstruction surgery include:
- Respiratory insufficiency
- Pneumothorax
- Hematoma formation
- Massive hemorrhage
- VAE
- Spinal cord injury
- Dislodgement of surgical instrumentation

Review Questions

1. Which nerve(s) can be injured if the patient's arms are abducted greater than 90 degrees during prone positioning?
   a. Ulnar
   b. Brachial plexus
   c. Radial
   d. Intercostal
2. The changes in lung volume that are associated with moderate to severe scoliosis include:
   a. Decreased vital capacity.
   b. Decreased residual volume.
   c. Increased total lung volume.
   d. Increased expiratory reserve volume.
3. Which monitoring modality is most sensitive for detecting a venous air embolus?
   a. Increased pulmonary artery pressures
   b. Decreased ETCO$_2$
   c. Increased end tidal nitrogen
   d. Precordial Doppler

4. The portion of the spinal cord that relays efferent motor responses is the:
   a. Anterior.
   b. Posterior.
   c. Dorsal.
   d. Lateral.
5. Inhaled anesthetic agents affect SSEP monitoring by:
   a. Increasing amplitude and decreasing latency.
   b. Decreasing amplitude and increasing latency.
   c. Decreasing amplitude and decreasing latency.
   d. Increasing amplitude and increasing latency.

Suggested Readings

Agarwal N, Hamilton DK, Ozpinar A, et al. Intraoperative neurophysiologic monitoring for adult patients undergoing posterior spinal fusion. *World Neurosurg* 2017;99:267-274.

Brull SJ, Prielipp RC. Vascular air embolism: a silent hazard to patient safety. *J Crit Care* 2017;42:255-263.

Chen Y, Wang BP, Yang J, Deng Y. Neurophysiological monitoring of lumbar spinal nerve roots: a case report of postoperative deficit and literature review. *Int J Surg Case Rep* 2017;30:218-221.

Cohen JL, Klyce W, Kudchadkar SR, et al. Respiratory complications after posterior spinal fusion for neuromuscular scoliosis: children with Rett syndrome at greater risk than those with cerebral palsy. *Spine* 2019;44(19):1396-1402.

Elisha S. Cardiovascular anatomy, physiology and pathophysiology. In: Nagelhout JJ, Elisha S, eds. *Nurse Anesthesia,* 6th ed. St. Louis, MO: Elsevier, 2018:441-478.

Gelalis ID, Papadopoulos DV, Giannoulis DK, et al. Spinal motion preservation surgery: indications and applications. *Eur J Orthop Surg Traumatol* 2018;28(3):335-342.

Grottke O. Intraoperative wake up test and postoperative emergence in patient's undergoing spinal surgery. *Anesth Analg* 2004;99(5):1521-1527.

Holt JB, Dolan LA, Weinstein SL. Outcomes of primary posterior spinal fusion for scoliosis in spinal muscular atrophy: clinical, radiographic, and pulmonary outcomes and complications. *J Pediatr Orthop* 2017;37(8):e505-e511.

Katranitsa L, Gkantsinikoudis N, Kapetanakis S, et al. Perioperative blood management in posterior instrumented fusion for adolescent idiopathic scoliosis: original study and short review of the literature. *Folia Med (Plovdiv)* 2018;60(2):200-207.

Li Y, Hong RA, Robbins CB, Gibbons KM, et al. Intrathecal morphine and oral analgesics provide safe and effective pain control after posterior spinal fusion for adolescent idiopathic scoliosis. *Spine* 2018;43(2):E98-E104.

Lonergan T, Place H, Taylor P. Acute complications after adult spinal deformity surgery in patients aged 70 years and older. *Clin Spine Surg* 2016;29(8):314-317.

Matsumoto M, Miyagi M, Saito W, et al. Perioperative complications in posterior spinal fusion surgery for neuromuscular scoliosis. *Spine Surg Relat Res* 2018;2(4):278-282.

Nickels TJ, Manlapaz MR, Farag E. Perioperative visual loss after spine surgery. *World J Orthop* 2014;5(2):100-106.

Othman Z. Hypotension-induced loss of intraoperative monitoring data during surgical correction of Scheuermann kyphosis. *Spine* 2004;29(12):258-265.

Roth S, Moss HE. Update on perioperative ischemic optic neuropathy associated with non-ophthalmic surgery. *Front Neurol* 2018; 9:557.

48

Anesthesia for Shoulder Arthroscopy

KEY POINTS

- An important aspect of the anesthetic course is intraoperative and postoperative pain relief provided by an interscalene block.
- Injuries that occur to the brachial plexus are reduced when patients are positioned in the beach chair position compared with the lateral decubitus position.
- In the beach chair position, when the blood pressure (BP) is taken on the arm, mean arterial pressure (MAP) is not reflective of the MAP in the brain.

- Patients in the beach chair position are at risk for an intraoperative stroke if low MAPs that are measured in the arm are assumed to be reflective of adequate cerebral and coronary perfusion due to gravity.

Case Synopsis

A 57-year-old man has been diagnosed with a torn right rotator cuff caused by a work-related injury. He is scheduled to have a shoulder arthroscopy and repair of his right rotator cuff.

Preoperative Evaluation and Demographic Data

Past Medical/Surgical History

- Smoker with a chronic cough
- Gastroesophageal reflux disease

List of Medications

- Celecoxib (Celebrex)
- Omeprazole (Prilosec)

Diagnostic Data

- Hemoglobin, 15 g/dL; hematocrit, 46%
- Glucose, 109 mg/dL; blood urea nitrogen, 18 mg/dL; creatinine, 1.3 mg/dL
- Electrolytes: sodium, 139 mEq/L; potassium, 4.2 mEq/L; chloride, 106 mEq/L; carbon dioxide, 26 mEq/L

Height/Weight/Vital Signs

- 180 cm, 113 kg
- BP, 114/73; heart rate, 61 beats per minute; respiratory rate, 21 breaths per minute; room air oxygen saturation, 97%; temperature, 36.6°C
- Electrocardiogram: normal sinus rhythm

Pathophysiology

Many advances have been made in orthopedic surgery in the last 30 years. Procedures that initially required hospitalization for several days are now performed via an arthroscopic approach, which is less invasive, and patients are routinely discharged from the hospital within 24 hours. The introduction of fiber-optics for visualization, smaller surgical instrumentation, and superior orthopedic techniques have led to the increasing popularity of less invasive arthroscopic shoulder surgery.

A rotator cuff injury involves one or more of the four muscles in the shoulder, as shown in Fig. 48.1. This may be an acute injury, such as from a fall or trauma. The trauma may lead to hemorrhage and inflammation of the bursa. The swelling that occurs with this process decreases the space available under the acromion. This may then lead to impingement with abduction of the shoulder. A vicious cycle begins as inflammation progresses.

The upper arm is connected to the shoulder joint by three bones: the clavicle, scapula, and humerus. Ligamentous support helps to stabilize the joint. Muscles of the rotator cuff (supraspinatus, infraspinatus, teres minor, and subscapularis) help keep the head of the humerus in place against the scapula, allowing it to lift and rotate. This network of muscles and tendons form a covering around the top of the humerus. The actual rotator cuff tear exists within the supraspinatus muscle and is the cause of pain for many adults, as is shown in Fig. 48.2.

Surgical Procedure

The type of surgery that is performed is dependent on the size and location of the tear. If the tendon is torn, it may

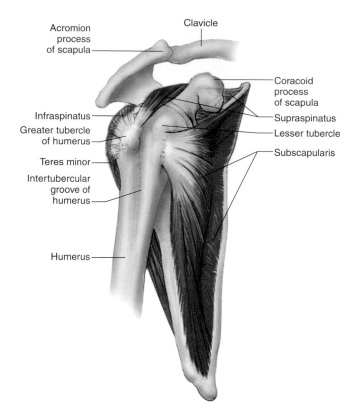

• **Fig. 48.1** Anatomy of the shoulder joint. (From Patton KT: *Anatomy & physiology*, ed 10, St. Louis, 2019, Elsevier.)

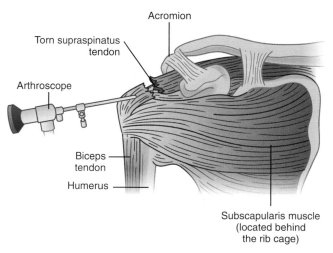

• **Fig. 48.2** Rotator cuff tear. (From Leonard PC: *Quick & easy medical terminology*, ed 9, St. Louis, 2020, Elsevier.)

require repair with suture via the arthroscope or by using an open technique. Sometimes the tendon may be torn away from the bone, and the intervention may require a direct repair of the tendon to the bone. The surgeon may also remove part of the acromion (connected to the scapula) due to impingement on the tendon, which could lead to a tear.

In the beach chair position, traction on the operative arm is frequently applied in order to improve the operating conditions.

• **BOX 48.1** **Complications and Benefits Related to Interscalene Blockade**

Complications
- Horner syndrome
- Brachial plexus injury
- Phrenic nerve injury
- Recurrent laryngeal nerve trauma
- Total spinal anesthetic
- Intravascular injection
- Intraneural injection
- Infection

Benefits
- Postoperative analgesia
- Shorter recovery time
- Rapid discharge time
- Unanticipated admission to the hospital for pain is reduced

---

The eyes must be protected from direct pressure, and the head is secured with a Velcro strap or tape. The ears of the patient must be checked to ensure they are not pinched by the strap. The anesthetist should periodically visualize the head and neck due to manipulation of the shoulder by the surgeon, assuring continuous alignment.

Anesthetic Management and Considerations

Preoperative Period

1. *Discuss the consent process for interscalene block for anesthetic management.*

    To gain an informed consent from the patient, explanation of the available anesthetic option of an interscalene block must be discussed. The patient needs to be informed of risks and possible complications, as well as expectations of the anesthetic procedure. Box 48.1 lists the complications and benefits associated with an interscalene block. A thorough history and a complete list of medications that the patient is taking should also be provided.

2. *Explain the nervous system innervation to the rotator cuff.*

    Innervation to the rotator cuff originates from the cervical plexus dividing into roots, trunks, divisions, cords, and branches. The supraspinatus and infraspinatus muscles of the rotator cuff are innervated by the suprascapular nerve, the teres minor muscle by the axillary nerve, and the subscapularis muscle by the subscapular nerve.

3. *Describe the method for placement of an interscalene block.*

    Before beginning a regional anesthetic of any type, check to see that emergency airway and resuscitation equipment is available and in working order. Also, observation of aseptic technique is essential.

To perform an interscalene block, the patient is positioned supine with the head facing away from the shoulder that is being anesthetized. The patient is asked to elevate the head slightly to bring the clavicular head of the sternocleidomastoid muscle into prominent view. The anesthetist's palpating finger is placed behind the sternocleidomastoid muscle, and the patient is told to relax the head lift. The palpable interscalene groove between the anterior and middle scalene muscle is palpated. The injection site in the interscalene groove lies at the level of the cricoid (C6), and this should be accomplished using ultrasound guidance.

Incremental local anesthetic injection, while intermittently aspirating to be sure that intravascular injection is not occurring, is accomplished. This method is used to decrease the potential for local anesthetic systemic toxicity (LAST). The symptoms associated with LAST most often begin with minor neurologic signs: lightheadedness, tinnitus, and metallic taste and then may progress to seizures, loss of consciousness, and respiratory arrest. The cardiovascular sign of severe LAST is associated with bradycardia followed by asystole. Thus the best treatment for LAST is to prevent the situation from occurring. The definitive pharmacologic treatment for LAST is the infusion of intralipids.

Intraoperative Period

4. *Describe the anatomic and physiologic changes that are associated with the beach chair position.*

Compared with the lateral position, surgeons often prefer the beach chair position for rotator cuff repair, which improves visualization, decreases distortion of the intraarticular anatomy, and minimizes the potential for brachial plexus injury. Significant physiologic changes occur when patients are in the upright position as gravity pulls blood downward away from the thorax. MAP, stroke volume (SV), cardiac output (CO), and PaO_2 all decrease. The alveolar–arterial oxygen gradient and pulmonary and vascular resistance all increase. When a patient is awake, these effects are compensated for by an increase in systemic vascular resistance (SVR) by up to 50% to 80%. However, this autonomic response is inhibited by general anesthetic medications, causing vasodilation and decreased CO.

Cerebral perfusion pressure (CPP) decreases by approximately 15% when a patient is in a sitting position, and this value is calculated as shown in the following equation:

$$CPP = MAP - ICP \ (or \ CVP)$$

CPP, Cerebral perfusion pressure; *CVP*, central venous pressure; *ICP*, intracranial pressure; *MAP*, mean arterial pressure.

General anesthetic agents cause vasodilation, myocardial depression, and impaired venous return, which can further impair cerebral blood flow. Inspiratory subatmospheric pressure during spontaneous ventilation increases venous return from the cerebral circulation, but this effect does not occur when positive pressure ventilation is initiated. Flexion of the head may obstruct the internal jugular veins and cause cerebral venous engorgement. Extension of the head may impair cerebral blood flow (CBF), resulting in cerebral ischemia.

The cerebral vasculature dilates and constricts to maintain constant blood flow to the brain. This concept—cerebral autoregulation—occurs when the patient's MAP is between 60 and 160 mm Hg. When the MAP is above or below these values, the degree of CBF becomes pressure dependent. However, with poorly controlled hypertensive patients, autoregulation of CBF is shifted to the right, requiring a higher MAP to ensure adequate cerebral perfusion. Some orthopedic surgeons request deliberate hypotension for shoulder arthroscopy, specifically rotator cuff repair. Decreasing the MAP to <60 mm Hg during deliberate hypotensive technique jeopardizes adequate CBF, especially in patients with chronic hypertension.

5. *Examine the correct location for a blood pressure cuff and state the physiologic significance.*

When placed in the supine position, the BP measured on the arm is similar to CPP in the absence of intracranial pressure (ICP). However, in the beach chair position, BP and MAP readings taken from the arm are higher than the CPP because blood flow from the heart must overcome the force of gravity. The difference in MAP when comparing the heart/arm and the brain will be equal to the hydrostatic pressure gradient. The mean brachial artery pressure obtained from a BP cuff may be 7 to 22 mm Hg lower than what is present in the brain.

If the BP at the heart/arm is 130/65 (MAP, 85 mm Hg) and the height of the external auditory meatus (representing the base of the brain) is 20 cm above the heart, the difference in BP at the heart compared with the brain will be 15 mm Hg. Thus the MAP at the base of the brain will be 70 mm Hg. There will be a greater disparity in BP and MAP if the cuff is placed on the patient's leg. During this surgery, placement of an arterial line is unnecessary.

In a series of patients having shoulder surgery in the beach chair position, BP significantly decreased, and severe hypotension was a likely cause of ischemic brain injury. It is recommended that MAP be maintained at a minimum of 60 mm Hg in healthy patients that are assumed to have normal cerebral vasculature. For elderly patients with hypertension and/or known cerebral vascular disease, the cerebral autoregulation curve is shifted to the right, and a higher MAP should be maintained.

Hypotension that occurs during arthroscopic surgery in the beach chair position should be aggressively treated. Treatment includes vigilant monitoring and titration of anesthetic gases, gradual position changes instead of abrupt changes, administration of intravenous (IV) fluid, and treatment with vasopressors as needed.

6. *Explain the rationale for why the external auditory meatus is utilized as the landmark for the circle of Willis.*

The auditory meatus is easily identifiable, and it is relatively constant as an indicator of the location of the base of the brain and the circle of Willis. Measurements or estimates of the MAP can be made once the patient is in the beach chair position. The critical variable is the vertical distance from the circle of Willis to the BP cuff.

7. *Discuss the importance of maintaining normocarbia for patients who are placed in the beach chair position.*

Hypocapnia significantly reduces internal carotid artery and CBF. This change will be exacerbated when the patient is placed in the sitting position. Hence, significant hypocapnia should be avoided whenever possible to decrease the potential for cerebral hypoperfusion.

Postoperative Period

8. *List potential postoperative complications that can occur after arthroscopic rotator cuff repair under general anesthesia with an interscalene block.*

Respiratory depression can occur in the postoperative period due to increased opioids administered during the surgical procedure. The anesthetist must be aware of the possibility of postoperative respiratory depression because analgesia provided by interscalene block results in decreased postoperative pain.

Review Questions

1. If a patient's CPP at the circle of Willis is 60 mm Hg, what is the corresponding CPP at the highest point in the brain?
   a. 69 mm Hg
   b. 60 mm Hg
   c. 51 mm Hg
   d. 55 mm Hg
2. The external auditory meatus is a landmark that:
   a. Estimates the position of the most cephalad position of the brain.
   b. Estimates the position of the base of the brain.
   c. Estimates the MAP of the brain.
   d. Estimates intracranial pressure.
3. Physical injury to the patient in the beach chair position for rotator cuff surgery:
   a. Can result and somatosensory evoked potential monitoring is recommended.
   b. Is a rare occurrence.
   c. Is most often associated with peroneal nerve injury.
   d. Can be prevented by assuring normal anatomic alignment throughout the procedure.

4. The brachial plexus originates as the cervical plexus at the spinal cord level of:
   a. C8–T1.
   b. C5–T1.
   c. C2–C8.
   d. C6–C8.
5. Hypocapnia that is associated with the sitting position:
   a. Causes minimal change in carotid blood flow.
   b. Causes increased cerebral blood flow.
   c. Causes a synergistic decrease in carotid blood flow.
   d. Causes increased blood flow velocity in the middle cerebral artery.

Suggested Readings

Aguirre JA, Etzensperger F, Brada M, et al. The beach chair position for shoulder surgery in intravenous general anesthesia and controlled hypotension: impact on cerebral oxygenation, cerebral blood flow and neurobehavioral outcome. *J Clin Anesth* 2019;53:40-48.

Bhatti MT, Enneking FK. Hypotensive technique and sitting position in shoulder surgery. *Anesth Analg* 2003;97:1199.

Bosco L, Zhou C, Murdoch JAC, et al. Pre- or postoperative interscalene block and/or general anesthesia for arthroscopic shoulder surgery: a retrospective observational study. *Can J Anaesth* 2017;64(10):1048-1058.

Brull SJ, Prielipp RC. Vascular air embolism: a silent hazard to patient safety. *J Crit Care* 2017;42:255-263.

Cullen DJ, Kirby RR. Beach chair position may decrease cerebral perfusion: catastrophic outcomes have occurred. *Anesthesia Patient Safety Foundation Newsletter* 2007;22:25-27.

Drummond JC. The lower limits of autoregulation: time to revise our thinking? *Anesthesiology* 1997;86:1431–1433.

Higgins JD, Frank RM, Hamamoto JT, et al. Shoulder arthroscopy in the beach chair position. *Arthrosc Tech* 2017;6(4):e1153-e1158.

Hussain N, Goldar G, Ragina N, et al. Suprascapular and interscalene nerve block for shoulder surgery: a systematic review and meta-analysis. *Anesthesiology* 2017;127(6):998-1013.

Hirsch MT. Anesthesia for orthopedics and podiatry. In: Nagelhout JJ, Elisha S, eds. *Nurse Anesthesia,* 6th ed. St. Louis, MO: Elsevier, 2018:947-958.

Kim YS, Han NR, Seo KH. Changes of intraocular pressure and ocular perfusion pressure during controlled hypotension in patients undergoing arthroscopic shoulder surgery: a prospective, randomized, controlled study comparing propofol, and desflurane anesthesia. *Medicine (Baltimore)* 2019;98(18):e15461.

Murphy GS, Greenberg SB, Szokol JW. Safety of beach chair position shoulder surgery: a review of the current literature. *Anesth Analg* 2019;129(1):101-118.

van Erp JHJ, Ostendorf M, Lansdaal JR. Shoulder surgery in beach chair position causing perioperative stroke: four cases and a review of the literature. *J Orthop* 2019;16(6):493-495.

49

Hip Arthroplasty

KEY POINTS

- Postoperative venous thromboembolism can be a devastating complication associated with total hip replacement. Interventions can be instituted to decrease the potential of thromboembolism.
- Advantages to providing regional anesthesia include decreased intraoperative blood loss, decreased perioperative deep vein thrombosis (DVT), and minimal need for airway manipulation or control.

- Because infection after total hip arthroplasty (THA) can be life threatening, confirmation and administration of antibiotics within 1 hour of incision is imperative.
- Respiratory compromise can occur in patients that are placed in the lateral decubitus position.
- Postoperative pain control will decrease sympathetic nervous system stimulation and allow for early ambulation.

Case Synopsis

An 86-year-old woman complained of right hip joint pain, which resulted in pain and difficulty walking. As a result of the x-ray, she is diagnosed as a right hip fracture, and THA is scheduled.

Preoperative Evaluation and Demographic Data

Past Medical/Surgical History

- Rheumatoid arthritis
- Shortness of breath
- Hypertension
- Obesity (body mass index [BMI] = 32 kg/m^2)

List of Medications

- Celecoxib (Celebrex)
- Nifedipine (Adalat CC)
- Atorvastatin (Lipitor)

Diagnostic Data

Hematology Report

- Hemoglobin, 10.9 g/dL; hematocrit, 32.7%
- Platelets: 62/mm^3
- White blood cells: 3.2/mm^3
- Lactate dehydrogenase, 224 units; erythrocyte sedimentation rate, 24 mm/hr
- Alkaline phosphatase, 14 units/dL

Pulmonary Function Test

- Forced vital capacity (FVC), 67% (predicted, 6 L; measured, 4 L)

- Forced expiratory volume (FEV$_1$), 40% (predicted, 5 L; measured, 2 L)
- FEV$_1$/FVC, 60% (predicted, 83%; measured, 50%)

Dobutamine Stress Echocardiography

- Left ventricle (LV) is normal in size and systolic function. EF = 55%. The LV appears normal in size. LV systolic function is normal. Baseline LV diastolic function is consistent with abnormal relaxation (stage 1).
- Right ventricle (RV) is normal in size and systolic function.
- Left atrium (LA)/pulmonary veins: the LA is normal; the LA cavity is mildly dilated.
- Right atrium (RA)/inferior vena cava/superior vena cava: the RA is normal.
- Mitral valve: there is trivial mitral regurgitation.
- Tricuspid valve (TV): normal with trivial regurgitation; regurgitant velocity is 243.0 cm/s, and estimated RV systolic pressure is 28 mm Hg.
- Aortic valve/left ventricular outflow tract: the peak gradient is 14.0 mm Hg; the mean gradient is 8 mm Hg; there is mild aortic regurgitation.

Height/Weight/Vital Signs

- 170 cm, 96 kg
- Blood pressure, 150/88; heart rate, 72 beats per minute; respiratory rate, 16 breaths per minute; room air oxygen saturation, 97%; temperature, 36.8°C
- Electrocardiogram (ECG): normal sinus rhythm (occasional premature ventricular contraction), left ventricular hypertrophy
- Cardiac Doppler: ejection fraction (EF) 55%

Pathophysiology

More than 200,000 total hip replacements are performed annually in North America. Progressively, severe arthritis of the hip joint, as seen in osteoarthritis (degenerative disease), is associated with aging and "wear and tear" of the joint over time. Patients scheduled for THA are usually older and often have preexisting medical conditions that may affect perioperative outcome. Osteoarthritis is the most common indication for hip arthroplasty, usually occurring after age 50 and often in individuals with a familial history of arthritis. The hip joint, which contains the spheroid femoral head and acetabular cavity, degenerates over time and prevents the smooth movement of these surfaces, causing pain. This process inhibits the ability of the patient to bear weight on the affected hip, and ambulation is frequently impaired. A comparison of the normal and abnormal hip joint is shown in Fig. 49.1. Other factors that lead to degenerative joint disease include congenital hip joint abnormalities, traumatic injuries, and rheumatoid arthritis.

Rheumatoid arthritis is an autoimmune disease that causes inflammation of the synovial membrane, producing greater amounts of synovial fluid than normal and damage to the articular cartilage, leading to pain and severe joint immobility. Inflammation associated with rheumatoid arthritis progression causes the formation of a mass known as a *pannus*, causing the invasion and destruction of soft tissue, cartilage, and bone. Traumatic arthritis can result from a severe injury to the hip, causing a condition known as *avascular necrosis,* which can further cause hip bone necrosis and death of the bone (aseptic necrosis). Patients with any one of these conditions might benefit from a THA to relieve chronic pain and improve functional status.

Surgical Procedure

The hip joint is a simple ball-and-socket joint formed by the femoral head and part of the pelvis called the *acetabulum.* When the cartilage is damaged and smooth movement is impeded, the joints become stiff and painful. THA, one of the most successful procedures in orthopedic surgery, is performed to improve mobility and relieve pain. Numerous hardware designs and materials are used for THA depending on surgeon preference. This procedure involves the dislocation of the femoral head from the acetabulum with excision of the arthritic femoral head and a portion of the femoral neck. The acetabulum is reamed to accept a cemented or cementless prosthetic metallic or plastic cup, and this process is repeated to the femur so that the modular femoral stem and head component (metal or ceramic) can be inserted (Fig. 49.2). Patients who have a BMI of greater than 50 kg/m^2 are at increased risk for developing postoperative complications. Box 49.1 lists the most common complications that are associated with THA.

Anesthetic Management and Considerations

Preoperative Period

1. *Describe the preoperative preparation for a patient having a THA.*

   Because THA is frequently an elective procedure, preparation of the patient should include a complete and comprehensive health and physical examination to assess the

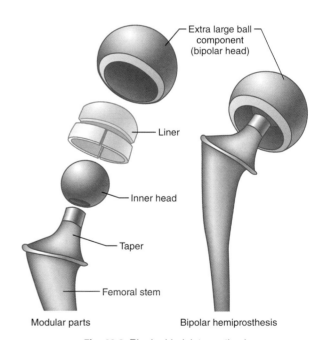

• **Fig. 49.2** Bipolar hip joint prosthesis.

Extra large ball component (bipolar head)
Liner
Inner head
Taper
Femoral stem
Modular parts
Bipolar hemiprosthesis

• **BOX 49.1** **Most Common Complications Associated With a Total Hip Arthroplasty**

- Infection
- Thromboembolism
- Nerve injury (femoral, obturator, lateral femoral cutaneous)
- Dislocation
- Implant failure
- Limb length discrepancy
- Periprosthetic fracture

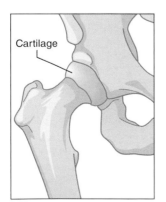
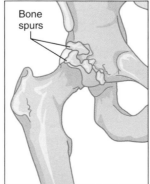

Cartilage

Bone spurs

• **Fig. 49.1** Normal and abnormal right hip joint.

health of the patient and to identify any comorbid conditions that would potentially interfere with the perioperative period. Laboratory tests will be ordered as indicated by the findings in the history and physical. Antiinflammatory medications will need to be discontinued at least 1 week before surgery to decrease the risks associated with platelet function and clotting. Additionally, preoperative radiographic examinations of the hip joint and cervical spine x-rays are taken to assess flexion and extension in patients known to have rheumatoid arthritis if general anesthesia is a possibility. Flexion and extension of the cervical region and temporomandibular joint mobility are major concerns in patients with severe arthritis, which can make airway management difficult or impossible. A thorough dental evaluation is necessary for all patients and especially for those with poor dentition. Although infection is uncommon with this procedure, bacteria accompanying dental disease can pose a major postoperative concern in these patients. Preoperative care or extraction of diseased teeth may be necessary before proceeding to surgery. Typing and cross-matching for the possibility of allogenic blood transfusion or preparation of autologous blood should be assured before administration of anesthesia. If the procedure is urgent, a cell-saver system should be readily available. Any coexisting disease factors should be medically controlled to ensure optimization before surgery.

2. *Discuss the preoperative concerns regarding this patient.*

Although the concern regarding the patient's rheumatoid arthritis is addressed during the preoperative preparation of the THA patient, the anesthetist must also remember that the systemic inflammatory disease arthritis can potentially affect every organ system in this patient. Preoperative evaluation for pericardial effusion and rhythm disturbances may require preoperative pacemaker (external) assistance. In addition to the routine preoperative history and physical, this patient needs to be queried more as to the etiology and severity of her hypertension, the current therapy, and to determine if end-organ damage that accompanies chronic hypertension has occurred. Hypertension commonly affects a considerable proportion of the world population. Preoperative antihypertensive therapy is indicated; however, there is a lack of consensus concerning the preoperative evaluation and perioperative care of hypertension for patients having noncardiac surgery.

This patient might also benefit from a thorough renal examination. Urinalysis, serum creatinine, and blood urea nitrogen (BUN) may be necessary to obtain information about the presence and extent of renal parenchymal disease. Oftentimes, THA is indicated in the treatment of osteonecrosis—a condition often seen in patients with chronic renal failure (CRF) and believed to be associated with steroid use.

Lastly, although age alone is not an indication of cognitive dysfunction, the patient presenting with THA may also be prone to dementia of unknown etiology (sometimes called *multi-infarct dementia*). This is a concern to the anesthetist because failure to assess cognitive integrity during the preoperative period may lead to complication during the postoperative period. Additionally, if there is any concern regarding the cognitive status of this patient, there should also be concerns regarding the importance of the "informed consent."

3. *Identify patient characteristics that increase the susceptibility to hip fracture.*

Depending on etiology, the sex of the patient may be a factor increasing the susceptibility to hip fracture. Likewise, advanced age and obesity have been suggested as positive risk factors. Increased BMI was found to be a risk factor for total hip replacement caused by osteoarthritis. The variables related to the surgeon's decision to suggest the need for THA were the presence or absence of severe cardiovascular disease, physical subscale score, and amount of joint space narrowing. More recently, younger patients and patients with severe anatomic deformities are receiving THA procedures to improve activities of daily living.

4. *Discuss the options for the anesthetic technique for THA.*

For patients scheduled for THA, the choice of a neuraxial anesthetic, general anesthesia, or a combination of techniques can be offered. For some patients, the mention of regional anesthesia provokes fear of the needle stick and anxiety associated with being "awake" during the procedure. A thorough explanation of the available sedatives and their effects can often relieve some of these concerns. Regardless of the type of anesthetic chosen, patients must be assured of adequate analgesia and relief of their anxiety from induction to recovery. The anesthetist must also be sure to include in the discussion the potential side effects of anesthetic medications and subsequent options available to the patient.

Intraoperative Period

5. *Choose the monitoring modalities that you would employ during surgery.*

Monitoring should include all routine vital sign measurements such as ECG, noninvasive blood pressure monitoring, pulse oximetry, and body temperature. In patients that are physiologically unstable or those with severe comorbid diseases, continuous intraarterial blood pressure monitoring may be indicated. However, an arterial line may be placed after the patient is anesthetized because there is no conclusive evidence that intraarterial blood pressure monitoring during the induction of anesthesia prevents intraoperative complications. This patient will benefit from the use of simultaneous leads II, V_5, and multiple-lead ST analysis to monitor ventricular ectopy because patients with hypertension may be at increased risk of developing myocardial ischemia. Aberrant conduction in the ventricles of this patient should be further investigated with blood gas sampling and diagnostic attention to cause and effect, with correction of factors contributing to the ectopy before the addition of more invasive procedures.

6. *Which anesthetic techniques would be appropriate for this procedure?*

The anesthetic technique that is most appropriate for this procedure would consider the patient's comorbid factors and acceptance after the informed consent process. General endotracheal anesthesia and regional anesthesia are both appropriate choices for this patient. With general anesthesia, the lateral position and her obesity necessitate the need for endotracheal intubation for airway management. Aggravation of cricoarytenoid arthritis in patients with rheumatoid arthritis can be minimized by using a smaller-diameter endotracheal tube. Careful positioning of the head and neck are a primary concern during induction and intraoperative maintenance to avoid the potential for cervical spine or brachial plexus injury.

Regional techniques cause a sympathectomy as a result of the inhibition of preganglionic *B* fiber transmission, which extends from the thoracic to the first or second lumbar vertebrae. Vascular dilation leads to decreased blood pressure that can range from mild to severe. It is important for the anesthetist to realize that fluid volume loading and administering vasopressors might be necessary to avoid hypotension. This response may be more pronounced in the elderly patient population. Initial positioning might be uncomfortable in patients who have sustained traumatic injuries to the hip or have osteoarthritis and limited joint mobility.

7. *Discuss the advantages of providing regional anesthesia for THA.*

The advantages of using a regional anesthetic technique for THA include decreased intraoperative blood loss, decreased perioperative DVT, and minimal need for airway manipulation or control. Spinal anesthesia for THA may be associated with a lower 30-day mortality rate compared with general anesthesia. Lumbar epidural anesthesia can be performed even in the patient with rheumatoid arthritis because the lumbar spine is frequently unaffected in these patients. Single-dose spinal anesthesia placed at the L3–L4 level with 0.75% bupivacaine (15 mg) combined with 0.2 mg of morphine offers the patient a rapid onset of analgesia for up to 24 hours. A mixture of 2% lidocaine with 1:200,000 epinephrine administered over 13 to 17 minutes (approximately 15 to 20 mL) via an epidural technique provides a slow onset and gives the anesthetist more time to treat hypotension compared with a spinal anesthetic. If epidural opioids are added to the solution, postoperative analgesia is also provided.

8. *Discuss the physiologic manifestations of unintended (subarachnoid) intrathecal injection during the administration of local anesthesia with an epidural technique.*

If an unintended intrathecal injection occurs, there will be a profound sensory and motor block shortly after injection. The brain is more susceptible than the heart to the effects of local anesthetic toxicity. Low plasma levels of local anesthetic result in minor neurologic symptoms, which include numbness of the tongue, a metallic taste in the mouth, blurred vision, and circumoral numbness. As the plasma concentration increases, more severe neurologic signs such as decreased level of consciousness and seizures can occur. Other complaints may include dyspnea as a result of the blockade of proprioceptive afferent nerves of the abdominal and intercostals muscles progressing to respiratory arrest if the block continues to spread. Box 49.2 lists the signs and symptoms associated with local anesthetic systemic toxicity (LAST). Box 49.3 provides a crisis checklist for LAST.

9. *Describe the anesthetic considerations regarding positioning during a THA procedure.*

Positioning of the patient undergoing THA is extremely important to prevent neurovascular complications. The lateral decubitus position is most often used to facilitate exposure for the surgeon. Meticulous padding of the extremities and the maintenance of a neutral neck position are essential. Once the patient is anesthetized, an indwelling urinary catheter may be placed if the

---

• BOX 49.2 The Signs and Symptoms of LAST

Signs and symptoms are listed from least severe to most severe:
- Lightheadedness
- Numbness of the tongue
- Metallic taste in the mouth
- Circumoral numbness
- Visual impairment
- Altered level of consciousness
- Seizures
- Coma
- Myocardial depression

• BOX 49.3 Treatment for LAST

Primary Actions

1. Call for help, obtain "crash cart," obtain intralipids
2. Stop LA injection
3. Administer 100% oxygen and manage airway as indicated
4. Circulation
   - Begin ACLS/PALS
   - Administer intralipids ASAP
   - Administer IV fluid bolus/epinephrine for hypotension and/or bradycardia
   - Administer a benzodiazepine for seizures

Medication Dosages

- Administer Intralipid 20%:
  - For patients >70 kg, administer 100 mL IV bolus of 2-3 minutes, then 200-250 mL IV infusion over 15-20 minutes.
  - For patients <70 kg, administer 1.5 mL/kg IV bolus, then 0.25-0.5 mL/kg/min IV infusion
- Maximum Intralipid dose 12 mL/kg
- For hypotension/bradycardia: Epinephrine <1 mcg/kg
- For severe/sustained bradycardia: Atropine 0.5–1.0 mg
- Avoid: Vasopressin, calcium channel blockers and beta-blockers, propofol, local anesthetics

procedure is expected to be prolonged. Padded pegs are positioned at the level of the patient's rib cage and pubic areas when using the fracture table. A bean bag and axillary roll may be necessary to stabilize the patient, avoid compression of the brachial plexus and vascular structures, and relieve the pressure on the femoral triangle when placed in the lateral decubitus position. The dependent arm should be abducted and placed on a padded arm rest.

Care must be taken in the elderly and obese patients when positioned in lateral decubitus position, as pulmonary function can become compromised. This position results in increased perfusion in the dependent lung and increased ventilation in the nondependent lung. Hence ventilation–perfusion mismatch will occur, resulting in shunting, which may lead to a decrease in PaO_2. The degree of ventilation–perfusion mismatch is most pronounced in patients with underlying lung disease.

10. *Discuss the importance of maintaining normothermia during THA.*

Humans are homeothermic; as such, there are minimal variations in core body temperature. Unintentional perioperative hypothermia is one of the most common complications experienced by surgical patients because warming techniques are insufficient to counteract thermal redistribution resulting from the ablation of thermoregulatory vasoconstriction associated with anesthesia. Hypothermia can lead to metabolic acidosis as a result of the accumulation of acids (other than CO_2) or loss of base, resulting in a decreased pH and decreased HCO_3. The resulting central nervous system (CNS) effects of acidosis can greatly depress neuronal activity and increase the seizure threshold. Shivering-induced hypothermia can also increase oxygen consumption by as much as 600% and reduce platelet function causing the potential for coagulopathy.

11. *Discuss the anesthetic considerations for a patient with obstructive sleep apnea (OSA).*

Although this patient is moderately obese, OSA may be a concern because obesity is the most important independent risk factor for OSA. A STOP BANG assessment for OSA should be considered. There is a relationship between obesity and decreases in the pharyngeal area as a result of adipose tissue deposition, causing a decrease in the patency of the pharynx and an increase in the likelihood of airway collapse. Additionally, pharyngeal patency is determined by the difference between the extraluminal and intraluminal (transmural) pressure across its wall and the compliance of the wall. Obese patients have higher extraluminal pressure exerted on the pharyngeal wall as a result of superficial fat deposition. If concerns about the ability to intubate exist, the anesthetist should consider video laryngoscopy as the initial method for intubation or, at a minimum, having the equipment available is warranted.

12. *Describe the concerns regarding blood and fluid requirements for this patient.*

Blood and fluid requirements for this patient are of paramount importance because THA procedures are usually accompanied by major blood loss. Red blood cell (RBC) transfusion is one of the few treatments that adequately restore tissue oxygenation when oxygen demand exceeds supply. Securing two 14- to 16-gauge intravenous catheters is ideal to ensure adequate vascular access. Lactated Ringer's solution or normal saline may be started at 4 to 8 mL/kg/hr and adjusted as needed. Although there continues to be controversy regarding the superiority of administering crystalloids compared with colloid, crystalloid solutions are usually adequate to sustain normal hemodynamic parameters. Proponents of crystalloid therapy believe that hypovolemic shock causes both intravascular and interstitial fluid losses that can be easily replaced with crystalloids, whereas proponents of colloid therapy state that resuscitation with colloids for hypovolemic shock requires less volume and maintains oncotic pressure, which decreases extravasation to the extravascular space.

Intraoperative RBC scavenging can play an important role as an adjunct to autologous blood transfusion and help reduce total transfusion requirement. However, vigilance must be maintained to ensure that cells have been adequately washed to minimize drops in blood pressure upon reinfusion of scavenged blood. In cases when an infection is present, this modality is contraindicated. Another method of controlling blood loss is the use of deliberate hypotension in appropriately selected patients to decrease blood loss if mean arterial pressure is maintained between 50 and 60 mm Hg.

13. *Identify the complications associated with cement fixation.*

Although the quality of the bone–cement interface helps to reduce bleeding and fixes the hardware to the bone during THA, profound hypotension and death may occur shortly after the cemented femoral prostheses is inserted. This complication is not as common as in prior years; however, it can still be a factor in certain patient populations because methyl methacrylate can cause precipitous drops in blood pressure secondary to vasodilation and decrease PaO_2 secondary to embolization. It has also been theorized that methylmethacrylate has an inhibitory effect on myocardial excitation–contractile coupling, resulting in direct cardiac depression. Embolization of fat, air, fragmented bone, and cement have all been shown to occur during THA. Providers must ensure that patients are adequately hydrated before the procedure and vasopressors are readily available if hypotension occurs.

Postoperative Period

14. *Describe methods to enhance postoperative pain control after THA.*

Postoperative pain management may be addressed in a number of ways. The use of patient-controlled epidural opioids such as hydromorphone is extremely effective and can be accomplished via the epidural catheter placed for anesthesia. Likewise, a psoas compartment block (a single injection technique used with a nerve stimulator for anesthesia of the lumbar plexus) placed at the time of surgery provides postoperative analgesia for patients undergoing THA and significantly reduces narcotic requirements.

15. *Discuss the methods to decrease the possibility of postoperative venous thromboembolism after THA.*

    Patients must be made aware of the potential for DVT, and measures should be taken to prevent this complication. Due to her obesity, this patient is at increased risk of thromboembolism. Elastic compression stockings are used to facilitate venous return and

> • BOX 49.4 **Methods Used to Decrease the Incidence of Venous Thromboembolism**
>
> - Adequate oral hydration
> - Compression stockings
> - Ambulation
> - Regional anesthesia
> - Low-molecular-weight heparin

improve circulation. Patients must be encouraged to actively exercise the lower extremities and continue to take their anticoagulants as prescribed. Box 49.4 lists interventions that can be used to decrease the incidence of thromboembolism.

Review Questions

1. An advantage to providing regional anesthesia for hip arthroplasty includes:
   a. Increased need for airway manipulation or control.
   b. Decreased intraoperative blood loss.
   c. A more controlled environment for the patient to communicate discomfort.
   d. Decreased need for prolonged recovery room stay.

2. Patients who have a body mass index of greater than _____ are at increased risk for developing postoperative complications.
   a. 30
   b. 40
   c. 50
   d. 60

3. Perioperative arrhythmias that occur during surgery are associated with:
   a. Aggressive use of crystalloids.
   b. Acute renal failure.
   c. Antihypertensive agents.
   d. Common peroneal nerve compression.

4. Regional techniques cause a sympathectomy as a result of the inhibition of:
   a. Preganglionic *B* fiber transmission.
   b. Angiotensin II release.
   c. Decreased secretion of norepinephrine and epinephrine.
   d. Postganglionic alpha-adrenergic blockade.

5. Shivering-induced hypothermia can:
   a. Increase oxygen consumption by as much as 600%.
   b. Increase platelet function.
   c. Improve enzyme action of the coagulation cascade.
   d. Cause a leftward shift in the oxyhemoglobin dissociation curve.

Suggested Readings

Bugada D, Bellini V, Lorini LF, Mariano ER. Update on selective regional analgesia for hip surgery patients. *Anesthesiol Clin* 2018; 36(3):403-415.

Donauer K, Bomberg H, Wagenpfeil S, et al. Regional vs. general anesthesia for total knee and hip replacement: an analysis of postoperative pain perception from the international PAIN OUT registry. *Pain Pract* 2018;18(8):1036-1047.

Hannon CP, Keating TC, Lange JK, et al. Anesthesia and analgesia practices in total joint arthroplasty: a survey of the American Association of Hip and Knee Surgeons membership. *J Arthroplasty* 2019;34(12):2872-2877.

Hebl JR, Dilger JA, Byer DE, et al. A pre-emptive multimodal pathway featuring peripheral nerve block improves perioperative outcomes after major orthopedic surgery. *Reg Anesth Pain Med* 2008;33(6):510-517.

Hirsch MT. Anesthesia for orthopedics and podiatry. In: Nagelhout JJ, Elisha S, eds. *Nurse Anesthesia,* 6th ed. St. Louis, MO: Elsevier, 2018:947-958.

Johnson RL, Kopp SL, Burkle CM, et al. Neuraxial vs general anaesthesia for total hip and total knee arthroplasty: a systematic review of comparative-effectiveness research. *Br J Anaesth* 2016;116(2): 163-76.

Memtsoudis SG, Cozowicz C, Bekeris J, et al. Anaesthetic care of patients undergoing primary hip and knee arthroplasty: consensus recommendations from the International Consensus on Anaesthesia-Related Outcomes After Surgery group (ICAROS) based on a systematic review and meta-analysis. *Br J Anaesth* 2019;123(3): 269-287.

Minville V, Lubrano V, Bounes V, et al. Postoperative analgesia after total hip arthroplasty: patient-controlled analgesia versus transdermal fentanyl patch. *J Clin Anesth* 2008;20(4):280-283.

Perlas A, Chan VW, Beattie S. Anesthesia technique and mortality after total hip or knee arthroplasty: a retrospective, propensity score-matched cohort study. *Anesthesiology* 2016;125(4):724-31.

50

Above-the-Knee Amputation

KEY POINTS

- The anesthetic management of the amputation patient depends largely on the coexisting diseases.
- Prevention of central sensitization and chronic pain requires a multimodal approach.

- The most frequent postoperative complication resulting from the procedure is phantom limb pain, with or without accompanying stump pain.

Case Synopsis

A 25-year-old man was injured in a motorcycle accident. The patient has had three limb salvage surgeries in the past 6 months in an effort to save his affected leg. He is now scheduled for a right above-the-knee amputation (AKA).

Preoperative Evaluation and Demographic Data

Past Medical/Surgical History

- Five-year cigarette smoking history, but has not smoked in 3 months since accident
- Appendectomy under general anesthesia, no complications
- Six months ago: right lower extremity (RLE) open reduction internal fixation (ORIF) tibia/fibula, general anesthesia, no complications
- One month ago: revision to RLE, general anesthesia, no complications
- Three months ago: hardware exchange RLE, general anesthesia, no complications

List of Medications

- Gabapentin
- Celecoxib
- Oxycodone (OxyContin)

Diagnostic Data

- Hemoglobin, 12.2 g/dL; hematocrit, 36.4%

Height/Weight/Vital Signs

- 180 cm, 82 kg
- Blood pressure, 138/70; heart rate, 88 beats per minute; respiratory rate, 18 breaths per minute; room air oxygen saturation, 97%; temperature, 36.6°C

Pathophysiology

Many patients who present for an AKA have significant coexisting diseases such as diabetes, peripheral vascular, and cardiovascular disease. However, there are also a significant number of patients who are otherwise healthy who present for amputation due to trauma to the lower extremity.

An understanding of the mechanisms that can lead to stimulation of the pain pathway is necessary in order to plan for this case. Pain is more complex than nociception; it is the experience of the sensation, which can be variable and is dependent on each individual. Psychological and sociocultural factors influence the perception of pain. The primary afferent neurons have terminals that are stimulated by either heat, cold, or a mechanical event, such as pressure. Many chemicals are released, depending on the degree or type of tissue injury and include bradykinins, serotonin, and histamine, among others. This process activates the arachidonic acid cascade resulting in inflammation. The end products of the inflammatory process are also capable of stimulating the peripheral nerve, amplifying the pain stimulus. The process of conversion of the mechanical stimulation to the electrical activity, or an action potential, is a process known as *transduction*.

Primary afferent fibers have been classified by the type of stimulus and size; however, most nociceptive fibers can be stimulated by more than one modality. The afferent fibers are classified as A, B, or C. The speed of conduction is influenced by the amount of myelination that is present on the distinct fiber, which is present in A and B fibers. The A fibers transmit pain described as "sharp" and, because of the myelination, information is transmitted to the brain very rapidly. The C fibers are not myelinated and transmit pain signals more slowly, which may be described by patients as "dull" or "aching." In normal physiologic conditions, the electrical impulse is conducted through a nerve by a process known as *transmission*.

Afferent nerves enter the dorsal horn and terminate in the lamina V or I. A branch of these nerves ends in the lamina II and III (substantia gelatinosa) where interneurons modulate pain by inhibitory neurons. Most axons ascend on the opposite side in the spinothalamic tract. These axons terminate in either the thalamus or the somatosensory cortex where pain is perceived. A diagrammatic description of central and peripheral pain transmission and medications used to treat pain is presented in Fig. 50.1.

Surgical Procedure

During an AKA, the leg is completely excised at a point along the distal one-third of the femur, preserving as much of the femur as possible. This procedure is generally performed due to chronic peripheral vascular disease and gangrene, uncontrolled infection, or traumatic injury. A stump is formed if there is no evidence of infection at the site by using the anterior and posterior musculature. The adductor tubercle is

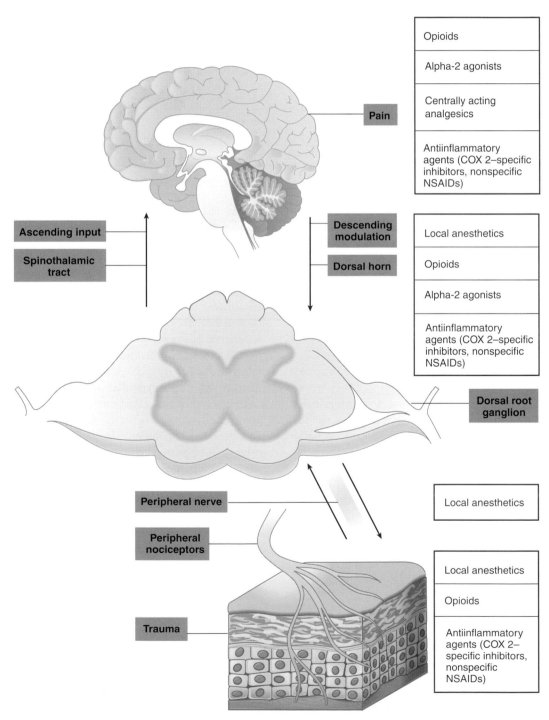

• **Fig. 50.1** Central and peripheral pain transmission. (From Waldman S, Terzic A: *Pharmacology and therapeutics: Principles to practice*, St. Louis, 2009, Saunders.)

frequently removed, so the adductor muscle or tendon is repaired to the femur to prevent unopposed abduction. The procedure is most often performed with the patient in the supine position. Blood loss is not usually significant when a tourniquet is used. The most frequent postoperative complication resulting from the procedure is phantom limb pain, with or without accompanying stump pain.

Anesthetic Management and Considerations

Preoperative Period

1. *Discuss the perioperative considerations for this patient.*

   The incidence of chronic pain resulting from amputation is reported to be as high as 80%. Therefore a primary consideration for this case involves a treatment plan to prevent the development of this debilitating condition. Recent evidence suggests that the prevention of the wind-up phenomenon is important because once this has occurred, it can result in intractable pain that is difficult to treat and may have long-lasting effects on many physiologic processes. Adequate treatment of the pain for this case involves a multimodal approach because the surgical trauma and resultant inflammation create significant afferent stimulation, which leads to central sensitization.

2. *Describe the process associated with central sensitization.*

   Acute pain, such as postoperative pain and the resultant inflammation, can have significantly long-lasting effects due to changes that occur in the peripheral and central nervous system. It has been well documented that the central nervous system has the capacity to be a dynamic system, a property known as plasticity. This dynamic system can result in a reduction of the threshold of peripheral neurons and other changes in the characteristics of the afferent neuron. This is generally thought to be caused by the inflammatory process. The barrage of sensory input from the periphery leads to an increase in the spinal neurons' excitability in the central nervous system. This peripheral and central sensitization has been called "wind-up," and once this has occurred, it can lead to intractable pain. Central sensitization involves physiologic changes in the nervous system that lead to symptoms such as allodynia, hyperalgesia, decreased pain threshold, and areas of referred pain. The underlying cause of these symptoms include:
   - Changes in the N-methyl-D-aspartate (NMDA) receptor
   - Ectopic neuronal firing
   - Changes in the gene expression of the sodium channel
   - Sensitization of the nociceptive receptor

3. *Explain the concept of multimodal analgesia.*

   Opioids are the mainstay for treating pain, but there are many undesirable side effects, including nausea and vomiting, respiratory depression, sedation, pruritus, urinary retention, and sleep disturbances. The goal of multimodal analgesia is to improve analgesia and reduce the prevalence of opioid-related side effects. This strategy targets different aspects of the pain pathway and utilizes the synergistic effects of combinations of medication to provide sufficient analgesia, while minimizing the side effects.

4. *Identify the consequences associated with prolonged opioid therapy.*

   Prolonged use of opioids is associated with the consequences noted earlier and beyond the side effects of the drug. Increasing dosages are often required to achieve the same level of analgesia—a process known as tolerance. Tolerance can be complicated by the fact that prolonged use of opioids is also associated with opioid-induced hypersensitivity. This phenomenon is not completely understood, but in animal studies the changes in the spinal cord after prolonged doses of opioids are similar to that of models of neuropathic pain. Prolonged use of opioids is also associated with hormonal changes and immunosuppression. Therefore minimizing the dosages and length of opioid therapy is desirable.

5. *What are the multimodal analgesic regimens for orthopedic surgery?*

   The multimodal analgesic regimens for orthopedic surgery include the use of local anesthetics, nonsteroidal antiinflammatory drugs (NSAIDs), acetaminophen, NMDA receptor antagonists, and opioids.

6. *Discuss the mechanism by which alpha-2 agonists facilitate analgesia.*

   Alpha-2 agonists have analgesic actions at peripheral, spinal, and brainstem sites where alpha-2 adrenoreceptors are located. However, the exact mechanism by which these medications reduce pain is not completely understood. Clonidine appears to enhance both peripheral and neuraxial blockade. Alpha-2 agonists are a valuable adjunct for treating sympathetically mediated pain by inhibiting the release of norepinephrine from the alpha-2 adrenoreceptors. When added to epidural infusion, clonidine has been shown to reduce the opioid requirement after orthopedic surgery. Dexmedetomidine is an alpha-2 agonist that is associated with sedation, but administering this drug can be useful to decrease the physiologic stress response associated with surgery and decrease postoperative pain.

7. *Discuss the mechanism by which ketamine or other NMDA receptor antagonists facilitate analgesia.*

   There has been great interest in ketamine as an adjunct for anesthesia after the mechanism of central sensitization has been elucidated. Although significant psychomimetic effects have been described with the use of ketamine, lower doses are not associated with these side effects and appear to provide excellent analgesic efficacy. Memantine is an alternative to ketamine that can be administered orally and has a lower incidence of undesirable side effects. The NMDA receptors are located on primary afferents, interneurons, and projection neurons.

8. *Discuss the mechanism by which gabapentin facilitates analgesia.*

Gabapentin is an anticonvulsant that was developed to be a gamma-aminobutyric acid (GABA) agonist, but it does not have an affinity for GABA. The binding site has been identified as the $\alpha 2\delta$ subunit of voltage-gated calcium channels. Gabapentin inhibits the calcium current in sensory neurons, and it is an important adjunct for preemptive analgesia. It is also thought to interact with the NMDA receptor complex, but this mechanism is still poorly understood.

9. *Discuss the mechanism of action of NSAIDs.*

Tissue injury causes activation of the arachidonic acid cascade, leading to the production of prostaglandins. These prostaglandins sensitize the nociceptors and can lead to hyperalgesia, or an increased response to stimuli. NSAIDs inhibit cyclooxygenase types 1 and 2 (COX-1 and COX-2), which decrease the production of prostaglandins. As shown in Fig. 50.2, all NSAIDs, with the exception of the COX-2–specific inhibitors such as celecoxib, which this patient is taking routinely, inhibit both COX-1 and COX-2 enzymes. The prostaglandins that are created by the COX-1 enzyme are necessary for homeostasis and contribute to adequate bronchial and renal vascular tone, normal platelet function, and the gastric barrier. Therefore when the prostaglandins necessary for physiologic functioning are inhibited, side effects such as bronchospasm, renal insufficiency, bleeding, and gastric ulceration can occur, especially if NSAIDs are taken at high doses and on a routine basis. The prostaglandins that are created by the COX-2 enzyme mediate pain and have been implicated in increasing edema formation resulting from surgical trauma.

NSAIDs inhibit the production of prostaglandins in the periphery as well as in the spinal cord, resulting in a reduction in inflammation and pain after surgery.

10. *Discuss the mechanism of action of acetaminophen.*

Recent evidence suggests that acetaminophen may inhibit the production of prostaglandins in the central nervous system. Theoretically, this effect is mediated by inhibition of a COX-3 receptor; however, this concept remains controversial. Multiple studies have demonstrated the efficacy of acetaminophen for decreasing pain and inflammation after surgery, without the side effects of the COX-2 inhibitors.

11. *Discuss the anesthetic considerations for this patient in the preoperative period.*

Administration of midazolam is recommended in the preoperative period because this procedure is associated with anxiety. It should be titrated to effect, and an opioid may also be considered. The regularly scheduled medications for this patient should be continued. This patient is already taking gabapentin 600 mg and celecoxib 200 mg twice daily. Unless contraindicated, neuraxial anesthesia is recommended for anesthesia and analgesia. Recent evidence suggests that an epidural catheter insertion followed by a 48-hour continuous bupivacaine infusion should be placed before the amputation procedure to improve postoperative outcomes.

Intraoperative Period

12. *Discuss the intraoperative considerations for this patient.*

A multimodal technique should be utilized in order to meet the anesthetic goals for this patient. Titration of medications is paramount to a successful anesthetic

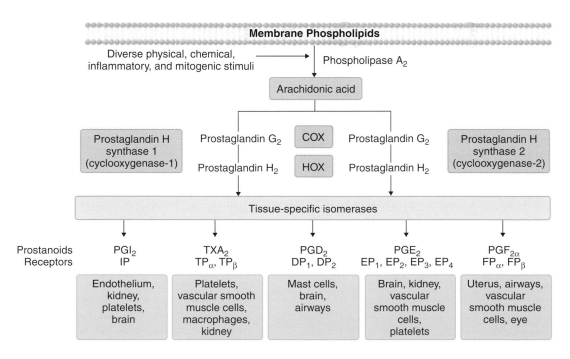

• **Fig. 50.2** Biologic formation of prostaglandins. (From Goldman L, Schafer AI: *Goldman-Cecil medicine*, ed 25, St. Louis, 2016, Elsevier.)

because this patient has been requiring opioids for an extended period. As part of a balanced anesthetic, the following adjuncts may be considered:

- Ketamine infusion: 0.1 to 0.3 mg/kg/hr intravenous (IV)
- Dexmedetomidine 0.5 to 1.0 mcg/kg IV
- Opioids: titrated to the observed analgesic effect

Postoperative Period

13. Discuss the postoperative considerations for this patient.

It is important to meet the psychological needs of the patient postoperatively. Providing a calm, quiet environment, especially if the patient exhibits signs of posttraumatic stress disorder, is vital. Multidisciplinary support, as well as family support, is optimal to aid the patient to deal with the significant emotional component of the loss of limb and loss of function.

The epidural infusion after surgery may contain a solution that will provide adequate sensory blockade: bupivacaine (0.125% to 0.25%) with or without adjuncts. Adjuncts to the epidural infusion include fentanyl 2 mcg/mL or hydromorphone 20 mcg/mL. The epidural infusion should be continued unless anticoagulation is required. If anticoagulation is planned and the epidural will be discontinued, a peripheral nerve catheter should be considered. A femoral nerve catheter and a sciatic catheter are required to provide

TABLE 50.1	Patient-Controlled Analgesia Settings		
	Bolus (mg)	Lockout (min)	Basal (mg/hr)
Fentanyl	0.015–0.05	3–10	0.02–0.1
Hydromorphone	0.1–0.5	5–15	0.2–0.5
Morphine	0.5–3	5–20	1–10
Methadone	0.5–3	10–20	—

adequate coverage for the amputee. The peripheral nerve catheters can be placed preoperatively, but if the epidural is to be used for the first 24 hours, the catheters can be placed on the first postoperative day.

Multimodal therapy should be resumed as soon as possible after surgery, with attention to the time frame that the patient is tolerating oral medications. IV agents should be utilized to maintain the multimodal therapy until the patient can take oral medications. If there is breakthrough pain, patient-controlled analgesia (PCA) may be necessary, and Table 50.1 includes recommendations for PCA settings. If significant opioid side effects are present (nausea, respiratory depression), it is possible to add ketamine to the PCA.

Review Questions

1. Which medication is not commonly used as a multimodal regimen for postoperative pain management?
   a. Dexmedetomidine
   b. Methadone
   c. Bupivacaine
   d. Celecoxib
2. Which is the primary pathway of the axons of second-order neurons on the contralateral side of the spinal cord?
   a. Spinothalamic tract
   b. Spinoreticular tract
   c. Spinomesencephalic tract
   d. Spinohypothalamic tract
3. Hydromorphone is _____ more potent than morphine.
   a. 2 times
   b. 3 times
   c. 5 times
   d. 15 times

4. Opioid-induced hyperalgesia is caused by:
   a. Improper dose escalation of opioids.
   b. Inadequate treatment of depression.
   c. Drug tolerance to the administration of opioids.
   d. Abnormal sensitivity after repeated exposure to opioids.
5. Which receptor is involved in central sensitization causing persistent pain?
   a. NMDA
   b. Mu opioid
   c. Kappa opioid
   d. Alpha-2 adrenergic

Suggested Readings

Alejandro S, Teasdall RD, Holden M, et al. Outcomes of below-the-knee amputations for chronic lower extremity pain. *J Surg Orthop Adv* 2017;26(4):200-205

Busse JW, Jacobs CL, Swiontkowski MF, et al. Complex limb salvage or early amputation for severe lower-limb surgery: a meta-analysis of observational studies. *J Ortho Trauma* 2007;21:70-76.

Ciufo DJ, Thirukumaran CP, Marchese R, Oh. Risk factors for reoperation, readmission, and early complications after below knee amputation. *Injury* 2019;50(2):462-466.

Cohen SP, Bhatia A, Buvanendran A, et al. Consensus guidelines on the use of intravenous ketamine infusions for chronic pain from the American Society of Regional Anesthesia and Pain Medicine, the American Academy of Pain Medicine, and the American Society of Anesthesiologists. *Reg Anesth Pain Med* 2018;43(5):521-546.

Glare P, Aubrey KR, Myles PS. Transition from acute to chronic pain after surgery. *Lancet* 2019;393(10180):1537-1546.

Hirsch MT. Anesthesia for orthopedics and podiatry. In: Nagelhout JJ, Elisha S, eds. *Nurse Anesthesia,* 6th ed. St. Louis, MO: Elsevier, 2018:947-958.

Kien NT, Geiger P, Van Chuong H, et al. Preemptive analgesia after lumbar spine surgery by pregabalin and celecoxib: a prospective study. *Drug Des Devel Ther* 2019;13:2145-2152.

Luo Y, Anderson TA. Phantom *limb pain: a review. Int Anesthesiol Clin* 2016;54(2):121-139.

Macone A, Otis JAD. Neuropathic pain. *Semin Neurol* 2018;38(6):644-653.

Nikolajsen L, Finnerup NB, Kramp S, et al. A randomized study of the effects of gabapentin on postamputation pain. *Anesthesiology* 2006;105:1008-1015.

Schwartzman RJ, Grothusen J, Kiefer TR, et al. Neuropathic central pain. *Arch Neurol* 2001;58:1547-1550.

St John E. Advances in understanding nociception and neuropathic pain. *J Neurol* 2018;265(2):231-238.

Wiech AK, Kiefer R, Topfner S, et al. A placebo-controlled randomized crossover trial of the N-methyl-D-aspartic acid receptor antagonist, memantine in patients with chronic phantom limb pain. *Anesth Analg* 2004;98:408-413.

Wylde V, Dennis J, Beswick AD, et al. Systematic review of management of chronic pain after surgery. *Br J Surg* 2017;104(10):1293-1306.

51

Bowel Resection for Necrotizing Enterocolitis

KEY POINTS

- Necrotizing enterocolitis (NEC) is one of the most common neonatal gastrointestinal emergencies, causing significant morbidity and mortality in this group.
- The anesthetic management for these patients is often complicated by multiple comorbidities and congenital anomalies.

- Relatively large volumes of intravenous (IV) crystalloid, colloid, blood, and blood products may be required.

Case Synopsis

A 10-day-old infant, who is in the neonatal intensive care unit (NICU), is scheduled to have an emergent laparotomy and bowel resection due to an intestinal perforation resulting from NEC. Your patient was born at 27 weeks' gestational age and has been suffering from worsening abdominal distention over the last 3 days. This patient also has a patent ductus arteriosus (PDA).

Preoperative Evaluation and Demographic Data

Current Treatment and Medications

- Currently this patient is in the NICU receiving total parenteral nutrition, a broad-spectrum antibiotic regimen, and oxygen via nasal prongs.

Diagnostic Data

- Hemoglobin, 9.8 g/dL; hematocrit, 29.4%; these values have been decreasing compared with previous measurements.
- Sodium, 140 mEq/L; potassium, 4.2 mEq/L; chloride, 104 mEq/L; bicarbonate, 27 mEq/L
- Calcium, 7.9 mg/dL; glucose, 70 mg/dL

Weight and Vital Signs

- Birth weight, 1450 grams
- Current weight, 1210 grams
- Blood pressure, 47/20; heart rate, 168 beats per minute; respiratory rate, 55 breaths per minute; temperature, 36.6°C (radiant warming); oxygen saturation of 92% with supplemental oxygen via nasal prongs

Pathophysiology

Although the exact causes of NEC are still the subject of debate, common predisposing factors include prematurity, sepsis, and formula feeding. The incidence of NEC is highest in low-birth-weight infants, often defined as birth weight less than 1500 grams. Some reviewers have supported the use of enteral supplementation of probiotics in premature infants who weigh greater than 1000 grams to reduce the risk of severe NEC. Extreme prematurity is defined as the gestational age between 24 and 30 weeks, extraordinarily small size, and underdeveloped organ systems. These characteristics provide a myriad of challenges independent of NEC that warrant consideration.

Several factors predispose low-birth-weight and premature neonates to developing NEC. Some of these causes include immune system and intestinal barrier immaturity, which increases the patient's susceptibility to bacterial translocation from the gastrointestinal lumen into systemic circulation. This process can lead to sepsis, increased risk of nosocomial viral or bacterial exposure, and the presence of other anatomic and physiologic anomalies. Hemodynamic instability, respiratory failure, coagulopathy, perinatal hypoxia, and hypoperfusion may also be contributing factors.

The most frequent finding on assessment of the neonate with NEC is abdominal distention. Sometimes the abdominal wall can become so distended that respiratory compromise and failure occur, necessitating ventilatory support. Metabolic acidosis is common, and it is believed to result from poor tissue perfusion. Thrombocytopenia and disseminated intravascular coagulation are present in many of these patients.

The abdominal radiographic findings that accompany NEC can include dilated loops of bowel, intraperitoneal fluid collection, and free air accompanying intestinal perforation. The hallmark sign of NEC is intramural gas collection. Currently, abdominal radiographs are used to determine the presence of intramural gas, portal venous gas, and free air within the abdomen. Sonography may improve the diagnostic ability of the surgeon, as fluid in the abdomen, increased bowel thickness, and bowel perfusion are not always easily appreciated on abdominal radiographs. Other findings may include poor skin turgor with a mottled appearance, diminished or absent peripheral pulses, and poor capillary refill. Decreasing blood pressure and urine output may indicate progressive intravascular hypovolemia.

Surgical Treatment

The effectiveness and survival rates of patients who are treated via laparotomy versus placement of a peritoneal drain at the bedside to decrease abdominal distention are comparable. The type of procedure (laparotomy versus peritoneal drainage) does not influence the survival or outcome of perforated NEC in low-birth-weight infants. Some have concluded that the difference in early mortality rates between cases of NEC treated with initial drain placement and laparotomy is not significant. The long-term outcomes in these groups are still under investigation.

Placement of a drain can be accomplished at the bedside by the surgeon in the NICU with minimal blood loss. Surgical exploration of these patients at the bedside or in the operating room is commonly accomplished via transverse laparotomy. The procedure can also be accomplished via a laparoscopic-assisted technique. After nonviable portions of bowel have been resected, a proximal stoma and distal mucus fistula are created, which can be reversed after the patient's condition improves. The combined experience of the anesthesia care team, surgeon, and neonatologist should decide on the best course of action. Additionally, communication among all team members is essential in order to facilitate high-quality patient care.

Anesthetic Management and Considerations

Preoperative Period

1. *Discuss the options that are available in order to optimize this patient for surgery.*

Several interventions can be beneficial to optimize the patient's condition before the surgical procedure. The operating room should be prepared by ensuring that the ambient temperature is increased, fluids are warmed, and forced-air warming devices are running before the arrival of the patient. Warming pads designed for use in neonates are available to minimize heat loss on the way to the operating room. Additionally, covering exposed body surface area with blankets or plastic will help maintain normothermia.

Ensuring adequate IV access can be extraordinarily challenging, especially during periods of hypovolemia and hypotension. Placing central lines, additional peripheral IV lines, or arterial lines as indicated by the patient's status before leaving the NICU, if time allows, can minimize operating room time while providing access for the infusion of fluids, blood products, or medications as needed during surgery. In situations where the patient is severely unstable or requires support difficult to maintain in the operating room such as an oscillating ventilator, bedside laparotomy can be undertaken in the NICU. Emergent laparotomy can also be performed at the bedside in situations in which the patient is too unstable to transport to the operating room. The patient may also require high-frequency oscillating ventilation.

2. *Describe the physiologic considerations affecting premature infants and their impact on anesthesia management.*

Many health problems are associated with premature infants independently of NEC, including the following:

- **Intraventricular hemorrhage:** Premature infants are often at high risk for intraventricular hemorrhage from a variety of causes, including hypoxia, hemodynamic instability, and acidosis. Intraventricular hemorrhage occurs commonly in premature infants, and many centers routinely screen extremely premature infants for this condition.

- **Cardiovascular immaturity:** The patient in this scenario has a PDA, and he is at increased risk for persistent left-to-right shunting and increased pulmonary blood flow resulting in pulmonary hypertension and congestive heart failure. Cardiovascular immaturity prevents effective compensation for blood loss and hypotension. Due to the functional immaturity of the heart, decreased ventricular elasticity limits contractility; therefore increases in cardiac output are dependent on increases in the heart rate. Bradycardia is poorly tolerated because hypoperfusion occurs despite immense metabolic demands. Fluid shifts that are associated with NEC can lead to intravascular depletion requiring significant volume replacement. Persistent fetal circulation and congenital cardiac defects necessitate meticulous inspection of IV lines for air bubbles.

The ductus arteriosus (DA), an opening between the pulmonary artery and aorta, normally undergoes functional closure between 15 hours and 4 days after birth. The DA will remain patent if hypoxemia or sepsis is present. The process of continuous shunting through a PDA can be a continuous cycle resulting in systemic hypoperfusion and severe hypoxemia. Shunting of blood through the PDA makes the bowel more susceptible to developing ischemia via hypoperfusion, which is thought to contribute to the incidence of NEC.

- **Hypothermia:** A large surface area to body weight ratio and diminished fat layer make premature infants prone to significant hypothermia, especially during laparotomy in the operating room. Many interventions can help maintain a relatively constant and warm environment, and these methods are listed in Box 51.1. Hypothermia will cause nonshivering thermogenesis to occur in pediatric patients who are less than 3 months of age. Blood flow will be redistributed to brown fat, and this process leads to the metabolism of triglycerides. Liberation of heat occurs as the triglycerides are broken into acetoacetic acid, beta-hydroxybutyric acid, and ketones that results in metabolic acidosis.

- **Fluid and electrolyte management:** Neonatal renal function is less efficient, predisposing them to sodium loss and less reliable reabsorption of sodium, glucose, bicarbonate, phosphates, and amino acids. During intraoperative management, neonates may require supplemental glucose; however, hyperglycemia should be avoided. These patients are frequently receiving total parenteral nutrition, and this therapy should be continued throughout the perioperative period.

- **Respiratory dynamics:** Respiratory function of the premature neonate is immature. In the case of the patient with NEC, this immature system can be severely compromised by increased work of breathing due to worsening abdominal distention, fatigue, hypoxia, and increased metabolic rate, which further decreases ventilatory reserves. Respiratory function also improves significantly if lung development is sufficient before birth. The younger the patient, the less viable the gas exchange mechanisms in the lungs and the more labile the intrinsic regulation of multiple physiologic processes like temperature management and blood sugar control.

High-frequency oscillating ventilation may be necessary to adequately oxygenate these patients during surgery. Effective means of providing additional supplemental oxygen, controlled ventilation, and intubation should be immediately available during transport to the operating room. The effect of increased oxygen consumption and diminished functional residual capacity complicated by sepsis and severe abdominal distention on the oxygen reserve of these patients dramatically increases the potential for rapid desaturation, hypoxemia, and acidosis. Additional equipment and personnel experienced in securing the airway should be immediately available before induction. The neonatologist is a valuable resource in helping to secure the airway in the NICU before departure for the operating room.

Intraoperative Period

3. *Discuss the factors that contribute to rapidly decreasing oxygen saturation during induction and intubation of a premature infant with NEC.*

   Neonatal hypermetabolism exacerbated by sepsis can combine to create a scenario where the patient is unable to compensate for periods of apnea or hypoxia. Additionally, respiratory compromise from lung immaturity and abdominal distention create a more fragile balance between oxygen supply and demand. These issues result in a state where the oxygen reserve of the patient is minimal and quickly exhausted. The oxygen exchange and reserve capacity of the lungs are diminished by the upward intrusion of abdominal distention and lung underdevelopment complicated by a lack of surfactant that facilitates alveolar collapse.

4. *Identify interventions that will aid in the successful placement of an endotracheal tube (ETT) for this patient.*

   There are several options for optimizing the airway management of this patient. Anesthetists and neonatologists familiar and experienced in intubating newborn patients should be present. Preoxygenation of any patient before intubation is appropriate. The head of a child is proportionately larger than that of an adult compared with the rest of the body. A small pad or towel under the shoulders can help overcome the tendency of the chin to move toward the chest and optimize the position for successful laryngoscopy. Small variations in the position of an ETT result in proper placement, extubation, and endobronchial intubation. Careful verification of proper placement is vital.

   Selecting the correct size ETT(s) and laryngoscope blade(s) for the patient is essential. If available, laryngoscope blades with the capacity to deliver in-line oxygen during laryngoscopy may help minimize the effect of apnea on oxygen saturation. Preoxygenation, immediately available help if needed, proper selection of equipment, and optimal positioning can all aid in providing an efficient and smooth induction and intubation.

5. *Discuss the pharmacologic and physiologic consequences to consider when providing anesthesia to the premature neonate.*

   Inhalation anesthetic agents can be safely used in this patient population, although the exact minimum alveolar concentration for this group is unknown. Premature infants experience an exaggerated hypotensive response to inhalational anesthetics due to their myocardial depressant and vasodilating properties and their potential to cause bradycardia. Hemodynamic stability will be dependent on the titration of the inhalation agents to the individual's response.

If the operation is to be performed in the NICU or the patient requires the use of a neonatal ventilator, IV anesthesia must be provided. Although many different IV agents have been used, opioid-based anesthesia coupled with neuromuscular blockade has been determined to provide a more stable hemodynamic profile. However, IV agents, including opioids and muscle relaxants, have the potential to exhibit significant pharmacokinetic variability when administered to these young patients. Many of these agents are metabolized by the liver by conjugation, hepatic function is immature, and medications can have a prolonged duration of effect. The choice of anesthetic agents that are to be used should be based on the individual patient's condition.

Opioid-based anesthesia often carries with it a prolonged respiratory depressant effect, contributing to delayed emergence and a requirement for postoperative mechanical ventilation. Given the significant preoperative respiratory compromise of these patients, postoperative mechanical ventilation is often electively continued, regardless of the anesthetic administered.

Immature metabolic processes and alterations in hepatic blood flow often contribute to the already wide variability in response to muscle relaxants. Neuromuscular transmission is immature, making titration of neuromuscular blockers difficult and can contribute to continued ventilatory support after surgery. The use of a nerve stimulator may be difficult and unreliable.

6. *Discuss some issues that may affect the choice of gas mixture administered to this patient during surgery.*

Continued administration of high concentrations of oxygen can contribute to visual impairment through the development of retinopathy of prematurity. Half of all low-birth-weight infants, less than 1500 grams, experience some degree of retinopathy of prematurity. This percentage increases to greater than 90% in the smallest premature infants. Retinopathy of prematurity is thought to result from a combination of factors, including hyperoxia. Experts suggest that titration of oxygen to maintain oxygen saturation between 87% and 92% is adequate. Maintenance of effective ventilation is challenging. Effective communication with the surgical team regarding the effects of abdominal packing and retraction can help balance the need for surgical exposure while minimizing ventilatory pressures.

The administration of nitrous oxide may contribute to further bowel distention; therefore its use is generally avoided. A mixture of air and oxygen titrated to the needs of the patient supplemented with low-volume percentages of an inhalation anesthetic as tolerated is often used.

7. *Discuss the fluid requirements of neonates undergoing laparotomy and bowel resection for NEC.*

The presence of gangrenous, perforated bowel coupled with exposure of the abdominal viscera to the environment can cause large amounts of third-space and evaporative fluid loss. Relatively large amounts of surgical blood loss combined with the presence of underlying coagulation abnormalities may necessitate the transfusion of large amounts of crystalloid, colloid, blood, and blood products. Correction of coagulation defects may require packed red blood cells, platelets, fresh frozen plasma, and cryoprecipitate. Preoperative anemia is common in premature neonates due to decreased red blood cell production. The need for preemptive transfusion before surgery should be considered. Transfusion in neonates is administered per kilogram of body weight. In these small patients, portions of a single unit of blood can be preordered and delivered to the operating room in prefiltered syringes. This serves multiple purposes. First, more exact volumes can be delivered. Second, this practice of splitting a unit into several smaller doses can allow a neonate who will receive several transfusions to be exposed to a smaller number of blood donors. One standard unit can often be used for multiple transfusions for one neonate before the unit expires.

The criteria for the delivery of blood to a patient should include the underlying normal hemoglobin value of the patient according to age, the overall condition of the patient, most current laboratory values, and both current and anticipated surgical blood loss. Hypovolemia and a compromised tissue oxygenation capacity are two indications for red blood cell administration.

Determining the circulating blood volume and estimated allowable blood loss can guide the anesthetist in determining when transfusion is appropriate and the volume of blood that may be required. The estimated circulating blood volume of the premature infant is approximately 90 to 100 mL/kg of body weight. Determining the volume of blood that should be transfused can be estimated in relation to total blood volume and hematocrit.

In this example, the patient is 1210 g or 1.21 kg and hematocrit is 29.4%. An absolute hemoglobin or hematocrit value necessitating the transfusion of blood has not been determined and should be based on the individual's condition. Consultation with the neonatal and surgical service should be considered when contemplating transfusion to attempt to meet the overall treatment goals of the patient. For the sole purpose of demonstrating the relevant equations, we will use an example of a low hematocrit of 25%.

- Blood volume:

$$1.21 \text{ kg} \times 95 \text{ mL/kg} = 114.95 \text{ mL}$$

- Red blood cell mass (Hct 29.4%):

$$114.95 \text{ mL} \times 0.294 = 33.75 \text{ mL}$$

- Red blood cell mass (Hct 25%):

$$114.95 \text{ mL} \times 0.25 = 28.73 \text{ mL}$$

- Allowable blood loss

$$33.79 \text{ mL} - 28.73 \text{ mL} = \text{approximately 5 mL}$$

This example demonstrates that a relatively small amount of blood loss can result in severe hypovolemia in these very small patients. The decision to transfuse must consider the overall situation, status of the patient, and surgical progress toward hemostasis. Transfusion of packed red blood cells is usually given in doses of 5 to 10 mL/kg of body weight per dose. These values provide only gross estimation because precise determination of surgical blood and fluid loss is difficult to ascertain. The effects of hemodilution by administration of crystalloid or colloid solutions must also be considered.

Laparotomy for bowel resection for NEC can require large-volume blood transfusions and the need for other blood components. Preoperative low platelet counts coupled with large-volume blood transfusions may indicate the need for platelet administration. Fresh frozen plasma is a blood product that can be considered when large amounts of packed red blood cells are transfused, as this can produce dilutional coagulopathy. Other information like coagulation studies can also guide transfusion decisions. Fresh frozen plasma, if indicated, is administered to improve plasma clotting factor availability and can be administered in 10 mL/kg infusions. The presentation of each patient and the operative course should be considered when the choice and volume of blood products is made.

Postoperative Period

8. *Consider the postoperative care of this patient in the NICU.*
   The choice of anesthetic administered will influence the need for postoperative mechanical ventilation. If neuromuscular blockade and opioid-based anesthesia are administered, it is likely than this patient will require a ventilator in the NICU. Massive volume transfusion and a difficult or prolonged surgical course may also lead the team to choose postoperative ventilatory support to aid in the care of the patient during the immediate postoperative period. If IV lines and ETT tubes are placed in the operating room, radiologic confirmation of correct placement may be helpful to the neonatal care team.

Review Questions

1. Which is the most common finding associated with necrotizing enterocolitis?
   a. Abdominal distention
   b. Hypotension
   c. Vomiting after feeding
   d. Lethargy
2. Which is a common radiographic finding associated with necrotizing enterocolitis?
   a. Poor bowel perfusion
   b. Pneumonia
   c. Pneumothorax
   d. Intramural gas
3. An intubated neonate that has NEC is at greatest risk for developing _____ during transportation to the operating room.
   a. blood loss
   b. third-space fluid loss
   c. hypothermia
   d. hypoxia

4. Which complication is most likely to occur during induction and intubation of a patient with NEC?
   a. Unrecognized difficult airway
   b. Esophageal intubation
   c. Dental injury
   d. Rapid desaturation
5. Which is a benefit to the patient of dividing one unit of blood into multiple transfusions for a patient with NEC?
   a. Cost containment
   b. Ease of dispensing
   c. Minimal donor exposures
   d. Conservation of scarce blood resources

Suggested Readings

Ahmed Z, Danielson L, Albeiruti R, et al. Blood transfusion in patients treated with surgery for necrotizing enterocolitis. *Paediatr Anaesth* 2015;25(2):196-199.

Alfaleh K, Bassler D. Probiotics for prevention of necrotizing enterocolitis in preterm infants. *Cochrane Database Syst Rev* 2008;111(5):1202-1204.

Bazacliu C, Neu J. Necrotizing enterocolitis: long term complications. *Curr Pediatr Rev* 2019;15(2):115-124.

Eaton S, Rees CM, Hall NJ. Current research on the epidemiology, pathogenesis, and management of necrotizing enterocolitis. *Neonatology* 2017;111(4):423-430.

Elisha S, Terry K. Neonatal anesthesia. In: Nagelhout JJ, Elisha S, eds. *Nurse Anesthesia*, 6th ed. St. Louis, MO: Elsevier, 2018:1093-1116.

Hackam D, Caplan M. Necrotizing enterocolitis: pathophysiology from a historical context. *Semin Pediatr Surg* 2018;27(1):11-18.

Michelet D, Brasher C, Kaddour HB, et al. Postoperative complications following neonatal and infant surgery: common events and predictive factors. *Anaesth Crit Care Pain Med* 2017;36(3):163-169.

Müller MJ, Paul T, Seeliger S. Necrotizing enterocolitis in premature infants and newborns. *J Neonatal Perinatal Med* 2016;9(3):233-42.

Neu J, Pammi M. Necrotizing enterocolitis: the intestinal microbiome, metabolome and inflammatory mediators. *Semin Fetal Neonatal Med* 2018;23(6):400-405.

Pierro A. The surgical management of necrotizing enterocolitis. *Early Hum Dev* 2005;81(1):79-85.

Subramaniam R. Anaesthetic concerns in preterm and term neonates. *Indian J Anaesth* 2019;63(9):771-779.

52

Infantile Hypertrophic Pyloric Stenosis

KEY POINTS

- Infantile hypertrophic pyloric stenosis (IHPS) is the most common cause of gastrointestinal obstruction in newborns and infants.
- The classic presentation includes nonbilious repeated emesis that can progress to projectile vomiting.
- IHPS occurs in 3% of live births, and it is more common among white males.

- Initial therapy for patients who have pyloric stenosis focuses on optimization of the patient's fluid volume and electrolyte status. Surgery is not performed on an emergency basis for pyloric stenosis.
- Preoperative management of fluid, electrolyte, and acid–base imbalances is imperative to the intraoperative and postoperative stability of the patient.

Case Synopsis

A 35-day-old infant boy is admitted for multiple episodes of projectile emesis after feedings, which began 48 hours ago. Diagnostic testing included an abdominal ultrasound, which confirmed the presence of pyloric stenosis. Surgery is scheduled for the next morning. Appropriate fluid, electrolyte, and acid–base balance management is instituted.

Preoperative Evaluation and Demographic Data

Past Medical/Surgical History

- None

List of Medications

- None

Diagnostic Data

- Sodium, 127 mEq/L; potassium, 2.5 mEq/L; chloride, 78 mmol/L; carbon dioxide, 36 mEq/L
- Blood urea nitrogen, 12 mg/dL; creatinine, 0.6 mg/dL
- Glucose, 55 mg/dL
- Arterial blood gas (ABG): pH, 7.49; PaO_2, 91 mm Hg; PCO_2, 41 mm Hg; HCO_3, 32 mm Hg; base excess, 28.0
- Palpable solid mass upper abdomen
- Abdominal ultrasound: hypertrophic pyloric muscle measuring 4.8 mm
- Upper gastrointestinal imaging (UGI) barium series if ultrasound nondiagnostic

Height/Weight/Vital Signs

- 57 cm, 5.3 kg
- Blood pressure, 70/38; heart rate, 172 beats per minute; respiratory rate, 40 breaths per minute; room air oxygen saturation, 97%; rectal temperature, 37.1°C
- Urine output (UOP), 1 mL/kg/hr

Pathophysiology

Pyloric stenosis occurs due to thickening of the smooth muscle of the pyloric valve, which is located at the junction between the stomach and small intestine, as shown in Fig. 52.1. This pathologic process is associated with a cleft palate and gastroesophageal reflux. Depending on the degree of gastric outlet obstruction, digestive contents are unable to move normally into the duodenum. This results in increased intragastric pressure, which causes vomiting immediately after feeding. Newborns are predisposed to rapidly developing hypovolemia, gastric aspiration, and electrolyte abnormalities that most commonly result in *hypokalemic, hypochloremic,* and *metabolic alkalosis.* This occurs due to the persistent vomiting and resulting decrease in fluid volume intake. Also, there is a high concentration of hydrogen ion and chloride present in gastric fluid that is lost. Although the etiology of pyloric stenosis is unknown, a possible relationship links thickening of the muscle of the pylorus to a deficiency in nitric oxide synthetase production.

Surgical Procedure

Pyloromyotomy can be performed using various techniques: laparoscopic, endoscopic, or open via a periumbilical or

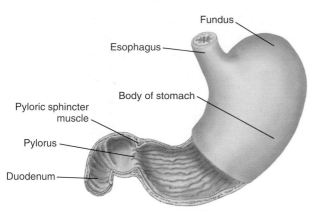

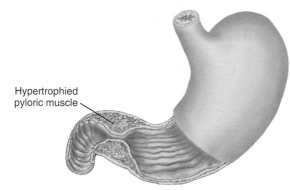

Normal pyloric opening

Pyloric stenosis

• **Fig. 52.1** Comparison of normal pyloric opening with evidence of pyloric stenosis. (From Ashwill JW, Droske SC: *Nursing care of children: Principles and practice*, ed 3, Philadelphia, 2007, Saunders.)

---

right upper quadrant incision. The laparoscopic technique utilizes a periumbilical telescope and two incision sites. The surgeon may make the incision in the duodenum that extends toward the stomach or from the stomach toward the duodenum in order to adequately spread the pyloric muscle.

The open technique uses a small incision that is made in the skin on the anterior abdominal wall. The layer of thickened muscle is then separated. The avascular part of the pylorus is identified, and a longitudinal incision is made to expose the mucosa. The separated muscle is brought up to the serous membrane, at which point closure of the area is initiated. The laparoscopic method allows quicker return to full feedings and has been associated with a more rapid hospital discharge compared with the open technique.

Anesthetic Management and Considerations

Preoperative Period

1. *Describe the population that is most likely to be diagnosed with pyloric stenosis.*

   IHPS is the most common cause of gastrointestinal obstruction in newborns and infants. Pyloric stenosis most commonly occurs among first-born males. The ratio of males to females is 4:1. It occurs in 2 to 3 per

---

• **BOX 52.1** Conditions Associated With Pyloric Stenosis

- Intestinal malrotation
- Urinary tract obstruction
- Esophageal atresia
- Omphalocele
- Cleft palate
- Gastroesophageal reflux

1000 live births and is predominant among whites. The typical age that the diagnosis is confirmed is at 3 to 6 weeks of life, but the pathologic process associated with pyloric stenosis can manifest as late as 12 weeks of age.

2. *Discuss pathologic conditions that are associated with pyloric stenosis.*

   Over 90% of infants that have pyloric stenosis are not associated with pathologic conditions; however, a list of anatomic and physiologic abnormalities that may accompany pyloric stenosis is listed in Box 52.1.

3. *Construct a preoperative strategy to optimize the patient condition before pyloromyotomy.*

   Pyloric stenosis may be a medical emergency due to the fluid loss, electrolyte, and acid–base imbalances caused by the repeated episodes of emesis over several days. Although it is well acknowledged that surgical repair is the definitive treatment, initial focus is placed on correction of the three areas mentioned previously.

   - An initial fluid bolus with crystalloids between 10 and 20 mL/kg depending on severity of dehydration and the patient's preoperative medical condition.
   - Fluids 1.5 to 2 times maintenance 5% dextrose and 0.25% normal saline with potassium chloride 2 to 4 mEq/100 mL only if UOP is greater than 1 mL/kg/hr.
   - Repeat blood gas measurements to ensure improved metabolic alkalosis with pH between 7.30 and 7.50 and sodium bicarbonate less than 30 mmol/l.
   - Repeat electrolytes to ensure stable sodium and potassium levels.
   - Check urine dipstick to assess specific gravity to be less than 1.02.
   - Ensure weighing of diapers for UOP greater than 1 mL/kg/hr.
   - Discuss antibiotic administration with surgeon; cefazolin 25 mg/kg.

Intraoperative Period

4. *Describe the induction plan most suitable for pyloric stenosis.*

   Rapid sequence induction (RSI) with cricoid pressure is the most suitable technique for this patient population. These patients have a gastric outlet obstruction and are at increased risk for aspiration. Stomach decompression with an orogastric tube is recommended in order to minimize the risk for aspiration.

Most of these patients have an intravenous (IV) catheter in place before surgery due to the need to balance their volume status. Typically, atropine 0.02 mg/kg (0.1 mg minimum) is administered before the induction of anesthesia to inhibit parasympathetic predominance resulting in bradycardia. Preoxygenation for several minutes followed by IV induction with propofol and rocuronium is indicated. Fentanyl may also be used to attenuate the response to laryngoscopy. If a difficult intubation is anticipated, an awake intubation should be planned.

5. *Construct a plan for maintenance and emergence.*

The surgical time for pyloromyotomy regardless of technique is between 30 and 60 minutes. If the surgical time is greater than 30 minutes, muscle relaxation may be maintained. An inhalation agent such as sevoflurane and air/O_2 is an appropriate option. Small amounts of opiates are considered to minimize the risk for postoperative apnea. Communication with the surgeon in relation to wound infiltration with local anesthetic should be discussed to guide the plan for pain management.

The abdominal contents are suctioned before awakening. Ondansetron is administered to decrease the potential for postoperative nausea and vomiting. Neostigmine and atropine are administered on a per kilogram weight basis for reversal of the muscle relaxant. The patient should be extubated when fully awake and meeting accepted extubation criteria.

6. *Specify the primary intraoperative complications associated with pyloric stenosis.*

- Increased risk for aspiration due to full stomach precautions. Preoperative medication to decrease gastric contents, gastric decompression, and placement of an endotracheal tube may decrease the risk, but do not prevent aspiration. Active inspiration and emesis may allow the passage of contents around the endotracheal tube, especially because uncuffed tubes are commonly used in this population.
- Initiation of the celiac reflex results from mesenteric traction stimulating afferent vagal nerve endings. Parasympathetic nervous system predominance will lead to bradycardia, apnea, and hypotension. Because neonates are dependent on a rapid heart rate to establish cardiac output, bradycardia results in decreased tissue perfusion and potentially cardiac arrest. The response usually resolves when the surgeon is asked to release tension on the mesentery or pressure on the intraabdominal organs or peritoneal cavity. Atropine can also be administered to help extinguish this response or treat recurring episodes of bradycardia.

- Duodenal perforation occurs in less than 5% of cases performed by pediatric surgeons. If the procedure is performed laparoscopically, the surgeon may decide to convert the case to open for repair.

Postoperative Period

7. *List the potential postoperative complications after pyloromyotomy.*
- Respiratory distress
- Hypoxemia/hypercarbia
- Hypoglycemia
- Hypothermia
- Pain
- Recurrent vomiting
- Electrolyte abnormality
- Inadvertent bowel perforation resulting in septicemia

8. *State two potential reasons for postoperative respiratory depression.*

Hypothermia is common among neonates and infants due to their increased body surface area (large head and chest) and small amount of subcutaneous fat tissue. It is vital to maintain a warm environment, cover the head, and utilize forced-air warming blankets intraoperatively and postoperatively. This patient population does not possess the concentration of muscle needed to shiver to increase heat production. If hypothermia exists in neonates and young infants, a process called nonshivering thermogenesis occurs as blood is shunted to anatomic areas where brown fat exists. The triglycerides that comprise the brown fat will be metabolized, and this process liberates heat. However, metabolic acidosis can rapidly occur due to the formation of acetone, β-hydroxybutyric acid, and acetoacetic acid.

The presence of hypoglycemia should be ruled out if apnea is noted in the postoperative period. These patients should receive IV fluids with dextrose until they are advanced to full feedings. It is common to restart feedings 8 hours after surgery.

9. *Discuss postoperative pain management for pyloromyotomy.*

The estimated pain score that is associated with pyloromyotomy is 4 to 5 on a 10-point scale.

Acetaminophen 10 to 15 mg/kg every 4 to 6 hours either by mouth or per rectum is a common treatment for postoperative pain management. A caudal block can also be performed.

Review Questions

1. Which is the most appropriate initial intervention for a patient with pyloric stenosis?
   a. Continue feeding; observe type, volume, and frequency of emesis
   b. Prepare for an emergency surgical procedure
   c. Manage fluid and metabolic deficits
   d. Schedule surgery for 6 hours after last breast milk intake

2. Which acid–base abnormality is associated with pyloric stenosis?
   a. Respiratory acidosis
   b. Metabolic acidosis
   c. Respiratory alkalosis
   d. Metabolic alkalosis

3. Which laboratory tests are most valuable to diagnose pyloric stenosis?
   a. CBC, PT, PTT
   b. Chemistry panel, calcium, and glucose
   c. ABG
   d. Both b and c
4. If a difficult intubation is not anticipated, which is the best technique for induction on a patient with pyloric stenosis?
   a. Intravenous induction
   b. Mask induction
   c. Awake fiber-optic intubation
   d. Rapid sequence induction with cricoid pressure

5. Which intraoperative complication is most likely to occur during pyloromyotomy?
   a. Hemorrhage
   b. Hypervolemia
   c. Aspiration
   d. Duodenal perforation

Suggested Readings

Allan C. Determinants of good outcome in pyloric stenosis. *J Pediatr Child Health* 2006;42(3):86-88.

Dalton BG, Gonzalez KW, Boda SR, et al. Optimizing fluid resuscitation in hypertrophic pyloric stenosis. *J Pediatr Surg* 2016;51(8):1279-82.

Elisha S, Terry K. Neonatal anesthesia. In: Nagelhout JJ, Elisha S, eds. *Nurse Anesthesia*, 6th ed. St. Louis, MO: Elsevier, 2018:1093-1116.

Galea R, Said E. Infantile hypertrophic pyloric stenosis: an epidemiological review. *Neonatal Netw* 2018;37(4):197-204.

Ibarguen-Secchia E. Endoscopic pyloromyotomy for congenital pyloric stenosis. *Gastrointest Endosc* 2005; 61(4):598-600.

Jobson M, Hall NJ. Contemporary management of pyloric stenosis. *Semin Pediatr Surg* 2016;25(4):219-224.

Kamata M, Cartabuke RS, Tobias JD. Perioperative care of infants with pyloric stenosis. *Paediatr Anaesth* 2015;25(12):1193-206.

Kelay A, Hall NJ. Perioperative complications of surgery for hypertrophic pyloric stenosis. *Eur J Pediatr Surg* 2018;28(2):171-175.

Lauriti G, Cascini V, Chiesa PL, et al. Atropine treatment for hypertrophic pyloric stenosis: a systematic review and meta-analysis. *Eur J Pediatr Surg* 2018;28(5):393-399.

Leclair M, Plattner V, Mirallie E, et al. Laparoscopic pyloromyotomy for hypertrophic pyloric stenosis: a prospective, randomized controlled trial. *J Pediatr Surg* 2007;42(4):692-698.

Wang JT, Mancuso TJ. How to best induce anesthesia in infants with pyloric stenosis? *Paediatr Anaesth* 2015;25(7):652-653.

53

Tracheoesophageal Fistula Repair

KEY POINTS

- The hallmark signs associated with tracheoesophageal fistula (TEF) include coughing, choking, cyanosis during feeding, and the inability to pass an oral catheter into the stomach.
- Although there are several variations of TEF, the most common is esophageal atresia with distal fistula (type C or IIIB).

- Positive pressure ventilation above the level of the fistula will inflate the stomach, increase the risk of aspiration, reduce the adequacy of ventilation, and can cause gastric rupture.
- Between 30% and 50% of patients with TEF have associated anomalies that must be evaluated before repair, most commonly VACTERL association.

Case Synopsis

A 2-day-old full-term infant boy has demonstrated coughing, choking, and cyanosis during feeding. After an inability to pass an orogastric tube into the stomach and radiologic evidence of air in the stomach, a diagnosis of TEF is made.

Preoperative Evaluation and Demographic Data

Past Medical/Surgical History

- Full gestational age male born at 37 weeks of age demonstrating polyhydramnios on ultrasound

List of Medications

- Pantoprazole
- D5 ½ NS infusion rate 12 mL/hr

Diagnostic Data

- Hemoglobin, 16.4 g/dL; hematocrit, 47.1%
- Electrolytes: sodium, 141 mEq/L; potassium, 3.4 mEq/L; chloride, 110 mEq/L; bicarbonate, 24 mEq/L; glucose, 96 mg/dL
- Chest–abdominal radiograph: orogastric tube placed in blind esophageal pouch, air in stomach, right upper lobe atelectasis.
- Transthoracic echocardiography (ECG): normal great vessels, small patent foramen ovale (PFO) with minimal left-to-right shunt, normal valves and function.

Height/Weight/Vital Signs

- 48 cm, 2.9 kg
- Blood pressure, 64/28; heart rate, 144 beats per minute; respiratory rate, 42 breaths per minute; room air oxygen saturation, 96%; temperature, 37.2°C

Pathophysiology

TEF occurs in approximately 1 in 3500 live births. Six primary anatomic variations of this congenital anomaly have been described by two overlapping classification systems, as shown in Fig. 53.1. The most common type of TEF is esophageal atresia with distal TEF, which accounts for almost 90% of all cases. The defect is an esophageal blind pouch (atresia) with a distal fistula connecting the stomach to the trachea. The lesion occurs because of incomplete separation of the trachea and esophagus that begins during the fourth to fifth week of embryo development. Survival of infants with TEF and no other congenital anomalies is greater than 95%. The presence of a TEF poses several severe risks to the infant: pulmonary aspiration is likely to occur, pneumonia and pneumonitis of the right upper lung are common, oral nutrition and fluids are not possible, and gastric distention with air can cause respiratory compromise.

Surgical Procedure

Surgical management for TEF includes locating and ligating the fistula and creating an anastomosis between the atretic segments of the esophagus. This is usually performed with the neonate in the left lateral decubitus position via a right thoracotomy. Thoracoscopic TEF repair is gaining popularity as surgeons become more adept with less invasive techniques. Thoracoscopic repair is usually performed in the prone position and has similar complication rates as the traditional open technique. In cases of severe congenital cardiac defects, chromosomal abnormalities, or extreme prematurity and low birth weight, primary correction of the TEF is difficult and is associated with significant risk. In high-risk cases, a gastrostomy is performed under local

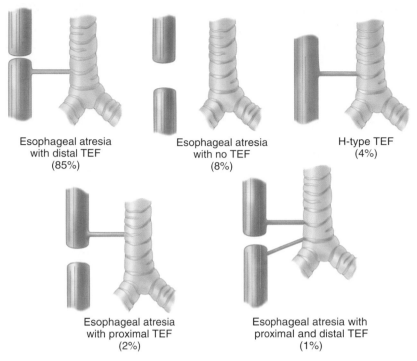

Esophageal atresia
with distal TEF
(85%)

Esophageal atresia
with no TEF
(8%)

H-type TEF
(4%)

Esophageal atresia
with proximal TEF
(2%)

Esophageal atresia with
proximal and distal TEF
(1%)

• **Fig. 53.1** Various types of tracheoesophageal fistulas *(TEF)* with relative frequency (%). (From Marcdante KJ, Kliegman RM: *Nelson essentials of pediatrics*, ed 8, St. Louis, 2019, Elsevier.)

anesthesia and definitive surgical correction of the TEF is deferred. The surgical correction is completed in stages for babies who demonstrate signs and symptoms associated with severe aspiration pneumonitis, as adequate oxygenation and ventilation during a thoracic surgery may be unattainable.

Anesthetic Management and Considerations

Preoperative Period

1. *Discuss the clinical presentation of a neonate with a TEF.*

    TEF is most frequently diagnosed during the first day of life when the neonate is unable to tolerate oral feeds without coughing, choking, and cyanosis. The suspicion of TEF is then confirmed with a chest radiograph showing a nasogastric tube coiled in the proximal esophagus. Oral contrast studies are no longer routinely done because of the risk of aspiration and associated fatality. Due to the inability of the fetus to swallow, the prenatal ultrasound often reveals polyhydramnios.

2. *Discuss the anatomic anomalies associated with TEF.*

    Over half of the babies born with TEF have other congenital anomalies or are born premature. Cardiac defects can be life threatening and must be ruled out with transthoracic echocardiography before TEF repair. Approximately 25% of those born with a TEF have cardiac defects, the most common being atrial or ventricular septal defects, coarctation of the aorta, and tetralogy of Fallot. TEF is also a component of VACTERL, which is

> **•BOX 53.1   Anomalies Associated With TEF**
>
> - **VACTERL:** Over 50% of patients with TEF have at least one additional anomaly
>   - **V**ertebral defects
>   - **A**nal atresia
>   - **C**ardiac defects (25% have a ventricular septal defect, atrial septal defect, tetralogy of Fallot, atrioventricular canal, or coarctation of the aorta)
>   - **T**racheoesophageal fistula
>   - **E**sophageal atresia
>   - **R**adial or renal anomalies
>   - **L**imb anomalies
> - Prematurity: 20%–40% are premature and weigh less than 2 kg
> - Cleft lip and genital abnormalities: 5% have additional midline defects

a combination of anomalies, as shown in Box 53.1. These defects were known as *VATERL syndrome* but were modified to include the common cardiac and limb anomalies. The specific gene or set of genes that causes VACTERL has not yet been identified, which is why it is considered an association as opposed to a syndrome.

3. *Identify the anatomic and physiologic changes to the pulmonary system that can be present with TEF.*

    The anesthetist can expect that some degree of pulmonary compromise has occurred. Even after the patient is no longer ingesting fluid by mouth, the potential for pulmonary aspiration is still high due to the fistula between the stomach and the trachea and the inability of the patient to manage their oral secretions. Right upper lobe pneumonia and aspiration pneumonitis commonly occur in patients with TEF. Additionally, the stomach can become full of air, inhibit diaphragmatic expansion, and compress the lungs. Emergent gastrostomy and intubation with one-lung ventilation could be lifesaving measures if extreme gastric insufflation of air occurs.

4. *Discuss preoperative patient medical management for TEF.*

TEFs must be repaired as soon as possible. Medical management of the patient focuses on prevention of aspiration pneumonitis that can preclude surgical correction. As soon as TEF is suspected, the child is given nothing by mouth and placed with their head elevated above their chest. The esophageal pouch is suctioned continuously via nasoesophageal tube. Intravenous (IV) fluids are given, and metabolic acidosis is corrected before surgery. Preoperative laboratory evaluation should include arterial blood gases (ABG), complete blood count (CBC), chemistry panel, type and crossmatch, and glucose. Transthoracic echocardiography and consultation from a pediatric cardiologist are also necessary before anesthesia. The presence of associated anomalies must be ruled out by examination, ultrasound, and radiography.

Intraoperative Period

5. *Discuss options of securing the airway.*

Correct placement of the endotracheal tube below the level of the fistula is crucial during endotracheal intubation and before ventilation. Maintaining spontaneous respirations during a mask induction with inhalation anesthetic agents prevents gastric insufflation from positive pressure. Alternatively, a rapid sequence IV induction without positive pressure mask ventilation can also be accomplished safely. In both methods, the endotracheal tube is advanced into the right mainstem bronchus and withdrawn slowly until bilateral breath sounds are heard. A flexible fiber-optic bronchoscope can be used to verify placement of the endotracheal tube and fistula. To further prevent the chance of gastric insufflation, the fistula can be occluded with a Fogarty balloon-tipped catheter from the trachea or from a gastrostomy. After confirmation of correct placement of the endotracheal tube, muscle relaxant can be used to assist with controlled ventilation. The endotracheal tube is in close proximity to the carina and fistula, and migration caudad can cause an endobronchial intubation; migration cephalad can cause insufflation of the stomach or inadvertent extubation. Therefore constant vigilance and reassessment are required throughout the perioperative period in order to deliver competent care.

6. *Describe appropriate monitoring and hemodynamic goals during TEF repair.*

In addition to the standard monitoring, patients having a TEF require unique considerations. Arterial blood pressure monitoring gives the anesthetist the advantage of continuous beat-to-beat assessment and access for blood gas/glucose monitoring. A left-sided precordial stethoscope alerts the anesthetist to a right mainstem intubation either from endotracheal tube migration or from surgical manipulation of the trachea.

This surgery is most often associated with minimal blood loss; however, due to the proximity of the surgical site to great vessels and vital organs, blood products should be available for infusion before incision. These patients will be receiving an IV fluid that contains glucose before surgery. It is necessary to continue this infusion along with maintenance fluids. Stopping the glucose solution can result in rapidly occurring hypoglycemia. It is prudent to monitor the glucose values during the perioperative period. Timely communication with the surgical team regarding the amount and speed of blood loss is essential. Consider replacing the blood loss 1:1 with 5% human albumin until the hematocrit falls below 30%.

The accuracy of end tidal carbon dioxide monitoring as a reflection of arterial carbon dioxide levels can be compromised by surgical retraction of lung tissue, compression of bronchi, aspiration pneumonia, atelectasis, small endotracheal tube size, and fresh gas flow rates, among many other factors. Therefore ABG should be routinely assessed at least every hour during surgical repair.

7. *Discuss anesthetic maintenance and intraoperative considerations.*

An adequate depth of anesthesia can be maintained with a combination of an inhalation anesthetic agent and opiates. The use of nitrous oxide for this surgical procedure and in this patient population is controversial. Nitrous oxide decreases the fraction of inspired oxygen, causes bowel distention, increases pulmonary vascular resistance, and inhibits methionine synthetase.

Muscle relaxation is usually required for surgical exposure and to facilitate in controlling ventilation. If vertebral defects are absent, a lumbar epidural catheter can be used for intraoperative anesthesia and/or postoperative analgesia. Maintaining appropriate temperature with a forced-air blanket is imperative because the increased body surface area in pediatric patients predisposes them to developing hypothermia.

8. *Discuss the challenge of maintaining adequate tissue oxygenation.*

A common difficulty during TEF repair is maintaining adequate oxygenation. Oxygen should be diluted with air to prevent arterial hyperoxia because of the increase in the risk of retinopathy of prematurity. Keeping the oxygen saturation between 95% and 99% and confirming the values via an ABG value is prudent. Precipitous oxygen desaturation is not uncommon and can occur from a variety of reasons. Before surgery, there may be atelectasis and secretions that cause shunting of pulmonary blood that can result in hypoxia and hypercarbia. This problem is compounded during surgery with retraction on lung tissue, bleeding, tracheal and bronchial compression, or endotracheal tube malposition. In the presence of arterial hypoxia, the surgeons may need to release traction and allow time for alveolar recruitment maneuvers. Frequent suctioning of blood and secretions may also be necessary to maintain satisfactory ventilation. Ventilator settings are frequently reassessed, as the peak inspiratory pressure and tidal volumes will vary during various stages of surgical repair.

> ●BOX 53.2   **Postoperative Complications Associated With Repair of TEF**
>
> - Apnea
> - Tracheal collapse or compression
> - Pneumothorax
> - Airway obstruction (blood or mucus)
> - Anastomosis leak
> - Hypoventilation
> - Recurrent laryngeal nerve damage
> - Atelectasis
> - Aspiration pneumonia

Postoperative Period

9. *Discuss extubation timing and options.*

Extubation in the operating room at the conclusion of surgery is desirable if spontaneous respiration is sufficient. Respiratory depression in the newborn can originate from hypothermia, hypoglycemia, or anemia, all of which must be addressed before extubation. The presence of the endotracheal tube can cause excessive pressure on the newly created anastomosis and increase the possibility of wound dehiscence. Moreover, reintubation can disrupt the surgical repair. Therefore the anesthetist must feel confident that the respiratory effort is sufficient before extubation. Although favorable, extubation is often precluded by poor pulmonary function, excessive secretions, and aspiration pneumonitis. Associated anomalies also complicate the clinical picture, and the child may require prolonged mechanical ventilation in the intensive care unit. Other postoperative complications associated with TEF are listed in Box 53.2.

10. *Discuss strategies that can be used to decrease postoperative pain.*

TEF repair is performed via thoracotomy or thoracoscopy, and adequate postoperative pain management is imperative. Opiate infusions are frequently used with close monitoring due to the potential for respiratory depression. Regional analgesia, in the form of lumbar or caudal epidural catheter, is particularly advantageous for postoperative pain control. Every TEF patient should be considered to have some degree of pulmonary insult, so avoiding the respiratory depressant effects of opiates is beneficial in the postoperative course.

11. *Discuss the clinical course and outcomes for survivors.*

Care of patients immediately after TEF repair should focus on the treatment of pulmonary insults and preventing pressure on the new anastomosis. During surgery, an orogastric tube is marked to the level of the anastomosis. Suction catheters should not be advanced past the TEF repair site. After surgery, every patient should be considered to have gastroesophageal reflux and be treated accordingly. A TEF is not a simple anomaly that can be completely treated by anastomosis and ligation. Upper gastrointestinal problems are chronic, and corrective or palliative treatments in the form of esophageal stricture dilation or Nissen fundoplication are often performed later in life. These patients will have a decreased number and integrity of their tracheal cartilages that can result in acute tracheal collapse after extubation or progressive tracheal compression. This population exhibits recurrent respiratory infections, reactive airway disease, and chronic restrictive and obstructive lung disease. The presence of associated congenital anomalies significantly increases the morbidity and mortality after TEF repair and can result in lifelong health problems.

Review Questions

1. What is an advantage of maintaining spontaneous respirations during the anesthetic induction of a patient with a TEF?
   a. Laryngeal muscles are relaxed for ease of endotracheal intubation.
   b. The need for positive pressure ventilation before securing the airway is reduced.
   c. Fiber-optic placement of a balloon catheter in the distal fistula is facilitated.
   d. There are no advantages to maintaining spontaneous respiration in this population.

2. The hallmark sign(s) of a patient with a TEF include:
   a. Impaired muscle tone and nasal flaring.
   b. Arterial oxygen desaturation with clear lung sounds.
   c. Coughing and choking during feeding.
   d. Orogastric tube placement in stomach confirmed by x-ray.

3. _____ is the congenital anomaly most commonly associated with TEF.
   a. Trisomy 21
   b. Goldenhar syndrome
   c. Cleft lip and palate
   d. VACTERL association

4. Which situation is an indication for definitive correction of a TEF for a 3-day-old infant?
   a. Atelectasis and infiltrates of the right upper lobe
   b. Tetralogy of Fallot
   c. Premature infant weighing 850 g
   d. Severe aspiration pneumonitis

5. The most common type of TEF accounting for almost 90% of patients is:
   a. Solitary esophageal blind pouch.
   b. Double fistulas between esophagus and right mainstem bronchus.
   c. Esophageal atresia with distal fistula.
   d. Tracheal fistula with upper and lower esophagus.

Suggested Readings

Daniel SJ, Smith MM. Tracheoesophageal fistula: open versus endoscopic repair. *Curr Opin Otolaryngol Head Neck Surg* 2016; 24(6):510-515.

Elisha S, Terry K. Neonatal anesthesia. In: Nagelhout JJ, Elisha S, eds. *Nurse Anesthesia*, 6th ed. St. Louis, MO: Elsevier, 2018:1093-1116.

Forero Zapata L, Pappagallo M. Esophageal atresia and tracheoesophageal fistula. *N Engl J Med* 2018;379(7):e11.

Ghaffaripour S, Souki FG, Martinez-Lu K, et al. Anesthetic approach for endoscopic repair of acquired tracheoesophageal fistula. *Semin Cardiothorac Vasc Anesth* 2017;21(4):357-359.

Gopal M, Woodward M. Potential hazards of contrast study diagnosis of esophageal atresia. *J Pediat Surg* 2007;42(6):E9–E10.

Ho AM, Dion JM, Wong JC. Airway and ventilatory management options in congenital tracheoesophageal fistula repair. *J Cardiothorac Vasc Anesth* 2016;30(2):515-520.

Holcomb GW III, Rothenberg SS, Bax KM, et al. Thoracoscopic repair of esophageal atresia and tracheoesophageal fistula: a multi-institutional analysis. *Ann Surg* 2005;242(3):422-430.

Krosnar S, Baxter A. Thoracoscopic repair of esophageal atresia with tracheoesophageal fistula: anesthetic and intensive care management of a series of eight neonates. *Pediatr Anesth* 2005;15(7):541-546.

Lee S. Basic knowledge of tracheoesophageal fistula and esophageal atresia. *Adv Neonatal Care* 2018;18(1):14-21.

Morini F, Conforti A, Bagolan P. Perioperative complications of esophageal atresia. *Eur J Pediatr Surg* 2018;28(2):133-140.

Shamji FM, Inculet R. Management of malignant tracheoesophageal fistula. *Thorac Surg Clin* 2018;28(3):393-402.

Sharma R, Dwivedi D, Choudhary R. Pneumothorax in a preterm during tracheoesophageal fistula repair: challenges in diagnosis and management. *Saudi J Anaesth* 2018;12(1):154-155.

54

Electroconvulsive Therapy

KEY POINTS

- Electroconvulsive therapy (ECT) is indicated for severe major depression and other psychiatric disorders that have no or a poor response to medical therapy.
- Approximately 100,000 patients receive ECT annually in the United States. The mortality rate is estimated to be 2 deaths per 100,000 treatments and usually occurs as a result of cardiovascular or pulmonary complications.
- General anesthesia is necessary to provide unconsciousness and muscle relaxation during the procedure.

- The major contraindications to providing ECT include pheochromocytoma, recent cerebrovascular accident (CVA), recent myocardial infarction (MI), increased intracranial pressure (ICP), and cervical spine instability.
- The disadvantages associated with ECT can include temporary or permanent cognitive impairment and memory loss.

Case Synopsis

A 68-year-old woman is scheduled for ECT. She has been treated for major depression for over 5 years and has become increasingly unresponsive to several psychotropic medications.

Preoperative Evaluation and Demographic Data

Past Medical/Surgical History

- Hypertension for 3 years
- Major depression for more than 10 years
- Cigarette smoking: 1 pack/day for over 25 years

List of Medications

- Sertraline (Zoloft)

Diagnostic Data

- Hemoglobin, 12.4 g/dL; hematocrit, 37%; glucose, 90 mg/dL
- Electrolytes: sodium, 140 mEq/L; potassium, 3.5 mEq/L; chloride, 106 mEq/L; carbon dioxide, 22 mEq/L
- Electrocardiogram (ECG): normal sinus rhythm; heart rate, 88 beats per minute; left ventricular hypertrophy; left anterior hemiblock

Height/Weight/Vital Signs

- 165 cm, 73 kg
- Blood pressure, 160/94; heart rate, 94 beats per minute; respiratory rate, 16 breaths per minute; temperature, 37.1°C; room air oxygen saturation, 97%

Pathophysiology

There is no single cause of depression; rather, a combination of genetic, biochemical, environmental, and psychological factors have been implicated in the disorder. It is more common among women, and it is theorized that the increased incidence of depression results from the variability of hormonal levels. Major depression is a chronic but treatable disorder, and early intervention is associated with the best outcome. Bipolar disorder (manic depressive disorder) is characterized by episodes of major depression and abnormally elevated mood (mania) or hypomania (less severe). The symptoms associated with depression and bipolar disorder are included in Boxes 54.1 and 54.2. The onset of depression typically presents during the late adolescent period or in early adulthood. However, it can occur in childhood as well as later in life.

Regardless of whether psychotherapy is instituted or not, the use of antidepressants is the primary intervention for treatment of depression. The most commonly used antidepressants are selective serotonin reuptake inhibitors (SSRIs) such as fluoxetine (Prozac), citalopram (Celexa), and sertraline (Zoloft). Serotonin and norepinephrine reuptake inhibitors (SNRIs) have similar effects as the SSRIs; examples include venlafaxine (Effexor) and duloxetine (Cymbalta). Both SSRIs and SNRIs have fewer side effects than older antidepressants such as the tricyclic antidepressants (TCAs) and monoamine oxidase inhibitors (MAOIs). However, for some individuals, TCAs (such as desipramine [Norpramin], doxepin [Sinequan], imipramine [Tofranil] and nortriptyline [Pamelor]) or MAOIs (such as isocarboxazid [Marplan]

For a diagnosis of depression, five of the following symptoms must be present nearly every day for at least 2 weeks:
- Feelings of sadness or emptiness
- Decreased interest or pleasure in activities
- Appetite change with weight loss or weight gain
- Decreased or increased sleeping
- Fatigue or loss of energy
- Feelings of worthlessness or guilt
- Agitation
- Difficulty in thinking or concentrating
- Recurrent thoughts of death or suicide

• BOX 54.2   **Symptoms of Mania (or a Manic Episode) in a Patient With Bipolar Disorder**

- Increased energy and activity, restlessness
- Euphoric mood
- Extreme irritability
- Fast speech patterns and flight of ideas
- Inability to concentrate
- Little need for sleep
- Unrealistic beliefs in one's abilities and powers
- Poor judgment
- Spending sprees
- A lasting change of behavior that is different from usual
- Increased sexual drive
- Drug abuse, especially cocaine, alcohol, and sedatives
- Provocative and/or aggressive behavior
- Denial
- Symptoms of psychosis, such as hallucinations and delusions, may also be present

and phenelzine [Nardil]) may be more effective than SSRIs or SNRIs. Regardless of the mechanism of action, antidepressants must be taken for 3 to 4 weeks before a full therapeutic effect is demonstrable. A relapse of the depression is possible if antidepressants are discontinued. For treatment of major depression, stimulants and antianxiety medications may be used in conjunction with an antidepressant. In addition to antidepressants, bipolar disorder is treated with mood stabilizers including lithium (Lithobid) and lamotrigine (Lamictal). Anticonvulsants such as valproate (Depakote) and carbamazepine (Tegretol) are beneficial for hard-to-treat bipolar episodes.

Surgical Procedure

ECT was introduced in the 1930s after it was observed that psychiatric symptoms in a schizophrenic patient appeared to decrease after a spontaneous seizure. Shortly after, ECT was discovered to be an effective treatment for depression and bipolar disorder. After its widespread use in the 1940s through the 1960s when it was administered without the benefits of anesthesia, ECT fell out of favor because of the untoward physical side effects associated

with the treatment such as awareness, bone fractures, broken teeth, myofascial pain, and memory loss. Indiscriminate use of the treatment, social stigma, and the introduction of antipsychotic and antidepressant drugs have also contributed to the decline. In the 1980s, there was renewed interest in ECT as an effective treatment for several psychiatric disorders, especially for those patients who did not respond to the new pharmacologic agents. At the same time, the need for general anesthesia and muscle relaxation was recognized. Although often stigmatized as a last treatment resort, ECT is an effective treatment and has several advantages for severe major (unipolar) depression, bipolar depression, acute mania, and catatonia. The response rate to ECT is greater and occurs much faster than the response rate to antidepressants, antipsychotics, or a combination of both antidepressants and antipsychotics. ECT is useful for treating schizophrenia that is unresponsive to medical antipsychotic therapy. It has also been used successfully to treat Parkinson disease and chronic pain, especially phantom limb pain. However, ECT is not an effective treatment for addiction, personality disorders, or somatization disorders. Most antipsychotic and antidepressant medications do not noticeably alter the patient's mood for 3 to 6 weeks. The rapid results obtained by ECT have been advantageous when treating patients who are acutely psychotic and suicidal. It is also considered an effective treatment alternative for mental illness during pregnancy. Older patients that have acute depression are the most likely group to benefit from ECT. The rate of recurring depression is high, and patients will need to continue taking their antidepressant medications after a series of ECT treatments. Maintenance ECT treatments do not appear to offer any advantage to medical management in preventing relapse.

During ECT, a brief pulse current is delivered via transcutaneous electrodes to one or both cerebral hemispheres with the intent of producing a generalized seizure. Electrodes are placed above each temple in bilateral ECT. When performing a unilateral ECT, electrodes are placed over one temple, usually the right (nondominant hemisphere), and near the vertex on the same side, this is referred to as a *right unilateral (RUL) ECT.* Approximately 800 milliamps of electrical energy are delivered for 1 to 6 seconds, producing a grand mal seizure with 10- to 15-second tonic and 30- to 60-second clonic phases.

Three waveforms can be used for ECT: sine wave, brief pulse wave, or an ultra-brief wave. Sine wave stimulus is associated with greater memory loss and is rarely used in the United States. The majority of ECT procedures utilize a brief pulse width of 0.5 to 1.0 msec. Regardless of the waveform that is administered, the strength of the stimulus must exceed the seizure threshold. Bilateral ECT delivers an electrical stimulus at 1.5 times the seizure threshold, whereas unilateral ECT may require a stimulus strength that is 6 to 12 times the seizure threshold. There is a significant increase in the seizure threshold with aging; to achieve a therapeutic seizure, a higher electrical stimulus may be required in elderly patients. In contrast to an RUL, bilateral ECT is associated with a rapid initial response and a longer remission of symptoms. RUL-ECT is associated with fewer cognitive side effects, especially for retention of verbal information, visual information, and autobiographical memory. When administered with an ultra-brief pulse width (0.3 msec), RUL-ECT appears to have less negative cognitive effects, especially on the retention of verbal information, visual information, and retrograde autobiographical memory. Regardless of the delivery method, the mechanism of action for the therapeutic effects of ECT is still unknown. Seizure duration of 30 to 60 seconds is desirable. Treatment efficacy appears to be dependent upon a minimum seizure duration of 25 seconds. Seizures that last less than 25 seconds in duration provide little, if any, benefit. During ECT, seizure duration is monitored by an unprocessed electroencephalogram (EEG) or by observation of seizure activity in an isolated limb. To observe isolated seizure activity, a tourniquet is applied (or a blood pressure cuff is inflated) before the administration of succinylcholine to limit distribution of the drug to the limb. This allows direct observation of the intensity and duration of the resultant seizure. A positive response to ECT is usually seen after three to five treatments, and a therapeutic effect is generally observed after a total of 400 to 700 seizure seconds. A typical ECT series includes two or three treatments per week for approximately 6 weeks; twice-weekly procedures are associated with a lower incidence of cognitive impairment. ECT may be repeated monthly for an additional 6 months.

The electrocardiographic changes associated with ECT, including atrioventricular dissociation, may occur. The hyperdynamic response to the electrical stimulus occurs within 2 minutes and is usually self-limiting. ECT causes a 100% to 400% increase in cerebral blood flow caused by the seizure-induced increase in cerebral metabolic rate and an increase in ICP. There is also an increase in intraocular and intragastric pressures during the procedure. The neuroendocrine response includes increased secretion of adrenocorticotropic hormone, cortisol, vasopressin, glucagon, epinephrine, and norepinephrine.

Anesthetic Management and Considerations

Preoperative Period

1. Describe the mechanisms of action of antidepressant medications.

Patients who present for ECT are frequently taking oral antidepressants such as TCAs, MAOIs, SSRIs, SNRIs, and lithium carbonate. TCAs block presynaptic reuptake of norepinephrine and serotonin but have little effect on reuptake of dopamine. MAOIs block the presynaptic metabolism of norepinephrine, serotonin, and dopamine. The SSRIs block the reuptake of serotonin, whereas the SNRIs block the reuptake of both serotonin and norepinephrine. The exact mechanism of action for

lithium is unknown. It has a narrow therapeutic index, and this drug should be discontinued before instituting ECT, as it increases the risk of delirium and prolongs the seizure duration. Lithium also potentiates the action of depolarizing and nondepolarizing muscle relaxants. Salt restriction or thiazide diuretics decrease renal clearance of lithium.

2. List the contraindications to having ECT.

Major contraindications to ECT include pheochromocytoma, recent CVA, recent MI, increased ICP, and unstable cervical spine. Relative contraindications include angina, congestive heart failure (CHF), aortic aneurysm, cerebral aneurysm, pregnancy, thrombophlebitis, major bone fracture, severe osteoporosis, glaucoma, retinal detachment, and automatic implantable cardioverter defibrillators (AICDs).

3. Discuss the preoperative testing indicated for patients undergoing ECT.

A baseline ECG is indicated for all patients having ECT. If the patient has a history of cardiovascular disease or a recent history of an acute cardiovascular event, a stress test or cardiac catheterization is indicated. Due to the potential increased risk of a second myocardial or cerebral ischemic event, ECT should be postponed for at least 6 to 8 weeks after an acute MI or CVA. Other preoperative tests are dependent on the individual patient and their medical history.

4. Discuss a typical ECT treatment plan.

ECT is administered two to three times per week for approximately 6 weeks. Maintenance ECT sessions may be continued monthly for an additional 6 months. Ideally, antidepressants and antipsychotics should be discontinued during the ECT treatments, especially lithium, which increases seizure duration and the incidence of postprocedure delirium. However, it is not always possible for antidepressants to be discontinued, and ECT has been safely administered to patients taking a variety of antidepressants and mood elevators.

Intraoperative Period

5. Discuss the anesthetic requirements for a patient undergoing ECT.

General anesthesia is required to provide a rapid loss of consciousness (LOC), amnesia, and muscle relaxation during the procedure. Ideally, the anesthetic agents that are administered will also attenuate the hyperdynamic response caused by the electrical stimulus and allow for the prompt return of consciousness and spontaneous ventilation. Patients should be NPO (nothing by mouth) for 6 to 8 hours, and patients who have cardiovascular disease should take their cardiovascular medication in the morning of the procedure (Box 54.3).

Because the effectiveness of ECT is dependent on the duration of the seizure activity, drugs that increase the seizure threshold (anticonvulsants,

- Verify signed informed consent.
- Perform a preanesthetic assessment.
- Ensure presence of emergency airway equipment, suction, medications, and cardiac defibrillator.
- Establish IV access.
- Administer ketorolac to patients at risk for posttreatment headache or myalgia.
- Apply monitors: ECG, pulse oximeter, BP.
- Apply tourniquet or second blood pressure cuff for observation of seizure activity.
- Administer glycopyrrolate for the antisialagogue effect.
- Preoxygenate patient: Administer induction agent (propofol, 0.75–1.5 mg/kg or etomidate, 0.15–0.3 mg/kg) and a muscle relaxant (succinylcholine 0.5–1 mg/kg).
- Insert bite block after loss of consciousness.
- Hyperventilate to decrease seizure threshold and prolong duration of seizure.
- Monitor duration seizure.
- Treat excessive sympathetic response with esmolol or labetalol.
- Treat emergence agitation with midazolam.
- Monitor recovery for ≥30 minutes.

benzodiazepines, lidocaine) should be discontinued before the treatment. Other drugs of concern include theophylline, which is associated with the development of status epilepticus during ECT and should be discontinued before treatment. Oral nonsteroidal antiinflammatory drugs (NSAIDs) can be administered before therapy to prevent posttreatment myalgia or headache. For patients who have a history of severe posttreatment myalgia or headache, ketorolac 30 mg intravenously (IV) can be administered before induction. Anesthetic management typically involves the use of an induction dose of an IV anesthetic followed by a short-acting muscle relaxant. Tracheal intubation is not necessary except for patients with a full stomach or in the last trimester of pregnancy.

ECT is usually administered in the postanesthesia care unit (PACU) or in a treatment room in a psychiatric treatment setting. Standard monitoring includes ECG, pulse oximetry, and BP measurement. After assessment of the patient's baseline vital signs, preoxygenation, and pretreatment with glycopyrrolate 0.2 mg IV, an induction agent and muscle relaxant is administered. After LOC, a bite block is inserted, and the patient is ventilated by mask using 100% oxygen. Hyperventilation will decrease the seizure threshold but may increase the hemodynamic response to stimulation. Ventilation is discontinued during administration of the electrical stimulus and the duration of the seizure noted by direct observation of the isolated limb. After return of consciousness and spontaneous ventilation, the patient should be monitored for at least 30 minutes. Midazolam can be administered to help treat emergence agitation.

6. Compare the effects of various induction agents on seizure activity.

Almost all IV anesthetics have anticonvulsant properties, and dosing is very important so as not to interfere with the therapeutic effect of the treatment. Larger-than-necessary dosages of IV anesthetics will shorten the seizure duration and reduce the efficacy of ECT, whereas inadequate dosing can result in awareness and recall.

Thiopental was the first IV anesthetic to be used for ECT. but methohexital (0.5 to 1 mg/kg) is an alternative for induction of ECT. Seizure duration with lower doses (0.75 mg/kg) of propofol is similar to the barbiturates. At higher doses (1 to 1.5 mg/kg), propofol can shorten the duration of seizure activity but does not appear to affect outcome of the treatment. Earlier recovery of cognitive function may be an advantage of propofol as an induction agent. Etomidate (0.15 to 0.3 mg/kg) prolongs the seizure duration, which may be beneficial in patients with seizure durations less than 25 seconds. However, it is associated with a greater hemodynamic response to electrical stimulation and a prolonged recovery period.

When used with lower doses of methohexital and propofol, both alfentanil (10 to 25 mcg/kg) and remifentanil (1 mcg/kg) are associated with a prolonged seizure duration and significant attenuation of the hyperdynamic cardiovascular response. With repeat ECTs, there appears to be a rise in seizure threshold during the treatment course when methohexital is used as the induction agent. Remifentanil can provide improved seizure response to ECT in patients who become refractory to seizure induction after a methohexital induction. As a sole agent or in combination with lower doses of methohexital or propofol, remifentanil is associated with lower seizure threshold, prolonged seizure duration, decreased hemodynamic response, and no increase in recovery time.

A pharmacodynamic property of benzodiazepines is prominent anticonvulsant activity. As a result, benzodiazepines significantly shorten the seizure duration and should be avoided before and during ECT. However, they may be required for termination of a prolonged ECT-induced seizure. The majority of ECT procedures are performed outside of the operating room; therefore inhalation anesthetics are rarely used. When used for ECT procedures, sevoflurane (1.7%) has a similar effect on seizure duration and hemodynamic response as thiopental, and higher concentrations are more effective in blunting the hemodynamic response. Sevoflurane is considered useful for women requiring ECT in the late stages of pregnancy, as it may reduce the incidence of ECT-stimulated uterine contractions.

Ketamine has been used for ECT, but concerns about increased ICP, increased sympathetic activity, and prolonged recovery has limited its use. However, ketamine is a racemic mixture, and there are significant differences in potency and side effects between the two isomers; increased potency and decreased psychomimetic effects are seen with the S isomer. The intense seizure activity provoked by ECT may cause excitotoxic neuronal damage mediated by glutamate via the N-methyl-D-aspartate (NMDA) receptor. This damage may account for the postoperative cognitive dysfunction associated with ECT. Ketamine is an NMDA antagonist and it may offer protection against this neuronal damage. Repeated electrocortical stimulation is associated with mossy fiber sprouting in the hippocampus, which correlates with ECT-induced memory impairment; ketamine appears to block the development of mossy fiber sprouting. Ketamine is associated with shorter reorientation times despite a longer elimination half-life.

7. *Describe the role of muscle relaxants when providing anesthesia for ECT.*

Muscle relaxants are used to prevent myalgia and other more serious musculoskeletal complications associated with ECT, including dislocations and fractures. The most commonly used muscle relaxant is succinylcholine. It can produce posttreatment myalgia secondary to muscular fasciculations. NDMR can be used as an alternative to succinylcholine in certain patients but does not appear to be as effective as succinylcholine in preventing muscle contractions during ECT. The NDMRs require a prolonged period of ventilatory support during the recovery period.

8. *Discuss the autonomic response to ECT.*

A brief period of parasympathetic nervous system predominance, which lasts less than 20 seconds, is the initial response to the electrical stimulus. The result includes increased salivation, severe bradycardia, hypotension, and the potential for brief episodes of asystole. This is followed by intense sympathetic stimulation, which can last for several minutes during which time tachycardia ($\geq$20% increase in heart rate), arrhythmias, and hypertension (30% to 40% increase in systolic pressure) will be present.

9. *Discuss management of the hemodynamic effects of ECT.*

The parasympathetic response to ECT can be limited or prevented by pretreatment with glycopyrrolate. It is effective as an antisialagogue and is associated with less tachycardia post-ECT than atropine. Atropine is used to treat bradycardia that persists during the procedure. Sympathetic effects such as tachycardia and hypertension are usually self-limiting. Lidocaine or esmolol can be used to reduce the incidence of tachycardia and hypertension before initiating ECT. Labetalol can also be used to blunt the cardiovascular response but is associated with a prolonged period of hypotension immediately after the treatment and in the early recovery period. Nifedipine provides more effective control of the hyperdynamic response, especially in elderly patients. In hypertensive patients, pretreatment with sublingual nifedipine may prevent or limit an increase in systemic vascular resistance (SVR) in response to electrical stimulation.

10. *Compare the different ECT techniques and their impact on cognitive function.*

In comparison to a sine wave stimulus, the use of a brief pulse stimulus (0.5 to 2 msec) is associated with a less negative effect on cognition. Ultra-brief pulse waveforms (less than 0.5 msec) may produce even fewer cognitive side effects. Although it requires the use of a higher dosage, RUL electrode placement is associated with a lower incidence of cognitive side effects. Treatments that occur twice a week are associated with a lower incidence of cognitive side effects compared with when they are prescribed three times a week. Rather than using a standard electrical stimulus, titrating the stimulus strength to the individual patient will allow dosing to minimally exceed the threshold, which is necessary to produce the therapeutic effect. When the electrical stimulus greatly exceeds the patient's seizure threshold, cognitive function is affected to a greater degree.

Postoperative Period

11. *List potential postoperative complications associated with ECT.*

During a standard course of ECT treatments, the overall mortality is less than 0.5%; the major causes of death are MI, CHF, and cardiac arrest. Complications include vertebral fracture, laryngospasm, myalgia, headache, confusion, memory loss, jaw pain, dental damage, and nausea and vomiting. Hemorrhagic and embolic stroke, prolonged seizure, postictal delirium, and brainstem herniation associated with a preexisting intracranial mass may also occur.

12. *Discuss the cognitive changes associated with ECT.*

Irrespective of the etiology, all seizures are associated with a period of cognitive impairment. Short-term effects include emergence agitation. Posttreatment disorientation (postictal confusion) lasting for minutes to hours is not uncommon; however, it occurs more frequently in the elderly population. Retrograde amnesia generally affects memories for weeks to months preceding the treatment. Memory loss gradually improves over time, usually within 7 months, but some patients complain of persistent or permanent memory loss. Antegrade amnesia can also occur immediately after the treatment, but these effects are short-lived and temporary compared with retrograde amnesia. Cognitive side effects appear to be more frequent in patients taking lithium. To minimize cognitive dysfunction, ECT should be administered to the nondominant hemisphere. The degree of long-term memory loss increases as the number of treatments increases.

13. *Describe the risk of awareness and recall during ECT.*

During ECT, awareness under anesthesia, recall of paralysis, and seizures can occur as a result of an inadequate dosage of the induction agent and/or premature administration of the muscle relaxant. LOC should be assured before administering succinylcholine and the electrical stimulus. Awareness and recall during ECT may be underreported because bilateral ECT tends to obliterate the memory of the ECT procedure. RUL-ECT, which is associated with less memory loss, may increase the incidence of recall if an inadequate induction dose is used or succinylcholine is administered before LOC.

14. Discuss the long-term outcome of ECT.

ECT is an effective short-term treatment for depression and other psychiatric disorders. However, relapse of symptoms is not uncommon. Patients who respond positively to a course of ECT will need to continue a treatment regimen with antidepressants after the prescribed series of ECT treatments. Some patients may require monthly maintenance ECT treatments for an extended period.

Review Questions

1. An advantage of ECT compared with antidepressant therapy for suicidal patients includes:
   a. Faster relief of symptoms.
   b. Retrograde amnesia of the suicidal thoughts.
   c. Lower mortality rate.
   d. Better patient compliance.
2. What electrical waveform is associated with the greatest degree of cognitive impairment?
   a. Ultra-brief pulse width
   b. Sine wave
   c. Brief pulse wave
   d. Delta wave
3. Which is the first hemodynamic response that occurs after the administration of the electrical stimulus?
   a. Tachycardia
   b. Hypertension
   c. Bradycardia
   d. Decreased cerebral blood flow

4. Which is an absolute contraindication to ECT?
   a. Increased intracranial pressure
   b. Angina
   c. Pregnancy
   d. Osteoporosis
5. Which medication is an NMDA antagonist?
   a. Propofol
   b. Etomidate
   c. Ketamine
   d. Diazepam

Suggested Readings

Andrad C, Thirthalli J, Gangadhar BN. Unilateral nondominant electrode placement as a risk factor for recall of awareness under anesthesia during electroconvulsive therapy. *J ECT* 2007;23(3):201-203.

Ding Z, White PF. Anesthesia for electroconvulsive therapy. *Anesth Analg* 2002;94(5):1351-1364.

Jankauskas V, Necyk C, Chue J, Chue P. A review of ketamine's role in ECT and non-ECT settings. *Neuropsychiatr Dis Treat* 2018;14:1437-1450.

Kadiyala PK, Kadiyala LD. ECT: a new look at an old friend. *Curr Opin Anaesthesiol* 2018;31(4):453-458.

Obbels J, Verwijk E, Bouckaert F, Sienaert P. ECT-related anxiety: a systematic review. *J ECT.* 2017 Dec;33(4):229-236.

Pinna M, Manchia M, Oppo R, Scano F, et al. Clinical and biological predictors of response to electroconvulsive therapy (ECT): a review. *Neurosci Lett* 2018;669:32-42.

Rasmussen KG. Propofol for ECT anesthesia a review of the literature. *J ECT* 2014;30(3):210-215.

Sobey R, Tracy A. Nonoperating room anesthesia. In: Nagelhout JJ, Elisha S, eds. *Nurse Anesthesia*, 6th ed. St. Louis, MO: Elsevier, 2018:1194-1215.

Soehle M, Bochem J. Anesthesia for electroconvulsive therapy. *Curr Opin Anaesthesiol* 2018;31(5):501-505.

Wojdacz R, Święcicki Ł, Antosik-Wójcińska A. Comparison of the effect of intravenous anesthetics used for anesthesia during electroconvulsive therapy on the hemodynamic safety and the course of ECT. *Psychiatr Pol* 2017;51(6):1039-1058.

55

Anesthesia for Office-Based Pediatric Dental Surgery

KEY POINTS

- Caries, or dental cavities, are the most prevalent chronic infection in early childhood and are a major cause of school absenteeism.
- Caries in children can cause intense pain, severe infection, and aesthetic embarrassment, as well as difficulties in eating, swallowing, and chewing.
- It is estimated that 56% of children between 2 and 3 years of age have caries, and 80% of children have experienced caries by age 17. The presence of dental caries has reached epidemic proportions in lower-income pediatric populations.
- Office-based anesthesia for dental surgery can be performed safely, conveniently, and cost-effectively.

Case Synopsis

A 7-year-old girl has presented to the dental office with complaints of pain in the teeth and jaw.

Preoperative Evaluation and Demographic Data

Past Medical/Surgical History

- Autism
- Obesity

List of Medications

- None

Diagnostic Data

- None

Height/Weight/Vital Signs

- 124 cm, 53 kg, BMI 35.4 kg/m²
- Blood pressure, 118/80; heart rate, 98 beats per minute; respiratory rate, 12 breaths per minute; room air oxygen saturation, 99%; temperature, 36.8°C

Pathophysiology

Dental caries is the most prevalent cause of chronic infections found in early childhood and is a major reason of school absenteeism. It occurs five to eight times more frequently than asthma. Caries in children can cause pain; aesthetic embarrassment; and difficulties in eating, swallowing, chewing, and speaking. This intraoral disease process has reached epidemic proportions in lower-income pediatric populations in North America. Early childhood caries has a lasting impact on both the child's primary dentition ("baby teeth") and their permanent dentition ("adult teeth") because infection in the primary teeth disrupts the development of the permanent teeth. It is estimated that 56% of children between ages 2 and 3 have caries and 80% of children have experienced caries by age 17.

Dental caries cause the molecular destruction of a part of or the entire calcified tooth structures (enamel, dentin, and cementum), which can progress into the dental pulp. Caries results in gradual loss of tooth structure, which can affect chewing and facial structure and cause infection if left untreated. Caries are caused by the acidic metabolites (low pH) of oral bacteria, principally the bacterium *Streptococcus mutans*. The oral microbiologic flora combined with liquid saliva, salivary proteins, and food debris forms a thick, sticky mass called *biofilm* or *dental plaque*.

Dental periodontal structures consist of the *gingiva* (gums), the *oral mucosal tissue*, the *periodontal membrane*, and the *bones* of the maxilla or the mandible. Biofilm, which adheres to exposed tooth structures, causes caries, periodontal tissue inflammation, and permanently destructive periodontal disease. Bacterial endotoxins that originate from oral bacteria can enter the bloodstream. These circulating endotoxins release inflammatory mediators that are transmitted to the coronary vasculature of the heart, causing coronary artery disease. Other long-term effects and serious illnesses resulting from untreated carious lesions include life-threatening systemic infections that can invade the fascial spaces of the head and neck, through the jawbones (osteomyelitis), and into the brain.

Pediatric dentists and pediatricians recommend the first dental visit at the first year of age. The oral flora of the infant develops from oral and bodily contact with primary caregivers, so careful and thorough oral hygiene is important.

Surgical Procedure

A dentist treats caries by careful and thorough excavation of caries from the tooth and then replaces the missing tooth structure with silver amalgam or glass-filled composite. In more extensive caries with pulpal invasion, the caries is carefully excavated, the pulpal remnants in the crown of the tooth are removed, and the remaining pulpal tissue is mummified with formocresol. The tooth is then restored with a stainless-steel crown. A root canal is not performed on primary teeth due to the potential for future exfoliation of the tooth with the eruption of the permanent adult teeth. The dental hand piece (drill) or dental laser uses copious amounts of water, which must be carefully suctioned by the dental assistant to prevent serious airway stimulation, which can cause coughing or laryngospasm.

Anesthetic Management and Considerations

Preoperative Period

1. *Restate the importance of daily oral hygiene for the pediatric patient.*

   It is essential for parent(s) or guardian(s) to remove the child's biofilm each day by brushing and flossing the teeth, because the child lacks the coordination to thoroughly cleanse their teeth with the needed proper and meticulous technique. Infants whose teeth have not yet erupted should have their mouth cleansed of biofilm at least daily with a clean wet washcloth, swabbing or wiping the entire inside of the mouth and the oral tissues. This process will have already been described and demonstrated by the dental team to the parent(s)/guardian(s) but can also be reinforced by the anesthesia provider.

2. *Discuss the relationship between autism and dental pathology.*

   Autism is a neurologic developmental disorder that may result in severe impairment of language, social interaction, behavior, and cognitive function. Most autistic patients function with a moderate degree of a mental deficit; however, autistic females may display severe mental dysfunction. Classic autism is prevalent in 10 to 20 cases per 10,000 births, and the male-to-female ratio is 3:1.

   The chronic pharmacologic treatment used to manage autism may have side effects that are of concern to dentists and anesthetists. Antipsychotic drugs may cause motor impairment affecting speech and swallowing, along with central nervous system depression and orthostatic hypotension, sialorrhea (excessive salivation), or xerostomia (dry mouth). Other common symptoms are dysgeusia

(altered taste), bruxism (teeth grinding along with clenching), stomatitis, and glossitis. Autistic patients can also present with gastroesophageal reflux disease (GERD) and a typical demand for low-textured foods, which easily adhere to teeth, resulting in significant dental disease. As a result, autistic patients can be challenging yet manageable candidates for office-based dental anesthesia.

3. *Identify indications and contraindications for office-based pediatric dental surgery.*

   Indications and contraindications for office-based anesthesia for pediatric dental surgery are listed in Boxes 55.1 and 55.2, respectively. The anesthetist, along with the dentist, must weigh such factors as the medical condition of the patient, the behavior of the patient, and the capabilities of the dentist/supporting staff to deal with the challenging pediatric patient and ensure patient safety.

4. *Describe the necessity of a presurgical consultation.*

   It is important to meet the patient, parent(s), or guardian(s) before the scheduled surgical appointment for a presurgical consultation. This gives the anesthetist the opportunity to perform a detailed examination of the patient's health history.

> **• BOX 55.1 Indications for Office-Based Anesthesia for Pediatric Dental Surgery**
>
> - Uncooperative/unmanageable behavior
> - Patient who requires immediate dental treatment
> - Unable to thoroughly examine
> - Unable to obtain intraoral dental radiographs
> - Necessity for little or no patient movement or no swallowing
> - Mentally challenged child or adult patients
> - Hypersalivation
> - Small mouth
> - Large tongue
> - Unable to attain intraoral local anesthesia
> - Claustrophobia
> - Need for comprehensive dental treatment needed in multiple quadrants
> - Need for tooth extraction(s)
> - Desire for convenience and significant cost savings

> **• BOX 55.2 Contraindications to Providing Office-Based Anesthesia for Pediatric Dental Surgery**
>
> - Severe allergies
> - Severe asthma
> - Severe cardiovascular pathology
> - Need for invasive monitoring
> - Inadequate facility or supporting staff
> - Craniofacial deformities
> - Aggressive or violent behavior
> - Severe seizure disorder
> - Severe claustrophobia
> - Physical status III or greater

• BOX 55.3 **Considerations for Postponement or Cancellation of Pediatric Office-Based Dental Surgery**

- Patient is not within accepted guidelines of nothing by mouth (NPO)
- Recent upper respiratory infection
- Unwilling or unable to allow premedication
- Systemic infection other than due to dental causes
- Inability to transfer or position the patient for dental surgery
- Inability to obtain intravenous access
- Inadequate number of needed assistants
- Parental or caregiver interference

• BOX 55.4 **Supplies Necessary for Pediatric Dental Surgery Anesthesia**

Utilities

- Backup power (uninterruptible power supply)

Equipment

- Patient monitor to include pulse oximeter, electrocardiogram, and blood pressure monitor with a selection of adequate-sized cuffs
- Liquid crystal body temperature stickers
- Emergency E cylinder oxygen tanks
- Positive pressure ventilation sources, including an ambu bag, with properly sized facemasks
- Defibrillator (charged) or AED
- Suction source or a suction machine, tubing, suction catheters, and Yankauer suctions; plan for emergency suction in the event of power failure
- Anesthesia cart to provide for organization of supplies, including endotracheal equipment, laryngeal mask airways, facemasks, nasal cannulas, disposable facemasks with oxygen tubing, oral and nasal airways, syringes (tuberculin, 3, 5, 10, 30, 60 mL), 18-gauge 1.5-inch needles, 20- and 22-gauge IV catheters, tourniquets, IV fluids and tubing, alcohol pads, adhesive tape, disposable gloves, and stethoscope
- Medication syringe pump
- Emergency medications to include, at a minimum, atropine, glycopyrrolate, epinephrine, ephedrine, phenylephrine, lidocaine, diphenhydramine, hydrocortisone, and a bronchial dilator inhaler such as albuterol

Additional Emergency Equipment and Supplies

- Cricothyrotomy kit

This appointment also allows the anesthetist to interact with the patient and gauge the temperament and challenges the patient could pose during the procedure. This meeting also gives the anesthetist time to discuss procedural rules such as strict nothing-by-mouth (NPO) policies, determine the need for physician consultation, and evaluate the risks and benefits of premedication.

5. *Demonstrate importance of the day-of-surgery anesthesia assessment.*

It is helpful to interview the parent(s) or guardian(s) and assess the patient the day of the dental surgery.

There are times that the anesthetic and the dental surgical procedure may necessitate cancellation as a result of the day-of-surgery anesthesia assessment. Box 55.3 lists some considerations that could postpone or cancel the dental surgical appointment due to a current medical condition(s) or an uncontrollable temperament of the patient. For patients with severe behavioral affect, the anesthetist should consider referral to a pediatric dentist (pedodontist) for treatment in an ambulatory surgical center or an operating room to be completed with general anesthesia.

6. *Describe the process of oral premedication for office-based dental treatment for the pediatric patient.*

Before administration of oral premedication, it is important to have the patient use the restroom to avoid patient movement after the onset of the premedication and to prevent soiling of the dental operatory. Preoperative sedation can be achieved using a variety of different medications; however, a common practice is to administer oral midazolam mixed with either liquid ibuprofen or liquid acetaminophen. Dosing should be based on the patient's ideal body weight. Before the administration of oral or intravenous (IV) agents, a complete anesthesia setup is necessary, and an example is included in Box 55.4. Any office-based anesthesia practice should comply with the Guidelines for Office-Based Anesthesia set forth by the American Association of Nurse Anesthetists.

Oral premedication is beneficial to decrease a patient's separation anxiety from the caregiver(s), insertion of the IV line, and for its amnestic effects. Vivid memories of a difficult dental visit could affect future dental care the patient could seek as they mature. Some patients require no premedication, and thus the anesthetist must decide whether premedication is beneficial to the individual patient.

The patient should rest only with the parent(s)/caregiver(s) in a quiet and nonstimulating room, away from the office reception area. Excessive stimulation could elicit unwanted behaviors and unnecessarily upset the patient. A warm blanket helps preserve body heat from the start and provides a sense of security for the patient. The anesthetist should assess the physiologic effects of the premedication and reassure the parent(s)/caregiver(s) as necessary.

Intraoperative Period

7. *Illustrate the anesthetic challenges that are present with an obese pediatric patient.*

It is estimated that approximately 30% of the pediatric patient population within the United States is presently considered obese, and the incidence is expected to increase in the future. Childhood obesity predisposes to a variety of pathologic disease processes in adulthood, which include type 2 diabetes mellitus, coronary artery disease, hypertension, cancer, joint disease, gallbladder disease, and pulmonary disease.

Calculating body mass index (BMI) for pediatric patients is based on data collected by the Centers for Disease Control and Prevention and accounts for the child's age, height, and weight. These factors are then compared with children considered to have ideal BMI. This patient's BMI is 35.4 kg/m^2, which places her in the ninety-ninth percentile for her age and places her into the category of obesity.

Several physiologic factors that may complicate the anesthetic course include:

- **Increased metabolic rate:** Because the metabolic rate in school-aged children is greater compared with an adult, short periods of hypoventilation or apnea will result in rapid desaturation.
- **Decreased functional residual capacity (FRC):** The FRC and specifically the residual volume (RV) are decreased in obesity. The RV acts a reservoir for oxygen during apnea. Patients with decreased FRC are prone to rapid desaturation during hypoventilation or apnea; therefore preoxygenation is imperative.
- **Redundant airway tissue:** Obesity increases the possibility of developing redundant airway tissue that can cause complete airway obstruction when anesthetic agents are administered.
- **Difficult ventilation/intubation:** Due to the presence of redundant airway tissue and other physical characteristics associated with obesity such as thick neck and a large tongue, difficult ventilation and intubation can cause an airway emergency, necessitating rapid airway intervention.

8. *Describe the anesthetic process for the office-based dental treatment for the pediatric dental patient.*
- **Positioning:** The dental chair is adjusted to accommodate the needs of the dentist. Small patients can be cushioned on a standard dental chair with a large pillow placed horizontally on the dental chair, along with a small dog bone–shaped travel pillow under the neck. Foam pads or rolled towels may also be used for padding the bony prominences and properly positioning the arms. The use of a blanket can be used to maintain cleanliness and to decrease heat loss.
- **Monitoring:** Before administration of anesthesia, it is imperative to apply electrocardiogram (ECG) leads, pulse oximetry, blood pressure cuff, precordial stethoscope, and a temperature monitor.
- **IV line insertion:** In order to decrease patient movement, inhalation of a nonhypoxic mixture of nitrous oxide and oxygen can be titrated to effect. Supporting the patient's head and face and assessing for possible patient movement is important. The anesthetist should consider using a subcutaneous bolus of 2% plain lidocaine, administered with a 29-gauge insulin syringe at the IV insertion site. The IV catheter is secured with tape and possibly gauze wrap to avoid inadvertent removal.
- **Induction:** Administration of an antisialagogue such as glycopyrrolate is used to decrease intraoral secretions. Suction must be available to evacuate saliva from the floor of the mouth and from the buccal vestibules. At this time, nitrous oxide is discontinued

- BOX 55.5 **Advantages of the Dental LMA for Office-Based Pediatric Anesthesia**

- Allows protection of the airway from dental debris, saliva, secretions, and blood
- Provides a secure airway
- Is easily placed
- Is relatively atraumatic to the patient's mouth, throat, and airway
- Can be adapted to work with dental nitrous oxide/oxygen machines
- Can work with an anesthesia machine
- Can be repositioned from side to side to allow the dentist better access to the patient's mouth
- Allows disconnection and reconnection at its midpoint to allow the dentist to check the occlusion (the bite) of the teeth

and oxygen at flow at 3 L/min via mask is for at least 5 minutes to avoid diffusion hypoxia. Sedation is achieved and maintained by administering propofol by infusion. Both eyes are carefully taped to avoid corneal abrasions.

A special dental laryngeal mask airway (LMA) is available to assist the anesthesia provider to maintain and safeguard the airway. The dental LMA can be adapted to work with dental nitrous oxide/oxygen delivery systems or attached to an anesthesia machine. Advantages associated with the dental LMA are listed in Box 55.5.

- **Maintenance:** Due to the increased metabolic rate that is characteristic of children, a propofol infusion is titrated to effect. Propofol infusion rates of 100 to 150 mcg/kg/min are frequently necessary to maintain unconsciousness. Patients experiencing stimulating dental procedures require noticeably higher maintenance infusion rates of propofol. Advantages to the use of propofol include ability to titrate, relatively short half-life, and potential antiemetic effects.

If the patient will require dental extractions, the anesthetist may consider administering incremental doses of fentanyl. Ketamine may also be titrated to help stabilize and control behaviorally agitated patients. Midazolam will help decrease the possibility of postoperative emergence delirium. Due to a synergistic anesthetic effect, the addition of these adjunctive agents will reduce the maintenance infusion rate of propofol. Dexamethasone is frequently administered to decrease postextraction swelling and inhibit nausea and vomiting. Additionally, a serotonin receptor antagonist such as ondansetron is used as nausea and vomiting prophylaxis. Ketorolac can be used to decrease postoperative pain.

Postoperative Period

9. *Explain the process of emergence from anesthesia after pediatric dental surgery.*

Even without the use of narcotics, emergence after a propofol infusion is frequently prolonged. This can be explained by the concept of context-sensitive half-time. As a lipid-soluble medication is administered by infusion, over time the drug is sequestered in tissue and accounts for the prolonged sedative effects. This effect is dependent on the duration of drug administration and the total dose administered. Continuing support of the airway and leaving the oral bite block in place allow for access to the posterior pharynx for suctioning. Gently supporting and reorienting the patient upon emergence is vital. It is prudent to consider bringing only one caregiver/parent to the operatory, after the patient has nearly emerged and is stable. Explaining to the caregiver that there is a possibility that the patient may exhibit emergence delirium is important.

10. *Correlate the modified Aldrete signs to the assessment of the patient during recovery.*

Recovery can be accomplished within the dental operatory or after transport of the patient to a well-equipped recovery area. The area should remain quiet and in the presence of a well-trained assistant. Hospital recovery room nurses commonly use modified Aldrete signs for postanesthetic assessment of the patient. The modified Aldrete score is obtained by assigning an objective score to assessment of the patient's activity, respirations, circulation, consciousness, and color. Discharge is appropriate when a patient is stable and has attained a minimum modified Aldrete score of 10.

Pediatric patients anesthetized in an office-based setting typically are discharged after approximately 20 to 30 minutes. If narcotics are administered for analgesia, discharge times are frequently increased.

Review Questions

1. Which is characteristic of advanced dental caries?
   a. Absence of intraoral inflammation and infection
   b. Minimal patient morbidity
   c. Pain and destruction of tooth structure
   d. Results from nonpreventable causes
2. Which patient should not be considered for office-based pediatric dentistry?
   a. ASA physical status classification III
   b. A cooperative 2-year-old patient
   c. An 11-year-old patient who refuses premedication
   d. A mentally challenged 55-year-old adult patient
3. The preoperative consultation and interview is:
   a. An unnecessary duplicity of the patient's health history.
   b. Performed only by the anesthesia provider.
   c. Completed several days before the patient's dental surgical appointment.
   d. Highlights concerns that could interfere with the anesthetic plan.

4. Which is the most appropriate statement regarding premedication of a pediatric patient presenting for dental surgery?
   a. Before setup of the anesthesia equipment and supplies
   b. In a quiet, nonstimulating environment
   c. With the parent(s)/guardian(s) and siblings present
   d. All pediatric patients should receive premedication
5. Which is false regarding the recovery of a pediatric patient after dental surgery?
   a. Can be performed in the dental chair
   b. Should occur with parent(s) or caregiver(s) present immediately after dental surgery
   c. Can be performed after transport to a well-equipped recovery room
   d. Requires the availability of a well-trained assistant

Suggested Readings

Campbell RL, Shetty NS, Shetty KS, Pope HL, Campbell JR. Pediatric dental surgery under general anesthesia: uncooperative children. *Anesth Prog* 2018;65(4):225-230.

Crall J. Improving oral health for individuals with special health care needs. *Pediatr Dent* 2007;29:98-104.

Elisha S, Terry K. Neonatal anesthesia. In: Nagelhout JJ, Elisha S, eds. *Nurse Anesthesia*, 6th ed. St. Louis, MO: Elsevier, 2018: 1093-1116.

Friedlander A, Yagiela J, Paterno V, et al. The neuropathology, medical management and dental implications of autism. *JADA* 2006; 137:1517-1527.

Gazal G, Fareed WM, Zafar MS, Al-Samadani KH. Pain and anxiety management for pediatric dental procedures using various combinations of sedative drugs: a review. *Saudi Pharm J* 2016;24(4): 379-85.

Keles S, Kocaturk O. Postoperative discomfort and emergence delirium in children undergoing dental rehabilitation under general anesthesia: comparison of nasal tracheal intubation and laryngeal mask airway. *J Pain Res* 2018;11:103-110.

Krishnan DG. Anesthesia for the pediatric oral and maxillofacial surgery patient. *Oral Maxillofac Surg Clin North Am* 2018;30(2): 171-181.

Lalwani K, Kitchin J, Lax P. Office-based dental rehabilitation in children with special care needs using a pediatric sedation service model. *J Oral Maxillofac Surg* 2007;65:427-433.

Moness Ali AM, Hammuda AA. Local anesthesia effects on postoperative pain after pediatric oral rehabilitation under general anesthesia. *Pediatr Dent* 2019;41(3):181-185.

Sebastiani FR, Dym H, Wolf J. Oral sedation in the dental office. *Dent Clin North Am* 2016;60(2):295-307.

Answers to Review Questions

Chapter 1

1. d. Bacterial tonsillitis is most commonly caused by group A beta-hemolytic streptococci.
2. c. Fluid administration is the initial concern with a patient presenting with hemorrhage postoperatively. Patients often present with hypovolemia due to the immeasurable amount of blood that has been oozing from the tonsillar bed site.
3. a. The primary goal of intraoperative management during a tonsillectomy is to obtund the oropharyngeal reflexes and prevent patient movement. Tonsillectomy is very stimulating; therefore a deep plane of anesthesia must be maintained in order to prevent patient movement during the surgical procedure.
4. a. An absolute indication for a tonsillectomy is recurrent hemorrhagic tonsillitis. Recurrent bleeding from prominent vessels of the tonsils or from the parenchyma due to recurrent tonsillitis or tonsillar hyperplasia can result in anemia and is an indication for tonsillectomy.
5. d. Ketorolac, an NSAID, inhibits platelet aggregation, thereby potentially increasing the risk of bleeding. The potential for bleeding is increased when subsequent doses are administered.

Chapter 2

1. d. Lymphatic metastasis is the most important mechanism of the recurrence, survival rates, and spread of head and neck squamous cell carcinoma from the primary sites. The risk of cervical lymphadenopathy varies depending on the site of origin, the size of the primary tumor, the histologic grade of the primary tumor, perineural invasion, perivascular invasion, and extracapsular spread.
2. a. The most common electrolyte disturbance for a patient undergoing RND is hyponatremia. This abnormality is usually dilutional. However, a subgroup of squamous cell cancers may result in paraneoplastic syndromes; the most common is the syndrome of inappropriate secretions of antidiuretic hormone (SIADH).
3. c. Although trapezium weakness can occur even when the spinal accessory nerve is preserved, these collective signs and symptoms are associated with surgical trauma to the spinal accessory nerve, resulting in the shoulder girdle mechanism deformity associated with painful "shoulder syndrome."
4. b. A hematoma is usually evident in the first few hours after the RND operation. Because blood under a flap accumulates rapidly, inspection is the best way to assess for hematoma formation.

Chapter 3

1. c. The risk factors that put this patient choice at highest risk for developing laryngeal cancer include history of smoking, alcohol abuse, gender, and advanced age (>50 years old).
2. b. The incidence of laryngeal cancer by region from the greatest to the least includes glottic to supraglottic to subglottic.
3. d. The assessment of laryngeal malignancy depends primarily on its location and the TNM staging of the tumor. The letters TNM represent tumor, node, and metastasis.
4. d. A combination of laryngoscopy with biopsies and CT scan are the diagnostic tests that best determine the staging of laryngeal carcinoma.
5. a. Although the anesthetist should be alert to all of the listed potential complications, the most important factors include airway protection and massive hemorrhage.

Chapter 4

1. c. Vocal cord polyps usually do not interfere with airway patency. Vocal cord polyps may interfere with vocal cord movement (vibration), causing changes in phonation. Vocal cord polyps are benign lesions caused by chronic exposure to stresses.
2. d. Lasers may cause burns and eye injury and ignite fires. The frequency of lasers is close to the visible light band and therefore does not expose operating room personnel to ionizing radiation such as gamma or x-rays.
3. b. Fire requires three components to occur: an ignition source, oxidizer, and fuel. A laser is an excellent ignition source; oxygen and nitrous oxide are oxidizers; and surgical drapes, alcohol disinfectants, and gauze sponges are all fuels. Carbon dioxide is not an ignitor, oxidizer, or fuel source.

4. a. Precautions to take during laser surgery include using the lowest concentration of oxygen (an oxidizer), avoiding nitrous oxide (an oxidizer), use of proper eye shields and protection, and being prepared to extinguish a possible fire.

5. c. Positive airway pressure, digital pressure with jaw thrust, and succinylcholine administration are all treatments for laryngospasm. Cricothyrotomy is not indicated for a laryngospasm that can be treated with less invasive interventions.

Chapter 5

1. d. Obstructive sleep apnea is a syndrome associated with periodic, partial, or complete obstruction of the upper airway during sleep that leads to episodes of apnea-hypopnea, frequent arousals, oxygen desaturation, and daytime hypersomnolence and hypercarbia.

2. c. Based on the ASA Clinical Practice Guidelines for OSA, an apnea-hypopnea index (AHI) of 25 indicates the patient has moderate OSA. Severe sleep apnea is defined as an AHI of 30 or 40 per the ASA Practice Guidelines.

3. a. Patients with OSA display poor upper airway control during sleep, which is associated with substantial decrements in pharyngeal dilator muscle activity; over time these muscles may develop neural/muscle damage, which further exacerbates the obstruction. OSA is associated with ventilatory control instability that results in increases and decreases in respiratory output to pharyngeal dilator muscles, which when combined with increased fat deposition in the airway and poor upper airway motor control may further contribute to episodes of obstruction.

4. b. Chronic repeated obstructive events of hypoxemia and hypercarbia cause sleep fragmentation, sympathetic hyperactivity, systemic inflammation with higher C-reactive protein and interleukin-6 levels, endothelial dysfunction, and metabolic dysregulation, all of which can increase the risk for cardiovascular, neuropsychologic, and endocrine disorders and an impaired quality of life.

5. b. Sleep architecture is altered after surgery with suppression of stage 3 and 4 REM and NREM sleep. Postoperative pain is highest in the first several days after UPPP surgery. Patients with OSA are at greater risk for life-threatening obstructive apnea secondary to respiratory depressive effects of opioids. After the third postoperative day, deep REM sleep rebounds and OSA patients are again at risk for life-threatening deep sleep-induced apnea.

Chapter 6

1. a. Signs that are associated with a bowel obstruction include constipation, abdominal distention, fever, and vomiting.

2. b. Advantages associated with laparoscopic bowel resection include decreased postoperative pain, decreased hospitalization time, decreased postoperative ileus, and rapid recovery of pulmonary function.

3. d. Contraindications to laparoscopic bowel resection include intestinal obstruction, bulky tumors, evidence of metastatic tumor growth in adjacent abdominal organs, and pregnancy.

4. b. Signs that are associated with a CO_2 gas embolus include hypotension, hypoxemia, decreased end tidal CO_2, and dysrhythmias.

5. c. Pain that is associated with laparoscopic bowel resection is most likely caused by subdiaphragmatic peritoneal irritation.

Chapter 7

1. d. Of the choices that are listed, deep venous thrombosis is the most common complication associated with the laparoscopic Roux-en-Y procedure.

2. c. Diabetes mellitus is a frequent coexisting disease that may rapidly resolve by successful weight loss postoperatively.

3. b. Creatinine levels are frequently normal, as obesity has limited negative effects on glomerular filtration, renal blood flow, and clearance. Advanced stages of diabetes can impair renal function, indicating the need for preoperative evaluation of renal function.

4. a and b. The overall effect of morbid obesity on the respiratory system is a decrease in total lung capacity, functional residual capacity and residual volume. The respiratory pattern on spirometry is similar to restrictive lung disease.

5. a. Abdominal pressures of 20 to 30 mm Hg can cause cardiovascular compromise as a result of decreased cardiac output, increased systemic vascular resistance, and decreased venous return.

Chapter 8

1. d. The perioperative administration of antibiotics is dependent on the individual patient's situation and whether the appendix has ruptured. Therefore the antibiotic regimen when comparing LA with OA will be the same. Advantages to an LA include improved aesthetic result, smaller incisions, decreased pain, less blood loss, less postoperative pulmonary impairment, a reduction in postoperative ileus, shorter hospital stays, faster postoperative recovery, fewer wound infections, and earlier return to daily functioning.

2. c. Nitrous oxide is a highly diffusible gas that can cause bowel distention, and this effect potentially makes the surgery more difficult to perform.

3. b. A vagal-mediated response initiated as a result of the celiac reflex can result in bronchospasm, bradycardia, and possibly asystole causing cardiovascular collapse. The primary intervention is to have the surgeon

evacuate the pneumoperitoneum immediately. Decreasing the amount of peritoneal stimulation can cause the reflex to immediately stop. Other interventions that should be instituted simultaneously include delivering 100% oxygen, increasing fluids, checking a blood pressure, and potentially administering glycopyrrolate/ephedrine and atropine for severe and continued bradycardia.

4. c. Respiratory acidosis most commonly occurs. The patient's functional residual capacity and vital capacity decrease due to cephalad diaphragmatic and abdominal contents displacement, leading to decreased pulmonary compliance, increased ventilation-perfusion mismatch, increased peak inspiratory pressure, and increased CO_2 that result in respiratory acidosis.

5. a. Durant maneuver entails placing the patient's head down below the level of the heart and into the left lateral decubitus position. It is one intervention that can be used to help restore blood flow through the heart during a venous CO_2 embolism.

Chapter 9

1. b. All of the following gases have been utilized during laparoscopic surgery; however, the safety profile of CO_2 allows its use during electrocautery and laser surgery. Carbon dioxide is also easily eliminated from the lungs.

2. d. Hemodynamic changes that occur with creation of a pneumoperitoneum include decreased venous return to the heart, decreased stroke volume, increased mean arterial pressure, and increased abdominal pressures.

3. d. Carbon dioxide insufflation during the creation of a pneumoperitoneum affects the pulmonary system by decreasing functional residual capacity, pulmonary compliance, and vital capacity. It will also result in an increased intrathoracic pressure.

4. c. Carbon dioxide insufflation during the creation of a pneumoperitoneum affects the renal system by increasing aldosterone and antidiuretic hormone secretion, decreasing urine output, and decreasing glomerular filtration rate.

5. d. Preoperative laboratory tests necessary for patients having a cholecystectomy include ALT, AST, bilirubin, albumin, and alkaline phosphatase.

Chapter 10

1. c. The refinement of immunosuppressant therapy has been instrumental in increasing the survival rates in patients undergoing OLT.

2. d. The major feature that is associated with NASH is fat deposition within the liver.

3. a. Hyperkalemia is a consequence of the progressive acidosis that can lead to cardiac dysrhythmias and asystole that is refractory to treatment.

4. b. Desmopressin (DDAVP) may be administered to help improve platelet function.

5. c. The most common period in which rejection occurs is during weeks 1 to 6 after the transplant.

Chapter 11

1. c. Of the choices, aminocaproic acid is the only option to decrease acute coagulopathy.

2. d. Corticosteroidogenesis is not a function that is performed by the liver.

3. d. Segments 2, 3, 4a, and 4b constitute the left lobe of the liver.

4. a. The factor that is most closely associated with increased early mortality after liver resection is severe blood loss.

5. d. Postoperative hypoglycemia is most commonly associated with liver resection.

Chapter 12

1. b. All of the symptoms listed can occur. However, the classic triad includes headache, diaphoresis, and tachycardia in the presence of hypertension.

2. d. The majority of extraadrenal pheochromocytomas (approximately 80%) are present in the abdomen.

3. a. Catecholamine synthesis occurs within the adrenal medulla. Under normal circumstances, the adrenal medulla secretes 80% epinephrine and 20% norepinephrine. However, pheochromocytomas that are composed of chromaffin cells secrete norepinephrine at a ratio of 9:1 compared with epinephrine.

4. b. The vital signs in choice b are within normal parameters. Proper alpha blockade followed by beta blockade must be accomplished. Hemodilution occurs after vasodilation and intravenous volume loading is established. The blood pressure should be less than 160/90 within 48 hours before surgery.

5. c. Tools used to diagnose the presence of a pheochromocytoma include diagnostic imaging, MIBG scanning, 24-hour urine test, plasma test, and clonidine suppression test. Urine tests include an elevation of metanephrines on three tests in a 24-hour period. Plasma tests include elevations in norepinephrine levels.

Chapter 13

1. b. The goal of anesthetic maintenance is to attenuate the sympathetic nervous system by maintaining an adequate depth of anesthesia and avoiding drugs that cause sympathetic stimulation.

2. d. Hypercarbia is not commonly associated with hyperthyroidism.

3. a. Thyrotropin-releasing hormone (TRH) is secreted by the hypothalamus, which stimulates the anterior

pituitary gland to produce thyroid-stimulating hormone (TSH), which directly causes the thyroid gland to synthesize T_3 and T_4.

4. a. Hyperthyroidism causes an increase in MAC of inhalational agents. Hyperthermia also increases MAC values.

5. d. Accidental removal of the parathyroid glands results in hypocalcemia.

Chapter 14

1. d. In all of these scenarios, the patient should be suspected of having an acute cervical spine injury until the possibility is definitively excluded by physical examination and radiologic evidence.

2. a. Succinylcholine can cause hyperkalemia due to acetylcholine receptor upregulation in a patient with a spinal cord injury after the first 24 to 48 hours and a patient with a crush injury. Succinylcholine is also a known triggering agent for malignant hyperthermia. Patients who have sustained a crush injury associated with muscle trauma are at risk of developing hyperkalemia.

3. d. It is estimated that carbon dioxide (CO_2) increases 6 mm Hg during the first minute and 3 to 4 mm Hg/minute while an adult patient is apneic. In this scenario, the CO_2 increases 6 mm Hg for the first minute and 4 mm Hg for every minute thereafter (3 minutes). The total increase for the time that the patient is apneic is 18 mm Hg, which when added to the existing $PaCO_2$ of 47 mm Hg (47 + 18) is 65 mm Hg.

4. b. The chemoreceptor reflex is initiated via the carotid and aortic bodies (peripheral chemoreceptors) in response to decreased PaO2, increased $PaCO_2$, and increased hydrogen ion concentration. The result is sympathetic nervous system activation.

5. c. The correct placement for needle decompression of a tension pneumothorax is opposite of the direction of the tracheal deviation in the second intercostal space at the midclavicular line.

Chapter 15

1. b and c. Hyperventilation and CSF drainage can used to decrease severely elevated ICP.

2. c. Cerebral perfusion pressure is determined by MAP and ICP.

3. a. A systolic blood pressure ≤100 mm Hg is associated with poor neurologic outcome in patients who have sustained an AHI.

4. c. Ringer's lactate should be avoided in patients presenting for craniotomy after AHI because it can increase brain swelling and it contains glucose. Due to worsening intracellular acidosis, hyperglycemia is associated with poor neurologic outcomes.

5. a. Headache, nausea, papilledema, unilateral pupillary dilation, abducens, and oculomotor palsies are all symptoms associated with increased ICP.

Chapter 16

1. a. RSI with cricoid pressure is the most correct method to induce and intubate a trauma patient due to increased possibility of aspiration. All trauma patients should be considered to have a full stomach.

2. d. Nitrous oxide is highly diffusible and accumulates in closed air spaces. The use of nitrous oxide could potentially increase the size of a pneumothorax or a pneumocephalus and cause bowel distention.

3. b. Acute ingestion of depressant substances decreases the anesthetic requirement. Depressants, such as alcohol, marijuana, and narcotics, have a synergistic depressant effect when combined with anesthetic agents and can lead to marked hypotension and bradycardia.

4. c. The liver is extremely vascular, and large vessels, such as the portal vein hepatic artery and hepatic vein, can be damaged. Injury to the liver or associated vasculature can result in the entrainment of air within the venous system, leading to a venous air embolism.

5. d. Low-velocity missiles have the potential to fragment and ricochet within the body, which, depending on the tissue or structures damaged, can lead to extensive tissue destruction.

Chapter 17

1. c. Pulmonary contusions are present in 70% of blunt thoracic injuries. The most definitive method for identification is a CT scan.

2. c. Lung volumes do not increase with body weight. Appropriate Tv ventilation should be based on the patient's ideal body weight. Although various methods can be used to determine ideal body weight, the formula 2.54 × height in inches − 100 = IBW. For the scenario described in question 2, the patient's ideal weight is near 84 kg (calculated at 82 kg). Based on this, tidal volumes should be between 6 and 8 mL/kg, as determined by the ARDSnet.

3. a. The plateau pressure is the longest period of alveolar distension. The ARDSnet demonstrated that plateau pressure (period of stretch) was most indicative of barotrauma.

4. d. Management of an aortic aneurysm requires blood pressure control to reduce transmural pressure on the lining of the blood vessels. Increased pressure can result in further dissection of the injured vasculature leading to rupture. Blood pressure control can occur via reductions in systemic vascular resistance (SVR) or cardiac output by reducing heart rate.

5. b. Hypercarbia and hypoxemia occur in patients with ARDS due to alveolar capillary edema and fibrosis, increased ventilation-perfusion mismatching, and atelectasis and decreased surfactant. Pulmonary hypertension occurs due to chronic hypoxia, which increases right ventricular pressure.

Chapter 18

1. a. Pulmonary resection procedures have been performed for a variety of etiologies, including (1) pulmonary masses, (2) malignant mesothelioma, (3) bronchiectasis, (4) tuberculosis, (5) and thoracic trauma. Pulmonary masses may present as benign or malignant pathology. Benign pathology includes carcinoid tumors, hemangiomas, bronchopulmonary sequestrations, and infection. The majority of pulmonary resection procedures are performed for the removal of malignant tissue (e.g., bronchogenic carcinoma).

2. a. Endocrinologic abnormalities and paraneoplastic neurologic syndromes are common in patients with SCLC. These syndromes include (1) SIADH, (2) Cushing syndrome, and (3) myasthenic syndrome (e.g., Eaton-Lambert syndrome). SIADH is present in up to 40% of patients with SCLC.

3. d. After fiber-optic bronchoscopy, correct placement and depth of insertion of a left-sided dual-lumen tube should reveal that the blue bronchial cuff is situated in the left mainstem bronchus and is visible just below the level of the carina without herniation.

4. a. During spontaneous respiration, the increased ventilation of the inferior/dependent areas of the lung is relatively matched to the increased perfusion in these same areas. However, with the institution of (1) anesthesia, (2) controlled ventilation, and (3) thoracotomy (e.g., open chest), the dependent lung in the lateral decubitus position undergoes a decrease in pulmonary compliance, while the nondependent lung undergoes a relative increase in ventilation. Due to the fact that perfusion does not change to the dependent area of the lung, a mismatch of ventilation and perfusion ensues.

5. c. Surgical clamping of the pulmonary artery inhibits arterial blood flow to the nonventilated lung. By eliminating intrapulmonary shunt from the nonventilated lung, physiologic shunt is decreased and hypoxemia is decreased in the process. Hemodynamic instability (e.g., due to the increase in right ventricular afterload and decrease in left ventricular preload) with clamping of the pulmonary artery prior to ligation is a contraindication to continuing with the pneumonectomy procedure.

Chapter 19

1. b. Eaton-Lambert syndrome is most often associated with oat-cell carcinoma, which is also known as small cell carcinoma of the lung.

2. a. Thymomas (tumors of the thymus gland) are commonly observed in patients with myasthenia gravis. These tumors play a role in the formation of antibodies that attack nicotinic acetylcholine receptors at the postsynaptic neuromuscular junction.

3. a. Mediastinoscopy would pose a severe risk for bleeding in the patient who has a coagulopathy, and therefore this surgical procedure is contraindicated.

4. c. The innominate artery is a branch of the thoracic aortic arch and gives rise to the right common carotid artery and the right subclavian artery. Compression of the innominate artery will decrease blood flow to the right arm by decreasing blood flow into the right subclavian artery.

5. a. A pneumothorax may result from inadvertent puncture of the pleura during a mediastinoscopy. Positive-pressure ventilation can cause the rapid accumulation of air within the pleural space, creating a tension pneumothorax, which results in cardiac and respiratory compromise.

Chapter 20

1. a. The incidence of mediastinal masses varies according to the age of the patient and location of the lesion. In adults, most mediastinal tumors occur in the anterior mediastinum. The two most common neoplasms of the anterior mediastinum are thymomas and lymphomas, which account for 30% of the pathology.

2. b. At the convergence of the superior, anterior, and middle mediastinum are (1) the middle portion of the superior vena cava, (2) the tracheal bifurcation, (3) the main pulmonary artery, (4) the aortic arch, and (5) the cephalad surface of the heart. Mediastinal masses are associated with direct cardiac and great vessel (i.e., aorta and main pulmonary artery) compression, superior vena cava syndrome, and tracheobronchial obstruction. Each of these complications is potentially life threatening and can result in death during surgery and anesthesia.

3. c. Despite adequate surgical resection of a mediastinal mass, the presence of tracheomalacia and inadequate cartilaginous tracheal support can cause tracheal collapse and necessitate postoperative intubation and ventilatory support.

4. c. The advantages associated with VATS compared with an open thoracotomy include decreased postoperative pain, reduction in the incidence of postoperative respiratory dysfunction, shorter postoperative course, and the promotion of a rapid recovery resulting in reduced length of hospital stay and cost.

5. a. Acute respiratory insufficiency is the most common and serious complication after pulmonary resection, which occurs in nearly 15% of patients after resection of bronchial carcinoma. Preexisting pulmonary pathology, pulmonary transudate, pulmonary trauma, and/or postoperative pain can precipitate inadequate respiratory effort.

Chapter 21

1. a. Thymic lymphocytes give rise to thymic lymphomas such as Hodgkin disease and non-Hodgkin lymphomas.

2. a, b, and c. Cholinergic crisis is associated with myosis and increased lacrimation and salivation.
3. b. Neostigmine (physostigmine) and pyridostigmine are also used for management of a myasthenic crisis, but steroids and surgery are indicated for chronic management of the myasthenic patient. Atropine is used in the treatment of a cholinergic crisis.
4. d. Thymomas are also associated with hypothyroidism and pernicious anemia. Lambert-Eaton myasthenic syndrome is associated with small cell carcinoma.
5. a. Partial DiGeorge syndrome is associated with an immune deficiency that improves over time. Complete DiGeorge syndrome is associated with athymia, severe immunodeficiency, and death before 2 years of age.

Chapter 22

1. c. The rule of 100 includes a PaO2 ≥100 mm Hg. It also includes SBP ≥100 mm Hg, urine output >100 mL/hour, and heart rate <100 beats per minute.
2. b. Diabetes insipidus presents with hypovolemia, hypernatremia, and hypokalemia. It causes hypotonic urine formation, occurs frequently with brain death, and is treated with IV vasopressin or desmopressin.
3. a. Viability of harvested organs is primarily dependent on the length of warm ischemic time. Organs are removed in the order of susceptibility to warm ischemia.
4. b. Anesthesia is required for DBD donors to eliminate spinal reflexes, which are activated by surgical stimulation. There is no perception of pain or awareness with brain death.
5. a. The OPO can direct end-of-life care without family consent for an individual with a signed driver's license or donor card.

Chapter 23

1. c. Regional anesthesia requires that the patient be awake and able to cooperate for the duration of the surgical procedure. Careful patient selection and preoperative education are essential because heavy sedation increases the incidence of intraoperative complications.
2. d. Stump pressures show a high degree of specificity but not sensitivity for the detection of cerebral hypoperfusion and ischemia.
3. c. The elimination half-time of heparin is approximately 1 hour, so only 3500 units of heparin should be circulating in the body 1 hour after administration. Because the dose of protamine is 1 mg/100 units heparin left in the body, the initial dose of protamine that should be administered is 35 mg.
4. a. Ipsilateral smile asymmetry is the result of cranial nerve damage. Contralateral facial asymmetry is the result of an intraoperative cerebral vascular event.
5. b. Ninety-five percent of all postoperative neurologic deficits are the result of thromboembolic events during carotid endarterectomy.

Chapter 24

1. d. Selective antegrade perfusion is utilized to prolong the amount of time that deep hypothermic circulatory arrest can be used.
2. a. Stanford type A aortic dissections include the aortic root, ascending aorta, and aortic arch.
3. c. The internal jugular vein is usually cannulated for retrograde cerebral perfusion.
4. b. Hypertension is the most common comorbidity present in the patient with acute aortic dissection.
5. b. Thrombocytopenia is a complication associated with deep hypothermic circulatory arrest.

Chapter 25

1. c. Compression of the conducting airways by a thoracic aneurysm may create a mediastinal mass effect and intolerance of the supine position. Such symptoms may have life-threatening consequences during induction of anesthesia. Careful evaluation and planning prior to surgery are imperative.
2. b. The anterior spinal artery is most commonly supplemented in the thoracic region by the artery of Adamkiewicz, a greater radicular artery that supplies most of the blood flow to the lower two-thirds of the anterior spinal cord.
3. a. The right radial artery is preferred because aortic cross-clamping is sometimes required proximal to the left subclavian artery during descending aortic repairs, making it impossible to use the left upper extremity for blood pressure monitoring.
4. d. Hypotension, hypothermia, and volatile anesthetics all produce decreases in amplitude and increases in latency with evoked potential monitoring, potentially mimicking spinal ischemia. Narcotics, including fentanyl, have a minimal inhibitory effect on evoked potential monitoring.
5. c. SCPP is defined as the difference between mean arterial pressure (MAP) and cerebrospinal fluid (CSF) pressure.

Chapter 26

1. b. Smoking is the single most independent risk factor for the development of AAA. It has been reported that 90% of all AAA patients have a history of nicotine abuse.
2. b. The initial response to aortic cross-clamping is arterial hypertension. Sodium nitroprusside, an arterial vasodilator, is the pharmacologic agent of choice. The anesthetist may also deepen the anesthetic agents to aid in decreasing the blood pressure.
3. c. Reactive hyperemia causes a transient decrease in blood pressure that results from the restoration of blood flow to ischemic tissues.

4. c. Myocardial infarction accounts for the highest post-operative morbidity in patients undergoing abdominal aortic aneurysm repair.

5. a. One major advantage associated with EVAR compared with an open approach to AAA repair is that it is unnecessary to apply an aortic cross clamp.

Chapter 27

1. c. Improved wound healing occurs due to the minimally invasive nature of the surgery and relatively small incisions compared with a traditional sternotomy.

2. a. The microvascular and macrovascular changes that are associated with diabetes predispose the patient for developing cardiovascular disease.

3. c. From these choices, aortic atherosclerotic disease is the only absolute contraindication to MIDCABG.

4. b. Employing transesophageal echocardiography for a patient with esophageal varices can result in severe esophageal hemorrhage and/or esophageal perforation.

5. d. Atenolol (Tenormin) is a beta-adrenergic receptor-blocking drug that causes increased myocardial oxygen supply, decreased myocardial oxygen demand, decreased myocardial contractility, and potentially bronchoconstriction from inhibition of B$_2$-adrenergic receptors in the lungs.

Chapter 28

1. c. The cranial vault consists of bone and establishes a fixed space in which blood, brain, and CSF occupy. Increases in blood, brain, or CSF volume will increase ICP. Decreasing the volume of any or all of these components will lower ICP.

2. b. Hyperventilation causes cerebral vasoconstriction, which lowers the total amount of blood in the cranial vault. The lower cranial vault blood volume lowers ICP. Hypoxia, hypercarbia, and VAAs cause cerebral vasodilatation, increasing the cranial vault volume, which increases ICP.

3. c. Cushing syndrome (hypercortisolism) is a hormonal disease marked by excessive cortisol. Cushing reflex is a physiologic response (increased blood pressure and reflexive decreased heart rate) to elevated ICP in reestablish adequate CPP. The Cushing triad is marked by the addition of irregular respirations to the Cushing reflex of hypertension and bradycardia. Confusion and lethargy are associated with elevated ICP.

4. b. Mannitol is an osmotic diuretic that pulls water out of intracellular and interstitial tissues into the vascular space for excretion. This lowers the amount of brain water (edema) and decreases the volume of brain tissue, lowering ICP. Mannitol is also a free radical scavenger. Mannitol has a greater affinity for free radicals and readily binds to them, thereby protecting tissues from the damaging effects.

5. c. The events associated with the greatest noxious stimulation are intubation, skin incision, glial resection and scraping, and emergence. The glial lining is the mesh of nerves and connective tissue that covers the skull under the scalp flap. Resection and scraping of this tissue are stimulating and may be associated with increased heart rate and blood pressure, as seen with other noxious events. Brain tissue is devoid of sensory nerve fibers and is not a stimulating procedure by itself. Skin closure is another noxious event and may unmask light anesthesia if anesthetics are weaned early; otherwise, emergence is the last event associated with noxious stimulation.

Chapter 29

1. b. Acromegaly typically develops over a period of years, and its onset of symptoms is gradual and subtle, making the initial diagnosis difficult.

2. b. Biventricular hypertrophy, insulin resistance, and sleep apnea commonly occur in patients with acromegaly. Excess growth hormone does not lead to fat deposition and obesity.

3. a. DI and SIADH may occur within the first 24 to 48 hours after surgery. Cranial nerve palsy, visual changes, and an altered level of consciousness can occur in the immediate postoperative period. These signs and symptoms are indications for the need for reexploration, CT scanning, or MRI.

4. a. Muscle relaxation should be used to ensure immobility, and for this reason, the use of a laryngeal mask airway is precluded. In the case of an acromegalic patient, laryngeal mask airway placement may be difficult because of anatomic changes. Short-acting medications should be used to expedite emergence so that an assessment can be performed immediately after extubation. Due to the prevalence of obstructive sleep apnea in this patient population, narcotics and benzodiazepines should be administered with caution. Transsphenoidal hypophysectomy involves a sublabial or endonasal approach, and access to the upper lip and nose is necessary. This is best achieved by placement of an oral endotracheal tube.

5. a. Nearly 80% of patients with Cushing disease have hypertension, and 50% have a diastolic blood pressure >100 mm Hg. Despite these findings, ECG abnormalities are common and include high-voltage QRS complexes and inverted T waves, possibly due to left ventricular strain and hypertrophy. Diastolic dysfunction is seen in over 40% of patients. The development of aortic stenosis is not specifically related to Cushing disease.

Chapter 30

1. d. Arguably, the single most important element in the successful asleep-awake craniotomy is a highly motivated, well-informed patient.

2. c. The anesthetist should determine the patient's wishes regarding abandoning the asleep-awake technique for a general anesthetic.
3. a. Cold irrigating solution applied to the cortex has been shown to stop seizure activity.
4. d. A light is placed under the drapes at the beginning of surgery to avoid the patient awakening in a dark and confined space.
5. b. Asleep-awake craniotomies are necessary in only a small percentage of patients—those in whom seizure focus may be suppressed during general anesthesia or that may be adjacent to an "eloquent" cortical function.

Chapter 31

1. d. The initial intervention for treating OCR is to notify the surgical team immediately and have the surgeon release traction or pressure, which frequently extinguishes the response.
2. d. During general anesthesia there will be a decrease in IOP and venous pressure and the eye will be relaxed. There is no drug that can reliably inhibit the OCR, nor can the incidence of OCR be predicted.
3. a. Regardless of the volatile anesthetic used, 1 MAC if the hemodynamic status permits is preferable for maintenance to prevent intraoperative patient awareness. If a patient has had RD repair with an unknown tamponading agent, it is prudent to avoid N_2O in order to prevent another RD or an increase in IOP.
4. a. Air is reabsorbed in 5 days, SF_6 in 10 days, and perfluoropropane in 30 days. Silicone oil is never reabsorbed and usually requires a second procedure to be removed.
5. c. Lying in the supine position and the administration of succinylcholine are the only options that increase IOP. Administration of succinylcholine raises IOP by 6 to 8 mm Hg, whereas lying in the supine position only increases IOP by 2 to 4 mm Hg. Both decreases in central venous pressure and deep inspiration decrease IOP.

Chapter 32

1. c. Succinylcholine is associated with a transient rise in IOP, which may theoretically cause loss of intraocular contents.
2. a. The presence of blood in the periorbital space may ameliorate the effect of local anesthetic by interfering with diffusion of molecules to the sensory nerves, and the volume of local anesthetic may elevate IOP.
3. d. Coughing or straining, which can be prevented by neuromuscular blockade, is associated with acute increases in IOP.
4. a. By relaxing the traction on extraocular muscles, the afferent limb (via the ophthalmic branch of CN V) is interrupted, decreasing vagal efferent impulses to the heart.

5. c. Many patients with open globe injury present for emergent surgical repair of the eye and may not have been fasting before induction of anesthesia. These patients are at risk for aspiration of stomach contents if they are extubated before return of protective reflexes.

Chapter 33

1. d. Femoral nerve injury results in a loss of sensation over the anterior thigh and medial aspect of the lower leg and motor weakness of the quadriceps muscle.
2. a. Blockade of the sensory dermatome at T4–T6 provides adequate anesthesia for an open hysterectomy.
3. b. Stroke volume is the only parameter of those listed that is decreased after creation of a pneumoperitoneum.
4. a. Peak inspiratory pressure is the only parameter of those listed that is increased after creation of a pneumoperitoneum.
5. d. Metoclopramide acts by blocking dopaminergic receptors located in the vomiting center, CTZ, and gastrointestinal tract.

Chapter 34

1. a. A low hemoglobin value facilitates the production of 2,3-diphosphoglycerate caused by anaerobic metabolism. This situation decreases the affinity of hemoglobin and oxygen by causing a confirmation change in the hemoglobin molecule.
2. c. The origin of the common peroneal nerve is on the outer surface of the fibula immediately below the knee. Damage to this nerve from pressure against the stirrup can result in foot drop and lower extremity paresthesia.
3. d. Progesterone inhibits the effects of motilin, thereby decreasing gastric motility.
4. c. A paracervical block anesthetizes the Frankenhauser ganglion and provides anesthesia to the uterus, cervix, and upper portion of the vagina.
5. a. Inhalation agents cause uterine atony that can increase blood loss. The degree of uterine atony is determined by the dose (concentration) of the inhalation agent that is administered. The greater the dose, the greater the inhibition of uterine contraction.

Chapter 35

1. a. The loss of deep tendon reflexes in parturients undergoing magnesium therapy typically occurs at 10 mEq/L.
2. c. Edema is not a reliable sign of preeclampsia, as it is present in approximately 30% of all parturients.
3. c. Cerebral N-methyl-D-aspartate receptors are thought to be the site of action of anticonvulsant properties associated with magnesium sulfate.

4. d. Phenylephrine, when used to treat maternal hypotension, may provide improved fetal acid–base balance compared with ephedrine.

5. b. Prostaglandin F2-alpha is associated with bronchospasm in asthmatic patients.

Chapter 36

1. a. Spinal anesthesia is the anesthetic technique of choice for cervical cerclage because it reduces the amount of intravenous medication administered and therefore its impact on mother and fetus is minimal.

2. c. The smooth muscle within vessel walls is relaxed by the hormones of pregnancy, resulting in a decrease in systemic vascular resistance and allowing the maternal vasculature to accommodate for the increase in cardiac output without increasing blood pressure.

3. d. Nonparticulate antacid should be given orally prior to any anesthesia administration to the parturient.

4. c. As pregnancy progresses, the intragastric pressure increases, but the rise in lower esophageal tone that would normally occur in response is prevented by the rotation and displacement of the gastroesophageal junction caused by the gravid uterus.

5. b. The difference between uterine arterial pressure and uterine venous pressure divided by uterine vascular resistance is the equation that is used to calculate UBF.

Chapter 37

1. a. A classical (longitudinal) uterine incision presents the greatest risk factor for uterine rupture in a patient undergoing VBAC because the orientation of the cut between muscle fibers does not lead to development of a strong scar. It also implies that the scar extends toward the fundus of the uterus, where the greatest tension is formed during contractions.

2. d. Uterine rupture would most likely be characterized by variable decelerations of the fetal heart rate and abdominal pain.

3. a. In contrast to other indications for emergency cesarean delivery, the optimal time for initiating a cesarean delivery for uterine rupture is within 15 minutes.

4. c. Staff availability to initiate a cesarean delivery rapidly is the most important asset to ensure safe management of a patient for VBAC. Rapid delivery is crucial to best ensure fetal survival after a catastrophic uterine rupture.

5. b. In the case of a bleeding mother and a compromised neonate, the professional *duty* of the anesthetist is to the mother primarily but may incorporate the neonate if required and if the mother is stable.

Chapter 38

1. c. Maternal desire for an epidural. Traditional approaches required that epidural analgesia not be initiated until the parturient had achieved a cervical dilation of at least 4 cm. This approach was borne of concern that epidural effects would inhibit labor. Although some studies have demonstrated a prolongation of labor in patients with an epidural, the degree of prolongation is not detrimental.

2. b. Bupivacaine 0.25%, although this strength also provides reliable analgesia.

3. c. T10–L1. Pain during the second stage is transmitted via S2–S4.

4. b. Placenta previa is characteristically not painful. The other choices should be considered in cases of breakthrough pain.

5. b. Postdural puncture headache. Backache and inadequate analgesia occur much more frequently. Nerve damage is a rare event.

Chapter 39

1. b. Because the uterine vasculature is not autoregulated, placental blood flow is directly dependent on the dynamic between perfusion pressure and vascular resistance.

2. d. Hyperventilation causes a left shift of the oxyhemoglobin disassociation curve, which inhibits oxygen release from maternal to fetal hemoglobin.

3. a. The absence of beat-to-beat variability is common when the fetus is exposed to general anesthetic agents and will resolve with cessation of the precipitating agent.

4. d. Warfarin is a known human teratogen.

5. d. Preterm labor accounts for 70% of perinatal morbidity and mortality.

Chapter 40

1. b. Labetalol is a nonspecific beta-1 and beta-2 antagonist that decreases myocardial contractility and heart rate. This medication is also an alpha-1 antagonist that decreases SVR and blood pressure.

2. c. Raising the patient's legs into the lithotomy position causes an increase in central blood volume. The predominant cardiovascular effect is increased preload, which causes an increase in myocardial oxygen consumption.

3. c. Robotic-assisted laparoscopic surgery for radical prostatectomy is associated with a decreased inflammatory mediator response, decreased blood loss, and slower heat loss compared with an open approach. The rate of infection is comparable for both procedures.

4. a. Both methylene blue and indigo carmine can produce allergic reactions that can result in anaphylaxis.

5. a. Hypothermia is associated with a decrease in metabolic rate resulting in decreased hepatic metabolism of medications. Postoperative shivering resulting from hypothermia dramatically increases myocardial oxygen consumption.

Chapter 41

1. a. Spinal anesthesia is the anesthetic technique of choice for TURP surgery because it allows the anesthetist to monitor the patient's neurologic function. Altered mental status may be indicative of dilutional hyponatremia.

2. c. TURP syndrome is associated with dilutional hyponatremia. Administering Lasix promotes diuresis, which decreases intravascular volume, restoring protein oncotic pressure. As a result, sodium returns from the interstitial space, restoring intravascular sodium concentration.

3. c. These signs and symptoms are associated with an intraperitoneal bladder perforation.

4. b. Although no one serum sodium value ensures specific signs and symptoms, a sodium value of 115 mEq/L is associated with confusion, widening QRS complex, and bradycardia.

5. b. Glycine is metabolized to ammonia, which is a direct myocardial depressant.

Chapter 42

1. a. Cardiac dysrhythmias may occur due to the mechanical stress exerted by the shock waves on the cardiac conduction system. Patients with a history of dysrhythmias or a cardiac pacemaker are at increased risk.

2. c. A patient who has had a myocardial infarction 2 years ago but is medically optimized and has been evaluated by a cardiologist can have ESWL. The other patient conditions are contraindications to this procedure.

3. d. A Bier block will not provide adequate analgesia during ESWL.

4. b. Shock waves in a gated ESWL should be timed to discharge 20 milliseconds after the R wave on the patient's ECG. This period corresponds with the absolute refractory period, minimizing the risk of cardiac dysrhythmias.

5. c. A T6 dermatome sensory block is necessary because the innervation to the kidney is from sympathetic nerves that arise from the T10–L1 spinal nerve distribution.

Chapter 43

1. c. Administration of adequate crystalloid is necessary in order to minimize intraoperative hemodynamic variability. Blood products should be administered judiciously if significant anemia exists. Anemia decreases oxygen-carrying capacity, and patients can develop a coagulopathy.

2. d. Bleomycin is an antitumor agent with known pulmonary toxic properties. Bleomycin-associated pulmonary toxicity occurs in 10% of patients, and the signs and symptoms manifest as a dry, hacking cough; dyspnea; tachypnea; and fever. Changes in pulmonary function tests occur in 20% of patients who receive bleomycin. Pulmonary complications include pulmonary fibrosis and interstitial pneumonitis. Arterial blood gas and chest x-ray analysis are important preoperative tests used to evaluate for potential pulmonary toxicity.

3. a. Intravenous line placement should be avoided on the side of lymph node dissection to help prevent the development of lymphedema. It is best to avoid placement of the IV line in the foot of a diabetic patient due to the potential for compromised wound healing and diabetic ulcers.

4. b. Women with the gene mutation *BRCA1* or *BRCA2* are considered very high risk for developing breast cancer.

5. b. Adequate blood supply to the flap is necessary for TRAM flap survival. Normothermia is important to prevent vasoconstriction associated with hypothermia. Normotension allows for adequate perfusion of the flap, preventing ischemia and flap death associated with hypotension. Normocarbia helps prevent vasoconstriction associated with hypocarbia.

Chapter 44

1. d. The tumescent technique reduces blood loss to 1% of the volume of aspirate.

2. b. An initial sign that is associated with local anesthetic toxicity is dizziness.

3. a. Decreased preload is associated with the prone position, caused by decreased venous return from pressure on the abdomen.

4. b. Pulmonary embolus is the greatest single cause of mortality in patients undergoing liposuction: 4.6 per 100,000 patients.

5. c. Lidocaine can potentiate nondepolarizing neuromuscular blocking medications.

Chapter 45

1. d. Each of the goals listed are among the indications for maxillofacial/orthognathic surgical procedures except for temporal arteritis.

2. c. A triangular fracture that extends above the bridge of the nose to below the zygomatic arches is consistent with a LeFort 2 fracture.

3. a. Elevating the patient's head will facilitate venous drainage and decrease venous pressure. This will lead to decreased blood loss. The other interventions listed may increase bleeding from the surgical site.

4. b. Epistaxis and turbinectomy are the most common complications associated with a nasal intubation. Cranial intubation can occur if extreme pressure is exerted on the endotracheal tube if a sphenoid sinus

fracture is present, such as with a LeFort 2 or 3 fracture. An esophageal intubation is not considered to be a complication during nasal intubation.

5. a. The relative restrictive nature of the surgical intervention, edema formation, and bandages may impede the ability of the anesthetist to control the patient's airway.

Chapter 46

1. b. Paresthesias of the neck, shoulders, arms, and sometimes the fingers are frequent symptoms of nerve root compression in the cervical vertebra. Irreversible paresthesias and/or paralysis may follow if allowed to persist. Conservative treatment can be initiated with medications, cervical injections, or traction. However, more severe symptoms are more aggressively treated with surgery.

2. b. Elevating and extending the head, which is necessary in order to achieve optimal alignment of the oral, laryngeal, and pharyngeal axes ("sniffing position"), is absolutely contraindicated in patients with suspected or actual cervical spine injuries, and acute spinal cord trauma can occur as a result of this maneuver.

3. c. Sympathetic nervous system denervation is caused by cervical spinal cord damage. The result is parasympathetic nervous system predominance, which includes bradycardia, hypotension, and hypothermia.

4. a. Providing a deep and superficial cervical plexus block can be used to decrease the postoperative pain associated with ACDF.

5. d. Damage to the carotid artery can cause acute dissection and damage to the intima of the vessel. Microemboli formation can occur and lodge in a cerebral vessel, resulting in decreased blood flow and an ischemic stroke.

Chapter 47

1. b. The brachial plexus originates from the fifth cervical vertebrae and extends through the first thoracic vertebrae. Motor or sensory deficits may be temporary or permanent if the patients are abducted greater than 90 degrees.

2. a. Due to the physical impingement of the thoracic cage on the lungs and the potential for impaired lung development, vital capacity measure during inspiration is decreased. Residual volume is increased, whereas both total lung volume and expiratory reserve volume are decreased.

3. d. Although the most sensitive monitor for detecting a VAE is transesophageal echocardiography, the next most sensitive monitor choice is a precordial Doppler.

4. a. The anterior or ventral portion of the spinal cord transmits motor information from the brain to the periphery.

5. b. The neurologic inhibitory effects of the inhaled agents decrease SSEP wave amplitude and increase latency in a dose-dependent manner.

Chapter 48

1. c. The cerebral perfusion pressure at the circle of Willis, or base of the brain, is 9 mm Hg lower in terms of gradient than the cephalad portion of the brain.

2. b. The external auditory meatus is easily recognized and represents the location of the base of the brain and the circle of Willis.

3. d. It is vital for the anesthetist to periodically assess the patient for normal anatomic alignment to prevent hyperextension of the neck, facial compression by surgical team, etc.

4. b. The brachial plexus stems from the ventral rami of C5–T1 nerve roots in most patients.

5. c. General anesthesia with hypocapnia alone can decrease internal carotid artery flow. Combined with the sitting position, this can decrease blood flow by an additional 18%.

Chapter 49

1. b. Advantages to providing regional anesthesia include decreased intraoperative blood loss, decreased perioperative DVT, and minimal need for airway manipulation or control.

2. c. Patients who have a body mass index of greater than 50 are at increased risk for developing postoperative complications.

3. c. Antihypertensive agents have different implications when anesthesia is administered. For instance, prolonged use of diuretics may lead to hypokalemia and hypomagnesemia and increase the risk of perioperative arrhythmias.

4. a. Regional techniques cause a sympathectomy as a result of the inhibition of preganglionic B fiber transmission, which extends from the thoracic to the first or second lumbar vertebrae. Vascular dilation leads to decreased blood pressure that can range from mild to severe.

5. d. Shivering-induced hypothermia can increase oxygen consumption by as much as 600%, cause a leftward shift in the oxyhemoglobin dissociation curve, increase cardiac irritability, reduce platelet function, and impair enzymes of the coagulation cascade.

Chapter 50

1. b. All of the medications with the exception of methadone are routinely used as a component part of a treatment plan utilizing various mechanisms of action for inhibiting the pain pathway. These agents target different points of transmission along the pain pathway.

2. a. Most second-order axons form the spinothalamic tract and send projections to the thalamus, the reticular formation, the nucleus raphe magnus, and the periaqueductal gray area. Because there are projections to the hypothalamus and reticular formation, it is probably responsible for the arousal response to painful stimuli. This tract is divided into lateral and medial aspects, with the lateral sending projections containing the information about the location and intensity of the pain, and the medial aspect is responsible for the autonomic and unpleasant emotional response to pain.

3. c. Hydromorphone is 5 to 7 times more potent than morphine. It is a useful alternative to morphine due to the potency and decreased incidence of nausea, pruritus, and sedation. It should be used with caution in patients with renal insufficiency due to the active metabolite hydromorphone-3-glucuronide that can produce neuroexcitation, including myoclonus and seizures.

4. d. Opioid–induced hyperalgesia has been described in both humans and animals. It is characterized by increased pain from a noxious stimuli (hyperalgesia) and pain from a previously nonpainful stimuli (allodynia). The cellular mechanism of opioid-induced hyperalgesia is similar to neuropathic pain, which is caused by changes to the NMDA receptor.

5. a. The NMDA receptor is thought to be involved in central sensitization. Antagonists that block the receptor reduce the excitatory neurotransmitter glutamate and block the input from C fibers and prevent the wind-up phenomenon.

Chapter 51

1. a. Abdominal distention is almost always present in cases of necrotizing enterocolitis.
2. d. Intramural gas is a hallmark finding of necrotizing enterocolitis.
3. c. Neonates are at increased risk of becoming hypothermic during transportation to the operating room.
4. d. A rapid decline in oxygen saturation can occur during brief periods of apnea during laryngoscopy in the compromised neonate.
5. c. The division of one unit of packed red blood cells by the blood bank per policy into small, weight-appropriate transfusions minimizes the number of donors to whom the patient is exposed. Although cost containment, ease of dispensing, and conservation may be true and helpful to the hospital, minimal donor exposure can be of benefit to the patient.

Chapter 52

1. c. Medical management is best achieved prior to surgical treatment in these patients. Immediate management involves regulation of fluid status, electrolytes, and acid–base imbalances.

2. d. Due to the repeated episodes of emesis, there is a deficit in hydrogen, chloride, sodium, and potassium. This results in hypovolemia and metabolic alkalosis.

3. d. The degree of electrolyte and glucose imbalance, as well as metabolic alkalosis, must be assessed in order to appropriately and efficiently guide the medical management of these patients before surgical intervention.

4. d. A rapid sequence induction is the best method because these patients are considered high risk for aspiration. Gastric decompression should be achieved prior to induction.

5. c. Full stomach precautions, including gastric decompression and endotracheal intubation, are standard of practice for pyloric stenosis. A histamine-2 blocker, such as ranitidine, and a gastrokinetic, such as metoclopramide, are commonly used in pediatrics for aspiration precautions. However, these interventions do not guarantee total protection or prevention of aspiration.

Chapter 53

1. b. Positive pressure ventilation above the level of the fistula can cause gastric insufflation, which increases the risk of aspiration, can compress the lungs, or can cause the stomach to rupture. Maintaining spontaneous respiration during induction limits the need for positive pressure mask ventilation.

2. c. The hallmark signs of a patient with a TEF are coughing, choking, and cyanosis during feeding; this is usually discovered in the first day of life. Lung sounds would not be clear due to recurrent aspiration.

3. d. The VACTERL association is the most common congenital anomaly that occurs with TEF. Over 50% of babies have one associated anomaly, and 25% have three.

4. a. A patient with a TEF will frequently have atelectasis of the right upper lobe. Primary repair of the closure should be postponed for severe associated anomalies, pneumonitis, or prematurity and weight less than 1 kg. These patients will usually have a gastrostomy under local anesthesia, and the thoracotomy is deferred until the procedure can be performed safely.

5. c. The most common type of TEF is esophageal atresia with distal fistula, also known as type C or IIIB.

Chapter 54

1. a. A faster relief of symptoms is a definite advantage of ECT for suicidal patients. Antidepressant medication can take 3 to 6 weeks to reach full therapeutic effect.

2. b. Sine wave ECT is associated with the greatest degree of cognitive impairment. Ultra-brief pulse width is associated with the least effect on cognitive function.

3. c. Parasympathetic activation, exhibited by bradycardia, is the initial response to electrical stimulation.

4. a. Increased intracranial pressure is an absolute contraindication to ECT. Angina, pregnancy, and osteoporosis are relative contraindications.

5. c. Ketamine is an NMDA antagonist.

Chapter 55

1. c. Initially, caries will cause almost unnoticeable destruction of the tooth structure. The patient may not even feel the sensation of pain, but the patient will probably notice sensitivity to touch, temperature, and when eating sugary foods. As time progresses, more severe pain and oral tissue destruction will occur.

2. a. Patients that present with compromised medical state, such as ASA physical status III or greater, are best treated in a hospital, where access to advanced medical personnel and equipment is present.

3. d. This important assessment provides a timely assessment of the patient's health on the day of surgery and gives the anesthesia provider a highlight of concerns that could interfere with the anesthetic on that day.

4. b. It is optimal to provide premedication in a quiet, nonstimulating environment promoting sedation rather than causing activity and agitation.

5. b. Continuous vigilance is required during the recovery phase. As a result, a well-equipped and well-staffed environment is necessary. Due to the possibility of emergence delirium, it is necessary to be prepared to protect the patient from physical harm.

Index

Page numbers followed by *f* indicate figures, *t* indicate tables, *b* indicate boxes.